Quick Reference (QR) Video Access

The images below are QR codes. Each code corresponds to a video from *Minor Emergencies.* For fast and easy video access, right from your mobile device, follow these instructions. The videos are also available on Expertconsult.com.

What You Need

- **A mobile device, such as a smartphone or tablet, equipped with a camera and Internet access.**
- **A QR code reader application (if you do not already have a reader installed on your mobile device, look for free versions in your app store.)**

How It Works

- **Open the QR code reader application on your mobile device.**
- **Point the device's camera at the code and scan.**
- **Each code opens an individual video player for instant viewing; no log-on required.**

Video 1: Epley or (Canalith) Otolith Repositioning Maneuver

Video 4: Symmetric Palpation of the Facial Bones

Video 2: Eyelid Eversion with Cotton-tipped Applicator

Video 5: Ear Irrigation Technique

Video 3: Slit Lamp Examination: Normal Anterior Chamber

Video 6: Initial Management of Epistaxis

Video 7: Stitch for Laceration of Vermilion Border

Video 8: Diagnosing a Rib Fracture Clinically with Indirect Stress

Video 9: Granulated Sugar for Stopping Hiccups

Video 10: Foreign Body Removal: Lost Vaginal Tampon

Video 11: Sacroiliac Joint Injection

Video 12: Trigger Point Injection

Video 13: Reduction: Patellar Dislocation

Video 14: Calf Squeeze Test

Video 15: Reduction of Shoulder Dislocation: Modified Kocher Maneuver or External Rotation Technique

Video 16: Buddy Taping After Reduction of Dislocated Second Toe

Video 17: Fishhook Removal: Needle Technique

Video 18: Fishhook Removal: Push Through or Advance and Cut Method

Video 19: Fishhook Removal: Retrograde or Modified String Technique

Video 20: Fishhook Removal: String Technique

Video 21: Fishhook Removal: Treble Fishhook

Video 22: Removal of a Minor Impaled Object

Video 23: Foreign Body Removal: Needle in Foot

Video 24: Draining Acute Paronychia Without Invasion of Skin

Video 25: Pencil Point Puncture Tattoo Removal

Video 26: Ring Removal–Compression: Exsanguination Technique

Video 27: Ring Removal: Ring Cutter

Video 28: Ring Removal–Traction: Countertraction

Video 29: Ring Removal: Orthopedic Pin Cutter

Video 30: Ring Removal: Pin Cutter-Cast Spreader Technique

Video 31: Foreign Body Removal: Superficial Wooden Sliver

Video 32: Producing a Bloodless Field

Video 33: Subcutaneous Foreign Body Removal: Probe Technique

Video 34: Removal of Traumatic Tattoos from Abrasions

 Video 35: Entrapped Zipper Removal: Attempting to Cut the Slide Apart

 Video 37: Fingertip Dressing

 Video 36: Zipper Entrapment Removal Techniques: Lubrication and Opening Zipper from Rear

 Video 38: Homemade Fingertip Dressing

Minor
Emergencies

3RD EDITION

Minor Emergencies

Philip Buttaravoli, MD FACEP

Fellow of the American College of Emergency Physicians
Adjunct Assistant Professor in the Department of Emergency Medicine
Fletcher Allen Health Care
Burlington, Vermont

Stephen M. Leffler, MD FACEP

Fellow of the American College of Emergency Physicians
Professor of Emergency Medicine
University of Vermont College of Medicine
Fletcher Allen Health Care
Burlington, Vermont

ELSEVIER
SAUNDERS

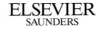

1600 John F. Kennedy Blvd.
Ste 1800
Philadelphia, PA 19103-2899

MINER EMERGENCIES

ISBN: 978-0-323-07909-9

Copyright © 2012 by Saunders, an imprint of Elsevier Inc.
Copyright © 2007, 2000 by Mosby, Inc., an affiliate of Elsevier Inc.

Notice

Knowledge and best practice in this field are constantly changing. As new research and experience broaden our understanding, changes in research methods, professional practices, or medical treatment may become necessary.

Practitioners and researchers must always rely on their own experience and knowledge in evaluating and using any information, methods, compounds, or experiments described herein. In using such information or methods they should be mindful of their own safety and the safety of others, including parties for whom they have a professional responsibility.

With respect to any drug or pharmaceutical products identified, readers are advised to check the most current information provided (i) on procedures featured or (ii) by the manufacturer of each product to be administered, to verify the recommended dose or formula, the method and duration of administration, and contraindications. It is the responsibility of practitioners, relying on their own experience and knowledge of their patients, to make diagnoses, to determine dosages and the best treatment for each individual patient, and to take all appropriate safety precautions.

To the fullest extent of the law, neither the Publisher nor the authors, contributors, or editors assume any liability for any injury and/or damage to persons or property as a matter of products liability, negligence or otherwise, or from any use or operation of any methods, products, instructions, or ideas contained in the material herein.

Library of Congress Cataloging-in-Publication Data
Buttaravoli, Philip M., 1945-
  Minor emergencies / Philip Buttaravoli, Stephen M. Leffler. — 3rd ed.
     p. ; cm.
  Includes bibliographical references and index.
  ISBN 978-0-323-07909-9 (pbk. : alk. paper)
  I. Leffler, Stephen M. II. Title.
  [DNLM: 1. Critical Care. 2. Emergencies. 3. Wounds and Injuries. WX 218]
  616.02'5—dc23
                                                                          2011049148

Senior Content Strategist: Kate Dimock
Content Development Strategist: Angela Rufino
Publishing Services Manager: Patricia Tannian
Senior Project Manager: Claire Kramer
Designer: Louis Forgione
Cover Illustrator: Esao Andrews

Printed in China

Last digit is the print number: 9 8 7 6 5 4 3 2 1

To Holly Lindsey

—*Philip Buttaravoli*

To my wife, Robyn, and my children, Zack and Emily, thank you for your love and support. To my colleagues in the Fletcher Allen Emergency Department, thank you for your efforts and hard work on this book and for the outstanding care you deliver to your patients on a daily basis. To Phil Buttaravoli, thank you for the opportunity to participate in the third edition of *Minor Emergencies.*

—*Stephen M. Leffler*

Contributors

Andrew Bushnell, MD
Associate Professor of Surgery
Division of Emergency Services
University of Vermont College of Medicine
Burlington, Vermont

Philip Buttaravoli, MD FACEP
Fellow of the American College of Emergency Physicians
Adjunct Assistant Professor in the Department of Emergency Medicine
Fletcher Allen Health Care
Burlington, Vermont

Maj Eisinger, MD
Associate Professor of Surgery
Division of Emergency Services
University of Vermont College of Medicine
Burlington, Vermont

Page Hudson, MD
Assistant Professor of Surgery
Division of Emergency Services
University of Vermont College of Medicine
Burlington, Vermont

Steve Hulsey, MD
Associate Professor of Surgery
Division of Emergency Services
University of Vermont College of Medicine
Burlington, Vermont

Wendy James, MD
Assistant Professor of Surgery
Division of Emergency Services
University of Vermont College of Medicine
Burlington, Vermont

Ray Keller, MD
Associate Professor of Surgery
Division of Emergency Services
University of Vermont College of Medicine
Burlington, Vermont

Stephen M. Leffler, MD FACEP
Fellow of the American College of Emergency Physicians
Professor of Emergency Medicine
University of Vermont College of Medicine
Fletcher Allen Health Care
Burlington, Vermont

Wayne Misselbeck, MD
Professor of Surgery
Division of Emergency Services
University of Vermont College of Medicine
Burlington, Vermont

Laurel Plante, MD
Assistant Professor of Surgery
Division of Emergency Services
University of Vermont College of Medicine
Burlington, Vermont

Alfred Sacchetti, MD FACEP
Chief Emergency Services
Our Lady of Lourdes Medical Center
Camden, New Jersey
Assistant Clinical Professor of Emergency Medicine
Thomas Jefferson University
Philadelphia, Pennsylvania

Michael Sheeser, MD
Assistant Professor of Surgery
Division of Emergency Services
University of Vermont College of Medicine
Burlington, Vermont

Mario Trabulsy, MD
Associate Professor of Surgery
Division of Emergency Services
University of Vermont College of Medicine
Burlington, Vermont

Katherine Walsh, MD
Assistant Professor of Surgery
Division of Emergency Services
University of Vermont College of Medicine
Burlington, Vermont

Daniel Wolfson, MD
Assistant Professor of Surgery
Division of Emergency Services
University of Vermont College of Medicine
Burlington, Vermont

Kevin Wyne, PA-C
Clinical Instructor
Department of Surgery
Division of Emergency Services
University of Vermont College of Medicine
Burlington, Vermont

Foreword

Patients do not experience emergencies that are "minor"; instead, acute care problems and minor urgent problems are "major" to patients, who expect accurate and timely decision making. Moreover, minor emergencies become a challenge to providers if they require an update on management or they need additional information to give the patient the very best care. This textbook details a full repertoire of minor emergencies and is an extremely effective resource in the acute care setting.

Minor Emergencies is a straightforward resource that will aid clinicians on the front line of medicine. The clinical problems are organized by system and are identifiable in the table of contents. Readers will find that it is easy to review a problem, as well as pinpoint and excerpt areas for further consideration. The highlighted discussions succinctly review the pathophysiology or injury mechanism, in addition to the clinical prognosis.

Each section is carefully referenced and contains relevant illustrations, diagrams, and images. Each chapter provides important cautions and highlights steps and strategies for the provider to consider while offering the highest quality care. Each section reflects experience from clinical practice and teaching sessions for learners of acute care medicine. The narrative contains up-to-date scientific approaches that are interwoven with practical strategies. The appendixes contain important protocols and references that will be useful in minor or major emergencies. *Minor Emergencies* is an extraordinary acute care tool for medical students, as well as experienced physicians.

My practice experience ranges from primary care offices in student health settings to athletic fields and the backcountry wilderness and from urgent care settings to the emergency room. On the basis of my experience, I fully recommend this book for the "go-to" shelf of your references. The text is quick, accurate, comprehensive, and effective.

Thomas C. Peterson, MD
Professor and Chair of Family Medicine
University of Vermont College of Medicine
Burlington, Vermont

Preface

Preface to the Second Edition

"Good judgment comes from experience, and a lot of that comes from bad judgment."
—Will Rogers

As a medical student at the University of Vermont in the late 1960s interested in emergency room care (this was considered peculiar at the time), I found myself disappointed that my medical education (excellent in every other way) was lacking when it came to the treatment of simple minor emergencies. I had this in mind when, in 1975, as the medical director of the emergency service at George Washington University Medical Center (and the first residency-trained emergency physician in the Washington, DC, area), I was given the opportunity to present a 1-hour lecture to their medical students on emergency medical care—"Common Simple Emergencies." (At that time, 1 hour was considered very generous for covering all of emergency medicine.)

I eventually expanded this slide show and lecture to a 6-hour series, which I presented regularly at the Georgetown University Medical Center Emergency Department. Even though there were still few published data on most of the topics covered in the lecture series, in 1985, with the help of emergency medicine attending physician Dr. Thomas Stair, I turned "Common Simple Emergencies" into a 300-page book. For the most part, the information contained within this publication was based on common practice and personal experience.

Fifteen years later, with more published data available, the book was again published under the present title and was expanded to 500 pages. The general format ("What To Do/What Not To Do") was maintained. Even with the greater volume of information, the book remained a practical guide.

Today, in stark contrast to when the original edition was published in 1985, there is a plethora of scientific data on most of the subject covered in *Minor Emergencies*. The book has now grown to over 800 pages. In the face of the sometimes overwhelming volume of data now available, I have endeavored to continue to present these topics on minor emergencies in a manner that will still allow this larger text to be a useful and practical guide.

I have maintained the simple basic format used in the previous edition and have continued to use bold font to bring the reader's eye to the key information in each chapter. I have added red font to help identify different topics within the text. The discussions are now highlighted and compressed using small font and double columns. These changes have allowed me to make the book more complete and comprehensive and yet still allow it to remain useful at a glance.

The clinical material has all been updated, new topics have been added, and I have used evidence-based data whenever available. Many more photographs and drawings have been added (in color) to benefit the reader. In addition, I have personally reviewed the index to help ensure its usefulness and have attempted to include many identifying symptoms in the index to help users find the topic they are searching for.

I have done all of this so that you as a clinician can have more fun with your patients. When emergencies are minor, it gives you an opportunity to lighten up and enjoy the art of healing. Patients appreciate a confident clinician with a good sense of humor who can stop the pain and/or the worry, fix the problem in a compassionate way, and also make them laugh. This book can provide you with the information that you need to perform competently and to relax when presented with the minor emergencies that patients will always need your help with. (You will have to supply the humor.) You will be greatly rewarded for your treatment by seeing their smiling faces and hearing their expressions of gratitude after happily making them well.

Philip M. Buttaravoli, MD FACEP

Preface to the Third Edition

To incorporate an academic element to the latest edition of *Minor Emergencies,* I have returned to my alma mater, the University of Vermont, thereby bringing the book full circle to its earliest origins. I asked Emergency Department Medical Director Stephen M. Leffler, MD, whether he and the rest of the emergency department medical staff would be interested in updating the clinical material in *Minor Emergencies* and bringing the book into the digital age with an electronic publication that would include video displays.

Steve, along with his department staff, accepted the challenge enthusiastically.

With their involvement, this latest edition of *Minor Emergencies* should prove to be more accurate and convenient for the user. There will be periodic updates of the electronic version, and this will maintain a continuous renewal of clinical information.

The book title of this third edition has been shortened with the elimination of the subtitle *Splinters to Fractures.* This subtitle was thought to be more misleading than informative, and the new abbreviated title better reflects the book's true essence.

It is my hope that this new edition will continue to provide support for all of the clinicians out there who are caring for the public's minor emergencies on a daily basis.

Philip Buttaravoli, MD FACEP

A note from the authors:

We have no relationships with or financial interests in any commercial companies that pertain to any of the products mentioned in this publication.

Any comments, suggestions, and/or questions can be directed to Drs. Buttaravoli and Leffler at e-med@juno.com and Stephen.Leffler@vtmednet.org under the subject heading Minor Emergencies.

Philip Buttaravoli, MD FACEP
(Butter ah'voli)
Stephen M. Leffler, MD FACEP

Acknowledgments

I have enjoyed the special opportunity to work with Kate Dimock, who has always been a delight to work with and has been most informative and supportive in the creation of this third edition. In addition, it has been a pleasure working with the extremely competent, efficient, and hardworking assistance of Kate Crowley, Angela Rufino Claire Kramer, and Michael Fioretti, as well as all the other contributors to this project at Elsevier.

Also, special thanks to the emergency department staff at Fletcher Allen Health Care and the University of Vermont.

Contents

PART 3
Ear, Nose, and Throat Emergencies   97
■ Philip Buttaravoli and Steve Hulsey

PART 4
Oral and Dental Emergencies   161
■ Philip Buttaravoli and Daniel Wolfson

PART **8**
Gynecologic Emergencies 331

■ Philip Buttaravoli and Wendy James

PART **9**
Musculoskeletal Emergencies 367

■ Philip Buttaravoli, Laurel Plante, and Wayne Misselbeck

PART 10
Soft Tissue Emergencies 527

■ Philip Buttaravoli, Michael Sheeser, and Kevin Wyne

PART **11**
Dermatologic Emergencies 639

■ Philip Buttaravoli and Page Hudson

Appendixes

Video Contents

See expertconsult.com

Minor
Emergencies

PART 1

Neurologic Emergencies

■ Philip Buttaravoli ■ Mario Trabulsy

Dystonic Drug Reaction

Presentation

The patient arrives at the emergency department (ED) or clinic with peculiar posturing, facial grimacing and distortions with a variety of involuntary muscle movements, and/or difficulty speaking. The patient is usually quite upset and worried about having a stroke. Pain is minimal, if at all. The jaw, tongue, lip, throat, and neck muscles are frequently involved. Hyperextension and lateral deviation of the neck along with upward gaze are the classic presentations. Often no history is offered. The patient may not be able to speak, may not be aware that he or she took any phenothiazines or butyrophenones (e.g., Haldol that has been used to cut heroin), may not admit that he or she takes illicit drugs or psychotropic medication, or may not make the connection between the symptoms and drug use (e.g., one dose of Compazine given to treat nausea or vomiting). The drugs that are most likely to produce a classic dystonic reaction are prochlorperazine (Compazine), haloperidol (Haldol), chlorpromazine (Thorazine), promethazine (Phenergan), and metoclopramide (Reglan). Acute dystonias usually present with one or more of the following types of symptoms:

> Buccolingual—protruding or pulling sensation of the tongue
> Torticollic—twisted neck or facial muscle spasm
> Oculogyric—roving or deviated gaze
> Tortipelvic—abdominal rigidity and pain
> Opisthotonic—spasm of the entire body

These acute dystonias can resemble partial seizures, the posturing of psychosis, or the spasms of tetanus, strychnine poisoning, or electrolyte imbalances. More chronic neurologic side effects of phenothiazines, including the restlessness of akathisia, tardive dyskinesias, and parkinsonism, do not usually respond as dramatically to drug treatment as do the acute dystonias (Figure 1-1). Onset of oculogyric crisis and torticollis reactions usually occurs within a few minutes or hours but may occur 12 to 24 hours after treatment with a high-potency neuroleptic, such as haloperidol.

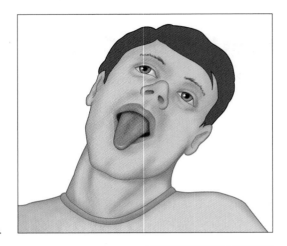

Figure 1-1 Patient with dystonic drug reaction.

What To Do:

✓ **Administer 1 to 2 mg of benztropine (Cogentin) or 25 to 50 mg of diphenhydramine (Benadryl) IV,** and watch for improvement of the dystonia over the next 5 minutes. Usually, the medication begins to work within 2 minutes of intravenous administration, and the symptoms completely resolve within 15 minutes. **This step is both therapeutic and diagnostic.** Benztropine produces fewer side effects (mostly drowsiness) and may be slightly more effective, but diphenhydramine is more likely to be on hand in the ED or physician's office. Benztropine may be given to children older than 3 years of age at the dose of 0.01 to 0.02 mg/kg IV, IM, or PO.

✓ **Instruct the patient to discontinue use of the offending drug** and arrange for follow-up if medications must be adjusted. **If the culprit is long acting, prescribe benztropine 2 mg or diphenhydramine 25 mg PO q6h for 24 to 72 hours to prevent a relapse.**

What Not To Do:

✗ Do not do any diagnostic workup when findings are typical. Administer benztropine or diphenhydramine first to see if symptoms completely resolve.

✗ Do not confuse dystonia with tetanus, seizures, stroke, hysteria, psychosis, meningitis, or dislocation of the mandible. None of these will resolve with IV benztropine or diphenhydramine.

✗ Do not persist with treatment if the response is questionable or there is no response. Continue with the workup to find another cause for the dystonia (e.g., tetanus, seizures, hypomagnesemia, hypocalcemia, alkalosis, muscle disease).

✗ Do not use IV diazepam first because it relaxes spasms resulting from other causes and thus leaves the diagnosis unclear.

Discussion

Dystonic reactions have been reported in 10% to 60% of patients treated with a neuroleptic medication, most commonly when patients just start or increase the dose of the drug. Patients with a family history of dystonia, patients with recent use of cocaine or alcohol, younger patients, male patients, and patients already being treated with agents such as fluphenazine or haloperidol are at higher risk for dystonic reaction.

Dystonia is idiosyncratic, not the result of a drug overdose. The extrapyramidal motor system depends on excitatory cholinergic and inhibitory dopaminergic neurotransmitters, the latter being susceptible to blockage by phenothiazine and butyrophenone medications. Anticholinergic medications restore the excitatory–inhibitory balance. One IV dose of benztropine or diphenhydramine is relatively innocuous, rapidly diagnostic, and probably justified as an initial step in the treatment of any patient with a dystonic reaction. IM administration may take as long as 30 minutes before an effect is seen.

Suggested Readings

Jhee SS: Delayed onset of oculogyric crisis and torticollis with intramuscular haloperidol, *Ann Pharmacother* 37:1434–1437, 2003.

Lee AS: Treatment of drug-induced dystonic reactions, *JACEP* 8:453–457, 1979.

Heat Illness

(Heat Edema, Heat Syncope, Heat Cramps, Heat Exhaustion)

Presentation

Heat illnesses are a spectrum of illnesses resulting from failure of the body's normal thermoregulatory mechanisms after exposure to excessive heat. Most heat-related illness is mild; however, severe hyperthermia associated with heat stroke, neuroleptic malignant syndrome, or serotonin syndrome is a severe, life-threatening condition and should not be overlooked.

The milder forms of heat-related illness include heat edema, heat syncope (or presyncope), or heat cramps. These illnesses are usually found after prolonged exposure to excessive heat and humidity in patients who are unable to remove themselves from the situation.

Heat edema is dependent edema of the hands and feet that may last for a few weeks.

Heat syncope is postural syncope or presyncope related to excessive heat exposure.

Heat cramps are painful muscle cramps after vigorous exertion in hot environments (often several hours later) in the calves, thighs, and/or shoulders.

Heat exhaustion is a slightly more severe form of heat illness, although it too is usually self-limited if treated appropriately. Elderly patients (without air-conditioning on a hot, humid day), workmen, or athletes (exerting themselves in a hot climate while taking in an inadequate amount of fluid) may be more symptomatic, with fatigue, weakness, lightheadedness, headache, nausea, and vomiting in addition to orthostatic hypotension and painful muscle spasms. The patient may have a normal temperature, or the temperature may be elevated to 40° C (104° F), with tachycardia, clinical evidence of dehydration, and, often (especially with exertion), profuse sweating. **Mental status is normal.**

The severe forms of heat-related illness are **characterized by alteration in mental status** associated with hyperthermia (temperature greater than 40° C). Neuroleptic malignant syndrome and serotonin syndrome are not classified as heat-related illnesses but present with severe hyperthermia and altered mental status and can be easily confused with heat stroke.

What To Do:

✅ **Assess and monitor all patients with minor heat illness for the development of heat stroke.** This is a much more serious form of heat illness, **which is accompanied by a core temperature of more than 40° C and altered mental status manifested by delirium, seizures, or coma.**

✅ Remove patients with any form of heat illness from the hot environment. Most of the clothing should be removed to promote cooling, and a **rectal temperature should be determined.**

✓ Obtain a careful history from the patient or witnesses, with special attention to the type and length of heat exposure, any underlying medical problems, and any medications being used that might predispose the patient to developing heat illness.

✓ Perform a physical examination, looking for abnormal vital signs, associated medical illness, dehydration, and diaphoresis.

✓ **For heat edema,** inform patients of the benign nature of this problem, and let them know that they can anticipate having this swelling for a few weeks. Advise them to keep their extremities elevated above the level of their heart as much as possible and, in severe cases, to use compressive stockings.

✓ **For heat syncope or presyncope, patients should rest and receive oral or intravenous rehydration.** They should be thoroughly evaluated for any injury resulting from a fall, and **all potentially serious causes of syncope should be considered** (see Chapter 11).

✓ **For heat cramps** alone, provide muscle stretching and massage, and administer an oral electrolyte solution (½ tsp table salt in 1 quart of water) or intravenous normal saline for rapid relief.

✓ **For true heat exhaustion, provide intravenous rehydration with normal saline or a glucose-in-hypotonic saline solution (1 L over 30 minutes). Obtain serum sodium, potassium, glucose, magnesium, calcium, and phosphorus levels, as well as hematocrit, blood urea nitrogen, and creatinine levels. Electrolyte abnormalities should be corrected appropriately.** Rapid correction of hypernatremia can cause cerebral edema.

✓ **When there is hyperthermia, the patient should be sprayed or sponged with tepid or warm water (to prevent shivering) and then fanned to enhance evaporation and cooling.** Ice water immersion is more effective in rapid cooling but poorly tolerated in most patients (especially elderly patients).

✓ If not treated properly, **heat exhaustion may evolve into heatstroke, which is a major medical emergency that may lead to cardiac arrhythmias, rhabdomyolysis, serum chemistry abnormalities, disseminated intravascular coagulation, irreversible shock, and death.** Physical examination and laboratory analysis should provide the correct diagnosis.

✓ When patients with minor forms of heat illness respond successfully to treatment, with vital signs returning to normal and symptoms relieved, they may be discharged with instructions on how to avoid future episodes and advised to continue adequate fluid intake over the next 24 to 48 hours. Elderly and mentally ill patients should be encouraged to maintain adequate fluid intake in the future, to prevent recurrence. People engaged in strenuous exercise in hot weather should be encouraged to drink water more frequently than thirst dictates. Runners should drink 100 to 300 mL of water or a hypotonic glucose-electrolyte solution (Gatorade and others) 10 to 15 minutes before beginning a race and should drink about 250 mL every 3 to 4 kilometers. Those who must work in a hot environment with high humidity should be encouraged to acclimate themselves over several weeks. Successive increments in the level of work performed in a hot environment result in adaptations that eventually allow a person to work safely at levels of heat that were previously intolerable or life threatening.

✓ Elderly patients and their caretakers, as well as parents of small children, should be educated about high-risk situations and instructed about putting limits on activity during hot and humid days.

✓ **Admission should be considered for elderly patients who have chronic medical problems, significant electrolyte abnormalities, or risk for recurrence. All patients who are treated but do not have a complete resolution of their symptoms over several hours should also be admitted.**

What Not To Do:

✗ Do not do a comprehensive laboratory workup on young, healthy patients with minimal symptoms or minor heat-related illness.

✗ Do not use pharmacologic agents that are designed to accelerate cooling. None have been found to be helpful. The role of antipyretic agents in heat illness has not been evaluated.

✗ Do not continue therapeutic cooling techniques after the temperature reaches 38.5° C. Beyond this point, continued active cooling may result in hypothermia.

✗ Do not recommend salt tablets to prevent heat illness. Fluid losses during exercise are much greater than electrolyte losses.

✗ Do not overlook the possibility of neuroleptic malignant syndrome and serotonin syndrome with patients who have recently begun taking neuroleptic drugs or serotonergic agents.

✗ Do not allow overhydration in athletes who are trying to prevent heat illness (especially women and slow runners). Severe cases of hyponatremia that resulted from excessive water consumption have been reported.

Discussion

Control of thermoregulation resides within the hypothalamus, which stimulates cutaneous vasodilation and sweating through the autonomic nervous system in response to elevation of blood temperature. Blood flow to the skin may increase 20-fold. Cooling normally occurs by transfer of heat from the skin by radiation, convection, and evaporation. As the ambient temperature exceeds the body's temperature, a rise in body temperature may occur in response to radiation and convection of heat from the environment. When the humidity rises, the body's ability to cool through evaporation is diminished.

Dehydration and salt depletion impair thermoregulation by reducing the body's ability to increase cardiac output needed to shunt heated blood from the core circulation to the dilated peripheral circulation. Cardiovascular disease and use of medications that impair cardiac function can also result in increased susceptibility to heat illness.

Although athletes are commonly thought to be most at risk for heat illness, children and the elderly, poor, and socially isolated are particularly vulnerable.

Compared with adults, children produce proportionately more metabolic heat, have a greater surface area-to-body mass ratio (which causes a greater heat gain from the environment on a hot day), and have a lower sweating capacity, which reduces their ability to dissipate heat through evaporation. These facts emphasize the danger of leaving a child unattended in a car during hot weather. A fatal event can occur within 20 minutes if normal heat loss mechanisms become overwhelmed.

(continued)

Discussion continued

Both children and young adults (most often athletes and laborers) are associated with exertional heat illness, where there has been intense strenuous activity in a hot, humid environment. Elderly, chronically ill, or sedentary adults, as well as small children, are associated with nonexertional heat illness. Environmental conditions, along with a predisposition for impaired thermoregulation, lead to heat illness in these patients. The elderly and infirm may have diminished cardiac output, a decreased ability to sweat, and decreased ability to vasoregulate. Medications may predispose them to heat illness because of negative effects on cardiac output (beta-blockers) or on sweating (anticholinergics) or because of volume depletion (diuretics). Nonexertional heat illness may be indolent in its onset and may be associated with significant volume depletion.

Heatstroke is the deadliest of heat illnesses. Treatment, especially aggressive cooling procedures and fluid replacement, must begin immediately to help ensure survival. Morbidity and mortality are directly associated with the duration of elevated core temperature. More intensive evaluation and treatment are required for these patients than is covered in this chapter. The most serious complications of heat stroke are those falling within the category of multiorgan dysfunction syndrome. They include encephalopathy, rhabdomyolysis, acute renal failure, acute respiratory distress syndrome, myocardial injury, hepatocellular injury, intestinal ischemia or infarction, pancreatic injury, and hemorrhagic complications, especially disseminated intravascular coagulation, with pronounced thrombocytopenia.

Suggested Readings

American Academy of Pediatrics: Climatic heat stress and the exercising child and adolescent, *Pediatrics* 106 (1 Pt 1):158–159, 2000.

Bouchama A, Knochel JP: Heat stroke, *N Engl J Med* 346:1978–1988, 2002.

Wexler RK: Evaluation and treatment of heat-related illnesses, *Am Fam Physician* 65:2307–2314, 2319–2320, 2002.

Hyperventilation

Presentation

The patient is anxious and complains of shortness of breath and an inability to fill the lungs adequately. The patient also may have palpitations, dizziness, intense anxiety, fear, chest or abdominal pain, tingling or numbness around the mouth and fingers, and possibly even flexor spasm of the hands and feet (carpopedal spasm) (Figure 3-1). The patient's respiratory volume is increased, which may be apparent as increased respiratory rate, increased tidal volume, or frequent sighing. The remainder of the physical examination is normal. The patient's history may reveal an obvious precipitating emotional cause (such as having been caught stealing or being in the midst of a family quarrel or any other form of stress during work or normal life). The patient may experience alternating periods of hypoventilation or brief periods of apnea as her body tries to allow carbon dioxide (CO_2) levels to drift back up to the normal range. If this occurs, the pattern is usually abrupt onset of transient apnea without a drop in O_2 saturation, immediately preceded and followed by profound hyperventilation.

What To Do:

⊘ Perform a brief physical examination, checking especially that the patient's mental status is good; there is no unusual breath odor; there are good, equal excursion and breath sounds in both sides of the chest; and there is no swelling, pain, or inflammation of the legs or other risk factors for pulmonary emboli.

⊘ **Measure pulse oximetry,** which should be between 98% and 100%.

⊘ **Calm and reassure the patient.** Explain to the patient the cycle in which rapid, deep breathing can cause physical symptoms upsetting enough to cause further rapid, deep breathing. Repeat a cadence ("in… out… in…") to help the patient voluntarily slow her breathing, or have her voluntarily hold her breath for a while.

⊘ If the patient cannot reduce her ventilatory rate and volume, **provide a length of tubing through which she can breathe** (Figure 3-2), **or use a reservoir bag with O_2, keeping the pulse oximetry monitor on to avoid hypoxia.** This will allow the patient to continue moving a large quantity of air but will provide air rich in carbon dioxide (CO_2), allowing the blood partial CO_2 (P_{CO_2}) to rise toward normal. (Carbogen gas [5% CO_2] also may be used, if available.) **Administration of 50 to 100 mg of hydroxyzine (Vistaril) IM or lorazepam (Ativan) 1 to 2 mg SL, IM, or IV often helps to calm the patient, allowing her to control her respirations.**

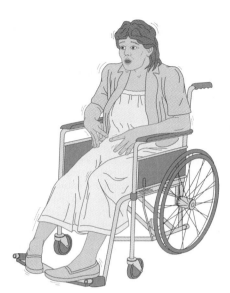

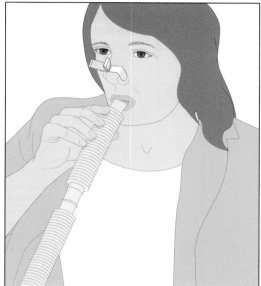

Figure 3-1 The patient experiences anxiety and shortness of breath and feels as though she is unable to fill her lungs, leading to carpopedal spasm.

Figure 3-2 Instruct the patient to breathe through a length of tubing to increase the percentage of inspired CO_2.

✅ **If these symptoms cannot be reversed and respiratory effort cannot be reduced in this manner within 15 to 20 minutes, double check the diagnosis by obtaining arterial blood gas measurements and looking for a metabolic acidosis or hypoxia indicative of underlying disease.**

✅ Reexamine the patient after hyperventilation is controlled. Identify the psychological stressor that prompted the attack.

✅ Ensure that the patient understands the hyperventilation syndrome and knows some strategies for breaking the cycle next time. (It may be valuable to have the patient reproduce the symptoms voluntarily). Arrange for follow-up with a primary care physician or psychiatric counselor as needed.

What Not To Do:

❌ Do not overlook the true medical emergencies, including pneumothorax, asthma, chronic obstructive pulmonary disease (COPD), pneumonia, pulmonary embolus, hyperthyroidism, diabetic ketoacidosis, liver disease, salicylate overdose, sepsis, uremia, substance abuse, sympathomimetic toxidrome, myocardial infarction, congestive heart failure (CHF), and stroke, which also may present with hyperventilation.

❌ Do not use the traditional method of breathing into a paper bag to increase the concentration of inspired CO_2. This increases the potential for inadvertently causing hypoxia and is no longer considered to be appropriate therapy.

Ⓧ Do not do an extensive laboratory and imaging study workup when the history and physical examination are convincingly consistent with psychogenic hyperventilation syndrome. However, be suspicious of an organic cause when the patient has risk factors or does not improve as expected.

Discussion

The acute respiratory alkalosis of hyperventilation causes transient imbalances of calcium, potassium, and perhaps other ions, with the net effect of increasing the irritability and spontaneous depolarization of excitable muscles and nerves. First-time victims of the hyperventilation syndrome are the most likely to visit the emergency department or doctor's office, and this is an excellent time to educate them about its pathophysiology and the prevention of recurrence. Repeat visitors may be overly excitable or may have emotional problems and need counseling.

During recovery after hyperventilation, the transition from hypocapnia to normocapnia is associated with hypoventilation. Be aware that patients may experience significant hypoxemia after hyperventilation. Some investigators believe that there is no benefit in having a patient rebreathe her own exhaled air and that any benefit provided is the result of the reassurance of "instructional manipulation" and the patient's belief in the treatment rather than the elevated fractional concentration of CO_2 in inspired gas ($FiCO_2$).

Suggested Readings

Callaham M: Hypoxic hazards of traditional paper bag rebreathing in hyperventilating patients, *Ann Emerg Med* 18:622–628, 1989.

Chin K, Ohi M, Kita H, et al: Hypoxic ventilatory response and breathlessness following hypocapnic and isocapnic hyperventilation, *Chest* 112:154–163, 1997.

Demeter SL, Cordasco EM: Hyperventilation syndrome and asthma, *Am J Med* 81:989–994, 1986.

Saisch SGN, Wessely S, Gardner WN: Patients with acute hyperventilation presenting to an inner-city emergency department, *Chest* 110:952–957, 1996.

Hysterical Coma or Pseudoseizure

Presentation

The patient is unresponsive and brought to the emergency department on a stretcher. There is usually a history of recent emotional upset: an unexpected death in the family, school or employment difficulties, or the breakup of a close relationship. There may be a history of sexual abuse, eating disorders, depression, substance abuse, anxiety disorders, or personality disorders. Hysterical coma and pseudoseizures rarely occur in social isolation. The patient may be lying still on the stretcher or demonstrating bizarre posturing or even asynchronous or dramatic thrashing with prolonged seizure-like movements. Head turning, from side to side, and pelvic thrusting are typical of psychogenic seizures. A patient with true seizures usually has abdominal contractions but lacks corneal reflexes, whereas a patient with pseudoseizures usually has corneal reflexes but lacks abdominal contractions. The patient's general color and vital signs are normal, without any evidence of airway obstruction. Consciousness is often partially preserved and sometimes regained very quickly after the convulsive period. Commonly, the patient is fluttering his or her eyelids or resists having his or her eyes opened. With eyelids closed, a patient with rapid (saccadic) eye movements is awake. On the other hand, a patient with slow, roving eye movements has a true depressed level of consciousness. Tearfulness during the event argues against true epileptic seizure. With pseudoseizures, there should not be fecal or urinary incontinence, self-induced injury, or lateral tongue biting. Most true seizures are accompanied by a postictal state of disorientation and altered level of arousal and responsiveness. During an epileptic seizure, the plantar response is often extensor, whereas during a psychogenic nonepileptic seizure, it is usually flexor.

A striking finding in hysterical coma is that the patient may hold his or her breath when the examiner breaks an ammonia capsule over the patient's mouth and nose. (Real coma victims usually move the head or do nothing.) A classic finding in hysterical coma is that when the patient's apparently flaccid arm is released over his or her face, it does not fall on the face but drops off to the side. The patient may show remarkably little response to painful stimuli, but there should be no true focal neurologic findings, and the remainder of the physical examination should be normal.

What To Do:

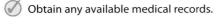 Obtain any available medical records.

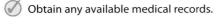 **Perform a complete physical examination, including a full set of vital signs and O$_2$ saturation. Patients under the stress of real illness or injury sometimes react with hysterical or histrionic behavior.** This is especially true in patients with a history of psychiatric illness, substance abuse, or sociopathic behavior. Therefore always fully investigate any suspicion of true underlying pathology.

✓ **Check glucose with a bedside finger stick.**

✓ **When organic illness is unlikely, do not allow any visitors, and place the patient in a quiet observation area, minimizing any stimulation until the patient "awakens." Check vital signs every 30 minutes.**

✓ **When there is significant emotional stress involved, administer a mild tranquilizing agent, such as hydroxyzine pamoate (Vistaril) 50 to 100 mg IM or lorazepam (Ativan) 1 to 2 mg IV or IM.**

✓ Consider obtaining a drug screen and investigating for possible sexual abuse. **In women, consider ordering a pregnancy test.**

✓ **If a generalized seizure is questionable, verify with a lactate level or blood gas analysis, which would show metabolic acidosis with a true tonic-clonic seizure.**

✓ When the patient becomes more responsive, reexamine him or her, obtain a more complete history, explain the apparent emotional cause of the symptoms, and offer follow-up care, including psychological support, if appropriate. Keep in mind that pseudoseizures are commonly associated with sexual abuse, eating disorders, depression, substance abuse, anxiety disorders, and personality disorders.

✓ **If the patient is not awake, alert, and oriented after about 90 minutes, begin a more comprehensive medical workup.** Illnesses to consider include Guillain-Barré syndrome, myasthenia gravis, electrolyte disorders, hypoglycemia, hyperglycemia, renal failure, occult neoplasm, dysrhythmias, systemic infection, toxins, and other neurologic disorders.

What Not To Do:

✗ Do not become angry with the patient and torture him or her with painful stimuli in an attempt to "wake" the patient.

✗ Do not administer anticonvulsants when pseudoseizures are suspected.

✗ Do not perform expensive workups routinely.

✗ Do not ignore or release the patient who has not fully recovered. Instead, the patient must be fully evaluated for an underlying medical problem, which may require hospital admission.

Discussion

Pseudoseizures and hysterical coma are more common in women than men. True hysterical coma is an unconscious manifestation of psychosocial distress that the patient cannot control. Antagonizing the patient often prolongs the condition, whereas ignoring the patient seems to take the spotlight off of the peculiar behavior, allowing the patient to recover. Some psychomotor or complex partial seizures are difficult to diagnose because of dazed confusion or fuguelike activity and might be labeled a pseudoseizure or psychogenic disorder. If the diagnosis is not obviously hysteria, the patient might require an electroencephalogram (EEG), administered during sleep, and deserves a referral to a neurologist. Psychiatric disorders as potential causes of syncope or coma should be suspected in young patients who faint frequently, patients in whom syncope does not cause injury, and patients who have many symptoms (e.g., nausea, lightheadedness, numbness, fear, dread).

Suggested Readings

Benbadis SR: Photo quiz: the value of tongue laceration in the diagnosis of blackouts, *Am Fam Physician* 70: 1757–1758, 2004. Available at http://www.aafp.org/afp/20041101/photo.html.

Dula DJ, DeNaples L: Emergency department presentation of patients with conversion disorder, *Acad Emerg Med* 2:120–123, 1995.

Glick TH, Workman TP, Gaufberg SV: Suspected conversion disorder: foreseeable risks and avoidable errors, *Acad Emerg Med* 7:1272–1277, 2000.

Kaufman KR: Pseudoseizures and hysterical stridor, *Epilepsy Behav* 5:269–272, 2004.

Reuber M, Baker GA, Smith DF, et al: Failure to recognize psychogenic nonepileptic seizures may cause death, *Neurology* 62:834–835, 2004.

Idiopathic Facial Paralysis

(Bell's Palsy)

Presentation

The patient with this condition is often frightened by his facial disfigurement or fear of having had a stroke. He complains of a sudden onset of numbness, a feeling of fullness or swelling, periauricular pain, or some other change in sensation on one side of the face—a crooked smile, mouth "drawing," or some other asymmetric weakness of facial muscles; an irritated, dry, or tearing eye; drooling out of the corner of the mouth; or changes in hearing or taste. Symptoms develop over several hours or days. Often there will have been a viral illness 1 to 3 weeks earlier, or there may have been another trigger, such as stress, fever, dental extraction, or cold exposure. On initial observation of the patient, it is immediately apparent that he is alert and oriented, with a partial or complete unilateral facial paralysis that includes one side of the forehead (Figure 5-1).

What To Do:

⊘ Perform a thorough neurologic examination of the cranial and upper cervical nerves and limb strength, noting which nerves are involved and whether unilaterally or bilaterally. **Ask the patient to wrinkle his forehead, close his eyes forcefully, smile, puff his cheeks, and whistle, observing closely for facial asymmetry. Central or cerebral lesions result in relative sparing of the forehead** because of cross-innervation of the orbicularis oculi and frontalis muscles. Check tearing, ability to close the eye and protect the cornea, corneal desiccation, hearing, and, when practical, taste. Examine the ear canal and pinna for herpetic vesicles and the tympanic membrane for signs of otitis media or cholesteatoma.

⊘ **Patients with facial paralysis accompanied by acute otitis media, chronic suppurative middle-ear disease, mastoiditis, otorrhea, or otitis externa require emergent otolaryngologic consultation.** Facial weakness progressing to paralysis over weeks to months, progressive twitching, or facial spasm suggests a neoplasm affecting the facial nerve. When facial paralysis is associated with pulsatile tinnitus and hearing loss, suspect a glomus tumor or cerebellar pontine angle tumor. Diplopia, dysphagia, hoarseness, facial pain, or hypesthesia suggests involvement of cranial nerves other than the seventh and calls for neurologic consultation with early magnetic resonance imaging (MRI).

⊘ If there is a history of head trauma, obtain a computed tomography (CT) scan of the head (including the skull base) or an MRI to rule out a temporal bone fracture.

⊘ MRI with medium contrast of the skull shows a marked increase in the ability to reveal lesions, even of small dimensions, inside the temporal bone and at the cerebellopontine angle.

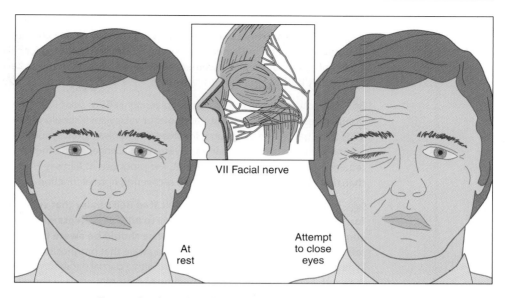

VII Facial nerve

At
rest

Attempt
to close
eyes

Figure 5-1 Partial or complete unilateral facial paralysis that includes one side of the forehead.

✅ **If there are no absolute contraindications to steroid use** (i.e., upper gastrointestinal [GI] bleeding, tuberculosis, acquired autoimmune deficiency syndrome [AIDS], or immunosuppression), **begin therapy with prednisone, 60 mg qd, for 7 days.** For patients with relative contraindications (i.e., hypertension, diabetes), consider giving prednisone in only those patients with a complete paralysis, because they are at higher risk for permanent disability. Prednisone is the only treatment shown to reduce the risk for long-term sequelae of Bell's palsy.

✅ Although there is only controversial data to support its efficacy—but because the most widely accepted cause of a true Bell's palsy, at present, is a neuropathy induced by herpes simplex virus—**when a patient presents within 7 to 10 days of the onset of acute paresis (or paralysis) and symptoms are severe and no other cause is suspected, it is reasonable to prescribe a 10-day course of either acyclovir (Zovirax) (200 to 400 mg) 5 times per day, or 7 days of the more expensive valacyclovir (Valtrex) (1000 mg bid).** There is some evidence to suggest that treatment within 3 days of the onset of symptoms with combined acyclovir and prednisone therapy may be beneficial. Again, this is most likely to have the most gain in patients with a complete lesion, because they have a higher risk for prolonged facial weakness or other sequelae.

✅ **If the cornea is dry or likely to become dry or injured as a result of the patient's inability to produce tears and blink, protect it by patching. If patching is not necessary, recommend that the patient wear eyeglasses, apply methylcellulose artificial tears regularly during the day, and use a protective bland ointment or tape the eyelid shut at night.**

✅ If the patient resides in or has traveled to a tick-endemic area, send a serum specimen for acute-phase Lyme disease titers, if available, because this is another treatable disorder that can present as a facial neuropathy. When there is a history of a tick bite or rash that is consistent with erythema migrans, a lumbar puncture may be required to make a more rapid, definitive diagnosis. **In areas where Lyme disease is endemic, a 10-day course of tetracycline or doxycycline may be indicated.** Amoxicillin is usually substituted for children younger than 8 years of age or for pregnant women. Cefuroxime and erythromycin have also been used successfully but are generally less effective.

✓ If the cause appears to be herpes zoster-varicella or shingles of the facial nerve (e.g., grouped vesicles on the tongue), acyclovir or valacyclovir should still be effective (see Chapter 170). If the geniculate ganglion is involved (i.e., Ramsay-Hunt syndrome, with vesicles in or around the ear, decreased hearing, severe otalgia, encephalitis, meningitis), the patient may require hospitalization for IV treatment. The prognosis of Ramsay-Hunt syndrome is much worse than that of Bell's palsy, with only 10% recovering normal function.

✓ **Inform the patient with uncomplicated Bell's palsy that symptoms may progress for 7 to 10 days. Reassure him that 70% to 80% of patients with Bell's palsy recover completely within a few weeks but that he should be aware that some patients are left with permanent facial weakness.** Be aware that prognosis is linked to the severity of symptoms. Although most (94%) patients with a partial paralysis recover fully, approximately 40% with a complete paralysis at the time of presentation have some residual weakness. Provide for definite follow-up and reevaluation.

✓ Provide appropriate specialty referral, when there is a mass in the head or neck or a history of any malignancy.

What Not To Do:

✗ Do not overlook alternative causes of facial palsy that require different treatment, such as cerebrovascular accidents and cerebellopontine angle tumors (which usually produce weakness in limbs or defects of adjacent cranial nerves), multiple sclerosis (which usually is not painful, spares taste, and often produces intranuclear ophthalmoplegia), and polio (which presents as fever, headache, neck stiffness, and palsies).

✗ Do not order a CT scan unless there is a history of trauma or the symptoms are atypical and include such findings as vertigo, central neurologic signs, or severe headache.

✗ Do not make the diagnosis of Bell's palsy in patients who report gradual onset of facial paralysis over several weeks or facial paralysis that has persisted for 3 months or more. These patients require further evaluation by a neurologist or an otolaryngologist.

Discussion

Idiopathic nerve paralysis is a common malady, affecting 20 per 1 million people every year, especially diabetic or pregnant patients and those between the ages of 15 and 45 years. Up to 10% of patients have a recurrence on the same or other side of the face. The facial nerve is responsible for facial muscle innervation; lacrimal, nasal, and submandibular gland innervation; taste for the anterior two thirds of the tongue; and sensation of the external auditory canal, pinna, and tympanic membrane. Although Bell's palsy was described classically as a pure facial nerve lesion, and physicians have tried to identify the exact level at which the nerve is compressed, the most common presenting complaints are related to trigeminal nerve involvement. The mechanism is probably a

Discussion continued

spotty demyelination of several nerves at several sites caused by reactivated herpes simplex virus. Genetic, metabolic, autoimmune, vascular, and nerve entrapment etiologies have been proposed without definitive proof. It should also be noted that for patients with Bell's palsy, a benefit from steroids or acyclovir has not been definitively established. However, available evidence suggests that steroids are probably effective, and acyclovir (combined with prednisone) is possibly effective in improving facial functional outcomes.

Suggested Readings

Adour KK, Ruboyianes JM, Von Doersten PG, et al: Bell's palsy treatment with acyclovir and prednisone compared with prednisone alone: a double-blind, randomized, controlled trial, *Ann Otol Rhinol Laryngol* 105:371–378, 1996.

Austin JR, Peskind SP, Austin SG, et al: Idiopathic facial nerve paralysis: a randomized double-blind controlled study of placebo versus prednisone, *Laryngoscope* 103:1326–1333, 1993.

Baringer JR: Herpes simplex virus and Bell's palsy (editorial), *Ann Intern Med* 124:63–65, 1996.

Baumgarten KL, Lopez AA, Pankey GA: Rash, Bell's palsy, and back pain following a flu-like illness, *Infect Med* 16: 370-372, 378–379, 1999.

Becelli R: Diagnosis of Bell palsy with gadolinium magnetic resonance imaging, *J Craniofac Surg* 14:51–54, 2003.

Grogan P, Gronseth G: Practice parameter: steroids, acyclovir, and surgery for Bell's palsy (an evidence-based review). Report of the quality standards subcommittee of the American Academy of Neurology, *Neurology* 56:830–836, 2003.

Hato N, Matsumoto S, Kisaki H, et al: Efficacy of early treatment of Bell's palsy with oral acyclovir and prednisolone, *Otol Neurotol* 24:948–951, 2003.

Murakmi S, Mizobuchi M, Nakashiro Y, et al: Bell's palsy and herpes simplex virus: identification of viral DNA in endoneural fluid and muscle, *Ann Intern Med* 124:27–30, 1996.

Ronthal M: Bell's palsy: prognosis and treatment. [*UptoDate* website]. Available at http://www.uptodate.com. Accessed May 5, 2011.

Stankiewicz JA: A review of the published data on steroids and idiopathic facial paralysis, *Otolaryngol Head Neck Surg* 97:481–486, 1987.

Migraine Headache

Presentation

Migraine headache may occur with or, more commonly, without aura. The patient, more commonly female, complains of a pulsating, severe unilateral headache lasting 4 to 72 hours, usually with photophobia and nausea, with or without vomiting and aggravated by moderate physical activity (e.g., walking or climbing stairs). Less commonly, the headache may be bilateral and pressing, and it may follow ophthalmic or neurologic symptoms that resolved as the headache developed. Scintillating castellated scotomata in the visual field, corresponding to the side of the subsequent headache, form the classic aura pattern, but fully reversible visual loss, sensory symptoms (pins and needles and/or numbness), or dysphasia may occur. Basilar-type migraine may be associated with fully reversible dysarthria, vertigo, tinnitus, decreased hearing, double vision, or ataxia. Unlike other headaches, migraines are especially likely to wake the patient in the morning. There may be a family or personal history of similar headaches, and onset during the patient's teens or 20s is common. Primary headaches, which include migraine, tension-type headache, and cluster headache, are benign; these headaches are usually recurrent and not caused by organic disease. Secondary headaches are caused by underlying organic diseases, ranging from sinusitis to subarachnoid hemorrhage.

What To Do:

✅ **Migraine headaches (and similar recurrent primary headache syndromes, with or without nausea and vomiting) are usually treated successfully with IV prochlorperazine (Compazine), 10 mg (0.15 mg/kg up to 10 mg for pediatric migraine headaches), or metoclopramide (Reglan), 10 mg,** with or without a bolus of saline to counteract vasodilatation and orthostasis. **To help prevent mental and motor restlessness (akathisia), administer diphenhydramine (Benadryl), 12 to 25 mg IV, along with the prochlorperazine or metoclopramide.**

✅ If the migraine is of recent onset, the patient has not already taken ergotamines, and starting an IV line may be difficult, treatment should be begun with sumatriptan (Imitrex), 6 mg SC, or dihydroergotamine (DHE 45), 0.25 to 1 mg IM, in a single dose. These drugs are more expensive than prochlorperazine and metoclopramide and can have adverse cardiovascular effects. If DHE is administered IV, pretreatment with an antiemetic, such as prochlorperazine, is necessary.

✅ If the pain has been present most of the day and has precipitated a secondary muscle headache, evinced by muscle tenderness at bony insertions, add ketorolac (Toradol), 60 mg IM, or ibuprofen (Motrin), 800 mg PO for a nonsteroidal anti-inflammatory drug (NSAID) effect (see Chapter 9).

✓ **If the pain persists and the clinician wants to avoid the use of narcotic analgesics, some treatments to try, which have inconclusive evidence but are inexpensive and have few side effects, include intranasal lidocaine and IV magnesium sulfate.**

✓ **Administer intranasal 4% lidocaine (Xylocaine).** Use a 1-mL syringe. Have the patient lie supine with the head hyperextended 45 degrees and rotated 30 degrees toward the side of the headache, and drip 0.5 mL (10 drops) of the lidocaine solution into the ipsilateral nostril over 30 seconds. The patient should remain in this position for 30 minutes. If the headache is bilateral, repeat on the other side. Another technique is to take 4% lidocaine jelly, apply it to a long cotton pledget, and slide it down the nasal canal using bayonet forceps, posterior to the middle turbinate on the side of the headache. The clinician should be aware that the evidence for the effectiveness of intranasal lidocaine in the acute treatment of migraine is inconsistent.

✓ Another relatively benign and inexpensive alternative to narcotics that may be added to regimens including either prochlorperazine or metoclopramide is an **IV infusion of magnesium sulfate, 1 to 2 g in a 10% solution over 5 to 10 minutes.**

✓ If the pain remains severe and drug dependency has been considered, **add a narcotic analgesic (e.g., hydromorphone [Dilaudid], 1 to 2 mg, or morphine sulfate, 4 to 10 mg IV)** and have the patient lie down in a dark, quiet room. It can be cruel to attempt to obtain a complete history and physical examination (and it is unrealistic to expect the patient to cooperate) before some pain relief has been achieved.

✓ After 20 minutes, when the patient is feeling a little better, take the history and perform a physical examination that includes a funduscopic and a complete neurologic examination. **If there are persistent changes in mental status, fever, or stiff neck, or, on neurologic examination, focal findings such as diplopia or unilateral hyperreflexia, paresthesias, weakness, or ataxia, proceed with CT examination, lumbar puncture (LP), or both, to rule out intracranial pathology or infection as the cause of the "migraine."**

✓ **Other danger signals that should trigger a more intensive diagnostic workup, looking for secondary disorders, include hyperacute onset of a new, severe headache ("the worst ever"); a progressive history of seizures; onset with exertion, cough, bending, or sexual intercourse; onset during pregnancy (cerebral venous thrombosis) or during or after middle age; and the presence of a systemic malignant disease, infection, compromised immune system, any new neurologic findings or papilledema on funduscopic examination.**

✓ In patients who are older than the age of 50, consider the possibility of temporal arteritis and obtain an erythrocyte sedimentation rate (ESR). If temporal arteritis is present, there should be jaw claudication and tenderness over the temporal artery. The ESR should be found elevated to more than 50 mm per hour.

✓ **If the presentation is indeed consistent with a migraine or other primary headache, allow the patient to sleep in the emergency department (ED) or clinic undisturbed except for a brief periodic neurologic examination. Typically, the patient will awaken after 1 to 3 hours, with the headache completely resolved or much improved and with no neurologic residua.**

✓ For future attacks, if acetaminophen or NSAIDs have been ineffective and there are no cardiovascular risks, prescribe a self-injector preloaded with 6 mg of sumatriptan. If the patient prefers to take medication orally, try tablets of ergotamine, 1 mg, and caffeine, 100 mg (Cafergot)—two at the first sign of the aura, then one every half hour up to a total daily dosage of six tablets with a maximum of 10 per week. If nausea and vomiting prevent the use of oral medication, Cafergot is also available in rectal suppositories at the same dosage, but one or two suppositories are usually sufficient to relieve a headache. Both oral and rectal absorption of ergotamine is erratic. Sumatriptan can also be administered as a nasal spray. Use the lowest effective dose, either one or two 5-mg sprays or one 20-mg spray. The dose may be repeated once after 2 hours, not to exceed a total daily dose of 40 mg. Rizatriptan (Maxalt, Maxalt MLT—absorbable wafer) can be given, 5 to 10 mg orally every 2 hours, to a maximal dosage of 30 mg per day. Frovatriptan (Frova) and almotriptan (Axert) and eletriptan (Relpax) are oral triptans approved by the US Food and Drug Administration (FDA). There have been few head-to-head trials of the triptans and none since the reformulation of the oral form of sumitriptan to a faster-acting form in 2004. According to one study, prior to the reformulation of sumitriptan, rizatriptan (10 mg), eletriptan (80 mg), and almotriptan (12.5 mg) provide the "highest likelihood of consistent success" for acute migraine. Individual patient responses may vary, and there is no clear indication to choose one over another.

✓ **Parenteral administration of dexamethasone (10 to 25 mg IV) has been shown to prevent early recurrence of migraine headaches** within 24 to 72 hours, in a meta-analysis of several studies (number needed to treat = 9). Oral administration of prednisone does not provide any benefit. Dexamethasone does not provide any relief of the acute headache. **For patients who are not frequently being treated with dexamethasone, but who commonly have early recurrence of headache, this appears to be a good option to add to the standard abortive therapy.** Frequent treatment with dexamethasone may result in adrenal suppression.

✓ **Instruct the patient to return to the ED if there is any change in or worsening of the usual migraine pattern, and make arrangements for medical follow-up. First-time migraine attacks warrant a thorough elective neurologic evaluation to establish the diagnosis.** Long-term prophylaxis may include nonprescription plain magnesium gluconate (200 to 400 mg tid), antidepressants, calcium channel antagonists, NSAIDs, beta-blockers, or anticonvulsants. Lifestyle changes, such as eliminating caffeine, smoking, and certain food triggers, may also be indicated.

What Not To Do:

✗ Do not initiate a comprehensive laboratory workup and perform neuroimaging when the patient presents with a typical benign primary headache with no neurologic deficits.

✗ Do not prescribe medications containing ergotamine, caffeine, or barbiturates for continual prophylaxis. They will not be effective used this way, and withdrawal from these drugs may produce headaches.

✗ Do not omit follow-up, especially for first attacks.

✗ Do not overlook possible meningitis, subarachnoid hemorrhage, glaucoma, or stroke, conditions that may deteriorate rapidly if undiagnosed. Patients with subarachnoid hemorrhage who have normal mental status on presentation are at highest risk for misdiagnosis. Do not talk yourself out of doing a CT/LP in any patient with sudden onset (hyperacute) of the worst headache of their life just because the patient looks good or has a normal examination.

Discussion

Unilateral pain is even more characteristic of migraine than is the aura. ("Migraine" is a corruption of "hemicranium.") The pathophysiology is probably unilateral cerebral vasospasm (producing the neurologic symptoms of the aura), followed by vasodilation (producing the headache). Neurologic symptoms may persist into the headache phase, but the longer they persist, the less likely it is that they are caused by the migraine. Cluster headaches and other trigeminal-autonomic cephalalgias are characterized by trigeminal activation coupled with parasympathetic activation. These headaches are intermittent, short lasting, sharp, excruciating, and unilateral, accompanied by lacrimation and rhinorrhea. Attacks occur in clusters lasting from 7 days to 1 year, and during the pain, patients are usually agitated and restless. The treatment of an attack is usually the same as that for migraines.

Acute migraine headaches are self-limited and respond well to placebos, and, therefore, several different therapies are effective. No single drug or class of drug has clearly emerged as the best treatment for acute migraine. The wide variability in patient needs and responses means that many agents will continue to play important roles. Although butalbital-containing compounds are often used to treat migraine, their use should be limited because of the risk of overuse and consequent medication overuse headache and withdrawal problems. Be cautious in the use of ergot or serotonin agonists to treat any patient who has angina, focal weakness, or sensory deficits. It is possible to precipitate ischemia of the brain or heart in such patients by using preparations that act by causing vasoconstriction. Sumatriptan should not be administered to postmenopausal women, men older than 40 years, and patients with vascular risk factors, such as hypertension, hypercholesterolemia, obesity, diabetes, smoking, or a strong family history of vascular disease. Sumatriptan also should not be used within 24 hours of administration of an ergotamine-containing medication.

Patients with aneurysms or arteriovenous malformations can present clinically as migraine patients. If there is something different about the severity or nature of this headache, consider the possibility of a subarachnoid hemorrhage. Headaches that are always on the same side and in the same location are very suspicious for an underlying structural lesion (e.g., aneurysm, arteriovenous malformation).

To help reassure patients, it can be noted that isolated headache was the first and only clinical symptom in just 8.2% of patients with an intracranial tumor.

Many patients seeking narcotics have learned that faking a migraine headache is even easier than faking a ureteral stone, but they usually do not follow the typical course of falling asleep after being given a shot and waking up a few hours later with pain relief. It is a good policy to limit narcotics for treatment of migraine headaches to one or two shots and avoid prescribing oral narcotics in the ED or doctor's office.

Suggested Readings

Aukerman G, Knutson D, Miser WF: Management of the acute migraine headache, *Am Fam Physician* 66:2123-2130, 2140–2141, 2002.

Bajwa Z, Sabaha A: Acute treatment of migraine in adults. [*UptoDate* website]. Available at http://www.uptodate.com. Accessed February 18, 2011.

Brousseau DC, Duffy SJ, Anderson AC, et al: Treatment of pediatric migraine headaches: a randomized, double-blind trial of prochlorperazine versus ketorolac, *Ann Emerg Med* 43:256–262, 2004.

Cameron JD, Lane PL, Speechley M: Intravenous chlorpromazine vs intravenous metoclopramide in acute migraine headache, *Acad Emerg Med* 2:597–602, 1995.

Clinch CR: Evaluation of acute headaches in adults, *Am Fam Physician* 63:685–692, 2001.

Coppola M, Yealy DM, Leibold RA: Randomized, placebo-controlled evaluation of prochlorperazine versus metoclopramide for emergency department treatment of migraine headache, *Ann Emerg Med* 26:541–546, 1995.

Corbo J, Esses D, Bijur PE, et al: Randomized clinical trial of intravenous magnesium sulfate as an adjunctive medication for emergency department treatment of migraine headache, *Ann Emerg Med* 38:621–627, 2001.

Demirkaya S, Dora B, et al: Efficacy of intravenous magnesium sulfate in the treatment of acute migraine attacks, *Headache* 41:171–177, 2001.

Drotts DL, Vinson DR: Prochlorperazine induces akathisia in emergency patients, *Ann Emerg Med* 34:469–475, 1999.

Ferrari MD, et al: Oral triptans (serotonin 5-HT 1B/1D agonists) in acute migraine treatment: a meta-analysis of 53 trials, *Lancet* 358:1668, 2001.

Frank LR, Olson CM, Shuler KB, Gharib SF: Intravenous magnesium for acute benign headache in the emergency department, *Can J Emerg Med* 6:327–332, 2004.

Huff JS: What is a migraine, anyway, and when is it gone? *Acad Emer Med* 5:561–562, 1998.

Kabbouche MA, Vockell AB, LeCates SL, et al: Tolerability and effectiveness of prochlorperazine for intractable migraine in children, *Pediatrics* 107:E62, 2001.

Kao LW, Kirk MA, Evers SJ, et al: Droperidol, QT prolongation, and sudden death: what is the evidence? *Ann Emerg Med* 41:546–558, 2003.

Klapper JA, Stanton J: Current emergency treatment of severe migraine headaches, *Headache* 33:560–562, 1993.

Lipton RB, Bigal ME, Steiner TJ, et al: Classification of primary headaches, *Neurology* 63:427–435, 2004.

Maizels M, Scott B, Cohen W, et al: Intranasal lidocaine for treatment of migraine, *JAMA* 276:319–321, 1996.

Matchar DB: Acute management of migraine. Paper presented at the 55th Annual meeting of the American Academy of Neurology, Honolulu, Hawaii, April 8, 2003.

Mauskop A, Altura BT, Cracco RQ, et al: Intravenous magnesium sulfate rapidly alleviates headaches of various types, *Headache* 36:154–156, 1996.

Miner JR, Fish SJ, Smith SW, et al: Droperidol vs prochlorperazine for benign headaches in the emergency department, *Acad Emerg Med* 8:873–879, 2001.

Salomone JA, Thomas RW, Althoff JR, et al: An evaluation of the role of the ED in the management of migraine headaches, *Am J Emerg Med* 12:134–137, 1994.

Seim MB, March JA, Dunn KA: Intravenous ketorolac vs intravenous prochlorperazine for the treatment of migraine headaches, *Acad Emerg Med* 5:573–576, 1998.

Silvers SM, Simmons B, Wall S, et al: Clinical policy: critical issues in the evaluation and management of patients presenting to the emergency department with acute headache, *Ann Emerg Med* 39:108–122, 2002.

Vinson DR: Treatment patterns of isolated benign headache in US emergency departments, *Ann Emerg Med* 39:215–222, 2002.

Vinson DR, Drotts DL: Diphenhydramine for the prevention of akathisia induced by prochlorperazine: a randomized, controlled trial, *Ann Emerg Med* 37:125–131, 2001.

Weaver CS, Jones JB, Chisholm CD: Droperidol vs. prochlorperazine for the treatment of acute headache, *J Emerg Med* 26:145–150, 2004.

Seizures (Convulsions, Fits), Adult

Presentation

The patient experiencing seizures may be found in the street, the hospital, or the ED. The patient may complain of an "aura," feel he is "about to have a seizure," experience a brief petit mal "absence," exhibit the repetitive stereotypical behavior of complex partial seizures, display the whole-body tonic stiffness or clonic jerking of generalized (grand mal) seizures, or simply be found in the gradual recovery of the postictal confusion and lethargy. Patients experiencing generalized tonic-clonic seizures can injure themselves, most often by biting the tongue laterally or by having an unprotected fall.

What To Do:

If the patient is having a generalized tonic-clonic seizure, stand by him for a few minutes, until the jerking movements subside, to guard against injury or airway obstruction. Usually, only suctioning or turning the patient on his side is required, but breathing will be uncoordinated until the tonic-clonic phase is over.

Watch the pattern of the seizure for clues to the cause. (Did clonus start in one place and "march" out to the rest of the body? Did the eyes deviate one way throughout the seizure? Was there any staring or focal motor symptoms? Did the whole body participate?) If the seizure is over get a careful description of the event from an eyewitness, if possible.

If the seizure lasts more than 5 minutes or recurs before the patient regains consciousness (status epilepticus), it has overwhelmed the brain's natural buffers, and drugs should be initiated to stop the seizure. Give 2 to 4 mg of IV lorazepam (Ativan) at 2 mg/min (recommended treatment),

> or give 5 to 10 mg of IV diazepam (Valium) at 2 to 5 mg/min,
> > or **give 0.02 mg/kg diazepam rectally (gel or IV form may be used) when IV access cannot be obtained,**
> > or **give 5 mg (0.07 mg/kg) of IM midazolam (Versed) when IV access cannot be obtained.**

With a prolonged seizure, this treatment should be followed by loading with phenytoin (Dilantin) or fosphenytoin (Cerebyx) to prevent recurrence of seizures. Give phenytoin, 10 to 15 mg/kg IV over 30 minutes—at less than 50 mg/min. (The patient should be on cardiac monitoring during administration, and a Dilantin level should be checked first if the patient is thought to be taking the drug.) Alternatively, give fosphenytoin, 15 to 20 mg/kg IV or IM at a maximum IV rate of 150 mg PE (phenytoin sodium equivalents)/min with an initial maintenance dose of 4 to 6 mg/min. (Although much more expensive than phenytoin, fosphenytoin can be given more quickly over 15 minutes, or, if IV access is absent, this drug can be given IM; it does not have the tissue toxicity of extravasated phenytoin if IV access is questionable.)

✓ Status epilepticus is defined as a generalized tonic-clonic seizure in an adult that lasts more than 5 minutes or intermittent convulsions, without recovery of baseline level of consciousness between seizures.

✓ **In all cases of status epilepticus, check the patient's blood glucose level (especially if he is wearing a "diabetes" MedicAlert bracelet or medallion) by performing a quick finger stick test and administering IV glucose if the level is below normal.**

✓ If the patient arrives in the postictal phase, examine thoroughly for injuries and signs of systemic disease that can provoke seizures. Elevated temperature can be a sign of meningitis or encephalitis. Nuchal rigidity strongly suggests either central nervous system (CNS) infection or subarachnoid hemorrhage. Record a complete neurologic examination, the results of which are apt to be bizarre. Repeat the neurologic examination periodically, looking for findings suggestive of focal brain disease.

✓ If the patient is indeed recovering, you may be able to obviate much of the diagnostic workup by waiting until he is lucid enough to give a history. Postictal inability to arouse may last 10 minutes after a generalized tonic-clonic seizure, with confusion typically lasting less than 30 minutes.

✓ If the patient arrives awake and oriented after a presumed seizure, corroborate the history through witness accounts or the presence of injuries, such as a scalp laceration, a bitten tongue, or the presence of urinary or fecal incontinence.

✓ Doubt a generalized tonic-clonic seizure if there is no typical postictal recovery period.

✓ Investigate for alcohol or substance abuse; withdrawal from alcohol, benzodiazepines, or barbiturates can provoke seizures.

✓ If the patient has a history of seizure disorder or is taking anticonvulsant medications, check his records and determine current and past frequency of seizures. Speak to his physician, and find out whether a cause has been determined and what studies have been performed (e.g., CT, MRI, EEG). Look for reasons for this relapse (e.g., poor compliance with medications, infection, ethanol poisoning, or lack of sleep).

✓ **If the seizure is clearly related to alcohol withdrawal, give 2 mg of IV lorazepam (Ativan) and ascertain why the patient reduced consumption of alcohol.** Reasons for decreasing alcohol consumption may include inability to afford alcohol, suffering from pancreatitis or gastritis causing inability to consume alcohol (requiring further evaluation and treatment), or, the patient may have decided to try to stop drinking, realizing it is bad for him. If the patient is requesting detoxification, he should be supported in this decision both medically and emotionally, and additional recovery resources should be discussed.

✓ If a patient is demonstrating signs of delirium tremens, such as tremors, tachycardia, and hallucinations, withdrawal should be medically supervised and treated with benzodiazepines.

✓ Initial treatment with IV lorazepam has been shown to produce a significant reduction in the risk for recurrent seizures related to alcohol.

✓ Because many alcoholics are malnourished, ED physicians will often presumptively treat alcohol withdrawal symptoms with an IV infusion containing glucose, 100 mg of thiamine, 2 g of magnesium, 1 mg of folic acid, and multivitamins, even though there is no convincing evidence that this regimen is of any true benefit in isolated alcohol withdrawal. However, thiamine has been shown to be beneficial in preventing coma and death as a result of Wernicke encephalopathy in patients presenting with altered mental status. Administration of thiamine and vitamins is inexpensive, and has very few side effects. Given this, it is advisable to treat alcoholic patients presenting with acute delirium for both alcohol withdrawal and thiamine deficiency.

✓ **If the seizure is a new event, obtain a serum glucose level (to confirm a rapid bedside test result) as well as serum electrolyte concentrations (sodium, calcium, magnesium), renal function tests, hepatic function tests (if liver impairment is suspected), complete blood cell count (if infection is suspected), and urine toxicology screen (if drugs of abuse are suspected). In women of childbearing age, test for pregnancy.**

✓ **With new-onset seizures, a brain CT scan should be performed to rule out intracranial hemorrhage, ischemic stroke, or tumor. MRI is the gold standard in evaluating seizure disorders and should be obtained when available.**

✓ Lumbar puncture should be performed when fever, persistent altered mental status, or nuchal rigidity indicates a possibility of meningitis or encephalitis. Suspicion of subarachnoid hemorrhage should also prompt lumbar puncture, even when head CT scans are normal. A lumbar puncture should also be performed on immunocompromised patients.

✓ About 50% of all patients with a new onset of seizure require hospitalization. Most of these patients can be identified by abnormalities evident on physical examination, head CT scan, toxicology studies, or the other tests mentioned earlier.

✓ **If the patient has an established seizure disorder, blood tests are not routinely needed when the patient has a single breakthrough seizure. Anticonvulsant drug levels should be checked when toxicity or noncompliance is suspected.** The dose should be adjusted to keep the level above the breakthrough point. Finding a level below the reported therapeutic range should not prompt a dose increase in a patient who has been seizure free for a prolonged period. Neuroimaging and lumbar puncture are unnecessary unless there are new findings to cause suspicion for tumor, intracranial hemorrhage, or CNS infection.

✓ **A neurologist should be consulted before antiepileptic drug treatment is initiated for brief new-onset seizures.** Many neurologists think it is in the patient's best interest to withhold long-term anticonvulsant therapy until a second seizure occurs. The neurologist may want to make a detailed evaluation of the patient and counsel him regarding risk for seizure recurrence, the advantages and disadvantages of anticonvulsant therapy, and the psychosocial effect of another seizure. **Patients with a single, brief, uncomplicated seizure, a normal neurologic examination, no comorbidity, and no known structural brain disease need not be started on any antiepileptic drug prior to outpatient referral.**

✓ High risk for recurrence is present when there is a history of brain insult, when an EEG demonstrates epileptiform abnormalities, and when MRI demonstrates a structural lesion.

✅ **Patients with generalized seizures should be advised to avoid dangerous situations. They should take showers rather than baths, not swim without supervision, and not work at heights. Driving should also be restricted until an appropriate seizure-free period has elapsed, specified 6 to 12 months in most states.**

✅ **If the neurologist recommends phenytoin loading in a stable awake patient, an acceptable oral regimen can be prescribed. Give 1 g of phenytoin capsules divided into three doses (400 mg, 300 mg, 300 mg) administered at 2-hour intervals.**

What Not To Do:

❌ Do not forget to check blood glucose at the bedside.

❌ Do not stick anything in the mouth of a seizing patient. The ubiquitous padded throat sticks may be nice for a patient to hold and to bite on at the first sign of a seizure, but they do nothing to protect the airway and are ineffective when the jaw is clenched.

❌ Do not rush to give IV diazepam to a seizing patient. Most seizures stop within a few minutes. It is diagnostically useful to see how the seizure resolves without medication aid; also, the patient will awaken sooner if he has not been medicated.

❌ Do not wait 30 minutes before initiating anticonvulsant therapy for a patient having a continuous seizure or not awakening between intermittent seizures (old definition of status epilepticus). For practical purposes, a seizure lasting longer than 5 minutes should be treated as generalized convulsive status epilepticus, because a generalized tonic-clonic seizure lasting longer than 5 minutes is unlikely to stop spontaneously.

❌ Be careful not to assume an alcoholic cause. Ethanol abusers sustain more head trauma and seizure disorders than does the population at large.

❌ Do not treat alcohol withdrawal seizures with phenobarbital or phenytoin. Both are ineffective (and unnecessary because the problem is self limiting) and can themselves produce withdrawal seizures.

❌ Do not rule out alcohol withdrawal seizures on the basis of a high serum ethanol level. The patient may actually be withdrawing from an even higher baseline.

❌ Do not be fooled by pseudoseizures. Even patients with genuine epilepsy occasionally fake seizures for various reasons, and an exceptional performer can be convincing. Amateurs may be roused with ammonia or smelling salts, and few can simulate the fluctuating neurologic abnormalities of the postictal state. Probably no one can voluntarily produce the pronounced metabolic acidosis or serum lactate elevation of a grand mal seizure (see Chapter 4).

❌ Do not release a patient who has persistent neurologic abnormalities before a head CT scan or specialty consultation has been obtained.

❌ Do not allow a patient who experienced a seizure to drive home.

Discussion

Seizures are time-limited paroxysmal events that result from abnormal, involuntary, rhythmic neuronal discharges in the brain. Except for rare instances, seizures are not predictable and can occur at inconvenient, embarrassing, or even dangerous times. Seizures are usually short, lasting less than 5 minutes, but can be preceded by a prodromal phase and followed by a long postictal phase, during which there is a gradual return to baseline.

Seizures have been referred to as either grand mal seizures (convulsive movements) or petit mal seizures (staring without convulsive movements). Currently, more precise terminology is preferred.

Epilepsy is a disease characterized by spontaneous recurrence of unprovoked seizures. Provoked seizures result from transient alterations in brain metabolism in an otherwise normal brain. Some factors that can trigger such seizures are hypoglycemia, hyponatremia, hypocalcemia, alcohol and illicit drug withdrawal, meningitis, encephalitis, stroke, and certain toxins and toxic drugs.

The new terminology for seizures divides them into two classes: generalized seizures and partial seizures. With generalized seizures, there is a complete loss of consciousness at onset of the seizure. Partial seizures are characterized by retention of consciousness, because they begin in a limited brain region. Partial seizures can secondarily generalize.

There are seven types of generalized seizures, which start throughout the entire cortex at the same time and, therefore, cause loss of consciousness. They are the following:

- Generalized tonic-clonic (grand mal) seizures with a tonic phase of whole-body stiffening, followed by a clonic phase of repetitive contractions.
- Tonic seizures, which consist of only the stiffening phase.
- Clonic seizures, which consist of only the repetitive contractions.
- Myoclonic seizures, characterized by brief, lightning-like muscular jerks.
- Absence (petit mal) seizures, which are manifested as brief (1 to 10 seconds) episodes of staring and unresponsiveness. These seizures, unlike complex partial seizures, are rarely found in adults, are very brief, do not produce postictal confusion, and occur very frequently (up to 100 per day).
- Atypical absence seizures, which are similar to absence seizures but last longer and often include more motor involvement.

- Atonic seizures, characterized by sudden loss of muscle tone and subsequent falling or dropping to the floor unprotected (drop attacks). These seizures must be differentiated from syncope. (see Chapter 11).

Partial seizures are divided into simple and complex. In simple partial seizures, only one neurologic modality is affected during the seizure. The resulting symptoms depend on the area of the brain cortex from which the seizure arises. Motor (focal) seizures may produce clonic hand movements. Sensory, autonomic, and psychiatric symptoms may be expressed as visual phenomena, olfactory sensations (usually unpleasant), déjà vu phenomena, and formed hallucinations or memories. These "auras" are merely simple partial seizures.

Complex partial seizures (psychomotor or temporal lobe seizures) are associated with alteration, but not loss, of consciousness. The patient is awake and staring blankly but is not responsive to external stimuli. These seizures may be accompanied by automatism (repetitive, purposeless movements, such as lip smacking and chewing, hand wringing, patting, and rubbing) and last 30 to 50 seconds. They are followed by postictal confusion and occur weekly to monthly.

Generalized tonic-clonic seizures are frightening and inspire observers to "do something," but usually it is necessary only to stand by and prevent the patient from injury.

The age of the patient is associated with the probable underlying cause of a first seizure and therefore is a factor in disposition. In the 12- to 20-year-old patient, the seizure is probably "idiopathic," although other causes are certainly possible. In the 40-year-old patient experiencing a first seizure, neoplasm, posttraumatic epilepsy, and withdrawal must be excluded. In the 65-year-old patient experiencing a first seizure, cerebrovascular insufficiency must also be considered. With elderly patients, the possibility of an impending stroke, in addition to the other possible causes, should be kept in mind during treatment and workup.

Also, patients should be discharged for outpatient care only if there is full recovery of neurologic function, should possibly be given a full loading dose of phenytoin, and should make clear arrangements for follow-up or return to the ED if another seizure occurs. An EEG can usually

(continued)

Discussion continued

be done electively, except in cases of status epilepticus. A toxic screen may be needed to detect the many drug overdoses that can present as seizures, including overdoses of drugs such as amphetamines, cocaine, isoniazid, lidocaine, lithium, phencyclidine, phenytoin, and tricyclic antidepressants.

Suggested Readings

Diazepam. [*Lexi-Comp* website]. Available at www.Lexi.com. Accessed February 18, 2011.

D'Onofrio G, Rathlev NK, Ulrich AS, et al: Lorazepam for the prevention of recurrent seizures related to alcohol, *N Engl J Med* 340:915–919, 1999.

Eisner RF, Turnbull TL, Howes DS, et al: Efficacy of a "standard" seizure workup in the emergency department, *Ann Emerg Med* 15:33–39, 1986.

Henneman PL, DeRoos F, Lewis RJ: Determining the need for admission in patients with new-onset seizures, *Ann Emerg Med* 24:1108–1114, 1994.

Parzirandeh S, Burns DL: Overview of water-soluble vitamins. [*UptoDate* website]. Available at http://www.uptodate.com. Accessed February 18, 2011.

Schachter S: Evaluation of first seizures in adults. [*UptoDate* website]. Available at http://www.uptodateonline.com. Accessed February 18, 2011.

Shneker BF, Fountain NB: Epilepsy, *Dis Mon* 49:426–478, 2003.

Towne AR, DeLorenzo RJ: Use of intramuscular midazolam for status epilepticus, *J Emerg Med* 17:323–328, 1999.

Seizures (Convulsions, Fits), Febrile and Pediatric

Presentation

Parents who are frightened and concerned bring in their child who has just had a generalized seizure with jerking tonic-clonic movements and loss of consciousness, followed by a period of postictal obtundation that gradually resolves within 30 minutes. The patient has completely recovered by the time he is brought to your attention. The parents may have been horrified by the sight of their child becoming cyanotic with breathing difficulty, unresponsiveness, and jerking eye movements during the seizure. The child may be found to have a fever, and there may be a family history of febrile seizures. A vaccination with diphtheria and tetanus toxoids and whole-cell pertussis vaccine may have been administered earlier in the day or 1 to 2 weeks following a measles, mumps, and rubella vaccination.

What To Do:

In the nonfebrile child:

✅ Obtain a history of possible precipitating factors, such as trauma or toxin or drug ingestion. Inquire into recent condition(s) and medical history, as well as any family history of seizure disorders.

✅ Have witnesses describe the event in detail, including the type of motor and eye movements, changes in breathing and skin color, and whether or not there was complete loss of consciousness or incontinence. Determine the duration of the seizure and the length of the postictal period.

✅ Perform a physical examination that includes evaluation of pupil size and reactivity, along with funduscopy to look for retinal hemorrhage, which would suggest intentional injury. After the patient has experienced full recovery from the postictal state, the physical examination should be entirely normal.

✅ In children older than 6 months of age, in the absence of a history of illness, vomiting or diarrhea, or suspected ingestion, routine laboratory testing is not needed.

✅ **Infants younger than 6 months of age require immediate glucose testing to rule out hypoglycemia. Serum sodium, calcium, and magnesium levels should also be determined to rule out low levels of these electrolytes. Toxicology screening should be considered if there is suspicion of toxin exposure.**

✅ A computed tomography (CT) scan should be obtained if there are findings of head trauma, focal (partial) seizure, seizure longer than 5 minutes, focal postictal deficits not rapidly resolving (Todd paralysis), persistently altered level of consciousness, sickle cell disease, bleeding disorders, malignancy, or human immunodeficiency virus (HIV) infection. **For most children, immediate neuroimaging is not indicated.**

✅ **Children who have just one unprovoked seizure—for whom there is no suspicion of trauma, infection, or intoxication—and who have returned to their baseline state, may be discharged with appropriate medical follow-up. Antiepileptic drugs are usually not prescribed.**

✅ Parents should be appropriately reassured and informed that 60% of such children never have a recurrence. Discharge instructions should describe what to do if the seizure recurs.

✅ **If seizure activity persists for more than 5 minutes, consider bag-valve-mask ventilation or intubation if there is significant respiratory compromise. An IV line should be placed, and a bedside glucose test should be performed. If the patient is hypoglycemic, 0.5 to 1 g/kg of glucose should be given as a bolus (2 mL/kg of 25% dextrose in water or, in neonates, 5 mL/kg of 10% dextrose in water).**

With IV or IO (intraosseous) access:
— **give lorazepam (Ativan), 0.1 mg/kg IV over 2 to 5 minutes; may repeat in 5 to 10 minutes up to a 4-mg dose (recommended treatment)**
— or give diazepam (Valium), 0.2 to 0.5 mg/kg IV every 15 to 30 minutes to a maximum 5-mg dose.

Without IV or IO access:
— **give lorazepam, 0.1 mg/kg rectally up to a 4-mg dose**
— or give diazepam gel (Diastat), 0.5 mg/kg rectally up to a 10-mg dose.
— or give midazolam (Versed), 0.1 to 0.2 mg/kg IM × 1 up to a 10-mg dose.

✅ **All children who present in status epilepticus should be considered for treatment with a long-acting antiepileptic drug, such as:**

— **phenytoin (Dilantin), 20 mg/kg IV at less than 1 mg/kg/min up to 1000 mg**
— **or fosphenytoin (Cerebyx), 20 mg/kg PE (phenytoin sodium equivalents) up to 1000 mg at less than 3 mg/kg/min (safety and efficacy not established for pediatric patients)**
— or phenobarbital, 10 to 20 mg/kg IV up to 1000 mg at less than 1 to 2 mg/kg/min.

In the febrile child:

✅ A careful history and physical examination should be done to identify a possible source of the fever and to rule out any evidence of trauma.

✅ **Children between the ages of 6 months and 5 years who have simple febrile seizures (generalized, lasting less than 5 minutes and occurring only once in a 24-hour**

period) carry few risks for complications and do not require any routine diagnostic studies.

✓ **Children with fever without an identifiable source should be evaluated for urinary tract infection.**

✓ In patients whose level of consciousness has not returned to baseline; who have a bulging fontanel, a positive Kernig or Brodzinski sign, photophobia, severe headache, or pretreatment with antibiotics; or who are lethargic or irritable, lumbar puncture should be performed to exclude meningitis. Children who are younger than 6 months of age must be evaluated for metabolic abnormalities, underlying neurologic disorders, meningitis, and encephalitis.

✓ **Antibiotics are only indicated for focal infections.**

✓ **Antipyretics have not been found to be effective in preventing the recurrence of febrile seizures. Benzodiazepines are also probably of no practical benefit when used for prophylaxis.**

✓ **There is no evidence that children with simple febrile seizures have any difference in cognitive outcomes than children without such seizures, and although these seizures appear frightening, they are generally harmless. Parents should be reassured and given written, detailed information about febrile seizures and then referred back to their primary care physician for follow-up.**

✓ Febrile seizures that are focal, last more than 10 minutes, or recur within 24 hours are complex febrile seizures that require a more intensive investigation and are associated with a greater risk for later epilepsy.

What Not To Do:

✗ Do not perform a lumbar puncture on an afebrile child who has returned to normal mental status and has no meningeal signs.

✗ Do not do routine neuroimaging on children with first-time afebrile seizures or febrile seizure patients who have a normal neurologic examination with full postseizure recovery.

✗ Do not do routine laboratory testing on children who are older than 6 months of age who have not been ill without vomiting or diarrhea and where there is no suspicion of a toxic ingestion.

✗ Do not start antiepileptic drugs on patients with simple febrile seizures or first-time, unprovoked, uncomplicated seizures.

✗ Do not try using "around-the-clock" acetaminophen or ibuprofen to prevent the recurrence of febrile seizures. It may only contribute to the parents' fever phobia.

Discussion

Seizures are either generalized or partial (focal). Generalized seizures can be of several types: absence, atonic, tonic-clonic, tonic, myoclonic, or infantile spasms. Partial seizures are classified as simple (simple partial), in which consciousness is preserved, or complex (complex partial), in which consciousness is impaired. Secondarily generalized seizures are partial seizures that become generalized.

Paroxysmal nonepileptic disorders that may be mistaken for seizures include syncope (which may include a brief seizure with immediate awakening), breath-holding spells (which usually occur with crying until there is a noiseless state of expiration, color change, loss of consciousness, and postural tone with occasional body jerking and urinary incontinence), and night terrors (in which a 2- to 6-year-old child awakens suddenly within 4 hours of falling asleep, appears frightened or confused, cries, and becomes diaphoretic, tachycardic, and tachypneic and then falls asleep and is amnesic regarding the event the following morning). Other disorders that can mimic seizures are migraine headaches (which can be accompanied by an aura, motor dysfunction, and clouding of consciousness), apparent life-threatening events (ALTE) (which are episodes characterized by some combination of infant apnea, color change, choking, gagging, and loss of muscle tone), and pseudoseizures (most commonly occurring in teenage girls and usually consisting of bilateral, thrashing motor activity and rarely result in injury) (see Chapter 4).

Febrile seizures are defined as those that occur in febrile children who are 6 months to 5 years of age who do not have evidence of intracranial infection or known seizure disorder.

Because most febrile seizures occur during the first 24 hours of illness, the seizure is the first sign of a febrile illness in approximately 25% to 50% of cases. Although children with febrile seizures have high mean temperatures (39.8° C), they are not at high risk for serious bacterial illness.

Most clinicians now define status epilepticus to be continuous or repetitive seizure activity for longer than 5 minutes. Because almost all self-limited seizures stop within 5 minutes, antiepileptic drug therapy should be initiated for any patient with a seizure lasting longer than 5 minutes. Seizure duration of longer than 1 hour, especially with hypoxia, has been associated with permanent neurologic injury.

Overall, the risk for recurrent febrile seizures is increased in younger patients (younger than 12 months old) with a first-time febrile seizure, patients with lower temperatures (less than 40° C) on presentation of their first seizure, patients with shorter duration of fever before the seizure (less than 24 hours), and patients with a family history of febrile seizures.

In the general population, the risk for development of epilepsy by the age of 7 years is approximately 1%. Children who have had one simple febrile seizure have a slightly higher risk for developing epilepsy. Children who were younger than 12 months of age at their first simple febrile seizure or those who have had several simple febrile seizures have a 2.4% risk for developing epilepsy. The risk for developing epilepsy increases to 30 to 50 times that of the general population in patients who have had one or more complex febrile seizures, particularly seizures with focal features in a child with abnormal neurologic development.

Suggested Readings

El Radhi AS: Do antipyretics prevent febrile convulsions? *Arch Dis Child* 88:641–642, 2003.

Freedman SB, Powell EC: Pediatric seizures and their management in the emergency department, *Clin Pediatr Emerg Med* 4:195–206, 2003.

Shah SS, Alpern ER, Zwerling L, et al: Low risk of bacteremia in children with febrile seizures, *Arch Pediatr Adolesc Med* 156:469–472, 2002.

Trainor JL, Hampers LC, Krug SE, et al: Children with first-time simple febrile seizures are at low risk of serious bacterial illness, *Acad Emerg Med* 8:781–787, 2001.

Valencia I, Sklar E, Blanco F, et al: The role of routine serum laboratory tests in children presenting to the emergency department with unprovoked seizures, *Clin Pediatr* 42:511–517, 2003.

Warden CR, Zibulewsky J, Mace S, et al: Evaluation and management of febrile seizures in the out-of-hospital and emergency department settings, *Ann Emerg Med* 41:215–222, 2003.

Tension-Type (Muscle Contraction) Headache

Presentation

The patient complains of a mild to moderate, dull, steady (nonpulsating) pain, described as a pressing, tightening, squeezing, or constricting band, located bilaterally anywhere from the eyes to the occiput, perhaps including the neck or shoulders. Often the headache is a bilateral tightness or sensation of pressure around the temples. Most commonly, the headache develops near the end of the day or after some particularly stressful event. There is usually no photophobia, nausea, or vomiting, although photophobia and phonophobia can occur (but not both), and the patient may be anorexic. These headaches may also be associated with lightheadedness and feeling tired. Tension-type headache pain can last from 30 minutes to several days and can be continuous in severe cases. It is classified as infrequent episodic (<1 day per month), frequent episodic (1 to 14 days per month), and chronic (>15 days per month and can occur with or without muscle spasm). The pain may improve with rest or administration of nonsteroidal anti-inflammatory drugs (NSAIDs), acetaminophen, or other medications. The physical examination is unremarkable, except for possible cranial or posterior cervical muscle spasm or tenderness and difficulty relaxing.

What To Do:

✅ Obtain a complete general history (including environmental factors and foods that precede the headaches) and perform a physical examination (including a neurologic and funduscopic examination).

✅ If the patient complains of a sudden onset of the "worst headache of my life"—a thunderclap headache that reaches maximal intensity within 1 minute or a headache accompanied by any change in mental status, weakness, seizures, stiff neck, or persistent neurologic abnormalities— suspect a cerebrovascular cause, especially a subarachnoid hemorrhage, intracranial hemorrhage, aneurysm, or arteriovenous malformation. The usual initial diagnostic test for these is CT. Other indications for a CT scan are changes in frequency, severity, or clinical features of the headaches or a new, daily, persistent headache.

✅ A CT scan is also needed in evaluating the first headache in a patient 35 years old or older, or when exertion precipitates a headache that persists after the exertion stops, or when pain awakens the patient from sleep, or when the headache pain is unilateral or focal.

✅ If the headache is accompanied by fever and stiff neck or change in mental status, rule out bacterial meningitis as soon as possible by performing a lumbar puncture (LP).

✅ If there is a history or suspicion of head injury, especially in elderly patients or those on anticoagulants or with a bleeding diathesis, obtain a CT scan to rule out an intracranial hemorrhage. Chronic alcoholic patients must be presumed to be coagulopathic in these circumstances.

✅ If the headache is nonspecific or was preceded by ophthalmic or neurologic symptoms that are now resolving, which is suggestive of a migraine headache, try prochlorperazine, sumatriptan, or ergotamine therapy (see Chapter 6). If vasospastic neurologic symptoms persist into the headache phase, the cause may still be a migraine, but it becomes more important to rule out other cerebrovascular causes.

✅ If the headache follows prolonged reading, driving, or television watching, and decreased visual acuity is improved when the patient looks through a pinhole, the headache may be the result of a defect in optical refraction, which is correctable with new eyeglass lenses.

✅ If the temporal arteries are tender, check for visual defects, jaw claudication, myalgias, and an elevated erythrocyte sedimentation rate, which accompany temporal arteritis.

✅ If there is a history of recent dental work or grinding of the teeth, tenderness anterior to the tragus, or crepitus on motion of the jaw, suspect arthritis of the temporomandibular joint.

✅ If there is fever, tenderness to percussion over the frontal or maxillary sinuses, purulent drainage visible in the nose, or facial pain exacerbated by lowering the head, consider sinusitis.

✅ If pain radiates to the ear, inspect and palpate the teeth for tenderness. Dental pain is a common cause of such headache pain.

✅ Finally, **after checking for all other causes of headache, palpate the temporalis, occipitalis, and other muscles of the calvarium and neck to look for areas of tenderness and spasm that sometimes accompany muscle tension headaches. Watch for especially tender trigger points** (Figure 9-1) **that may resolve with gentle pressure, massage, or trigger-point**

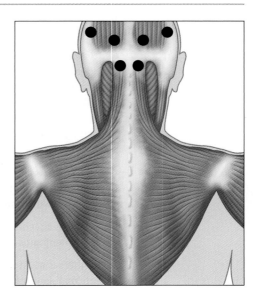

Figure 9-1 Tension headache trigger points.

injection (see Chapter 123). Such **trigger-point injection** may completely relieve symptoms within 5 to 10 minutes. Pain relief helps to make the diagnosis more certain.

✅ **If there are no contraindications, prescribe anti-inflammatory analgesics (e.g., ibuprofen, naproxen) which, in recent studies, have been shown to be more efficacious than acetaminophen. Recommend rest, and have the patient try applying cool compresses and massaging any trigger points. If NSAIDS are contraindicated, acetaminophen may also be effective.**

✅ Explain the cause and treatment of muscle spasm of the head and neck.

✅ Tell the patient that there is no evidence of other serious disease (if this is true); especially inform him that a brain tumor is unlikely. (Often this fear is never voiced.)

✅ Arrange for follow-up. Instruct the patient to return to the emergency department or contact his own physician if symptoms change or worsen.

What Not To Do:

❌ Do not discharge the patient without providing follow-up instructions. Many serious illnesses begin with minor cephalgia, and patients may postpone necessary early follow-up care if they believe that they were definitively diagnosed on their first visit.

❌ Do not obtain CT scans for patients who have long-term recurrent headaches with no recent change in pattern, no history of seizures, and no focal neurologic findings.

❌ Do not overlook possible subarachnoid hemorrhage or meningitis. Most CT scans and LP results should be normal. LP may be more sensitive than CT for detecting subarachnoid hemorrhage within 12 hours of the onset of headache.

❌ Do not prescribe analgesics combined with butalbital (Fioricet) or opiates. Initially, they may be useful, but they increase the risk for chronic daily headache.

❌ Do not prescribe sumatriptan or ergotamine without knowledge of the patient's previously prescribed medications, nor without arranging appropriate follow-up.

❌ Do not treat with muscle relaxants. There are no data to support their use, and there are side effects and habituation.

Discussion

Headaches are common and usually benign, but any headache brought to medical attention deserves a thorough evaluation. Screening tests are of little value; a laborious history and physical examination are required.

Tension-type headache is not a wastebasket diagnosis of exclusion but a specific diagnosis. (*Tension* refers to muscle spasm more than life stress.) Although tension-type headaches are common, the pathophysiology and likely mechanism remain unclear. The cause of these headaches is most likely multifactorial, including myofascial factors and heightened sensitivity of nerve fibers, both centrally and peripherally. Tension-type headache is often dignified with the diagnosis of "migraine" without any evidence of a vascular cause and is often treated with minor

(continued)

Discussion continued

tranquilizers, which may or may not help. It should be appreciated that migraine and tension-like headaches share some features that may make it difficult to distinguish one from the other. In fact, there seems to be support for the theory that tension-type headache and migraine are distinct entities, as well as for the suggestion that these disorders are the extremes of a continuum.

Focal tenderness over the greater occipital nerves (C2, C3) can be associated with an occipital neuralgia or occipital headache and can be secondary to cervical radiculopathy resulting from cervical spondylosis. This tends to occur in older patients and should not be confused with tension headache.

Thunderclap headaches have been described with both ruptured and unruptured intracranial aneurysms. Even if a CT scan and LP are normal, magnetic resonance angiography is needed to rule out an unruptured aneurysm.

Other causes of headache include carbon monoxide exposure from wood-burning heaters, fevers and viral myalgias, caffeine withdrawal, hypertension, glaucoma, tic douloureux (trigeminal neuralgia), and intolerance of foods containing nitrite, tyramine, or xanthine.

Suggested Readings

ACEP Clinical Policies Committee: Clinical policy for the initial approach to adolescents and adults presenting to the emergency department with a chief complaint of headache, *Ann Emerg Med* 27:821–844, 1996.

Brofeldt BT: Pericranial injection of local anesthetics for the management of resistant headaches, *Acad Emerg Med* 5:1224–1229, 1998.

Kaniecki RG: Migraine and tension-type headache: an assessment of challenges in diagnosis, *Neurology* 58(9 Suppl 6): S15–S20, 2002.

Millea PJ, Brodie JJ: Tension-type headache, *Am Fam Physician* 66:797–804, 805, 2002.

Taylor F: Tension-type headaches in adults. [*UptoDate* website]. Available at http://www.uptodate.com. Accessed December 3, 2010.

Trivial, Minimal, and Minor Head Trauma

(Concussion)

Presentation

Trivial or minimal head injuries are those that occur when an individual has been struck by a lightweight stick, has banged his head on the underside of a cabinet, or has fallen forward and struck his forehead on an object. There may or may not be an associated laceration, small hematoma, mild headache, or transient nausea or drowsiness. There is no loss of consciousness, amnesia, disorientation, vomiting, or seizure. The patient or family may be alarmed by the deformity caused by a rapidly developing scalp hematoma or "goose egg."

Minor head injuries or concussion may present after a sports injury, such as a forceful collision with an opponent or stationary object or any unprotected fall onto a hard floor.

Grade 1 concussions cause no loss of consciousness but may cause brief confusion or alteration in mental status that resolves within 15 minutes. Posttraumatic amnesia lasts less than 30 minutes.

Grade 2 concussions cause no loss of consciousness or brief loss of consciousness (less than 5 minutes), but confusion or mental status changes last longer than 15 minutes. Posttraumatic amnesia lasts longer than 30 minutes.

Grade 3 concussions cause loss of consciousness lasting longer than 5 minutes or post-traumatic amnesia lasting longer than 24 hours.

Patients with concussion may appear dazed or demonstrate a change in typical behavior or personality. They may report headache, nausea, dizziness, or feeling "foggy" or "not sharp." There may also be irritability or inappropriate emotional reaction (laughing, crying).

What To Do:

✓ Corroborate and record the history as given by witnesses. Ascertain why the patient was injured (was there a seizure or sudden weakness?), **and rule out particularly dangerous types of head trauma.** (A blow inflicted with a brick or a hammer is likely to produce a depressed skull fracture; a pedestrian who has been struck by a vehicle or who is victim of a violent assault is more likely to have a serious intracranial lesion.)

✓ Perform and record a physical examination of the head, looking for signs of a skull fracture, such as hemotympanum, posterior auricular or periorbital ecchymosis (Battle and Raccoon signs), or bony depression, and examine the neck for spasm, bony tenderness, limited range of motion, and other signs of associated injury.

✓ Consider the possibility of child abuse when there are other injuries, especially fractures and facial injuries, particularly if the child is younger than 1 year of age, if the family has a poor support system or resources, or if an unstable family situation exists.

✓ Perform and record a neurologic examination, paying special attention to mental status, cranial nerves, strength, and deep tendon reflexes to all four limbs. A funduscopic examination should be performed, looking for retinal hemorrhages, whenever child abuse is suspected.

✓ **If the history or physical examination suggests a clinically significant intracranial injury, obtain a noncontrast CT scan of the head. Criteria for obtaining a CT scan for an adult include documented loss of consciousness, amnesia, severe headache, persistent nausea and vomiting, cerebrospinal fluid leaking from the nose or ear, blood behind the tympanic membrane or over the mastoid (Battle sign), confusion, stupor, coma (a Glasgow Coma Scale score of 14 or less), physical evidence of significant trauma above the clavicles, or any focal neurologic sign. A CT scan should also be ordered if the patient is elderly (older than 60 years of age), is taking anticoagulant medications, has a known or suspected bleeding diathesis, or appears to be abusing alcohol or other drugs, or when there is a dangerous mechanism or previous neurosurgery or epilepsy. A CT scan is also indicated in patients with concerning findings, those who have no one to observe them or are unreliable.**

✓ If the history or physical examination suggests a clinically significant depressed skull fracture, such as a blow inflicted with a heavy object, suspected skull penetration, or palpable depression, obtain a CT scan to confirm or rule out the diagnosis. If a depressed skull fracture is discovered, arrange for neurosurgical consultation.

✓ **Criteria for obtaining a CT scan for a child include abnormal mental status (i.e., a Glasgow Coma Scale score or pediatric Glasgow Coma Scale score of less than 15 or confusion, somnolence, or repetitive or slow verbal communication), clinical signs of skull fractures (i.e., a palpable depressed fracture, retroauricular bruising, periorbital bruising, hemotympanum, or cerebrospinal fluid otorrhea or rhinorrhea), a history of vomiting or complaint of headache, and, in children aged 2 years or younger, a scalp hematoma.**

✓ **If the injury is considered trivial or minimal or fits the criteria for a category 1 or category 2 concussion, and no criteria for obtaining a CT scan (as mentioned earlier) have been met, then there is no longer a clinical indication for obtaining a CT scan.** Explain to the patient and concerned family and friends why radiographic images are not being ordered. Many patients expect radiograph or CT examinations but will gladly forego them once they understand that they probably would be of little value and not worth the significant risk from ionizing radiation exposure. Also, provide reassurance as to the benign nature of a scalp hematoma, despite the sometimes frightening appearance.

✓ Explain to the patient and a responsible family member or friend that the more important possible sequelae of head trauma are not always diagnosed by reading radiographs but rather by noting certain signs and symptoms that occur later. **Ensure that they understand and are given written instructions to seek immediate emergency care if any abnormal behavior, increasing drowsiness or difficulty in rousing the patient, headache, neck stiffness, vomiting, visual problems, weakness, or seizures are noted.**

✅ Recommend the appropriate length of time to abstain from sports participation **after concussion. With a** Grade 1 concussion, an athlete may return to play on the same day if there is a normal clinical examination at rest and after exertion. If the athlete becomes symptomatic, he may return to play in 7 days if he remains asymptomatic at rest and with exertional provocative testing (e.g., sit-ups).

✅ With a Grade 2 concussion, an athlete may return to play in 2 weeks if he remains asymptomatic at rest and with exertion for 7 days.

✅ **Parents should be informed about the possibility of postconcussive syndrome,** characterized by persistent headache, lightheadedness, easy fatigability, irritability, or sleep disturbance. No player should return to playing sports unless he is completely asymptomatic both at rest and with exertion. **If an athlete has persistent symptoms after 1 week, a CT scan or magnetic resonance imaging (MRI) scan is recommended.**

✅ **Second and third concussions require more extended time before allowing the patient to return to play,** and the athlete may have to be removed for the entire season.

What Not To Do:

❌ Do not skimp on the neurologic examination or its documentation.

❌ Do not obtain a head CT scan for isolated loss of consciousness without other signs or symptoms that meet the criteria for CT imaging.

Discussion

There is no universal agreement on the definition of a concussion. One of the most popular working definitions is a trauma-induced alteration in mental status that may or may not be accompanied by a loss of consciousness. Its pathophysiologic basis remains a mystery. It is unclear whether concussion is associated with lesser degrees of diffuse structural change seen in severe traumatic brain injury or if the entire mechanism is caused by reversible functional changes.

Published grading scales for concussion are not validated and represent a view from various experts, not a consensus of scientific evidence. The only exception is the Glasgow Coma Scale.

Good clinical judgment and the ability to identify postconcussion signs and symptoms will ensure that athletes do not return to play while symptomatic. It should be noted that second-impact syndrome, although rare, is a fatal, uncontrollable diffuse brain swelling that occurs after a blow to the head that is sustained before full recovery from a previous injury to the head. Previous concussions may also be associated with slower recovery of neurologic function.

A head CT scan is recommended in all elderly patients with minor head trauma. Known physiologic changes with aging may make the geriatric brain more susceptible to injury. Reduction in overall brain weight increases the space between the brain and the skull, which increases the risk for shearing and tearing of the bridging vessels. This also allows expansion of intracranial pressure and the classic symptoms expected with this pathophysiology.

Loss of consciousness alone is not predictive of significant head injury and is not an absolute indication for head CT. Most children sustaining blunt head trauma do not have traumatic brain injury. The benefits of information gained by CT imaging must be balanced by its disadvantages, which include exposure to ionizing radiation (which may have a significant impact on future cognition and cancer risk), transport of the child

(continued)

Discussion continued

away from the ED, the frequent requirement for pharmacologic sedation, additional healthcare costs, and increased time spent in the hospital. When there is no abnormality in mental status, no clinical signs of skull fracture, no history of vomiting, no headache, or no scalp hematoma (in children 2 years of age or younger), careful observation at home is an acceptable approach, with reevaluation and CT scanning for persistent or worsening symptoms. Children who are awake, alert, and asymptomatic (except when child abuse is suspected in children 2 years of age or younger) do not require special imaging.

Because of the risks for late neurologic sequelae (e.g., subdural hematoma, seizure disorder, meningitis, postconcussion syndrome), good follow-up is essential after any head trauma, but most patients without findings on initial examination do well. It is probably unwise to describe to the patient all of the subtle possible long-term effects of head trauma, because many may be induced by suggestion. Concentrate on explaining the danger signs that patients should watch for over the next few days. If postconcussion symptoms occur, a more formal neuropsychologic evaluation can delineate any subtle cognitive changes associated with the injury.

There is no universally accepted rule for determining whether CT head scanning is necessary. The criteria for ordering a CT scan suggested earlier represent a conservative but not scientifically proven approach.

Adults and pediatric patients with minor head injuries who meet the criteria for a CT scan but have a normal scan and neurologic examination may be safely discharged and sent home. One exception is with elderly anticoagulated patients, who require at least 6 hours of observation. The risk for delayed deterioration is low, but not zero, in any head-injured patient who is discharged to home. It is therefore mandatory that written discharge instructions be provided to competent caretakers regarding signs and symptoms of complications of head trauma and that these caretakers are able to bring the patient back to medical care if necessary. The patient may be given acetaminophen for headache, but more potent analgesics are best avoided so that any progression of symptoms can be detected. Postdischarge indications for return to the ED include confusion or impaired consciousness, abnormal gait, alteration in behavior, difficulty with eyesight, vomiting, worsening headache, unequal pupil size, or any other worrisome abnormality. Cold packs may be recommended to reduce the swelling, and the patient may be reassured that the hematoma will resolve in a few days to weeks. Patients should be considered for hospital admission for all but minimal or trivial injuries if there is no competent observer at home. Other indications for admission are intractable headache, nausea or other progressive symptoms, alcohol or drug intoxication, and any abnormalities in the neurologic examination.

Suggested Readings

Bergman DA: The management of minor closed head injury in children, *Pediatrics* 104:1407–1415, 1999.

Borczuk P: Predictors of intracranial injury in patients with mild head trauma, *Ann Emerg Med* 25:731–736, 1995.

Collins MW, Lovell MR, McKeag DB: Current issues in managing sports-related concussion, *JAMA* 282:2283–2285, 1999.

Cook LS, Levitt MA, Simon B, et al: Identification of ethanol-intoxicated patients with minor head trauma requiring computed tomography scans, *Acad Emerg Med* 1:227–234, 1994.

Davis RL, Hughes M, Gubler D, et al: The use of cranial CT scans in the triage of pediatric patients with mild head injury, *Pediatrics* 95:345–349, 1995.

Hall P, Adami HO, Trichopoulos, et al: Effect of low does of ionizing radiation in infancy on cognitive function in adulthood: Swedish population-based cohort, *BMJ* 328:19, 2004.

Holmes JF, Baier ME, Derlet RW, et al: Failure of the Miller criteria to predict significant intracranial injury in patients with a Glasgow Coma Scale score of 14 after minor head trauma injury, *Acad Emerg Med* 4:788–792, 1997.

Madden C, Witzke DB, Sanders AB, et al: High-yield selection criteria for cranial computed tomography after acute trauma, *Acad Emerg Med* 2:248–253, 1995.

McCrory PR, Berkovic SF: Concussion: the history of clinical and pathophysiological concepts and misconceptions, *Neurology* 57:2283–2289, 2001.

Miller EC, Derlet RW, Kinser D: Minor head trauma: is computed tomography always necessary? *Ann Emerg Med* 27:290–294, 1996.

Miller EC, Holmes JF, Derlet RW, et al: Utilizing clinical factors to reduce head CT scan ordering for minor head trauma patients, *J Emerg Med* 15:453–457, 1997.

Mitchell KA, Fallat ME, Raque GH, et al: Evaluation of minor head injury in children, *J Ped Surg* 29:851–854, 1994.

Palchak MJ: A decision rule for identifying children at low risk for brain injuries after blunt head trauma, *Ann Emerg Med* 42:492, 2003.

Poirier MP: Concussions: assessment, management, and recommendations for return to activity, *Clin Pediatr Emerg Med* 4:179–185, 2003.

Reynolds FD: Time to deterioration of the elderly, anticoagulated, minor head injury patient who presents without evidence of neurologic abnormality, *J Trauma* 54:492–496, 2003.

Rubin DM, Christian CW, Bilaniuk LT, et al: Occult head injury in high-risk abused children, *Pediatrics* 111:1382–1386, 2003.

Schunk JE, Rogerson JD, Woodward GA: The utility of head computed tomographic scanning in pediatric patients with normal neurologic examinations in the emergency department, *Pediatr Emerg Care* 12:160–165, 1996.

Schutzman SA, Greenes DS: Pediatric head trauma, *Ann Emerg Med* 37:65–74, 2001.

Shackford SR, Wald SL, Ross SE, et al: The clinical utility of computed tomographic scanning and neurologic examination in the management of patients with minor head injuries, *J Trauma* 33:385–394, 1992.

Stiell IG, Wells GA, Vandemheen K, et al: Variation in ED use of computed tomography for patients with minor head injury, *Ann Emerg Med* 30:14–22, 1997.

Vasovagal or Neurocardiogenic or Neurally Mediated Syncope

(Faint, Swoon)

Presentation

The patient experiences a brief loss of consciousness, preceded by a sense of warmth and nausea and awareness of passing out, with weakness and diaphoresis. The patient may or may not experience ringing in the ears or a sensation of tunnel vision. First, there is a period of sympathetic tone, with increased pulse and blood pressure, in anticipation of some stressful incident, such as bad news, an upsetting sight, or a painful procedure. Immediately after or during the stressful occurrence, there is a precipitous drop in sympathetic tone and/or surge in parasympathetic tone, resulting in peripheral vasodilatation or bradycardia, or both, leading to hypotension and causing the victim to lose postural tone, fall down, and lose consciousness.

Once the patient is in a horizontal position, normal skin color, normal pulse, and consciousness return within seconds. This time period may be extended if the patient is maintained in an upright sitting position.

Transient bradycardia and a few myoclonic limb jerks or tonic spasms (syncopal convulsions) may accompany vasovagal syncope, but there are no sustained seizures, incontinence, lateral tongue biting, palpitations, dysrhythmias, or injuries beyond a minor contusion or laceration resulting from the fall. Ordinarily, the victim spontaneously revives within 30 seconds, suffers no sequelae, and can recall the events leading up to the faint.

The whole process may transpire in an ED or a clinic setting, or a patient may have fainted elsewhere, in which case the diagnostic challenge is to reconstruct what happened to rule out other causes of syncope.

What To Do:

✓ To prevent potential fainting spells, arrange for anyone anticipating an unpleasant experience to sit or lie down prior to the offensive event.

✓ If an individual faints, catch her so she will not be injured in the fall, lay her supine on the floor or stretcher for 5 to 10 minutes, protect her airway, record several sets of vital signs, and be prepared to proceed with resuscitation if the episode becomes more than a simple vasovagal syncopal episode.

✓ **If a patient is brought in after fainting elsewhere, obtain a detailed history. Ask about the setting, precipitating factors, descriptions given by several eyewitnesses, and sequence of recovery. Look for evidence of painful stimuli (i.e., phlebotomy), emotional stress, or other unpleasant experiences, such as the sight of blood.**

✅ **Consider other benign precipitating causes, such as prolonged standing (especially in the heat), recent diarrhea and dehydration, or Valsalva maneuver during urination, defecation, or cough.**

✅ **Determine if there were prodromal symptoms consistent with benign neurocardiogenic syncope, such as lightheadedness, nausea, and diaphoresis.**

✅ In patients in whom there is no clearly benign precipitating cause, inquire whether the collapse came without warning or whether there was seizure activity with a postictal period of confusion, or ask if there was diplopia, dysarthria, focal neurologic symptoms, or headache. Also find out if there was any chest pain, shortness of breath, or palpitations or if the syncope occurred with sudden standing. Is there any reason for dehydration, evidence of gastrointestinal bleeding, or recent addition of a new drug?

✅ Obtain a medical history to determine if there have been previous similar episodes or there is an underlying cardiac problem (i.e., congestive heart failure [CHF], arrhythmias, valvular heart disease) or risk factors for coronary disease or aortic dissection. Look for previous strokes or transient ischemic attacks as well as gastrointestinal hemorrhage. Also note if there is a history of psychiatric illness.

✅ Ask about a family history of benign fainting or sudden death. (There is a familial tendency toward syncope.)

✅ **Check to see which medications the patient is taking and if any of these drugs can cause hypotension, arrhythmias, or QT prolongation.**

✅ **The performance of the physical examination should start with vital signs, to include an assessment of orthostatic hypotension.** (To make the diagnosis of orthostatic hypotension as the cause of syncope, it is helpful if the patient has a true reproduction of symptoms on standing.)

✅ Other important features of the physical examination include neurologic findings, such as diplopia, dysarthria, papillary asymmetry, nystagmus, ataxia, gait instability, and slowly resolving confusion or lateral tongue biting, as well as cardiac findings, such as carotid bruits, jugular venous distention, rales, and a systolic murmur (of aortic stenosis or hypertrophic obstructive cardiomyopathy).

✅ **Do an ECG. The value of this study is not its ability to identify the cause of syncope but, by identifying any abnormality, its ability to provide clues to an underlying cardiac cause.** Because an ECG is relatively inexpensive and essentially risk free, it should be done on virtually all patients with syncope, with the possible exception of young, healthy patients with an obvious situational or vasovagal cause.

✅ For patients in whom a clear cause of syncope cannot be determined after history and physical examination, initiate cardiac monitoring.

✅ Routine blood tests rarely yield diagnostically useful information. In most cases, blood tests serve only to confirm a clinical suspicion. **If acute blood loss is a possibility, obtain hemoglobin and hematocrit measures (although examination of stool for blood may be more accurate).**

✅ **Pregnancy testing should be done for all women of childbearing age, because ectopic pregnancy can be a dangerous cause of syncope.**

✅ **A head CT scan should only be obtained in patients with focal neurologic symptoms and signs or new-onset seizure activity or to rule out hemorrhage in patients with head trauma or headache.**

✅ **Admit patients with any of the following to the hospital:**

○ A history of congestive heart failure or ventricular arrhythmias

○ Associated chest pain or other symptoms compatible with acute coronary syndrome, aortic dissection, or pulmonary embolus

○ Evidence of significant congestive heart failure or valvular heart disease on physical examination

○ ECG findings of ischemia, arrhythmia (either bradycardia or tachycardia), prolonged QT interval, or bundle branch block (BBB)

○ Concomitant conditions that require inpatient treatment

✅ Consider admission for patients with syncope and any of the following:

○ Age older than 60 years

○ History of coronary artery disease or congenital heart disease

○ Family history of unexpected sudden death

○ Exertional syncope in younger patients without an obvious benign cause for the syncope

○ A complaint of shortness of breath

○ A hematocrit of less than 30%

○ An initial systolic blood pressure of less than 90 mm Hg or severe orthostatic hypotension

✅ Patients not requiring admission should be referred to an appropriate follow-up physician and should be instructed to avoid precipitating factors, such as extreme heat, dehydration, postexertional standing, alcohol, and certain medications. It is also reasonable to recommend an increase in salt and fluid intake to decrease syncopal episodes in the younger patient.

✅ Referral for tilt-table testing is appropriate when there has been recurrent, unexplained syncope without evidence of organic heart disease or after a negative cardiac workup.

✅ **After full recovery, explain to the patient with classic vasovagal syncope that fainting is a common physiologic reaction and that, in future recurrences, she can recognize the early lightheadedness and prevent a full swoon by lying down or sitting and putting her head between her knees.**

✅ Consider restricting unprotected driving, swimming, and diving for those with severe and recurrent episodes of vasovagal syncope without a trigger.

What Not To Do:

❌ Do not allow family members to stand while being given bad news, do not allow parents to stand while watching their children being sutured, and do not allow patients to stand while being given shots or undergoing venipuncture.

(X) Do not traumatize the fainting victim by using ammonia capsules, slapping, or dousing with cold water.

(X) Do not obtain a head CT scan unless there are focal neurologic symptoms and signs, unless there has been true seizure activity, or unless you want to rule out intracranial hemorrhage.

(X) Do not refer patients for EEG studies unless there were witnessed tonic-clonic movements or postevent confusion.

(X) Do not obtain routine blood tests unless there is a clinical indication based on the history and physical examination.

(X) Do not refer patients with obvious vasovagal syncope for tilt-table testing.

(X) Do not discharge syncope patients who have a history of coronary artery disease, congestive heart failure, or ventricular dysrhythmia; patients who complain of chest pain; patients who have physical signs of significant valvular heart disease, congestive heart failure, stroke, or focal neurologic disorder; or patients who have electrocardiographic findings of ischemia, bradycardia, tachycardia, increased QT interval, or BBB.

Discussion

Syncope is defined as a transient loss of consciousness and muscle tone. It is derived from the Greek word *synkoptein,* "to cut short." Presyncope is "the feeling that one is about to pass out."

Most commonly, the cause of syncope in young adults is vasovagal or neurocardiogenic. Observation of the sequence of stress, relief, and fainting makes the diagnosis, but, better yet, the whole reaction can usually be prevented. Although most patients suffer no sequelae, vasovagal syncope with prolonged asystole can produce seizures and rare incidents of death. The differential diagnosis of loss of consciousness is extensive; therefore loss of consciousness should not immediately be assumed to be caused by vasovagal syncope.

Several triggers may induce neurally mediated syncope, including emotional stress (anxiety; an unpleasant sight, sound, or smell) or physical stress, such as pain, hunger, dehydration, illness, anemia, and fatigue. In adolescents, symptoms of syncope may be related to the menstrual cycle or be associated with starvation in patients with eating disorders. Situational triggers include cough, micturition, and defecation.

Orthostatic hypotension is the second most common cause of syncope after neurocardiogenic syncope and is most frequently seen in the elderly. There are many causes of orthostatic hypotension, the most common of which are hypovolemia (vomiting, diarrhea, hemorrhage, pregnancy) and drugs (antihypertensives, angiotensin-converting enzyme [ACE] inhibitors, diuretics, and phenothiazines).

Neurologic causes of syncope include seizures, transient ischemic attacks, and migraine headaches, as well as intracranial hemorrhage.

Cardiac-related syncope is potentially the most dangerous form of syncope. Patients with known cardiac disease who also experience syncope have a significantly increased incidence of cardiac-related death. The patients at risk have ischemic heart disease, most significantly congestive heart failure, congenital heart disease, and valvular heart disease (particularly aortic valvular disorder) or are taking drugs that produce QT prolongation or are known to induce torsades de pointes (i.e., amiodarone, tricyclics, selective serotonin-reuptake inhibitors [SSRIs], phenothiazines, macrolides, quinolones, and many antifungals—becoming very dangerous in combination with one another).

Brugada syndrome is a rare but potentially lethal familial dysrhythmic syndrome characterized by an ECG that shows a partial right BBB with elevation of ST segments in leads V_{1-3}, which have a peculiar downsloping with inverted T waves (Figure 11-1).

Danger signs for cardiac-related syncope include sudden onset without warning or syncope—preceded by palpitations as well as associated chest pain, shortness of breath—and illicit drug use. Other danger signs are postexertional syncope (think about

(continued)

45

Discussion continued

fixed cardiac lesions) and syncope that occurred while the patient was seated or lying down.

Other serious causes of syncope that should be considered (and are usually accompanied by distinctive signs and symptoms) are aortic dissection and rupture, pulmonary embolism, ectopic pregnancy with rupture, and carotid artery dissection.

Elderly patients have a higher percentage of underlying cardiovascular, pulmonary, and cerebrovascular disease, and therefore, syncope in the elderly is more often associated with a serious problem than it is in younger patients. Myocardial infarction, transient ischemic attack, and aortic stenosis are examples of this. Carotid sinus syncope (secondary to, for example, tight collars, head turning, and shaving) is almost exclusively a disease of the elderly. If suspected, carotid sinus massage can confirm the diagnosis but should not be attempted if the patient has carotid bruits, ventricular tachycardia, or recent stroke or myocardial infarction. Arrhythmias, particularly bradyarrhythmias, are also more common in the elderly. For these reasons, elderly patients more often require hospitalization for monitoring and further diagnostic testing.

It should also be appreciated that elderly patients are more prone to abnormal responses to common benign situational stresses, including postural changes, micturition (exacerbated by prostatic hypertrophy in men), coughing (especially in patients with chronic obstructive pulmonary disease), and defecation associated with constipation. These abnormal responses are compounded by the effects of underlying illnesses and medications, including anticholinergics, antihypertensives (including eye drops with beta-blocker activity), and central nervous system (CNS) depressants.

Often, no single cause of syncope in the elderly can be identified. Patients improve after several small changes, however, including discontinuance of unnecessary medications, avoidance of precipitating events, and the use of support stockings or fludrocortisone (Florinef acetate), 0.05 to 0.4 mg PO qd (usual: 0.1 mg PO qd), for postural hypotension (off label).

Tilt-table testing has become a common component of the diagnostic evaluation of syncope. The accuracy of tilt testing is unknown, and a positive tilt test only diagnoses a propensity for neurocardiogenic events. Despite these limitations, referral for tilt-table testing can be useful in patients with recurrent, unexplained syncope and a suspected neurocardiogenic cause (a patient having typical vasovagal symptoms) but without a clear precipitant; in patients without cardiac disease or in whom cardiac testing has been negative; and in patients in whom testing clearly reproduces the symptoms.

Many pharmacologic agents have been used in the treatment of recurrent neurocardiogenic syncope. The relatively favorable natural history of neurocardiogenic syncope, with a spontaneous remission rate of 91%, makes it difficult to assess the efficacy and necessity of these drugs.

Psychiatric evaluation is recommended in young patients with recurrent, unexplained syncope without cardiac disease who have frequent episodes associated with many varied prodromal symptoms as well as other complaints.

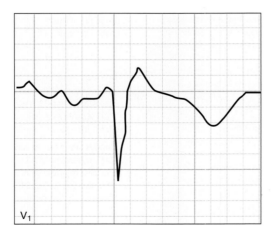

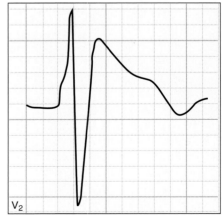

Figure 11-1 Brugada syndrome (V_1 and V_2).

Suggested Readings

Alegria JR, Gersh BJ, Scott CG: Comparison of frequency of recurrent syncope after beta-blocker therapy versus conservative management for patients with vasovagal syncope, *Am J Cardiol* 92:82–84, 2003.

Farwell DJ: Does the use of syncope diagnostic protocol improve the investigation and management of syncope? *Heart* 90:52, 2004.

Feinberg AN, Lane-Davies A: Syncope in the adolescent, *Adolesc Med* 13:553–567, 2002.

Graham DT, Kabler JD, Lunsford L: Vasovagal fainting: a diphasic response, *Psychosom Med* 6:493–507, 1961.

Lin JTY, Ziegler DK, Lai CW, et al: Convulsive syncope in blood donors, *Ann Neurol* 11:525–528, 1982.

Linzer M, Yang EH, Estes M, et al: Diagnosing syncope. I. Value of history, physical examination, and electrocardiography, *Ann Intern Med* 126:989–996, 1997.

Linzer M, Yang EH, Estes M, et al: Diagnosing syncope. II. Unexplained syncope, *Ann Intern Med* 127:76–86, 1997.

Massin MM, Bourguignont A, Coremans C: Syncope in pediatric patients presenting to an emergency department, *J Pediatr* 145:223–228, 2004.

Quinn JV, McDermott D, Stiell IG, et al: Prospective validation of the San Francisco syncope rule to predict patients with serious outcomes, *Ann Emerg Med* 47:448–454, 2006.

Quinn JV, Stiell IG, McDermott DA, et al: Derivation of the San Francisco syncope rule to predict patients with short-term serious outcomes, *Ann Emerg Med* 43:224–232, 2004.

Sarasin FP: Prevalence of orthostatic hypotension among patients presenting with syncope in the ED, *Am J Emerg Med* 20:497–501, 2002.

Schnipper JL, Kapoor WN: Cardiac arrhythmias: diagnostic evaluation and management of patients with syncope, *Med Clin North Am* 85:423–456, 2001.

Theopistou A, Gatzoulis K, Economou E: Biochemical changes involved in the mechanism of vasovagal syncope, *Am J Cardiol* 88:376–381, 2001.

Vertigo

(Dizziness, Lightheadedness)

Presentation

The patient who has dizziness may have a nonspecific complaint that must be further differentiated into either an altered somatic sensation (giddiness, wooziness, disequilibrium), orthostatic lightheadedness (sensation of fainting), or the sensation of the environment (or patient) spinning (true vertigo). Vertigo is a symptom produced by asymmetric input from the vestibular system because of damage or dysfunction of the labyrinth, vestibular nerve, or central vestibular structures of the brain stem. Vertigo is a symptom, not a diagnosis. It is customarily categorized into central and peripheral causes. Peripheral causes account for 80% of cases of vertigo, with benign positional vertigo, vestibular neuritis, and Meniere disease being most common. Peripheral causes tend to be more severe and sudden in onset but more benign in course when compared to central causes. Vertigo is frequently accompanied by nystagmus, resulting from ocular compensation for the unreal sensation of spinning. Nausea and vomiting also are common accompanying symptoms of true vertigo.

What To Do:

✓ **Clarify the type of dizziness.** Have the patient express how he feels in his own words (without using the word *dizzy*). Determine whether the patient is describing true vertigo (a feeling of movement of one's body or surroundings), has a sensation of an impending faint, or has a vague, unsteady feeling. Ask about any factors that precipitate the dizziness and any associated symptoms, as well as how long the dizziness lasts. Ask about drugs or toxins that could be responsible for the dizziness.

✓ If the symptoms were accompanied by neurologic symptoms, such as diplopia, visual deficits, sudden collapse, or unilateral weakness or numbness, consider a transient ischemic attack (TIA) as a possible cause and consider MRI and neurologic consultation.

✓ If the problem is near-syncope or orthostatic lightheadedness, consider potentially serious causes, such as heart disease, cardiac dysrhythmias, and blood loss or possible medication effects (see Chapter 11).

✓ With a sensation of disequilibrium or an elderly patient's feeling that he is unsteady and going to fall, look for diabetic peripheral neuropathy (lower-extremity sensory loss) and muscle weakness. These patients should be referred to their primary care physicians for management of underlying medical problems and possible adjustment of their medications.

✓ If there is lightheadedness that is unrelated to changes in position and posture and there is no evidence of disease found on physical examination and laboratory evaluation, refer these patients to their primary care physicians for evaluation for possible depression or other psychological conditions.

✓ **If the patient is having true vertigo, try to determine if this is the more benign form of peripheral vertigo or the potentially more serious form of central vertigo.**

✓ Peripheral vertigo (vestibular neuritis [the most common form of peripheral vertigo], labyrinthitis, and benign paroxysmal positional vertigo [BPPV]) is generally accompanied by an acute vestibular syndrome with rapid onset of severe symptoms associated with nausea and vomiting, spontaneous unidirectional horizontal nystagmus, and postural instability. Romberg testing, when positive, will show a tendency to fall or lean in one direction only, toward the involved side.

✓ Central vertigo (inferior cerebellar infarction, brain stem infarction, multiple sclerosis, and tumors) is generally less severe—with vertical, pure rotatory, or multidirectional nystagmus—and is more likely to be found in elderly patients with risk factors for stroke. It is possibly accompanied by focal neurologic signs or symptoms, including cerebellar abnormalities (asymmetric finger-to-nose and rapid alternating movement examinations) and the inability to walk caused by profound ataxia.

✓ **When examining the patient for nystagmus, have the patient follow your finger with his eyes as it moves a few degrees to the left and then to the right (not to extremes of gaze)** (Figure 12-1), and note whether there are more than the normal two to three beats of nystagmus before the eyes are still. Determine the direction of the nystagmus (horizontal, vertical, or rotatory) and whether or not fixating the patient's gaze reduces the nystagmus (a peripheral finding).

✓ Benign paroxysmal positional vertigo is the most common cause of vertigo in the elderly. Nystagmus may be detected when the eyes are closed by watching the bulge of the cornea moving under the lid.

✓ **Examine ears for cerumen, foreign bodies, otitis media, and hearing loss.** Ideally, check for speech discrimination. (Can the patient differentiate between the words *kite, flight, right?*) Abnormalities may be a sign of an acoustic neuroma.

✓ **Examine the cranial nerves and perform a complete neurologic examination that includes testing of cerebellar function (using rapid alternating movement, finger-to-nose, and gait tests when possible).** Check the corneal blink reflexes and, if absent on one side in a

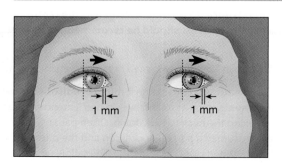

Figure 12-1 The eye should only move a few degrees to the left or right when examining for nystagmus.

patient who does not wear contact lenses, again consider acoustic neuroma. Complete the rest of a full general physical examination.

✓ Decide, on the basis of the aforementioned examinations, whether the cause is central (brain stem, cerebellar, multiple sclerosis) or peripheral (vestibular organs, eighth nerve). Suspicion of central lesions requires further workup, MRI (the most appropriate imaging study in these cases) when available, otolaryngologic or neurologic consultation, or hospital admission.

✓ **Peripheral lesions,** on the other hand, although more symptomatic, are more likely to be treatable and managed on an outpatient basis. Always consider how well the patient is tolerating symptoms after therapy and what the social conditions are at home before sending the patient home.

✓ **When peripheral vestibular neuronitis or labyrinthitis is suspected, because of sudden onset of persistent, severe vertigo with nausea, vomiting, and horizontal nystagmus with gait instability but preserved ability to ambulate, treat symptoms of vertigo with IV dimenhydrinate 50 mg (Dramamine) or meclizine (Antivert) 25 mg PO. Benzodiazepines, such as Valium or lorazepam (Ativan), may be used to potentiate the effects of the antihistamine. These symptom controlling medications should only be used for the first 48 to 72 hours. Remember that there are no confirmatory tests for vestibular neuritis and many of the symptoms overlap with those of posterior infarction; so, have a low index of suspicion to obtain an MRI to rule out central causes in elderly patients (older than 60 years old), anyone with other neurologic signs or symptoms, or patients with accompanying headache or an atypical course.**

✓ **Nausea may be treated with ondansetron (Zofran) or prochlorperazine (Compazine). If there are no contraindications (e.g., glaucoma), a patch of transdermal scopolamine (Transderm Scōp) can be worn for 3 days.** Some authors recommend hydroxyzine (Vistaril, Atarax), and **others suggest that corticosteroids (methylprednisolone [Solu-Medrol], prednisone) significantly improve recovery in patients with vestibular neuronitis.** Nifedipine (Procardia) had been used to alleviate motion sickness but is no better than scopolamine patches and should not be used for patients who have postural hypotension or who take beta-blockers.

✓ **If the patient does not respond, he may require hospitalization for further parenteral treatment and evaluation.**

✓ **After discharge, treat persistent symptoms of peripheral vertigo with lorazepam, 1 to 2 mg qid; meclizine (Antivert), 12.5 to 25 mg qid; or dimenhydrinate, 25 to 50 mg qid. Prochlorperazine suppository, 25 mg bid, or ondansetron (Zofran) PO or ODT can be used for persistent nausea, and bed rest should be recommended as needed until symptoms improve.**

✓ Arrange for follow-up in all patients treated in the outpatient setting.

✓ **BPPV is associated with brief (less than 1 minute) episodes of severe vertigo that are precipitated by movements,** such as rolling over in bed, extending the neck to look upward, or bending over and flexing the neck to look down. Often patients can recall a short period between the time they assumed a particular position and the onset of the spinning sensation. The diagnosis can be confirmed by performing the Dix-Hallpike maneuver.

✅ **When symptoms are consistent with BPPV, when there are no auditory or neurologic symptoms, and when the patient is no longer symptomatic, perform a Dix-Hallpike (formerly Nylen-Barany) maneuver** (Figure 12-2, *A* and *B*) **to confirm the diagnosis and determine which ear is involved.**

✅ To perform the Dix-Hallpike maneuver, have the patient sit up for at least 30 seconds, then lie back, and quickly hang his head over the end of the stretcher, with his head turned 45 degrees to the right. Wait 30 seconds for the appearance of nystagmus or the sensation of vertigo. Repeat the maneuver on the other side. When this maneuver produces positional nystagmus after a brief latent period lasting less than 30 seconds, it indicates benign paroxysmal positional vertigo. **The ear that is down when the greatest symptoms of nystagmus are produced is the affected ear, which can be treated using canalith-repositioning maneuvers.** An equivocal test is not a contraindication to performing canalith-repositioning maneuvers.

✅ **To prevent nausea and vomiting when these symptoms are not tolerable for the patient, premedicate him with an antiemetic such as metoclopramide (Reglan), 10 mg IV, or ondansetron (Zofran), 4 mg IV.** These maneuvers can be performed quickly at the bedside, thereby moving semicircular canal debris to a less sensitive part of the inner ear (utricle). This can produce rapid results, often providing much satisfaction to both patient and clinician.

 ✅ **The most well studied of these maneuvers is the Epley maneuver. With the patient seated, the patient's head is rotated 45 degrees toward the affected ear. The patient is then tilted backward to a head-hanging position, with the head kept in the 45-degree rotation. The patient is held in this position (same as the Dix-Hallpike position with the affected ear down) until the nystagmus and vertigo abate (at least 20 seconds, but most clinicians recommend 4 minutes in each position). The head is then turned 90 degrees**

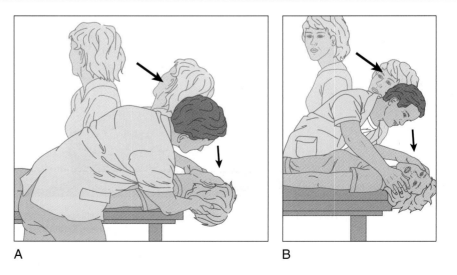

A   B

Figure 12-2 A, The patient's head is 30 degrees below horizontal. With her head turned to the right, quickly lower the patient to the supine position. **B,** Repeat with her head turned to the left.

toward the unaffected ear and kept in this position for another 3 to 4 minutes. With the head remaining turned, the patient is then rolled onto the side of the unaffected ear. This may again provoke nystagmus and vertigo, but the patient should again remain in this position for 3 to 4 minutes. Finally, the patient is moved to the seated position, and the head is tilted down 30 degrees, allowing the canalith to fall into the utricle. This position is also held for an additional 3 to 4 minutes (Figure 12-3).

Contraindications to these maneuvers include severe cervical spine disease, unstable cardiac disease, and high-grade carotid stenosis.

Most authors recommend that the patient remain upright or semi-upright for 1 to 2 days and avoid bending over after a successful canalith repositioning. To help the patient keep from tilting his head or bending his neck, you can fit him with a soft cervical collar for the rest of the day. (The patient can sleep on a recliner with his head no lower than 45 degrees.) The patient may continue to feel off-balance for a few days and should not drive home from the medical facility.

The maneuvers can be repeated several times if the symptoms do not resolve on the first attempt. If the initial findings are somewhat unclear, no harm is done if the canalith-repositioning maneuver is performed on the apparently unaffected ear.

If a patient has a complete resolution of symptoms with repositioning, other causes for the vertigo become less likely. If symptoms persist or are atypical, referral to an otorhinolaryngologist or neurologist is appropriate.

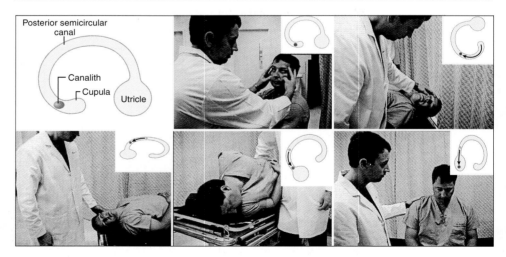

Figure 12-3 Epley maneuver. **Top** (*left to right*), The first window is a legend for the *inset*, which is a simplified representation of a posterior semicircular canal. This figure shows the Epley canalith-repositioning maneuver for the left semicircular canal. The patient's head is turned 45 degrees toward the affected ear, with the patient holding the physician's arm for support. The patient is then lowered to a supine position. The patient's head remains turned 45 degrees and should hang off the end of the bed. **Bottom,** In the third position, the patient's head is rotated to face the opposite shoulder. Next, the patient is rolled onto his side, taking care to keep the head rotated. The patient is now returned to a seated position with the head tilted forward. (Adapted from Koelliker P, Summers R, Hawkins B: Benign paroxysmal positional vertigo. *Ann Emerg Med* 37:392-398, 2001, with permission from The American College of Emergency Physicians.)

What Not To Do:

Ⓧ Do not expect to determine the exact cause of dizziness for all patients who present for the first time. Make every reasonable attempt to determine whether or not the origin is benign or potentially serious, and then make the most appropriate disposition.

Ⓧ Do not attempt provocative maneuvers if the patient is symptomatic with nystagmus at rest. Prolonged symptoms are inconsistent with BPPV, which is the only indication for doing such provocative maneuvers.

Ⓧ Do not go through the Epley maneuvers too rapidly. Success depends on holding the patient in each position for 3 to 4 minutes.

Ⓧ Do not give antivertigo drugs to elderly patients with disequilibrium or orthostatic symptoms. These medications have sedative properties that can worsen the condition. These drugs will also not help depression if this is the underlying cause of lightheadedness.

Ⓧ Do not give long-term vestibular suppressant drugs to patients with BPPV unless you are unable to perform repositioning maneuvers and the patient's symptoms are severe.

Ⓧ Do not make the diagnosis of Meniere disease (endolymphatic hydrops) without the triad of paroxysmal vertigo, sensorineural deafness, and low-pitched tinnitus, along with a feeling of pressure or fullness in the affected ear that lasts for hours to days. With repeat attacks, a sustained low-frequency sensorineural hearing loss and constant tinnitus develop.

Ⓧ Do not proceed with expensive laboratory testing or unwarranted imaging studies, especially with signs and symptoms of benign peripheral vertigo. Remember, CT will not rule out posterior fossa disease. Most causes of dizziness can be determined through obtaining a complete patient history and clinical examination. If radiographic studies are needed, MRI is the most sensitive for posterior fossa and brain stem abnormalities.

Ⓧ Do not prescribe meclizine, scopolamine, and other vestibular suppressants for more than a few days during acute vestibular hypofunction caused by vestibular neuritis and labyrinthitis. These drugs may actually prolong symptoms if given on a long-term basis, because they interfere with the patient's natural compensation mechanisms within the denervated vestibular nucleus.

Discussion

Vertigo is an illusion of motion, usually rotational, of the patient or the patient's surroundings. The clinician responsible for evaluating this problem should consider a differential diagnosis, with special attention to whether the vertigo is central or peripheral in origin. A large number of entities cause vertigo, ranging from benign and self-limited causes, such as vestibular neuritis and BPPV, to immediately life-threatening causes, such as cerebellar infarction or hemorrhage. In general, the more violent the sensation of vertigo and the more spinning, the more likely that the lesion is peripheral. Central lesions tend to cause less intense vertigo and more vague symptoms. Peripheral causes of vertigo or nystagmus include irritation of the ear (utricle, saccule, semicircular canals) or the vestibular division of the eighth cranial (acoustic) nerve caused by toxins, otitis, viral infection, or cerumen or a foreign body lodged against the tympanic membrane. The term *labyrinthitis* should be reserved for vertigo with hearing changes, and the term *vestibular neuronitis* should be reserved for the common, transient vertigo, without hearing changes, that

(continued)

Discussion continued

is sometimes associated with upper respiratory tract viral infections. Paroxysmal positional vertigo may be related to inappropriate particles (free-floating debris or otoliths) in the endolymph of the semicircular canals. If it occurs after significant trauma, suspect a basal skull fracture with leakage of endolymph or perilymph, and consider otolaryngologic referral for further evaluation.

The vestibular nerve is unique among the cranial nerves in that the neurons in this nerve, on each side, are firing spontaneously at 100 spikes/sec with the head still. With sudden loss of input from one side, there is a strong bias into the brain stem from the intact side. This large bias in neural activity causes nystagmus. The direction of the nystagmus is labeled according to the quick phase, but the vestibular deficit is actually driving the slow phase of nystagmus.

Vestibular neuritis is preceded by a common cold 50% of the time. The prevalence of vestibular neuritis peaks at 40 to 50 years of age. Vestibular neuritis is probably similar to Bell's palsy and is thought to represent a reactivated dormant herpes infection in the Scarpa ganglion within the vestibular nerve. Viral labyrinthitis can be diagnosed if there is associated hearing loss or tinnitus at the time of presentation, but the possibility of an acoustic neuroma should be kept in mind, especially if the vertigo is mild.

Central causes include multiple sclerosis, temporal lobe epilepsy, basilar migraine, and hemorrhage or infarction or tumor in the posterior fossa. Patients with a slow-growing acoustic neuroma in the cerebellopontine angle usually do not present with acute vertigo but rather with a progressive, unilateral hearing loss, with or without tinnitus. The earliest sign is usually a gradual loss of auditory discrimination.

Vertebrobasilar arterial insufficiency can cause vertigo, usually with associated nausea, vomiting, and cranial nerve or cerebellar signs. It is commonly diagnosed in dizzy patients who are older than 50 years of age, but more often than not the diagnosis is incorrect. The brain stem is a tightly packed structure in which the vestibular nuclei are crowded in with the oculomotor nuclei, the medial longitudinal fasciculus, and the cerebellar, sensory, and motor pathways. It would be unusual for ischemia to produce only vertigo without accompanying diplopia, ataxia, or sensory or motor disturbance. Although vertigo may be the major symptom of an ischemic attack, careful questioning of the patient commonly uncovers symptoms implicating involvement of other brain stem structures. Objective neurologic signs should be present in frank infarction of the brain stem.

Nystagmus occurring in central nervous system (CNS) disease may be vertical and disconjugate, whereas inner-ear nystagmus never is. Central nystagmus is gaze directed (beats in the direction of gaze), whereas inner-ear nystagmus is direction fixed (beats in one direction, regardless of the direction of gaze). Central nystagmus is evident during visual fixation, whereas inner-ear nystagmus is suppressed.

A peripheral vestibular lesion produces unidirectional postural instability with preserved walking, whereas an inferior cerebellar stroke often causes severe postural instability and falling when walking is attempted.

If vertebrobasilar arterial insufficiency is suspected in an elderly patient who has no focal neurologic findings, it is reasonable to place such a patient on aspirin and provide him with prompt neurologic follow-up.

Either central or peripheral nystagmus can be caused by toxins, most commonly alcohol, tobacco, aminoglycosides, minocycline, disopyramide, phencyclidine, phenytoin, benzodiazepines, quinine, quinidine, aspirin, salicylates, nonsteroidal anti-inflammatory drugs (NSAIDs), and carbon monoxide.

Vertigo in an otherwise healthy young child is usually indicative of benign paroxysmal vertigo that may be a migraine equivalent, especially when associated with headache.

Suggested Readings

Epley JM: Positional vertigo related to semicircular canalithiasis, *Otolaryngol Head Neck Surg* 112:154–161, 1995.

Froehling DA, Silverstein MD, Mohr DN, et al: Does this patient have a serious form of vertigo? *J Am Med Assoc* 271:385–388, 1994.

Herr RD, Zun L, Matthews JJ: A directed approach to the dizzy patient, *Ann Emerg Med* 18:664–672, 1989.

Hotson JR, Baloh RW: Acute vestibular syndrome, *N Engl J Med* 339:680–685, 1998.

Koelliker P, Summers RL, Hawkins B: Benign paroxysmal positional vertigo: diagnosis and treatment in the emergency department, *Ann Emerg Med* 37:392–398, 2001.

Marill KA, Walsh MJ, Nelson BK: Intravenous lorazepam versus dimenhydrinate for treatment of vertigo in the emergency department: a randomized clinical trial, *Ann Emerg Med* 36:310–319, 2000.

Radtke A, van Brevern M, Tiel-Wilck K, et al: Self-treatment of benign paroxysmal positional vertigo: Semont maneuver versus Epley procedure, *Neurology* 63:150–152, 2004.

Ravid S, Bienkowski R, Eviatar L: A simplified diagnostic approach to dizziness in children, *Pediatr Neuro* 29:317–320, 2003.

Strupp M, Zingler VC, Arbusow V, et al: Methylprednisolone, valacyclovir, or the combination for vestibular neuritis, *N Engl J Med* 351:354–361, 2004.

Tusa RJ: Vertigo, *Neurol Clin* 19:23–55, 2001.

Weakness

Presentation

An older patient, complaining of isolated "weakness" or an inability to carry on her usual activities or care for herself, comes to an acute care clinic or ED, often brought in by family members.

What To Do:

✓ Obtain as much of the history as possible. Speak to available family members or friends, as well as the patient, and ask for details. Are there any new medications that can produce weakness (also consider toxins)? Is the patient weak before certain activities (suggests depression)? Is the weakness located in the limb girdles (suggests polymyalgia rheumatica when there is symmetric joint pain or painful myopathy) (see Chapter 127)? Is the weakness mostly in the distal muscles (suggests neuropathy)? Is the weakness caused by repetitive actions (suggests myasthenia gravis)? Is the weakness unilateral, with slurring of speech or confusion (suggests cerebrovascular accident)?

✓ **Obtain a thorough medical history and complete physical examination,** including a review of symptoms (e.g., headaches, weight loss, cold intolerance, change in appetite or bowel habits), with a full set of vital signs; also include testing for strength of all muscle groups (graded on a scale of 1 to 5), deep tendon reflexes, and neurologic status. Do a rectal examination for occult stool blood. **Order a head CT scan if there is an unexplained change in mental status or there are abnormal neurologic findings. Obtain an MRI or CT with contrast if a structural cord lesion is suspected.**

✓ **Obtain a spectrum of laboratory tests that include pulse oximetry and/or arterial blood gases, chest radiograph, ECG, cardiac enzymes, urinalysis, blood cell counts, sedimentation rate, and glucose, blood urea nitrogen, and electrolyte levels,** which may disclose hypoxia, hypercarbia, myocardial infarction, anemia, infection, diabetes, uremia, polymyalgia rheumatica, hyponatremia, or hypokalemia, which are the most common causes of "weakness." Tests determining serum phosphate and calcium levels may also be valuable.

○ **Weakness is frequently the only complaint in elderly patients with acute myocardial infarction. Weakness or fatigue is the most common atypical complaint for women with acute myocardial infarction.**

○ **Weakness is one of the most common complaints in the elderly with acute urinary tract infection.**

✅ If no cause for weakness can be found, probe the patient, family, and friends once again for any hidden agenda (i.e., no one to look after "Granny" while the family goes on vacation), and if none is found, take the patient seriously, be sympathetic, and assure her that serious illnesses have been ruled out at this time. Send the patient home and make arrangements for definite follow-up and further testing if necessary.

What Not To Do:

❌ Do not order any laboratory tests that will not yield results quickly. Stick to tests that will return results while the patient is in the ED or clinic, and defer any long-term investigations to a follow-up physician. Obtaining laboratory results that will never be interpreted or acted on is worse than obtaining none at all.

❌ Do not insist on making the diagnosis in the ED or acute care clinic in every case. The goals during the first visit are to rule out acute, life-threatening conditions and then make arrangements for further evaluation. The primary care physician providing follow-up may consider disorders such as hyperthyroidism, hypothyroidism, chronic fatigue syndrome (or chronic Epstein-Barr virus infection), chronic parvovirus B19 infection, and Lyme disease.

Discussion

The complaint of weakness should not be considered a "minor emergency" until all other significant causes are ruled out. Therefore approach the patient with "weakness" with an open mind, and be prepared to take some time with the evaluation. Demonstrable localized weakness usually points to a specific neuromuscular cause, and generalized weakness is the presenting complaint for a multitude of ills. In young patients, weakness may be a sign of psychological depression, whereas in older patients, in addition to depression, it may be the first sign of a subdural hematoma, pneumonia, urinary tract infection, diabetes, dehydration, malnutrition, heart attack, heart failure, or cancer.

When a patient's weakness is suspected to be a psychiatric problem, consider the somatoform disorders, such as hypochondriasis, anxiety and sleep disorders, malingering, depression, and factitious illness (e.g., Munchausen syndrome). (These diagnoses should be avoided until all other organic causes have been ruled out.)

It is important to exclude Guillain-Barré syndrome, which is one of the critical, life-threatening causes of weakness. The pattern is not always an ascending paralysis or weakness but usually does depress deep-tendon reflexes. **Botulism is another condition that must be excluded** through the history or observation. Patients suffering from these sorts of neuromuscular weakness are in danger when they cannot breathe. Pulmonary function studies, such as pulse oximetry, capnography, blood gases, peak flow, or vital capacity, can be helpful in identifying patients who might be close to severe respiratory compromise.

PART 2

Ophthalmologic Emergencies

■ Philip Buttaravoli   ■ Ray Keller

Conjunctivitis

(Pink Eye)

Presentation

Conjunctivitis is the most common diagnosis in patients with a red eye and discharge, but not all red eyes are the result of conjunctivitis. With bacterial conjunctivitis, the patient complains of a red, irritated eye, and perhaps a gritty or foreign-body sensation; a thick, purulent discharge that continues throughout the day; and crusting or matting of the eyelids on awakening (Figure 14-1). It is most often unilateral. With viral conjunctivitis, the complaint may be of a similar discomfort or burning, with clear tearing, preauricular lymphadenopathy, or symptoms of upper respiratory tract infection (Figure 14-2). On the other hand, with allergic conjunctivitis, the main complaint may be itching, with minimal conjunctival injection, seasonal recurrence, and cobblestone hypertrophy of the tarsal conjunctivae or bubble-like chemosis of the conjunctiva covering the sclera (Figure 14-3). Ocular symptoms are usually accompanied by nasal symptoms, and there may be other allergic events in the patient's

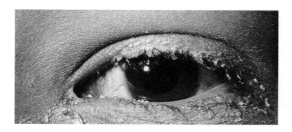

Figure 14-1 Bacterial conjunctivitis. (Adapted from Palay DH, Krachmer JH: *Primary Care Ophthalmology,* ed 2. St Louis, 2005, Mosby.)

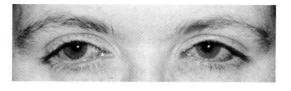

Figure 14-2 Viral conjunctivitis. (Adapted from Palay DH, Krachmer JH: *Primary Care Ophthalmology,* ed 2. St Louis, 2005, Mosby.)

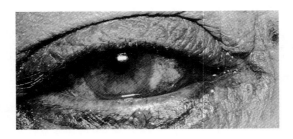

Figure 14-3 Allergic conjunctivitis. (Adapted from Palay DH, Krachmer JH: *Primary Care Ophthalmology,* ed 2. St Louis, 2005, Mosby.)

history that support the diagnosis of ocular allergy. Examination discloses generalized injection of the conjunctiva, with thinning out toward the cornea. (Localized inflammation suggests some other diagnosis, such as presence of a foreign body, an inverted eyelash, episcleritis, or a viral or bacterial ulcer.)

Vision and pupil reactions should be normal, and the cornea and anterior chamber should be clear. Any discomfort should be temporarily relieved by the instillation of topical anesthetic solution.

If few symptoms are present on awakening but discomfort worsens during the day, dry eye is probable. Eye-opening during sleep, which leads to corneal exposure and drying, results in ocular redness and irritation that is worse in the morning.

Physical and chemical conjunctivitis, caused by particles, solutions, vapors, and natural or occupational irritants that inflame the conjunctiva, should be evident from the history.

Deep pain, pain not relieved by topical anesthetic, severe pain of sudden onset, photophobia, vomiting, decreased vision, and injection that is more pronounced around the limbus (ciliary flush) suggest more serious involvement of the cornea or the globe's internal structures (e.g., corneal ulcer, keratitis, acute angle–closure glaucoma, uveitis) and demand early or immediate ophthalmologic consultation.

What To Do:

✓ **Instill proparacaine (Alcaine, Ophthaine, Ophthetic) anesthetic drops to allow a more comfortable examination and to help determine whether the patient's discomfort is limited to the conjunctiva and cornea.** If there is no pain relief, the pain comes from deeper eye structures.

✓ Examine the eye, including assessment of visual acuity (correct for any refractive error and record results) and pupil reaction and symmetry, inspection for foreign bodies, estimation of intraocular pressure by palpating the globe above the tarsal plate, and examination with a slit lamp (when available), and fluorescein staining and ultraviolet or cobalt blue light to assess the corneal epithelium.

✓ Ask about and look for signs of any rash, arthritis, or mucous membrane involvement, which could point to Stevens-Johnson syndrome, Kawasaki syndrome, Reiter syndrome, or some other syndrome that can present with conjunctivitis.

✓ **For bacterial conjunctivitis, instruct the patient to begin therapy by applying warm or cool compresses (for comfort and cleansing) q4h, followed by instillation of ophthalmic antibiotic solutions, such as trimethoprim plus polymyxin B (Polytrim) 10 mL,**

1 to 2 drops q2-6h; azithromycin 1% (AzaSite) 2.5 mL, 1 drop bid for 2 days, then 1 drop qd for 5 more days; or **ciprofloxacin 0.3% solution (Ciloxan) 5 mL, 1 to 2 drops q2-4h;** or instillation under the lower lid of topical antibiotic ointments (which transiently blur vision and may be cosmetically unacceptable), such as erythromycin 0.5% (Ilotycin), bacitracin–polymyxin B (Polysporin), or tobramycin 0.3% (Tobrex), 3.5 g each, with oral analgesics as needed.

✓ No clinical sign or symptom can adequately distinguish all viral from bacterial infections. Therefore, if it is unclear whether the problem is viral or bacterial, it is safest to treat it as bacterial.

✓ Continue therapy for approximately 5 days or for at least 24 hours after all signs and symptoms have cleared. It should be noted that several studies suggest that bacterial conjunctivitis is self limiting and will resolve without any antibiotics in most patients. Therefore it is reasonable to use the less expensive topical preparations on the less severe cases (i.e., polymyxin B/trimethoprim–generic).

✓ **With contact lens wearers (in whom *Pseudomonas* is more likely to be a problem), it is more justifiable to use a more expensive fluoroquinolone (i.e., moxifloxacin [Vigamox] 0.5% solution 3 mL, 1 to 2 drops tid, or gatifloxacin [Zymar] 0.3% solution 5 mL, 1 to 2 drops every 2 hours when awake, then taper to 1 to 2 drops qid).**

✓ **For mild to moderate viral and chemical conjunctivitis, apply cold compresses and weak topical vasoconstrictors, such as naphazoline 0.1% (Naphcon), every 3 to 4 hours,** unless the patient has a shallow anterior chamber that is prone to acute angle–closure glaucoma with mydriatics. Inform the patient or parents about the self-limited nature of most cases and the lack of benefits (with some risk for complications) from topical antibiotics. You could reassure them further by offering a delayed prescription that they could get filled if the symptoms have not resolved after 5 days. If necessary, provide mild systemic analgesics.

✓ **For allergic conjunctivitis, apply cold compresses and prescribe ketotifen fumarate 0.025% (Zaditor) [over the counter] or azelastine hydrochloride 0.05% (Optivar), 1 drop bid.** These are H_1-antihistamines and mast cell stabilizers. The antihistaminic effect of ketotifen occurs within minutes after administration and has a duration of up to 12 hours. **Combining this topical therapy with systemic antihistamines may give the maximal symptomatic relief.** Topical corticosteroid drops provide dramatic relief, but prolonged use increases the risk for opportunistic viral, fungal, and bacterial corneal ulceration; cataract formation; and glaucoma. **When a steroid is required, loteprednol (Alrex) 0.2% suspension, 1 drop qid, reportedly does not cause cataract or glaucoma.** Ophthalmologic consultation is recommended. If a severe contact dermatitis is suspected, a short course of oral prednisone is indicated (see Chapter 160).

✓ If the problem is dry eye (keratoconjunctivitis sicca), treat with artificial tear drops (Refresh Tears, Lacri-Lube, Gen Teal). If chlorine from a swimming pool is causing chronic red eye (student athletes and recreational swimmers), using a nonsteroidal anti-inflammatory drug (NSAID) eye drop (Ketorolac [Acular] 0.5%, 1 drop qid) may provide some comfort, but swimming goggles are the best solution.

✓ Instruct the patient to follow up with an ophthalmologist if the infection does not completely resolve within 2 days. Obtain earlier consultation if there is any involvement of

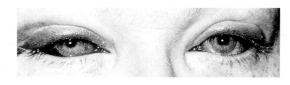

Figure 14-4 Epidemic keratoconjunctivitis. (Adapted from Palay DH, Krachmer JH: *Primary Care Ophthalmology,* ed 2. St Louis, 2005, Mosby.)

the cornea or iris, impaired vision, light sensitivity, inequality in pupil size, or other signs of corneal infection, iritis, or acutely increased intraocular pressure. In addition, refer patients who have had eye surgery, have a history of herpes simplex keratitis, or wear contact lenses to an ophthalmologist.

Return to school or daycare should parallel behavior in the common cold.

What Not To Do:

Do not forget to wash hands and equipment after examining the patient; herpes simplex or epidemic keratoconjunctivitis (Figure 14-4) can be spread to clinicians and other patients. For viral forms of conjunctivitis, do not forget to instruct the patient regarding the contagious nature of the disease and the importance of hand washing and use of separate towels and pillows for 10 days after the onset of symptoms.

Do not use ophthalmic neomycin, because of the high incidence of hypersensitivity reactions.

Do not patch an infected eye; this interferes with the cleansing function of tear flow.

Do not routinely culture an eye discharge. Cultures should only be obtained with neonatal conjunctivitis or when the infection does not respond to treatment.

Do not use topical antiviral drugs for simple cases of viral conjunctivitis. They are of no benefit.

Do not give steroids without arranging for ophthalmologic consultation, and never give steroids if a herpes simplex infection is suspected.

Do not make a diagnosis of conjunctivitis unless visual acuity is normal and there is no evidence of corneal involvement, iritis, or acute glaucoma.

Discussion

Warm or cool compresses are soothing for all types of conjunctivitis, but antibiotic drops and ointments should be used only when bacterial infection is likely. Neomycin-containing ointments and drops should probably be avoided because allergic sensitization to this antibiotic is common. Any corneal ulceration found with fluorescein staining requires ophthalmologic consultation. Most viral and bacterial conjunctivitis hosts will resolve spontaneously, with the possible exception of *Staphylococcus, Meningococcus,* and *Gonococcus* organism infections, which can produce destructive sequelae without treatment.

Most bacterial conjunctivitis in immunocompetent hosts is caused by *Streptococcus pneumoniae, Haemophilus influenzae, Staphylococcus aureus,* or *Moraxella catarrhalis.* Routine conjunctival cultures

Discussion continued

are seldom of value, but Gram's method should be used to stain and culture any copious yellow-green, purulent exudate that is abrupt in onset and quickly reaccumulates after being wiped away (findings with both *Neisseria gonorrhoeae* and *N. meningitidis*). *N. gonorrhoeae* infection confirmed by gram-negative intracellular diplococci requires immediate ophthalmologic consultation and treatment with IM ceftriaxone as well as topical antibiotics. Corneal ulceration, scarring, and blindness can occur in a matter of hours.

Chlamydial conjunctivitis will usually present with lid droop, mucopurulent discharge, photophobia, and preauricular lymphadenopathy. Small, white, elevated conglomerations of lymphoid tissue can be seen on the upper and lower tarsal conjunctiva, and 90% of patients have concurrent genital infection. In adults, doxycycline, 100 mg PO bid for 3 weeks, or azithromycin (Zithromax), 1 g PO × 1 dose, plus topical tetracycline (Achromycin Ophthalmic Ointment) 1%, q3-4h for 3 weeks should control the infection. (Also treat sexual partners.) Although it is somewhat difficult to culture, *Chlamydia* can be confirmed by monoclonal immunofluorescent antibody testing from conjunctival smears or by polymerase chain reaction (PCR) testing.

Newborn conjunctivitis requires special attention and culture of any discharge, as well as immediate ophthalmologic consultation. The pathogens of greatest concern are *N. gonorrhoeae, C. trachomatis,* and herpes simplex virus (HSV). *N. gonorrhoeae* infections usually begin 2 to 4 days after birth, whereas *C. trachomatis* infections start 3 to 10 days after birth. If conjunctivitis is noted on the first day of life, this is more likely to be a reaction to silver nitrate prophylaxis.

Epidemic keratoconjunctivitis is a bilateral, painful, highly contagious conjunctivitis usually caused by an adenovirus (serotypes 8 and 19). The eyes are extremely erythematous, sometimes with subconjunctival hemorrhages. There is copious watery discharge and preauricular lymphadenopathy. Treat the symptoms with analgesics, cold compresses, and, if necessary, corticosteroids

(loteprednol [Alrex], 0.2% suspension, 1 drop qid). Because the infection can last as long as 3 weeks and may result in permanent corneal scarring, provide ophthalmologic consultation and referral. Patients should be instructed on hand washing with soap, changing pillowcases, and not sharing household items. Patients should also be told to avoid communal activities (work, school, daycare) for 10 to 14 days or while there is a discharge, to avoid infecting others. These patients should also avoid wearing contact lenses. Nondisposable contacts should be sterilized, and patients with disposable contacts should use new lenses after 14 days.

Herpes simplex conjunctivitis is usually unilateral. Symptoms include a red eye, photophobia, eye pain, and blurred vision with a foreign-body sensation. There may be periorbital vesicles, and a branching (dendritic) pattern with bulbar terminal endings of fluorescein staining confirms the diagnosis. Treat with trifluridine 1% (Viroptic), 1 drop q2h, 9×/day, then reduce dose to 1 drop q4-6h after reepithelialization for another 7 to 14 days (maximum of 21 days of treatment). In addition, instill 1 cm of Vidarabine (Vira-A) ointment 5× daily at 3-hour intervals up to 21 days. Also give acyclovir, 800 mg PO 5× daily for 7 to 10 days, or valacyclovir (Valtrex), 1 g bid for 7 to 10 days. Analgesics and cold compresses will help provide comfort. Cycloplegics, such as homatropine 5% (1 to 2 drops bid to tid), may help control pain resulting from iridocyclitis. Topical corticosteroids are contraindicated, because they can extend duration of the infection. Because corneal herpetic infections frequently leave a scar, ophthalmologic consultation is required.

Herpes zoster ophthalmicus is shingles of the ophthalmic branch of the trigeminal nerve, which innervates the cornea and the tip of the nose. It begins with unilateral neuralgia, followed by a vesicular rash in the distribution of the nerve. Ophthalmic consultation is again required (because of frequent ocular complications), but topical corticosteroids may be used. Prescribe systemic acyclovir (Zovirax), 800 mg q4h (5× daily) for 7 to 10 days, or valacyclovir (Valtrex), 1 g PO tid for 7 to 10 days.

Suggested Readings

Abramaian FM: Outbreak of bacterial conjunctivitis at a college—New Hampshire, January-March 2002, *Ann Emerg Med* 40:524–527, 2002.

Bremond-Gignac D, Mariano-Kurkdjian P, et al: Efficacy and safety of azithromycin 1.5% eye drops for purulent bacterial conjunctivitis in pediatric patients, *Pediatr Infect Dis J* 29:3, 2010.

David SP: Should we prescribe antibiotics for acute conjunctivitis? *Am Fam Physician* 66:1649–1651, 2002.

Kowalski RP, Karenchak LM, Romanowski EG: Infection disease: changing antibiotic susceptibility, *Ophthalmol Clin North Am* 16:1–9, 2003.

Rose PW, Harnden A, Brueggemann AB, et al: Chloramphenicol treatment for acute infective conjunctivitis in children in primary care, *Lancet* 366:37–43, 2005.

Schiebel N: Use of antibiotics in patients with acute bacterial conjunctivitis, *Ann Emerg Med* 41:407–409, 2003.

Shaikh S, Ta CN: Evaluation and management of herpes zoster ophthalmicus, *Am Fam Physician* 66:1723–1730, 2002.

Sheikh A: Use of antibiotics in patients with acute bacterial conjunctivitis, *Ann Emerg Med* 41:407, 2003.

Yaphe J, Pandher KS: The predictive value of the penlight test for photophobia for serious eye pathology in general practice, *Fam Pract* 20:425–427, 2003.

Contact Lens Complications

Presentation

A patient who wears hard, impermeable, or rigid gas permeable contact lenses comes to the emergency department in the early morning complaining of severe eye pain after he has left his lenses in for longer than the recommended time period. Extended-wear soft contact lenses can cause a similar syndrome when worn for days or weeks and have become contaminated with bacteria and/or irritants. The patient may not be able to open his eyes for examination because of pain and blepharospasm. He may have obvious corneal injury, with signs of iritis and conjunctivitis, or may have no findings visible without fluorescein staining.

What To Do:

✓ **Instill topical anesthetic drops such as proparacaine (Alcaine, Ophthaine) to provide comfort for examination.**

✓ Perform a complete eye examination, including best-corrected visual acuity, assessment of pupil reflexes, examination with funduscopy, and inspection of conjunctival sacs. Use a slit lamp if available.

✓ With a bright light examination, note whether there are any hazy areas or ulcerations on the cornea.

✓ **Instill fluorescein dye** (use a single-dose dropper or wet a dye-impregnated paper strip and touch it to the tear pool in the lower conjunctival sac), have the patient blink, and examine the eye under cobalt blue or ultraviolet light, looking for the green fluorescence of dye bound to dead or areas of absent corneal epithelium. Rinse out the dye afterward.

✓ When a corneal defect is visualized, sketch the area of corneal injury on the patient record.

✓ When the symptoms consist of a mild burning, a foreign body sensation, and/or dryness, and examination with fluorescein staining shows mild punctate uptake (**superficial punctate keratitis;** Figure 15-1), **treatment consists of discontinuation of lens use and the instillation of fluoroquinolone drops—ciprofloxacin 0.3% (Ciloxan), 1 to 2 drops q1-6h (use more frequently for the first 2 to 3 days). Prescribe analgesics (e.g., naproxen, ibuprofen, oxycodone) as needed, and administer the first dose if appropriate.**

✓ Instruct the patient to avoid wearing his lenses until cleared by the ophthalmologist and to seek ophthalmologic follow-up within 1 day.

✓ **Contact lens–induced acute red eye (CLARE)** can occur with extended-wear contact lenses and has been defined as **an acute onset of a red eye associated with corneal**

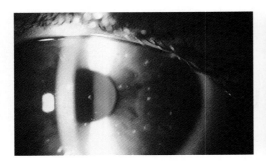

Figure 15-1 General appearance of superficial punctate keratitis under slit-lamp examination. (Adapted from Yanoff M, Duker JS: *Ophthalmology,* ed 2. St Louis, 2004, Mosby.)

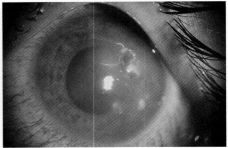

Figure 15-2 Microbial keratitis. Intraepithelial infiltration of the cornea by *Pseudomonas* organisms in a hydrophilic contact lens wearer. (Adapted from Yanoff M, Duker JS: *Ophthalmology,* ed 2. St Louis, 2004, Mosby.)

infiltrates. Typically, symptoms of ocular discomfort, foreign-body sensation, and redness are noted on awakening. These findings are usually unilateral, and, on examination, conjunctival injection, mild chemosis, and peripheral corneal infiltrates are seen. The corneal epithelium overlying the infiltrates may be intact, or a mild punctate keratopathy may be present. **Treatment consists of discontinuation of contact lens wearing until complete resolution has occurred. There is apparently no medical therapy indicated for this condition, but it would be considered reasonable and prudent to initiate the same treatment as that provided for superficial punctate keratitis.**

⊘ **When patients complain of severe pain, irritation, photophobia, and tearing associated with infiltrates and epithelial defects, they are at high risk for the most serious complication of contact lens wear** (**microbial keratitis;** Figure 15-2). The most commonly cultured organisms are gram negative, particularly *Pseudomonas aeruginosa*. The more severe the symptoms are, the larger the corneal epithelial defect (>1.5 mm), and the more central its location, the greater the morbidity is likely to be, with resultant permanent loss of vision. **These patients demand prompt ophthalmologic consultation, along with the initiation of treatment with the most potent topical antibiotics (i.e., a combination of either fortified cefazolin or vancomycin and fortified tobramycin or gentamicin).** Suspected microbial ulcers must be scraped and cultured and a Gram stain performed. Contact lens care solutions and the contact lens case should also be cultured along with the ulcer if possible. **Patients with less severe cases can be treated with moxifloxacin (Vigamox), 0.5% solution, 3 mL, 1 to 2 drops every 2 hours when awake or gatifloxacin (Zymar), 0.3% solution, 5 mL, 1 to 2 drops every 2 hours when awake then taper to 1 to 2 drops qid.** Ophthalmologic consultation with next-day follow-up is still very important.

⊘ **In the presence of minimal signs of inflammation in a patient with significant pain that is out of proportion to the findings, consider the possibility of Acanthamoeba keratitis.** This form of infection from overwearing of soft lenses can damage the eye rapidly and may require excision and hospitalization.

What Not To Do:

⊗ Do not discharge a patient with topical anesthetic ophthalmic drops for continued administration; they potentiate serious injury.

Ⓧ Do not let a patient reuse contaminated or infected lenses.

Ⓧ Do not patch eyes damaged by contact lens abrasions or early ulcerative keratitis.

Ⓧ Do not prescribe antibiotic ointments that do not provide prophylaxis against *Pseudomonas* organisms (e.g., erythromycin and sulfas).

Ⓧ Do not use drops or ointments containing steroids without an ophthalmologist's recommendation.

Discussion

Hard or rigid gas-permeable contact lenses and extended-wear soft lenses left in place too long deprive the avascular corneal epithelium of oxygen and nutrients that are normally provided by the tear film. This produces diffuse ischemia, which can cause an increase in bacterial binding to the corneal epithelium. Soft lenses can absorb chemical irritants, allergens, bacteria, and amoebas if they soak in contaminated cleaning solution.

Patient-related factors—such as alteration of the recommended wearing or replacement schedules and noncompliance with recommended contact lens care regimens for economic reasons, convenience, or in error—contribute to contact lens–related complications.

Studies have shown that the major risk for infection with conventional contact lenses is overnight wear. The risk for infection is still 5 times greater with extended-wear contact lenses compared with that for daily wear. Initial results of studies looking at silicone hydrogel contact lenses (Pure Vision) worn for extended periods are encouraging in that they appear to result in a lower incidence of microbial keratitis than seen with the standard extended-wear lenses.

There are millions of contact lens wearers in the United States. Adverse reactions range from minor transient irritation to corneal ulceration and infection that may result in permanent loss of vision caused by corneal scarring. *Pseudomonas* organism infection is most commonly associated with contact lens–related microbial keratitis. Thus the management of these cases should differ from the routine care of mechanical corneal abrasions that are not caused by contact lens wear. Occlusive patching and corticosteroid medications favor bacterial growth and are, therefore, not generally recommended for initial treatment in the setting of contact lens use.

Suggested Readings

Donshik PC: Extended wear contact lenses, *Ophthalmol Clin North Am* 16:79–84, 2003.

Schein OD: Contact lens abrasions and the nonophthalmologist, *Am J Emerg Med* 11:606–608, 1993.

Suchecki JK, Donshik P, Ehlers WH: Contact lens complications, *Ophthalmol Clin North Am* 16:471–484, 2003.

Corneal Abrasion

Presentation

The patient may complain of eye pain or a sensation of the presence of a foreign body after being poked in the eye with a finger, twig, or equivalent object. The patient may have abraded the cornea while inserting or removing a contact lens. Removal of a corneal foreign body produces some corneal abrasion, but corneal abrasion can occur without any identifiable trauma. There is often excessive tearing, blurred vision, and photophobia. Often the patient cannot open her eye for the examination because of pain and blepharospasm. Abrasions are occasionally visible during sidelighting of the cornea. Conjunctival inflammation can range from minimal to severe conjunctivitis with accompanying iritis.

What To Do:

✓ **Instill topical anesthetic drops to eliminate any pain or blepharospasm and thereby permit examination (e.g., proparacaine [Ophthetic], tetracaine [Pontocaine]).**

✓ Perform a complete eye examination (including assessment of best-corrected visual acuity, funduscopy, anterior chamber bright-light examination, and inspection of conjunctival sacs for a foreign body).

✓ **Perform the fluorescein examination** by wetting a paper strip impregnated with dry, orange fluorescein dye and touching this strip into the tear pool inside the lower conjunctival sac. After the patient blinks, darken the room and examine her eye under cobalt-blue filtered or ultraviolet light. (The red-free light on the ophthalmoscope does not work.) **Areas of denuded or dead corneal epithelium will fluoresce green and confirm the diagnosis.**

✓ If a foreign body is present, remove it and irrigate the eye.

✓ **When a corneal abrasion is present, treat the patient with antibiotic drops, such as trimethoprim plus polymyxin B (Polytrim), 10 mL, 1 drop q2-6h, while awake.** Some physicians prefer ophthalmic ointment preparations, which may last longer but tend to be messy. If ointment is preferred, erythromycin 0.5%, 3.5 g, or polymyxin B/bacitracin, 3.5 g, applied inside the lower lid (1- to 2-cm ribbon) qid is effective and least expensive. **In patients who wear contact lenses or who were injured by organic material (such as a tree branch), an antipseudomonal antibiotic (e.g., ciprofloxacin [Ciloxan] 0.3%, 1 to 2 drops q1-6h, or ofloxacin [Ocuflox] 0.3%, 1 to 2 drops q1-6h, should be used. Contact lens wearing should be discontinued until the abrasion is healed.**

✓ **Analgesic nonsteroidal anti-inflammatory drug (NSAID) eye drops of diclofenac (Voltaren), 0.1%, 5 mL, or ketorolac (Acular), 0.5%, 5 mL, 1 drop instilled qid, provide pain relief and do not inhibit healing.**

✓ If iritis is present (as evidenced by consensual photophobia or, in severe cases, an irregular pupil or miosis and a limbic flush in addition to conjunctival injection), consult the ophthalmologic follow-up physician about starting treatment with topical mydriatics and steroids (see Chapter 20).

✓ **Even when there are no signs of iritis, one instillation of a short-acting cycloplegic, such as cyclopentolate 1% (Cyclogyl), will relieve any pain resulting from ciliary spasm.**

✓ Although not likely to be available to the non–contact lens user, **a soft, disposable contact lens (e.g., NewVue, Acuvue) in combination with antibiotic and nonsteroidal anti-inflammatory drops can provide further comfort as well as the ability to see out of the affected eye.** As with any contact lens worn overnight, there is probably an increased risk for infectious keratitis; so, this should be provided in concert with an ophthalmologist.

✓ **Prescribe analgesics (e.g., oxycodone, ibuprofen, naproxen) as needed,** and administer the first dose when appropriate. Most abrasions heal without significant long-term complications; therefore pain relief should be our primary concern with uncomplicated abrasions. This treatment of pain should be guided by an individual patient's age, concomitant illness, drug allergy, ability to tolerate NSAIDs, potential for opioid abuse, and employment conditions, such as driving and machine operation.

✓ **Warn the patient that some of the pain will return when the local anesthetic wears off.**

✓ **Make an appointment for ophthalmologic or primary care follow-up to reevaluate the abrasion the next day.** If the abrasion has not fully healed, the patient should be evaluated again 3 to 4 days later, even if he feels well.

✓ Instruct patients about the importance of wearing eye protection. This is particularly needed for persons in high-risk occupations (e.g., miners, woodworkers, metalworkers, landscapers) and those who participate in certain sports (e.g., hockey, lacrosse, racquetball). Other preventive measures include keeping the fingernails of infants and children clipped short and removing objects such as low-hanging tree branches from the home environment.

What Not To Do:

✗ Do not be stingy with pain medication. The aforementioned treatments may not provide adequate analgesia, and supplementation with NSAIDs or narcotic analgesics may be necessary for a day.

✗ Do not give the patient any topical anesthetic for continued instillation.

✗ Do not miss anterior chamber hemorrhage or other significant eye trauma that is likely to cause immediate visual impairment.

✗ Do not use a soft contact lens if bacterial conjunctivitis, ulcer, or abrasions caused by contact lens overwear are present.

(X) Do not use an eye patch. Although eye patching traditionally has been recommended in the treatment of corneal abrasions, studies now show convincingly that patching does not help healing or pain, interferes with binocular vision, and may even hinder corneal repair.

Discussion

Corneal abrasions constitute a loss of the superficial epithelium of the cornea (Figure 16-1). They are generally painful because of the extensive innervation in the affected area. Healing is usually complete in 1 to 2 days unless the abrasions are deep, there is extensive epithelial loss, or there is underlying ocular disease (e.g., diabetes). Larger abrasions that involve more than half of the corneal surface may take 4 to 5 days to heal. Scarring will occur only if the injury is deep enough to penetrate the collagenous layer.

Fluorescein binds to corneal stroma and dead or denuded epithelium but not to intact corneal epithelium. Collections of fluorescein elsewhere—pooling in conjunctival irregularities and in the tear film—are not pathologic findings.

The traditional use of eye patching has been shown to be unnecessary for both corneal reepithelialization and pain relief. Prophylactic antibiotic treatment is used because concomitant infection can cause slower healing of corneal abrasions; however, there is no strong evidence for their use.

Continuous instillation of topical anesthetic drops can impair healing, inhibit protective reflexes, permit further eye injury, and even cause sloughing of the corneal epithelium.

With small, superficial abrasions, ophthalmologic follow-up is not required if the patient is completely asymptomatic within 12 to 24 hours. With deep or larger abrasions or with any worsening symptoms or persistent discomfort, ophthalmologic follow-up is necessary within 24 hours because of the risk for corneal infection or ulceration. Ophthalmologic follow-up is also required for recurrent corneal erosions—repeated spontaneous disruptions of the corneal epithelium. This can occur in corneal tissue weakened by abrasion months or years earlier. Symptoms are the same as those for corneal abrasions but occur spontaneously on awakening and opening the eyes or after simply rubbing the eyes. Lesions usually are found near the original abrasion.

Patients who wear contact lenses should also be reevaluated in 24 hours and again 3 to 4 days later, even if they feel well. Hard and soft contact lenses can abrade the cornea and cause a diffuse keratitis or corneal infiltrates and ulcers (see Chapter 15).

In follow-up examination of corneal abrasions, inspect the base of the corneal defect, ensuring that it is clear. If the base of the abrasion becomes hazy, it may indicate the early development of a corneal ulcer and demands immediate ophthalmologic consultation.

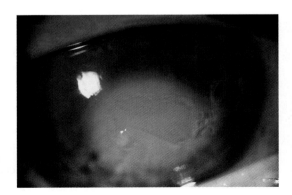

Figure 16-1 Corneal epithelial abrasion showing fluorescein uptake. (From Goldman L, Ausiello D: *Cecil Textbook of Medicine,* ed 22. Philadelphia, 2004, Elsevier.)

Suggested Readings

Arbour JD, Brunette I, Boisjoly HM, et al: Should we patch corneal erosions? *Arch Ophthalmol* 115:313–317, 1997.

Campanile TM, St. Clair DA, Benaim M: The evaluation of eye patching in the treatment of traumatic corneal epithelial defects, *J Emerg Med* 15:769–774, 1997.

Carley F: Mydriatics in corneal abrasion, *J Accid Emerg Med* 18:273, 2001.

Flynn CA, D'Amico F, Smith G: Should we patch corneal abrasions? A meta-analysis, *J Fam Pract* 47:264–270, 1998.

Kaiser PK, Pineda R: A study of topical nonsteroidal anti-inflammatory drops and no pressure patching in the treatment of corneal abrasions, *Ophthalmology* 104:1353–1359, 1997.

Kirkpatrick J: No eye pad for corneal abrasions, *Eye* 7:468–471, 1993.

Le Sage N, Verreault R, Rochette L: Efficacy of eye patching for traumatic corneal abrasions: a controlled clinical trial, *Ann Emerg Med* 28:129–134, 2001.

Michael JG, Hug D, Dowd MD: Management of corneal abrasion in children: a randomized clinical trial, *Ann Emerg Med* 40:67–72, 2002.

Salz JJ, Reader AL, Schwartz LJ, et al: Treatment of corneal abrasions with soft contact lenses and topical diclofenac, *J Refractive Corneal Surg* 10:640–646, 1994.

Szucs PA, Nashed AH, Allegra JR, Eskin B: Safety and efficacy of diclofenac ophthalmic solution in the treatment of corneal abrasions, *Ann Emerg Med* 35:131–137, 2000.

Weaver CS, Terrell KM: Update: do ophthalmic nonsteroidal anti-inflammatory drugs reduce the pain associated with simple corneal abrasion without delaying healing? *Ann Emerg Med* 41:134–140, 2003.

Wilson SA, Last A: Management of corneal abrasion, *Am Fam Physician* 70:123–130, 2004.

Foreign Body, Conjunctival

Presentation

Low-velocity projectiles, such as windblown dust particles, can be stuck under the upper tarsal plate, loose in the tear film, or lodged in a conjunctival sac. The patient will feel a foreign-body sensation but may not be very accurate in locating the foreign body by sensation alone. On examination, normally occurring white papules inside the lids can be mistaken for foreign bodies, and transparent foreign bodies can be invisible in the tear film (until outlined by fluorescein dye). Most particles are easily identified as dark specks, which are most often found under the upper eyelid.

What To Do:

✓ **Make sure that the mechanism of injury did not include high-velocity debris (e.g., hammering metal on metal, drilling, grinding, or exposure to explosive forces).**

✓ **Instill topical anesthetic drops** (proparacaine [Ophthaine, Alcaine, Ophthetic] or tetracaine [Pontocaine]). This should relieve discomfort and any uncontrollable blepharospasm.

✓ Perform a best-corrected visual acuity examination and funduscopy; examine the cornea, anterior chamber, and tear film with a bright light (best done with a slit lamp), and then examine the conjunctival sacs.

✓ To examine the lower sac, pull the lower lid down with your finger while the patient looks up (Figure 17-1).

 ✓ **To examine the upper sac; hold the proximal portion of the upper lid down with a cotton-tipped swab while pulling the lid out and up by its lashes, everting most of the lid, as the patient looks down. Push the cotton swab downward to help turn the upper conjunctival sac "inside out"** (Figure 17-2, *A* to *C*). The stiff tarsal plate usually keeps the upper lid everted after the swab is removed, as long as the patient continues looking downward. Looking up will reduce the lid to its usual position.

✓ **A loose foreign body usually will adhere to a moistened swab lightly touched to the surface of the conjunctiva and is thereby removed** (Figure 17-2, *D* and *E*), **or it can be washed out by copious irrigation with saline.**

✓ **Perform a fluorescein examination** to disclose any corneal abrasions caused by the foreign body. These vertical scratches occur when the lid closes over a coarse object and should be treated as described in Chapter 16.

✓ Follow with a brief saline irrigation to remove possible remaining fragments.

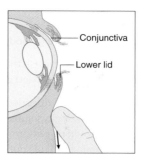

Figure 17-1 The patient looks up while the lid is pulled down.

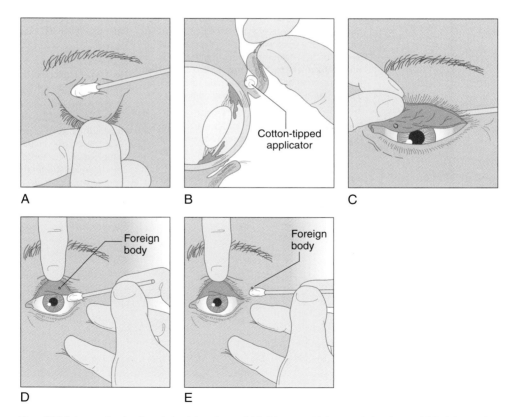

Figure 17-2 A, A cotton-tipped applicator is placed above the upper lid. **B,** Lid eversion with the patient looking downward. **C,** Push down on the applicator to reveal a foreign body hidden under the tarsal plate. **D** and **E,** The moistened applicator touches the foreign body, lifting it away.

What Not To Do:

(X) Do not overlook a foreign body lodged in the deep recesses of the upper conjunctival sac.

(X) Do not overlook an eyelash that has turned in and is rubbing on the surface of the eye. Sometimes a lash may be sticking out of the inferior lacrimal punctum. Extract any such lashes.

(X) Do not overlook an embedded or penetrating foreign body. Maintain a high index of suspicion with high-velocity injuries or when there is periorbital tissue damage. Radiography or CT examination should be performed for suspected metallic intraocular foreign bodies, whereas MRI should be obtained to rule out a nonmetallic object.

(X) Do not overlook a corneal abrasion. Fluorescein staining will uncover these superficial lesions.

Discussion

Good first aid (providing copious irrigation, pulling the upper lid down over the lower lid, and avoiding rubbing of the eyes) will take care of most ocular foreign bodies. The history of injury with a high-velocity fragment, such as a metal shard chipped off from a hammer or chisel, should raise suspicion of a penetrating foreign body, and radiographs or CT scans should be obtained.

The signs associated with an intraocular foreign body can be extremely subtle, causing only slight erythema and local discomfort. Visual acuity often is markedly decreased, but normal visual acuity is possible. There may be conjunctival chemosis, hyphema, localized cataract, or an iris injury with resultant pupil deformity. MRI should be used to locate radiolucent objects but should never be used to image magnetic foreign bodies.

Techniques for conjunctival foreign body removal can also be applied to locating a **displaced contact lens** (see Chapter 23), but be aware that fluorescein dye absorbed by soft contact lenses fades slowly.

When eyelids become glued shut with cyanoacrylate (Crazy Glue or Super Glue), it is usually impossible to perform a complete eye examination or even gently separate the eyelids. Simply apply an antibacterial ointment and, if more comfortable for the patient, patch the eye. Spontaneous opening will occur in 1 to 2 days, and a more thorough examination can be performed at that time if any discomfort persists.

Foreign Body, Corneal

Presentation

The patient's eye has been struck by a falling or an airborne particle, often a fleck of rust loosened while working under a car. Other possibilities include particles from metal grinding, windblown grit, and wood or masonry from construction sites. The patient will complain of a foreign-body sensation and tearing and, possibly over time, will develop constant pain, redness, and photophobia (posttraumatic iritis). Moderate- to high-velocity foreign bodies (fragments chipped from a chisel when struck by a hammer or spray from a grinding wheel) can be superficially embedded on the corneal surface or lodged deep in the corneal stroma, the anterior chamber, or even the vitreous. Superficial foreign bodies may be visualized by simple sidelighting of the cornea or by slit-lamp examination. Deep foreign bodies may be visible on funduscopy only as moving shadows, with a slight or invisible puncture in the sclera.

What To Do:

✅ **Instill topical anesthetic drops** (proparacaine [Ophthaine, Alcaine, Ophthetic] or tetracaine [Pontocaine]). This should relieve discomfort and any uncontrollable blepharospasm.

✅ Perform a best-corrected visual acuity examination, funduscopy (looking for shadows), and bright-light anterior-chamber examination (slit lamp is best), and check pupil symmetry and anterior chamber cell/flare (for iritis) and conjunctivae (for loose foreign bodies).

✅ **Under magnification, a superficial corneal foreign body (usually metal or grit, but occasionally paint or plastic) will be seen adherent to the corneal surface.** Often it is embedded within the corneal epithelium. With iron particles, there will be a halo of particulate debris and rustlike discoloration within the surrounding epithelial tissue (Figure 18-1).

✅ With more serious punctures through the anterior corneal surface penetrating into the anterior chamber, leakage of intraocular fluid from the puncture site might be seen. Streaming of fluorescein dye in this scenario is called the Seidel sign. Such a perforation requires immediate ophthalmologic intervention and application of a protective eye shield.

✅ **If there is any suspicion of a penetrating intraocular foreign body, because there was a high-velocity mechanism of injury, obtain special orbital radiographs or CT scans to locate it or rule it out.** At present, CT scans are considered the gold standard, and have the highest accuracy in diagnosis and localization. The physician should request 3-mm sections through the orbit, unless a foreign body was seen on plain radiography, in which case 6-mm sections are acceptable. **Ultrasonography (US)** is an increasingly popular modality for detecting intraocular foreign bodies because of its immediate availability for emergency physicians familiar with these

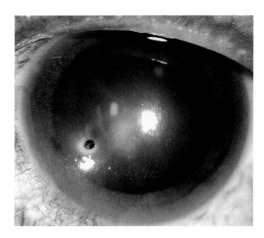

Figure 18-1 Small iron-containing corneal foreign body. (Adapted from Palay DA, Krachmer JH: *Primary Care Ophthalmology,* ed 2. St Louis, 2005, Mosby.)

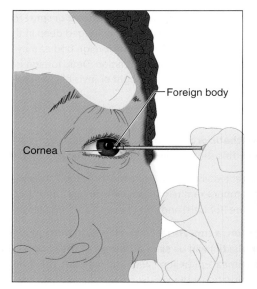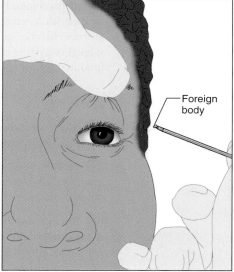

Figure 18-2 Removing a corneal foreign body with an 18-gauge needle.

techniques. **MRI should be used to locate a nonmetallic object. MRI should never be used if a magnetic foreign body is suspected.** If an intraocular foreign body is discovered, immediate ophthalmologic consultation and intervention must be obtained. Any intraocular foreign body can lead to infection and endophthalmitis, a serious condition that can lead to loss of the eye.

✓ **A loosely embedded corneal foreign body** might be removed by touching it with a **moistened swab,** as shown in Chapter 17, but **if the object is firmly embedded, it will have to be scraped off (under magnification, preferably with a slit lamp) with an ophthalmic spud or an 18-gauge needle** (Figure 18-2). Some emergency physicians recommend using a small

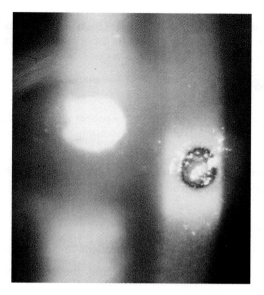

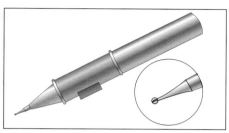

Figure 18-4 Battery-operated corneal burr for rust ring removal.

Figure 18-3 Iron-containing corneal foreign body after removal with a residual rust ring. (Adapted from Marx J, Hockberger R, Walls R: *Rosen's Emergency Medicine,* vol 6, ed 3. St Louis, 2006, Mosby.)

needle for scraping, to minimize the possibility of a corneal perforation, but with a tangential approach, the larger needle is less likely to cause harm.

Give the patient an object to fixate on so that he will keep his eye still; brace your hand on his forehead or cheek and approach the eye tangentially so that no sudden motion can cause a perforation of the anterior chamber with the needle. **Removal of the foreign body leaves a defect that should be treated as a corneal abrasion** (see Chapter 16).

If a rust ring is present, it may appear that a foreign body still remains adherent to the cornea after it has been picked away (Figure 18-3). **Use the needle to continue scraping away this rust-impregnated corneal epithelium. A corneal burr, if available, is preferable for this task** (Figure 18-4). This mechanical burr should be held in the same tangential manner as the needle, as described earlier. The operator's hand should also be braced against the side of the patient's face.

If the extent of the corneal defect is unclear, perform an additional fluorescein examination.

Any large corneal infiltrate or corneal ulcer or significant anterior chamber reaction should be managed as a bacterial keratitis (see Chapter 15).

Finish treatment with further irrigation to loosen possible remaining fragments and with instillation of drops of a mydriatic (homatropine 5%) when photophobia and signs of iritis are present (see Chapter 20).

Instill and prescribe a nonsteroidal anti-inflammatory drug (NSAID) ophthalmologic analgesic drop (diclofenac [Voltaren], 0.1%, 5 mL, or ketorolac [Acular], 0.5%, 5 mL, 1 drop qid).

✅ **Provide for antibiotic eye drops or ointment (polymyxin B/trimethoprim [Polytrim], 10 mL, 1 drop q2-6h while awake, or polymyxin B/bacitracin, 3.5 g, applied inside the lower lid [1- to 2-cm ribbon] qid).**

✅ **Oral analgesic medications should also be provided.** The first dose should be given before the patient is discharged from the medical facility.

✅ With deep central corneal foreign bodies, the patient should be advised of the possibility of unavoidable scar formation and subsequent vision impairment. This conversation should be documented.

✅ **Make an appointment for ophthalmologic follow-up in 1 to 2 days to evaluate for complete healing or any residual corneal staining.**

What Not To Do:

❌ Do not use MRI when there is a suspected magnetic intraocular foreign body.

❌ Do not overlook a foreign body lodged deep inside the globe; the delayed inflammatory response can lead to blindness or even loss of the eye.

❌ Do not leave an iron corneal foreign body in place without arranging for early ophthalmologic follow-up the next day.

❌ Do not allow a patient to leave without ophthalmologic consultation when there is diffuse or focal corneal opacity, abnormal shape of the pupil, or significant loss of visual acuity.

❌ Do not be stingy with pain medication. Large corneal abrasions resulting from foreign-body removal can be quite painful.

❌ If homatropine was instilled, do not forget to tell the patient that he will have blurred near vision and an enlarged pupil for 12 to 24 hours.

Discussion

Superficial corneal foreign bodies are much more common than deeply embedded corneal foreign bodies. Sometimes, the foreign body may not be present at the time of the eye examination. It may have spontaneously dislodged, leaving only the resultant rust ring and/or punctate corneal abrasion with pain and possible photophobia.

Generally, superficial foreign bodies that are removed soon after the injury leave no permanent scarring or visual defect. The deeper the injury, the more the corneal stroma is involved, and the longer the time interval between the injury and treatment, the greater the likelihood of complications. If infection develops, the prognosis will also worsen.

Suggested Reading

Mueller J, McStay C: Ophthalmologic procedures in the emergency department, *Emerg Med Clin North Am* 26:1, 2008.

Hordeolum

(Stye)

Presentation

The patient complains of redness, nodular swelling, and pain in the eyelid, perhaps at the base of an eyelash (stye or external hordeolum) or deep within the lid (meibomitis, meibomianitis, or internal hordeolum, which is best appreciated with the lid everted) and perhaps with conjunctivitis and purulent drainage. In some cases, the complaint may be that of generalized edema and erythema of the lid (cellulitis). There may be a history of similar problems.

Examination most commonly reveals a localized tender area of swelling, often with a pointing eruption on either the internal or the external side of the eyelid (Figure 19-1).

What To Do:

✓ Examine the eye, including assessment of best-corrected visual acuity and inversion of the lids (see Chapter 17 for technique). No corneal or intraocular disease should be found.

✓ **Show the patient how to instill antibiotic drops or ointment (e.g., polymyxin B/trimethoprim [Polytrim], 10 mL, 1 drop q2-6h, or polymyxin B/bacitracin, 3.5 g, 1- to 2-cm ribbon lower lid qid) into the lower conjunctival sac q2-6h.**

✓ **Instruct her to apply warm tap water compresses for approximately 15 minutes qid.**

✓ **If there are signs of spreading infection (e.g., tender lid edema and erythema with or without preauricular lymphadenitis), provide appropriate systemic antibiotic coverage (e.g., cephalexin [Keflex], 500 mg q6h; dicloxacillin [Dynapen], 500 mg q6h; or erythromycin, 333 mg tid for 7 days). Consider coverage for methicillin-resistant *Staphylococcus aureus* (MRSA) if it is prevalent in your community (e.g., doxycycline, 100 mg bid for 7 days).**

✓ Instruct the patient to consult an ophthalmologist or return to the ED or clinic if the problem is not clearly resolving in 2 days or if it gets any worse. Tell her not to squeeze the stye, because this may spread the infection into surrounding tissues. Also let her know that frequent recurrences are common.

✓ **If the abscess does not spontaneously drain or resolve in 2 days and if it is pointing, it may be incised with the tip of a No. 11 scalpel blade or 18-gauge needle. Drainage should be accomplished by making a small puncture at the point of maximum tissue thinning, where underlying pus is visible.** Again, instruct the patient to continue using warm compresses and then to consult an ophthalmologist or return to the ED or clinic if the problem is not clearly resolving in 2 days or if it gets any worse.

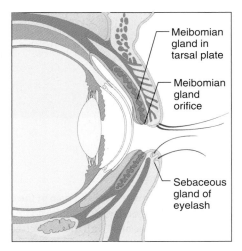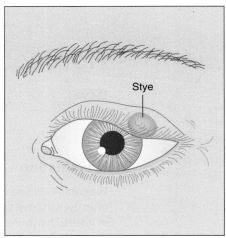

Figure 19-1 Stye of sebaceous gland (gland of Zeiss).

What Not To Do:

(X) Do not overlook orbital or periorbital cellulitis, which is a severe infection and requires aggressive systemic antibiotic treatment.

(X) Do not culture drainage from a stye unless MRSA is suspected. Eye cultures are usually of little clinical value, and they are costly.

(X) Do not make deep incisions along the lid or eyelash margins. This can lead to lid deformity or abnormal eyelash growth.

Discussion

The terminology describing the two types of hordeolum has become confusing. Meibomian glands run vertically within the tarsal plate, open at tiny puncta along the lid margin, and secrete oil to coat the tear film. The glands of Zeiss and Moll are the sebaceous glands opening into the follicles of the eyelashes. Either type of gland can become occluded and superinfected (S. aureus is the causative pathogen in 90% to 95% of cases), producing meibomianitis (internal hordeolum) or a stye (external hordeolum). The immediate care for both acute infections is the same.

A chronic granuloma of the meibomian gland is called a *chalazion;* it is painless, will not drain, and requires excision.

Most hordeola eventually point and drain by themselves. Therefore warm soaks (qid for 15 minutes) are the mainstays of treatment. When lesions are pointing, surgical drainage speeds the healing process.

If the patient appears to have diffuse cellulitis of the lid, fever, and/or painful or restricted extraocular movements, posterior extension (creating an orbital cellulitis) should be suspected. Such cases must be managed aggressively with IV antibiotics and immediate subspecialty consultation.

Iritis

(Acute Anterior Uveitis)

Presentation

The patient usually complains of the onset over hours or days of unilateral eye pain, blurred vision, and photophobia. He may have noticed a pink-colored eye for a few days, suffered mild to moderate trauma during the previous day or two, or experienced no overt eye problems. There may be tearing, but there is usually no discharge. Eye pain is not markedly relieved after instillation of a topical anesthetic. On inspection of the junction of the cornea and conjunctiva (the corneal limbus), a circumcorneal injection, which on closer inspection is a tangle of fine ciliary vessels, is visible through the white sclera. This limbal blush or ciliary flush is usually the earliest sign of iritis. A slit lamp with 10× magnification may help with identification, but the injection is usually evident merely on close inspection. As the iritis becomes more pronounced, the iris and ciliary muscles go into spasm, producing an irregular, poorly reactive, constricted pupil and a lens that will not focus. The slit-lamp examination should demonstrate white blood cells or light reflection from a protein exudate in the clear aqueous humor of the anterior chamber (cells and flare) (Figure 20-1).

What To Do:

✓ **Using topical anesthesia, perform a complete eye examination that includes best-corrected visual acuity assessment, pupil reflex examination, funduscopy, slit-lamp examination of the anterior chamber (including pinhole illumination to bring out cells and flare), and fluorescein staining to detect any corneal lesion.**

✓ Shining a bright light in the normal eye should cause pain in the symptomatic eye (consensual photophobia). Visual acuity may be decreased in the affected eye.

✓ **Attempt to ascertain the cause of the iritis.** (Is it generalized from a corneal insult or conjunctivitis, a late sequela of blunt trauma, infectious, or autoimmune?) Approximately 50% of patients have idiopathic uveitis that is not associated with any other pathologic syndrome. Idiopathic iritis should be suspected when there is acute onset of pain and photophobia in a healthy individual who does not have systemic disease.

✓ **When a patient presents with a first occurrence of unilateral acute anterior uveitis and the history and physical examination are unremarkable, there is no need for any diagnostic workup for systemic disease. With recurrent or bilateral acute uveitis, with or without suspicious findings historically or on physical examination, a diagnostic workup should be initiated at the time of the visit or by the ophthalmologist on follow-up. Unless history and physical examination indicate otherwise, this should include a complete blood count (CBC), an erythrocyte sedimentation rate (ESR), a Lyme titer, and a chest radiograph.**

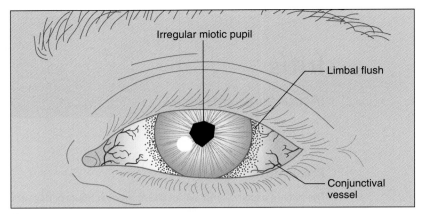

A

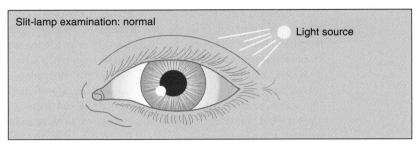

B

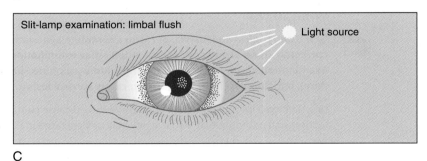

C

Figure 20-1 A, Early signs of iritis. **B,** Normal reflection of pinhole light from the cornea and iris. **C,** Cells and flare from iritis in highlight appear similar to what is seen when a light beam is projected through a dark, smoky room.

When possible, **determine intraocular pressure,** which may be normal or slightly decreased in the acute phase because of decreased aqueous humor production. An elevated pressure should alert you to the possibility of acute glaucoma.

Explain to the patient the potential severity of the problem; this is no routine conjunctivitis, but a process that can develop into blindness. You can reassure him that the prognosis is good with appropriate treatment.

✅ **Arrange for ophthalmologic follow-up within 24 hours, with the ophthalmologist agreeing to the treatment as follows:**

○ **Dilate the pupil and paralyze ciliary accommodation with 1% cyclopentolate (Cyclogyl) drops,** which will relieve the pain of the muscle spasm and keep the iris away from the lens, where miosis and inflammation might cause adhesions (posterior synechiae). **For a more prolonged effect (homatropine is the agent of choice for uveitis), instill a drop of homatropine 5% (Isopto Homatropine) before discharging the patient.**

○ **Suppress the inflammation with topical steroids, such as 1% prednisolone (Inflamase, Pred Forte), 1 drop qid.**

✅ Newer formulations of corticosteroids, such as loteprednol 0.2% (Alrex) or 0.5% (Lotemax), 5 mL, 1 drop qid, may reduce the risk for raising intraocular pressure, but they also appear to be less efficacious in reducing inflammation.

✅ **Prescribe oral pain medicine if necessary, including nonsteroidal anti-inflammatory drugs (NSAIDs) if tolerated.**

✅ **Ensure that the patient is seen the next day for follow-up.**

What Not To Do:

❌ Do not let the patient shrug off his "pink eye" and neglect to obtain follow-up, even if he is feeling better, because of the real possibility of permanent visual impairment.

❌ Do not give antibiotics unless there is evidence of a bacterial infection.

❌ Do not overlook a possible penetrating foreign body as the cause of the inflammation.

❌ Do not assume the diagnosis of acute iritis until other causes of red eye have been considered and ruled out.

❌ Avoid dilating an eye with a shallow anterior chamber and precipitating acute angle–closure glaucoma (Figure 20-2).

Discussion

Physical examination should focus on visual acuity; presence of pain; location of redness; shape, size, and reaction of the pupil; and the intraocular pressure, if it can be obtained safely. If a slit lamp is available, the diagnosis can be made more definitively.

Uveitis is defined as inflammation of one or all parts of the uveal tract. Components of the uveal tract include the iris, the ciliary body, and the choroids. Uveitis may involve all areas of the uveal tract and can be acute or chronic; however, it is the acute form—confined to the iris and anterior chamber

(iritis) or the iris, anterior chamber, and ciliary body (iridocyclitis)—that is most commonly seen in an ED or urgent care facility.

Iritis (or iridocyclitis) represents a potential threat to vision and requires emergency treatment and expert follow-up. The inflammatory process in the anterior eye can opacify the anterior chamber, deform the iris or lens, scar them together, or extend into adjacent structures. Posterior synechiae can potentiate cataracts and glaucoma. Treatment with topical steroids is the mainstay of therapy for acute anterior

(continued)

Discussion continued

uveitis, but this therapy can backfire if the process is caused by an infection (especially herpes keratitis); therefore the slit-lamp examination is especially useful. Topical steroids alone can also contribute to cataract formation as well as the development of glaucoma.

Iritis may have no apparent cause, may be related to recent trauma, or may be associated with an immune reaction. In addition to association with infections such as herpes, Lyme disease, and microbial keratitis, uveitis is found in association with autoimmune disorders, such as ankylosing spondylitis, Reiter syndrome (conjunctivitis, urethritis, and polyarthritis), psoriatic arthritis, and inflammatory bowel disease, as well as in association with underlying malignancies.

Sometimes an intense conjunctivitis or keratitis (see Chapters 14 and 15) may produce some sympathetic limbal flush, which will resolve as the primary process resolves and requires no additional treatment. A more definite, but still mild, iritis may resolve with administration of cycloplegics and may not require steroids. All of these conditions, however, mandate ophthalmologic consultation and follow-up.

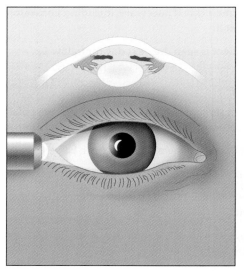

A

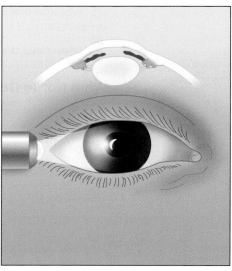

B

Figure 20-2 A, Normal iris. **B,** Domed iris casts a shadow. The shallow anterior chamber is prone to acute angle–closure glaucoma if the pupil is dilated.

Suggested Readings

Au YK, Henkind P: Pain elicited by consensual pupillary reflex: a diagnostic test for acute iritis, *Lancet* 2:1254–1255, 1981.

Patel H, Goldstein D: Pediatric uveitis, *Pediatr Clin North Am* 50:125–136, 2003.

Powdrill S: Ciliary injection: a differential diagnosis for the patient with acute red eye, *JAAPA* 23:50–54, 2010.

Periorbital and Conjunctival Edema

Presentation

The patient is frightened by facial distortion and itching that appeared either spontaneously or up to 24 hours after being bitten by a bug or coming in contact with some irritant. One or both eyes may be involved. The patient may have been rubbing her eyes; however, an allergen or chemical irritant may cause periorbital edema long before a reaction, if any, is evident on the skin of the hand. There may be minimal to marked generalized conjunctival swelling (chemosis), giving the sensation of fullness under the eyelid, but there is little injection (Figure 21-1). In extreme cases, this chemosis may appear as a large, watery bubble ("watch-glass chemosis"), which may be frightening to the patient but is actually quite harmless. Tenderness and pain should be minimal or absent, but pruritus may at times be intense. There should be little or no erythema of the skin and no photophobia or fever. Visual acuity should be normal, there should be no fluorescein uptake over the cornea, and the anterior chamber should be clear.

What To Do:

✓ Inquire about possible causes, including allergies and chemical irritants. Pollen, animal dander, neomycin-containing eye drops, insect protein (a gnat flying into the eye), cosmetics, hair sprays, and contact lens solutions, as well as the usual causes of contact dermatitis, are sources for these reactions (see Chapter 160).

✓ After completing a full eye examination, reassure the patient that this condition is not as serious as it looks.

✓ **Prescribe hydroxyzine (Atarax), 25 to 50 mg q6h, for mild to moderate periorbital swelling and a 3- to 5-day course of steroids (prednisone, 20 to 40 mg qd) for more severe cases.**

✓ Ophthalmic drops are soothing and reduce swelling when the conjunctiva is involved. **Prescribe olopatadine 0.1% (Patanol), ketotifen fumarate 0.025% (Zaditor) [now over the counter], or azelastine hydrochloride 0.05% (Optivar), 1 drop bid. These are H_1 antihistamines and mast-cell stabilizers and should be prescribed for 1 week, then prn thereafter.**

✓ **A short course of a topical steroid agent (loteprednol 0.02% [Alrex] or 0.05% [Lotemax], 1 drop qid) should be reserved for the more severe cases. This may be used for up to 1 week.**

✓ Instruct the patient to apply cool compresses to reduce swelling and discomfort.

✓ Warn the patient about the potential signs of infection.

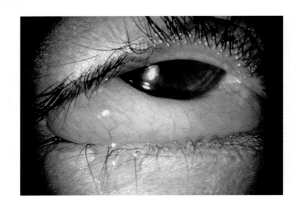

Figure 21-1 Spontaneous swelling and itching are common symptoms of periorbital and conjunctival edema. This represents an allergic conjunctivitis with chemosis secondary to an airborne allergen. (Adapted from Palay DH, Krachmer JH: *Primary Care Ophthalmology*, ed 2. St Louis, 2005, Mosby.)

What Not To Do:

(X) Do not apply heat; heat causes an increase in swelling and pruritus.

(X) Do not confuse this condition with orbital or periorbital cellulitis, which are serious infections manifested by pain, heat, and fever. Orbital cellulitis is more posterior, involves the ocular muscles (which causes painful extraocular movements), and calls for IV antibiotic therapy and hospital admission.

Discussion

The dramatic swelling that often brings a patient to the ED or the family doctor occurs because there is loose connective tissue surrounding the orbit. Fluid quickly accumulates when a local allergic response leads to release of histamine from mast cells, which causes increased capillary permeability, resulting in dramatic eyelid and periorbital swelling. The insect envenomation, allergen, or irritant responsible may actually be located some distance away from the affected eye, on the scalp or face, but the loose periorbital tissue is the first to swell. If the swelling is due to contact dermatitis (e.g., poison ivy) and the allergen is bound to the skin, oral steroids should be continued for 10 to 14 days, until the skin renews itself (see Chapters 160 and 182).

Periorbital Ecchymosis

(Black Eye)

Presentation

The patient has suffered blunt trauma to the eye, most often resulting from a blow inflicted during a fistfight, a fall, a sports injury, or a car accident, and he is alarmed because of the swelling and discoloration. Family or friends may be more concerned than the patient about the appearance of the eye. There may be an associated subconjunctival hemorrhage, but the remainder of the eye examination should be normal, and there should be no palpable bony deformities, diplopia, or subcutaneous emphysema (Figure 22-1).

What To Do:

✅ **Determine, as well as possible, the specific mechanism of injury.** A fist is much less likely than a line-drive baseball to cause serious injury.

✅ **Perform a complete eye examination,** including a bright-light examination to rule out an early hyphema (blood in the anterior chamber) or an abnormal pupil; a funduscopic examination to rule out a retinal detachment, vitreous hemorrhage, or dislocated lens; and a fluorescein stain to rule out corneal abrasion. Best-corrected visual acuity testing should always be performed and, with an uncomplicated injury, is expected to be normal. **All patients having contusions associated with visual loss, severe pain, proptosis, pupil irregularity, new visual "floaters," loss of red reflex, or extensive subconjunctival hemorrhage should be referred to an ophthalmologist immediately.**

✅ **Special attention should be given to ruling out a blow-out fracture of the orbital floor or wall.** Test extraocular eye movements, looking especially for restriction of eye movement or diplopia on upward gaze, and check sensation over the infraorbital nerve distribution. Paresthesia in the distribution of the infraorbital nerve suggests a fracture of the orbital floor. Enophthalmos usually is not observed, although it is part of the classic textbook triad associated with a blow-out fracture. Subcutaneous emphysema is a recognized complication of orbital wall fracture.

 ✅ **Symmetrically palpate the supraorbital and infraorbital rims as well as the zygoma, feeling for the type of deformity that would be encountered with a displaced tripod fracture.** A unilateral deformity will be obvious if your thumbs are fixed in a midline position while you use your index fingers to palpate the patient's facial bones, both left and right, simultaneously (Figure 22-2).

✅ **When there is a substantial mechanism of injury or if there is any clinical suspicion of an underlying fracture, obtain a CT scan of the orbit.** CT scans are more sensitive than plain radiographs and allow visualization of subtle fractures of the orbit and small amounts of orbital air.

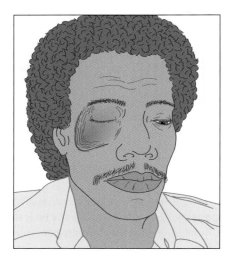

Figure 22-1 Blunt trauma to the eye.

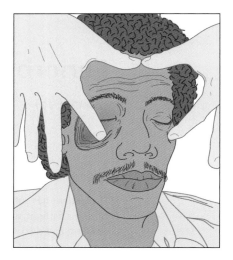

Figure 22-2 Proper hand placement for symmetrically palpating the supraorbital and infraorbital rims.

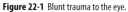

If a significant injury is discovered, consult an ophthalmologist. For diplopia resulting from a blow-out fracture, immediate surgical intervention is not required, and follow-up may be delayed for 7 to 10 days, after the edema has subsided. However, a patient with a hyphema should see an ophthalmologist within 24 hours. The patient should be instructed to rest with his head elevated. A protective metal shield should be placed over the eye, and the patient should be instructed to refrain from taking aspirin or nonsteroidal anti-inflammatory drugs (NSAIDs). Hospital admission is not required.

Consider the possibility of abuse; when suspected, obtain the appropriate consultations and make the appropriate referrals.

When a significant injury has been ruled out, reassure the patient that the swelling will subside within 12 to 24 hours, with or without a cold pack, and that the discoloration will take 1 to 2 weeks to clear. Acetaminophen should be sufficient for analgesia.

Instruct the patient to follow up with an ophthalmologist if there is any problem with vision or if pain develops after the first few days. Rarely, traumatic iritis, retinal tears, or vitreous hemorrhage may develop later, secondary to blunt injury.

With sports-related injuries, recommend protective eyewear made of polycarbonate. Polycarbonate lenses are available in prescription and nonprescription lenses in a sturdy sports frame.

What Not To Do:

Do not order unnecessary radiographs. For minor injuries, if the eye examination is normal and there are no palpable deformities, radiographs and CT scans are unnecessary.

Do not brush off bilateral deep periorbital ecchymoses ("raccoon eyes"), especially if caused by head trauma remote to the eye. This may be the only sign of a basilar skull fracture.

Discussion

Black eyes are usually nothing more than uncomplicated facial contusions. Patients become upset about them because they are so near to the eye, because they produce such noticeable facial disfigurement, and because the patient may seek retaliation against the person who hit him. Nonetheless, serious injury or abuse must always be considered and appropriately ruled out before the patient is discharged.

The extent of ocular damage depends on the size, hardness, and velocity of the blunt object causing the injury. A direct blow to the globe from a blunt object smaller than the eye's orbital opening is more likely to cause injury to internal ocular structures (e.g., iris injury, ruptured globe, hyphema, retinal hemorrhage, retinal detachment, and vitreous hemorrhage). Injury by a blunt object larger than the orbital opening exerts force on the floor of the orbit or the medial wall, which is more likely to result in fractures of the thin bones (e.g., blow-out fracture).

Sudden orbital swelling or inflation immediately after nose blowing is caused by air being forced from a paranasal sinus (most often the maxillary) to the orbit through a fracture, which may act as a one-way valve, increasing the orbital pressure and potentially leading to a compressive optic neuropathy.

Suggested Readings

Cook T: Ocular and periocular injuries from orbital fractures, *J Am Coll Surg* 195:831–834, 2002.

Corrales G, Curreri A: Eye trauma in boxing, *Clin Sports Med* 28:591–607, 2009.

Rodriguez JO, Lavina AM, Agarwal A: Prevention and treatment of common eye injuries in sports, *Am Fam Physician* 67:1481–1488, 2003.

Removal of Dislocated Contact Lens

Presentation

The patient may know that the lens has dislocated into one of the recesses of the conjunctiva and complains only of the loss of refractory correction, or he may have lost track of the lens completely, in which case the eye is a logical place to look first. Pain and blepharospasm suggest a corneal abrasion, perhaps resulting from attempts to remove an absent lens that was thought to be still in place.

What To Do:

⊘ **If pain and blepharospasm are a problem, topically anesthetize the eye.**

⊘ **Pull back the eyelids as if looking for conjunctival foreign bodies, invert the upper lid, and, if necessary,** instill fluorescein dye (a last resort with soft lenses, which absorb the dye tenaciously).

⊘ **If the lens is loose, slide it over the cornea, and let the patient remove it in the usual manner. Irrigation may loosen a dry, stuck lens.**

⊘ **For a more adherent hard lens, use a commercially available suction cup lens remover. Soft lenses may be pinched between the fingers, or a commercially available rubber pincer can be used** (Figure 23-1). **Another option is to take a Morgan irrigation lens attached to a 5-mL syringe filled with 2 mL of normal saline. Flush the Morgan lens with the saline, place the lens over the contact, aspirate on the syringe to produce suction, and remove the Morgan lens and the contact lens together from the conjunctival sac** (Figure 23-2).

⊘ Put the lens in a proper container with sterile saline.

⊘ Complete the eye examination, including best-corrected visual acuity assessment and bright-light and fluorescein examination. Treat any corneal abrasion as explained in Chapter 16.

⊘ Instruct the patient to refrain from wearing the lens until all symptoms have abated for 24 hours and to see his ophthalmologist if there are any problems.

What Not To Do:

ⓧ Do not give up on locating a missing lens too easily. Lost lenses have been excavated from under scar tissue in the conjunctival recesses years after they were first dislocated.

ⓧ Do not omit examination with fluorescein stain for fear of ruining a soft contact lens. The dye may take a long time to elute out, but it is most important to find the dislocated lens.

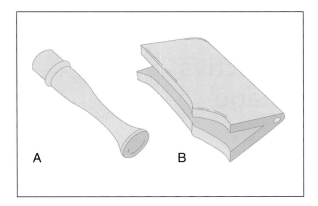

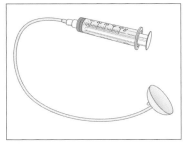

Figure 23-1 A, Rubber suction cup used for extracting hard lenses. **B,** Rubber pincer used for extracting soft lenses.

Figure 23-2 Morgan lens attached to a 5-mL syringe.

Discussion

The deepest recess in the conjunctiva is under the upper lid, but lenses can lodge anywhere; in extremely rare cases, lenses have perforated the conjunctival sac and migrated posterior to the globe. Be sure to evert the upper conjunctival sac by pushing down with a cotton-tipped applicator (see Chapter 17). Often, no lens can be found because the lens was missing from the start, through actual loss or forgetfulness.

Subconjunctival Hemorrhage

Presentation

This condition may occur spontaneously or may follow a minor trauma, coughing episode, vomiting, straining at stool, or heavy exercise. There is no pain or visual loss, but the patient may be frightened by the appearance of her eye and have some sensation of superficial fullness or discomfort. Often a friend or family member is frightened by the appearance and insists that the patient see a physician. This hemorrhage usually appears as a bright red area covering part of the sclera but contained by the conjunctiva (Figure 24-1). It may cover the whole visible globe, sparing only the cornea.

What To Do:

✓ **Look for associated trauma or other signs of a potential bleeding disorder, including overmedication with anticoagulants.** A history of significant trauma or evidence of recurrent hemorrhage or bleeding from other sites (e.g., hematuria, melena, ecchymosis, epistaxis) warrants a careful evaluation for ocular trauma or a bleeding diathesis.

✓ **Perform a complete eye examination** that includes (1) best-corrected visual acuity assessment, (2) conjunctival sac inspection, (3) bright-light examination of the anterior chamber, (4) extraocular movement testing, (5) fluorescein staining, and (6) funduscopic examination.

✓ **Reassure the patient that there is no serious eye damage; explain that the blood may continue to spread, but the redness should resolve in 2 to 3 weeks.**

What Not To Do:

✗ Do not do an extensive hematologic workup for isolated subconjunctival hemorrhage in healthy patients who are not taking anticoagulants.

✗ Do not neglect to warn the patient that the redness may spread during the next 2 days. If the patient is not warned, she may return, alarmed by the "growing hemorrhage."

✗ Do not ignore any significant finding discovered during the history or complete eye examination. Penetrating injuries, lacerations, and ruptured globes also present with subconjunctival hemorrhage, obscuring the damage beneath.

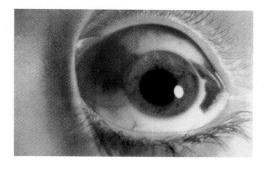

Figure 24-1 A bright red area covering part of the sclera.
(From Marx J, Hockberger R, Walls R: *Rosen's Emergency Medicine,* ed 6. St Louis, 2006, Mosby.)

Discussion

Although this condition looks serious, it is usually caused by a harmless leak in a superficial conjunctival blood vessel resulting from trivial trauma or a sudden Valsalva maneuver or coughing. Patients only need to be reassured that although it appears to be serious, this is actually a minor problem that will resolve spontaneously over time without any eye damage. Recurrent hemorrhage or evidence of other bleeding sites should prompt evaluation for a vasculitis or clotting disorder, with blood tests that should include an erythrocyte sedimentation rate, a complete blood count, platelet count, prothrombin time, partial thromboplastin time, and international normalized ratio (INR).

Suggested Readings

Incorvaia C, Costagliola C, Parmeggiani F: Recurrent episodes of spontaneous subconjunctival hemorrhage in patients with factor XIII Val34Leu mutation, *Am J Ophthalmol* 134:927–929, 2002.

Rajvanshi P, McDonald G: Subconjunctival hemorrhage as a complication of endoscopy, *Gastrointest Endosc* 53:251–253, 2001.

Sodhi PK, Jose R: Subconjunctival hemorrhage: the first presenting clinical feature of idiopathic thrombocytopenic purpura, *Jpn J Ophthalmol* 47:316–318, 2003.

Ultraviolet Keratoconjunctivitis

(Welder's or Tanning Bed Burn)

Presentation

The patient arrives in the ED or clinic complaining of severe, intense, burning eye pain, usually bilateral, beginning 6 to 12 hours after a brief exposure without eye protection to a high-intensity ultraviolet (UV) light source, such as a sunlamp or welder's arc. The eye examination shows conjunctival injection and tearing; fluorescein staining may be normal or may show diffuse superficial uptake (discerned as a punctate keratopathy under slit-lamp examination). The patient may also have first-degree burns on his skin.

What To Do:

✓ **Apply topical anesthetic ophthalmic drops (e.g., proparacaine [Ophthetic], tetracaine [Pontocaine]) once to permit examination.**

✓ Perform a complete eye examination, including best-corrected visual acuity assessment, funduscopy, anterior chamber bright-light examination, fluorescein staining, and conjunctival sac inspection. There may be mild visual impairment.

✓ **Prescribe cold compresses, rest, and analgesics (e.g., oxycodone, hydrocodone, ibuprofen, naproxen) to control pain.**

✓ Provide lubricating ophthalmic ointment (erythromycin 0.5%, 3.5 g, or polymyxin B/bacitracin, 3.5-g tube applied inside the lower lid [1- to 2-cm ribbon] qid), or, if drops are preferred, polymyxin B/trimethoprim (Polytrim), 10 mL, 1 drop q2-6h. However, no evidence supports this practice. **Use of a bland ointment (e.g., Lacri-Lube) may be all that is required to reduce pain.**

✓ **Prescribe analgesic nonsteroidal anti-inflammatory drug (NSAID) eye drops (diclofenac [Voltaren] 0.1%, 5 mL, or ketorolac [Acular] 0.5%, 5 mL, 1 drop qid).**

✓ **Administration of a short-acting cycloplegic drop (e.g., cyclopentolate 1%) may help relieve the pain of reflex ciliary spasm.**

✓ Warn the patient that pain will return when the local anesthetic wears off but that the oral medication and topical NSAID prescribed should help relieve it. Symptoms should resolve after 24 to 36 hours. Medications can be stopped after symptoms resolve.

What Not To Do:

(X) Do not give the patient a topical anesthetic for continued instillation, which can slow healing, blunt protective reflexes, and allow damage to the corneal epithelium.

(X) Do not use the traditional eye patches. These dressings have been found to be of no value and might actually delay reepithelialization. Moreover, some patients find the loss of sight and depth perception (in the case of single-eye patching) to be unacceptable and wearing the patches to be more uncomfortable.

(X) Do not be stingy with pain medications. This is a painful, albeit short-lived, injury.

Discussion

The history of brief exposure to a welder's arc torch or other source of UV light exposure may be difficult to elicit because of the long asymptomatic interval. Longer exposures to lower-intensity UV light sources may resemble a sunburn. Healing should be complete in 12 to 24 hours. If the patient continues to experience discomfort for longer than 48 hours, an ophthalmologist should be consulted.

Other sources of UV phototoxicity can be found in scientific research and manufacturing technology. Several epidemic outbreaks of UV keratoconjunctivitis have been reported as the result of exposure to UV light from broken high-intensity mercury vapor lamps, such as those found in community gymnasiums. **Another common source of UV phototoxicity is the intense sunlight exposure found in water sports and sunny snow conditions (known to the layperson as snow blindness).**

Suggested Reading

Kirschke DL, Jones TF, Smith NM, et al: Photokeratitis and UV-radiation burns associated with damaged metal halide lamps, *Arch Pediatr Adolesc Med* 158:372–376, 2004.

PART 3

Ear, Nose, and Throat Emergencies

■ Philip Buttaravoli ■ Steve Hulsey

Cerumen Impaction

(Earwax Blockage)

26

Presentation

The patient may complain of "wax in the ear," a "stuffed-up" or foreign-body sensation, pain, itching, decreased hearing, tinnitus, or dizziness. Symptoms may be sudden in onset, if the patient put a cotton-tipped applicator down the ear canal or placed something like mineral oil into the ear canal in an attempt to soften the wax. On physical examination, the dark brown, thick, dry, or pasty cerumen, which is perhaps packed down against the eardrum (where it does not occur normally), obscures further visualization of the ear canal and the tympanic membrane.

What To Do:

☑ When excessive cerumen causes pain, hearing loss, vertigo, or disequilibrium, it must be removed. Another indication for removal is when it obscures visualization of a symptomatic tympanic membrane.

☑ Irrigation and manual removal can increase risk of infection in immunocompromised or diabetic patients. Canal trauma can lead to hemorrhage or hematoma in patients on anticoagulants.

☑ There is no clear evidence in the literature that one method of removing cerumen impaction is superior. There are three options for cerumen removal: (1) cerumenolytic agents, (2) irrigation, and (3) manual removal. These methods may be used alone or in combination. There is no literature support for using cerumenolytics on the first visit and attempting removal with irrigation or manual removal on a second visit.

☑ A Cochrane review concluded that no specific cerumenolytic was superior, and none were superior to saline or water, but that most agents led to some clearing of cerumen. Some commercial cerumenolytics can cause side effects, such as local irritation of the canal.

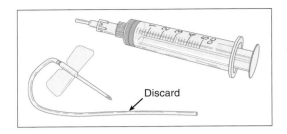

Figure 26-1 Five-mL syringe with short, soft catheter.

Procedure for Irrigation

✓ **First, explain the procedure to the patient. Ask about the possibility of eardrum perforation or myringotomy tubes, which are contraindications to irrigation. Instill warm (body temperature) water into the canal and let it sit for a few minutes.**

✓ Cover the patient with a waterproof drape and have him or her hold a basin or thick towel below the ear.

✓ **Fill a 5-mL syringe with body-temperature water, fit it with a short, soft-tubing catheter** (Figure 26-1). **Aim along the anterosuperior wall of the external canal while pulling the pinna posteriorly to straighten out the canal (do not occlude the whole canal), and squirt quickly to produce a jet lavage. Use a gentler pressure on small children. This irrigation usually needs to be repeated multiple times before the wax is finally flushed out.**

✓ Intermittently reexamine the ear to determine if the wax has been adequately cleared, and if so, grossly test the patient's hearing. If not, continue irrigating.

Procedure for Manual Removal

✓ **If irrigation is contraindicated, unsuccessful, or as an alternative technique, a cerumen spoon (ear curette) may be used.** Do not probe blindly into the canal. Perform manual removal under direct vision using an otoscope with the lens removed or using a headlamp. Warn the patient about potential discomfort or minor bleeding before using the curette. Metal curettes are more likely to cause canal trauma.

✓ **After irrigation or manual removal, a final rinse with an acetic acid otic solution (Vo Sol Otic) may help prevent secondary otitis.** This may be particularly important in older, diabetic, or immunocompromised patients.

✓ Finally, warn the patient that he or she may be required to have this procedure done again someday. In addition, warn him or her never to use swabs in the canal, which may increase the risk of future impaction or damage the ear.

What Not To Do:

ⓧ Do not irrigate an ear in which there is suspected or known tympanic membrane perforation or a myringotomy tube.

ⓧ Do not irrigate the ear with cold (or hot) solutions. This may cause severe vertigo with nausea and vomiting. Do not leave pooled water in the canal, which can lead to external otitis.

Discussion

This irrigation technique almost always works within 5 to 10 squirts. If the irrigation fluid used is at body temperature, it will soften the cerumen just enough to help it flush out as a plug. If the fluid is too hot or cold, it can produce vertigo, nystagmus, nausea, and vomiting.

A conventional syringe fitted with a large-gauge butterfly catheter (discard any needles) or standard IV extension tubing (J-loop)—either one with its tubing cut 1 cm from the hub—seems to work better than the big, chrome-plated syringes manufactured for irrigating ears. An alternative technique is to use a Water-Pik Oral Irrigator (at the lowest pressure setting).

Metal cerumen spoons or ear curettes can be dangerous and painful, especially for children, for whom this irrigation technique has proven more effective in cleaning the ear canal and allowing assessment of the tympanic membrane. If a cerumen spoon is required, use the soft, disposable, plastic variety.

Cerumen acidifies the ear canal with lysozymes, thereby inhibiting bacterial and fungal growth. It is also hydrophobic and repels water from the ear, further protecting it from infection.

Cerumen is produced by the sebaceous glands of the hair follicles in the outer half of the ear canal, and it naturally flows outward along these hairs. One of the problems associated with ear swabs is that they can push wax inward, away from these hairs, and against the eardrum, where the wax can then stick and harden. Cerumen is most likely to become impacted when it is pushed against the eardrum by these cotton-tipped applicators, hairpins, or other objects that people put down their ear canals, and also by hearing aids. Less common causes of cerumen impaction include overproduction of earwax and an abnormally shaped ear canal.

Advise patients that the best method of cleaning the external ear is to wipe the outer opening of the canal with a washcloth covering the patient's finger. Instruct them not to enter the ear canal itself.

Patients may ask about "ear candles" to remove wax. Candling, which involves burning a hollow candle inserted into the ear canal, is reported to create a negative pressure within the auditory canal, removing wax and other debris. On the contrary, though, it has been shown that candling does not create negative pressure or remove cerumen and has been found to cause ear injury. It is therefore not recommended.

Suggested Readings

Burton MJ, Doree CJ: Ear drops for the removal of ear wax (Cochrane Review). *The Cochrane Library,* Issue 2, 2007.

Robbins B: Randomized clinical trial of docusate, triethanolamine polypeptide, and irrigation in cerumen removal in children, *J Pediatr* 145:138–139, 2004.

Robinson AC, Hawke M: The efficacy of ceruminolytics: everything old is new again, *J Otolaryngol* 18:263–267, 1989.

Roland P, Smith TL, Schwartz RL, et al: Clinical practice guideline: cerumen impaction, *Otolaryngol Head Neck Surg* 139:S1–S21, 2008.

Roland PS, Easton DA, Gross RD, et al: Randomized, placebo-controlled evaluation of Cerumenex and Murine earwax removal products, *Arch Otolaryngol Head Neck Surg* 130:1175–1177, 2004.

Singer AJ, Sauris E, Viccellio AW: Ceruminolytic effects of docusate sodium: a randomized, controlled trial, *Ann Emerg Med* 36:228–232, 2000.

Epistaxis

(Nosebleed)

27

Presentation

The patient generally arrives in the ED or urgent care center with active bleeding from his nose, or he may be spitting up blood that is draining into his throat. There may be a report of minor trauma, such as sneezing, nose blowing, or nose picking. On occasion, the hemorrhage has stopped, but the patient is concerned because the bleeding has been recurrent. In rare instances, the bleeding may be brisk requiring resuscitation. Bleeding is most commonly present on the anterior aspect of the nasal septum, within the Kiesselbach area or on the inferior turbinate. Sometimes, especially with posterior epistaxis, a specific bleeding site cannot be determined.

What To Do:

✅ If significant blood loss is suspected, there are abnormal vital signs, or there is continued brisk bleeding, gain vascular access and administer crystalloid IV solution. Provide continuous cardiac monitoring and pulse oximetry. Ensure an adequate airway and oxygenation. Controlling significant hemorrhage should always take precedence over obtaining a detailed history or visualization of the specific bleeding site.

✅ With all nosebleeds, have the patient maintain compression on the nostrils by pinching with a gauze sponge, while all equipment and supplies are being assembled at the bedside. If the patient is unable to pinch the nostrils, a compression device can be made by taping two tongue blades together at one end and placing the other end across the soft portion of the nose. Commercially available nasal clips may also be used.

✅ Use of a headlight with a focused beam will allow you to have both hands free for examination and manipulation while ensuring good lighting and visualization.

✅ Have the patient sit upright (unless hypotensive). If necessary, sedate the patient with a mild tranquilizer, such as lorazepam (Ativan) or midazolam (Versed). Cover the patient and yourself to protect clothing. Follow universal precautions by using gloves and wearing protective eyewear and a surgical mask.

✅ **Prepare 5 mL of a solution to anesthetize and vasoconstrict the nasal mucosa. This can consist of 4% cocaine alone or a 1:1 mixture of 2% tetracaine and a vasoconstrictor such as 1% phenylephrine or 0.05% oxymetazoline.**

✅ **Form two elongated cotton pledgets (using ¼ of a cotton ball for each pledget), and soak them in the prepared solution.**

✓ **Instruct the patient to blow the clots from his nose, and then quickly inspect for a bleeding site using the nasal speculum and Frazier suction tip. Be sure to orient the nasal speculum vertically to avoid pain. Clear out any clots or foreign bodies** (Figure 27-1). The bleeding may be too brisk to indentify a bleeding site at this time, and therefore inspection may be delayed until vasoconstriction has slowed the hemorrhage.

✓ **Insert the medicated cotton pledgets as far back as possible into both nostrils (or one nostril, if the bleeding site is evident) using the bayonet forceps** (Figure 27-2).

✓ Allow the patient to relax with the pledgets in place for approximately 5 to 20 minutes, applying nose clips or having the patient pinch the anterior half of his or her nose.

✓ During this lull, inquire about the patient's history of nosebleeds or other medical problems, the pattern of this nosebleed, which side the bleeding seems to be coming from, use of any blood thinning medications or intranasal products (legal or illegal). Often, no cause for the bleeding can be identified, but when there is diffuse oozing, multiple bleeding sites, or recurrent bleeding, or if the patient is taking an anticoagulant, a hematologic evaluation should be performed (complete blood count [CBC] and international normalized ratio [INR]). Type and cross match the patient if significant blood loss is suspected.

✓ **In most cases, active bleeding will stop with the use of the vasoconstrictor alone. The cotton pledgets can be removed and the nasal cavity inspected using the nasal speculum and head lamp.** Gently inserting the nasal speculum and spreading the naris vertically will permit visualization of most anterior bleeding sources. If bleeding continues, insert another pair of medicated cotton pledgets, and repeat this procedure with more prolonged nasal compression. (Again, commercially available nasal clips can accomplish this for your patient.)

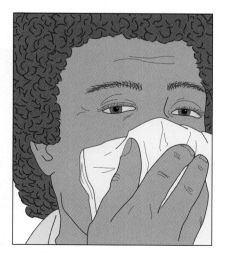

Figure 27-1 The patient must blow the clots from his nose prior to the insertion of medicated cotton pledgets.

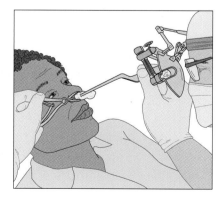

Figure 27-2 Insertion of medicated cotton pledgets.

✓ **Although infrequent, there are times when the patient is hemorrhaging so briskly that the nose must be tamponaded using a balloon catheter or other intervention without inspection, topical anesthesia, or attempted cautery.**

✓ **If the bleeding point can be located and the bleeding is not too brisk, attempt to cauterize a 0.5-cm area of mucosa around the bleeding site with a silver nitrate stick, and then cauterize the site itself.** If there is an individual vessel bleeding rapidly, hold the tip of the cautery stick on top of that vessel with pressure for up to 20 seconds or until the bleeding stops (Figure 27-3).

✓ **If the bleeding stops with cauterization, observe the patient for 15 to 30 minutes.** The cauterized area can then be covered with absorbable gelatin foam (Gelfoam), oxidized cellulose (Surgicel), or antibiotic ointment.

✓ **If the bleeding point cannot be located or if bleeding continues after cauterization, nonabsorbable or absorbable packing may be used.**

✓ **The two most common nonabsorbable packings are the sponge and the balloon.** The sponge is made of hydroxylated polyvinyl acetate, is compressed, and expands into a soft sponge when wet (**Merocel sponge,** Medtronic, Minneapolis, Minn.). **The balloon consists of an inflatable tube covered with a mesh of hemostatic carboxymethyl cellulose hydrocolloid (Rapid Rhino,** Arthro Care, Austin, Tex.).

✓ There are short and long varieties of the sponge and balloon, as well as balloons with anterior and posterior compartments. Longer packs can be used for patients suspected of posterior bleeding.

✓ **To use the sponge, coat it lightly with antibiotic ointment to provide some lubrication, and insert along the floor of the nasal cavity** into the already anesthetized nose. If you are having trouble fitting the sponge, it can be trimmed.

✓ Leave a bit of the sponge exposed to allow easy removal (some sponges have a string attached, which can be taped to the face). **Expand the sponge, after full insertion, with a small amount of saline. (You can also use the vasoconstricting solution for added hemostasis.)**

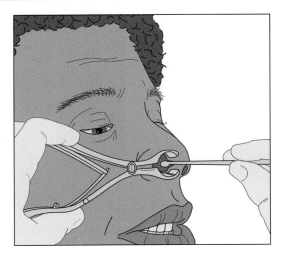

Figure 27-3 Cauterize mucosa with a silver nitrate stick.

✓ **The balloon pack** is less comfortable for the patient after insertion but can exert more local pressure to the bleeding site. **Possibly the most comfortable of these commercially available nasal tampons and the easiest to insert is the gel-coated, balloon-inflated Rapid Rhino nasal pack** (ArthroCare, Austin, Tex.).

✓ **To insert the nasal balloon,** choose the appropriate length and soak the balloon in water for 30 seconds to gel the colloid. **Insert the entire length of the balloon along the floor of the anesthetized nasal cavity.** If you do not insert the entire balloon into the nose, it will work its way out of the nose during inflation. **Inflate the balloon with air until the cuff feels firm or the patient experiences mild discomfort.** The air in the balloon may later be adjusted for patient comfort and control of bleeding. Tape the free end of the pilot cuff to the patient's cheek.

✓ An alternative anterior pack, though difficult and time consuming to place, can be made from up to 6 feet of ½-inch Vaseline gauze. Cover the gauze with antibiotic ointment and insert it with a bayonet forceps. Start with three or four layers in accordion fashion on the floor of the anesthetized nasal cavity, placing the gauze as far posterior as possible, pressing it down with each layer. This method should be reserved for situations in which the sponge, balloon and absorbable packing have failed or are not available (Figure 27-4).

✓ An alternative to using nonabsorbable packing is to use absorbable packing material. The advantages are that there is nothing to remove later, and there is more patient comfort. The disadvantages are a higher initial cost and lack of tamponading effect.

✓ Choices of absorbable packing material include oxidized cellulose (Surgicel, Johnson & Johnson, New Brunswick, N.J.), purified bovine collagen (Gelfoam, Pfizer, New York, N.Y.), both of which come in sheets and can be pressed against the bleeding site. Porcine gelatin (Surgiflo, Johnson & Johnson, New Brunswick, N.J.) and bovine gelatin–human thrombin (Floseal, Baxter, Deerfield, Ill.) are materials that can be mixed into a paste and applied to the nasal mucosa.

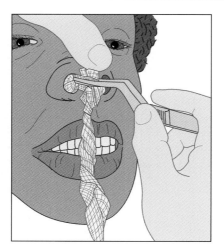 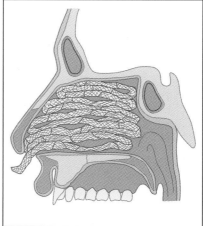

Figure 27-4 Packing the nasal cavity with ribbon gauze.

✓ If the hemorrhage does not stop after placing adequate packing anteriorly, unilateral or bilateral posterior packing or nasal balloons should be inserted. A lubricated double-balloon device (Epistat [Medtronic Xomed, Jacksonville, Fla.], Nasostat [Sparta, Pleasanton, Calif.]) (Figure 27-5) is passed into the affected nostril in that same way as the anterior balloon. The posterior balloon is inflated first with the manufacturer's recommended volume of normal saline, and the anterior portion of the device is withdrawn so that the posterior balloon seats snugly in the posterior nasal cavity to tamponade any bleeding. The anterior balloon is then inflated with the recommended volume of saline to prevent the posterior balloon from becoming unseated and possibly obstructing the airway.

✓ **If a commercial posterior balloon device is not available,** a 12-Fr Foley catheter may be used. Insert the catheter into the affected nasal cavity until the balloon is well into the posterior nasal cavity. Inflate the balloon with 5 to 7 mL of saline. Pull the partially inflated balloon anteriorly until it is snug against the posterior turbinates. Finish inflating the balloon with another 5 to 7 mL saline. If there is pain or displacement of the soft palate, remove some of the saline from the balloon. Secure the Foley anteriorly by placing an umbilical clamp over the catheter as it exits the nose. Make sure to pad the nose tissue with gauze to prevent pressure necrosis. An anterior Vaseline gauze pack may then be inserted.

✓ **If the bleeding cannot be controlled with all of the above measures, YOU NEED HELP!** Contact an ear-nose-throat (ENT) specialist or transfer the patient to a hospital with ENT care. The specialist may use electrocautery, transpalatal injection of vasoconstrictors, endoscopic cautery, surgical ligation, or embolization procedures. While the patient is awaiting specialist care, you must ensure hemodynamic stability using IV fluids or blood, if needed.

✓ **If on the other hand, as will most commonly occur, the bleeding has stopped with your interventions, observe the patient for 15 to 30 minutes. If there is no further bleeding from the nares or from the posterior pharynx, the patient may be discharged.** If the hemorrhage is suspected to have been large, determine that the patient is not symptomatically orthostatic, and check hemoglobin and hematocrit before discharging.

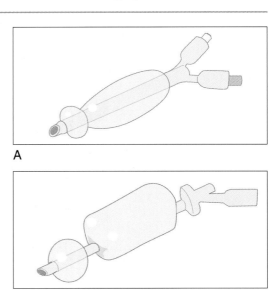

A

B

Figure 27-5 Double-balloon devices. **A,** Epistat. **B,** Nasostat.

✅ **If a nonabsorbable pack was inserted, the patient should be sent home on a regimen of antibiotics for 4 to 5 days to help prevent a secondary sinusitis and reduce the risk of toxic shock syndrome.** Choices of antibiotics include cephalexin (Keflex), amoxicillin/clavulanate (Augmentin), clindamycin (Cleocin), and trimethoprim/sulfamethoxazole (Bactrim).

✅ **The nonabsorbable packs should be removed in 2 to 5 days.** Packs for minor bleeds may be removed early; bleeds that are difficult to control or in patients on anticoagulants should be kept in the full 5 days.

✅ **Warn the patient about not sneezing with his mouth closed, bending over, straining, or picking his nose. Provide printed instructions regarding home care.**

✅ **Patients with simple nosebleeds can be referred to their primary care doctor for removal of the packing or for a recheck. If this is a recurrent bleeding episode, or there is concern for a nasal abnormality causing the bleeding, the patient should be referred to an ENT specialist.**

✅ If pain is a problem, Tylenol should be suggested and aspirin and other nonsteroidals avoided. Prescribe hydrocodone bitartrate/acetaminophen (Vicodin) if you think the pain will not be controlled with Tylenol.

✅ If the patient returns with mild oozing of blood from around an anterior pack, you may be able to stop the bleeding without removing the pack. Try injecting a vasoconstrictor directly into the sponge (not into the patient), or adding air to a nasal balloon pack.

✅ **When removing a compressed cellulose sponge pack, soften it with 1 to 2 mL of water or saline and wait 5 minutes,** thereby reducing trauma, pain, and the incidence of rebleeding.

What Not To Do:

Because of the nasopulmonary reflex, arterial oxygen pressure will drop about 15 mm Hg after the nose is packed. **Do not send home elderly patients or those with cardiac problems or chronic obstructive pulmonary disease (COPD)** without first checking their oxygen saturation. With packing in place, these patients are at risk for desaturation and may need admission.

❌ Do not waste time trying to locate a bleeding site if brisk bleeding is obscuring your vision in spite of vigorous suctioning. Have the patient blow out any clots and insert the medicated cotton pledgets immediately or go directly to anterior packing.

❌ Do not order routine clotting studies unless there is persistent or recurrent bleeding, use of anticoagulants or other evidence of an underlying bleeding disorder.

❌ Do not cauterize or place a painful device in the nose before providing adequate topical anesthesia unless rapid hemorrhaging requires it.

❌ Do not use an inadequate amount of gauze packing, if this method is chosen. It will only serve as a plug in the anterior nares rather than as a hemostatic pack.

❌ Do not discharge a patient as soon as the bleeding stops, but keep him for 15 to 30 minutes more. Look behind the uvula. If there is active blood flow, the bleeding has not been controlled adequately. Posterior epistaxis typically stops and starts cyclically and may not be recognized until all of the aforementioned treatments have failed.

Discussion

Epistaxis (Greek for nosebleed) affects people in all age groups but is most common and more troublesome in the elderly. Children tend to bleed secondary to nose picking; adolescents bleed secondary to facial trauma associated with athletic activity or fighting. Epistaxis in the middle-age patient is more often the harbinger of neoplastic disease. Nosebleeds in the elderly are generally the result of underlying vascular fragility in combination with blood-thinning medications.

Nosebleeds are more common in winter, no doubt reflecting the low, ambient humidity indoors and outdoors and the increased incidence of upper respiratory tract infections. In most cases, anterior bleeding is clinically obvious. In contrast, posterior bleeding may be asymptomatic or may present insidiously as nausea, hematemesis, anemia, hemoptysis, or melena.

Causes of epistaxis are numerous; dry nasal mucosa, nose picking, and vascular fragility are the most common causes, but others include trauma, foreign bodies, blood dyscrasias, nasal or sinus neoplasm or infection, septal deformity or perforation, atrophic rhinitis, hereditary hemorrhagic telangiectasis, and angiofibroma. Epistaxis that results from minor blunt trauma in healthy individuals rarely requires any intervention and will spontaneously subside with head elevation alone and avoidance of any nasal manipulation. (Always inspect for a possible septal hematoma.)

High blood pressure may make epistaxis more difficult to control; however, although it is often present with epistaxis, it is rarely the sole precipitating cause. Specific antihypertensive therapy is rarely required and should be avoided in the setting of significant hemorrhage.

Use of medications, especially aspirin, nonsteroidal anti-inflammatory drugs (NSAIDs), warfarin (Coumadin), heparin, enoxaparin (Lovenox), ticlopidine (Ticlid), dipyridamole (Persantine), and clopidogrel (Plavix), not only predisposes patients to epistaxis but also makes treatment more difficult.

Hereditary hemorrhagic telangiectasia is the most common systemic disorder of the vascular system that affects the nasal mucosa. Onset of symptoms is usually at puberty and progressively worsens with age.

Blood dyscrasias can be found in patients with lymphoproliferative disorders, immunodeficiency, systemic disease, or in the alcoholic patient. Thrombocytopenia can lead to spontaneous mucous membrane bleeding, with platelet counts of $10,000/mm^3$ to $20,000/mm^3$.

Platelet deficiency can be the result of chemotherapy agents, malignancies, hypersplenism, disseminated intravascular coagulopathy (DIC), drugs, and many other disorders. Platelet dysfunction can be seen in liver failure, kidney failure, and vitamin C deficiency as well as in patients taking aspirin and NSAIDs.

von Willebrand disease is the most common clotting factor abnormality that can result in frequent, recurring nosebleeds. Factor VIII deficiency (hemophilia A) and factor IX deficiency (hemophilia B) are also common primary coagulopathies.

One study of chronic nosebleeds in children showed that a third of these patients can be expected to have a coagulation disorder. The single best predictor of coagulopathy is family history.

Because of the nasopulmonary reflex, arterial oxygen pressure will drop about 15 mm Hg after the nose is packed, which can be troublesome in a patient with heart or lung disease and often requires hospitalization and supplemental oxygen.

Tumors or other serious diseases are infrequent causes of epistaxis. However, it is prudent for all patients who present with nosebleeds to have a complete nasopharyngeal examination by an ENT specialist in follow-up.

Suggested Readings

Gifford T, Orlandi R: Epistaxis, *Otolaryngol Clin N Am* 41:525–536, 2008.

Herkner H, Havel C, Müllner M, et al: Active epistaxis at ED presentation is associated with arterial hypertension, *Am J Emerg Med* 20:92–95, 2002.

Herkner H, Laggner A, Müllner M, et al: Hypertension in patients presenting with epistaxis, *Ann Emerg Med* 35:126–130, 2000.

Kucik CJ, Clenney T: Management of epistaxis, *Am Fam Physician* 71:305–311, 2005.

Manes P: Evaluating and managing the patient with nosebleeds, *Med Clin N Am* 94:903–912, 2010.

Pringle MB, Beasley P, Brightwell AP: The use of Merocel nasal packs in the treatment of epistaxis, *J Laryngol Otol* 110:543–546, 1996.

Roberts JR, Hedges JR, editors: *Clinical procedures in emergency medicine,* ed 3, Philadelphia, 1998, WB Saunders.

Sandoval C, Dong S, Visintainer P, et al: Clinical and laboratory features of 178 children with recurrent epistaxis, *J Pediatr Hematol Oncol* 24:47–49, 2002.

Singer AJ, Blanda M, Cronin K, et al: Comparison of nasal tampons for the treatment of epistaxis in the emergency department: a randomized controlled trial, *Ann Emerg Med* 45:134–139, 2005.

Thaha MA: Routine coagulation screening in the management of emergency admission for epistaxis: is it necessary? *J Laryngol Otol* 114:38–40, 2000.

Vaiman M, Martinovich U, Eviatar E: Fibrin glue in initial treatment of epistaxis in hereditary haemorrhagic telangiectasis, *Blood Coagul Fibrinolysis* 15:359–363, 2004.

Vaiman M, Segal S, Eviatar E: Fibrin glue: treatment for epistaxis, *Rhinology* 40:88–91, 2002.

Viducich RA, Blanda MP, Gerson LW: Posterior epistaxis: clinical features and acute complications, *Ann Emerg Med* 25:592–596, 1995.

Foreign Body, Ear

Presentation

Sometimes, a young child admits to putting something, such as a bead, a small stone, folded paper, or a bean, in his ear, or an adult may witness the act. At times, the history is not revealed, and the child simply presents with a purulent discharge, pain, bleeding, or hearing loss. An adult might have a pencil eraser or "Q-tip" come off in the ear canal while trying to remove earwax. Most dramatically, a panic-stricken patient arrives complaining of a "bug crawling around" in his ear. There may be severe pain if the object or insect has scratched or stung the canal or tympanic membrane.

What To Do:

✓ Use an otoscope to inspect the ear canal while pulling up and back on the pinna to help straighten the ear canal, thereby providing a better view.

✓ **If there is a live insect in the patient's ear, begin by filling the canal with a liquid to kill the insect. Mineral oil, 2% lidocaine (Xylocaine), or benzocaine/antipyrine (Auralgan) works well.** (Sterile 2% lidocaine would be most appropriate if there is a myringotomy tube in place or any other opening of the tympanic membrane [TM].) Instruct the patient to lie on his or her side, and then drip the liquid into the canal while pulling on the pinna and pushing on the tragus to remove air bubbles (Figure 28-1).

✓ **With a foreign body (FB) that is not too tightly wedged in the canal, and if tympanic membrane perforation or a myringotomy tube is not present, water irrigation is a very effective removal technique.** This can be accomplished with a syringe and scalp vein needle that has been cut short (Figure 28-2). Tap water at body temperature can be used to flush out the foreign body. Direct the stream along the wall of the canal and around the object, thereby flushing it out (Figure 28-3).

✓ **If a hard or spherical object remains tightly wedged in the canal, attempt to roll the foreign body out by getting behind it with a right-angle nerve hook, ear curette, or wire loop. (Alternatively, a Calgiswab can be bent into a right-angle hook and used in the same way.)** Use of these tools should be done under direct vision through an ear speculum. The patient's head should be firmly stabilized to prevent sudden movements. Whenever an instrument is used in the ear canal, warn the patient or parents beforehand that there may be a small amount of bleeding and pain because of the delicate lining of the ear canal (Figures 28-4 and 28-5).

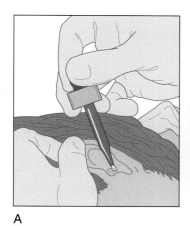
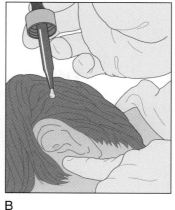

A   B

Figure 28-1 Drop mineral oil into the ear canal and squeeze out any air bubbles to kill any bug or insect in the ear.

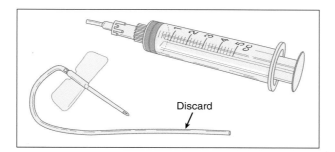

Discard

Figure 28-2 A short, soft catheter on a 5-mL syringe is safe and very effective for irrigating a loose foreign body out of the ear canal. *Note*: Discard the tubing after use.

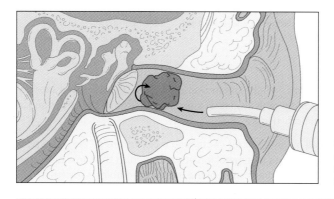

Figure 28-3 When irrigating a foreign body out of the ear, direct the stream of warm water toward an opening between the foreign body and the canal wall.

✓ **An alternative removal technique is to take a drop or two of cyanoacrylate (Super Glue, Dermabond), and place it on the end of the wooden shaft of a cotton swab. (Use the cotton end for irregular FBs.)** Then hold the wet glue against the foreign object until it hardens (approximately 30 seconds to a minute), and extract the foreign body from the canal.

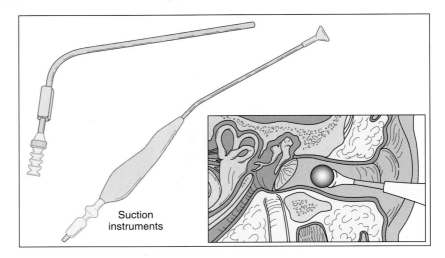

Figure 28-4 Various suction tips can be used to pull out a loose foreign body within the ear canal.

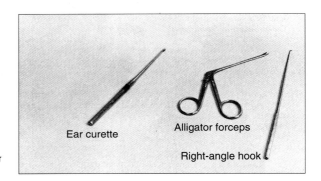

Figure 28-5 The right-angle hook is best suited for removing hard objects from the ear, whereas alligator forceps work best on soft objects.

Ear curette

Alligator forceps

Right-angle hook

If the object is light and moves easily, you can attempt to suction it out with a standard metal suction tip or (if available) a specialized flexible tip, by making an effective vacuum seal on the foreign body (Figure 28-6).

A small magnet or iron-containing metallic foreign body can be removed by touching a pacemaker magnet to a metal forceps and then, at the same time, touching the forceps to the foreign body, withdrawing all of the magnetized objects together.

Alligator forceps are good for grasping soft objects, such as cotton, paper, and certain insects.

There should be no delay in removing a foreign body in a canal when there is an obvious infection or when the foreign body is a disk or button battery. Do not irrigate or instill liquids into the ear canal, because on contact with moist tissue, the alkaline battery is capable of producing a liquefactive necrosis extending into deep tissues within hours. Be careful not to crush the battery. After removal of a battery, irrigate the canal to remove any alkali residue.

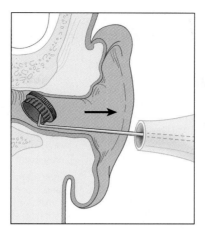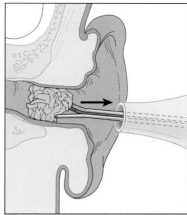

Figure 28-6 The various metal instruments that can be used to remove foreign bodies from an ear canal.

✓ **At any time, if a child becomes uncooperative, especially when using metal instruments, use procedural sedation as described in Appendix E.** Ketamine sedation appears to have a positive effect on the success rate of foreign body removal in children.

✓ **If the foreign body is tightly wedged in the canal and you cannot remove it, consult an ear-nose-throat (ENT) specialist.** If after removal, there is evidence of infection or perforation of the tympanic membrane, referral to an ENT specialist is also appropriate.

What Not To Do:

✗ Do not use a rigid instrument to remove an object from an uncooperative patient's ear without procedural sedation (see Appendix E). An unexpected movement might cause serious injury to the middle ear.

✗ Do not attempt to remove a large bug or insect without killing it first. They tend to be wily, evasive, and well-equipped for fighting in tunnels. In the heat of battle, the patient can become terrorized by the noise and pain.

✗ Do not attempt to irrigate a canal filled with a bean or other object that may swell with hydration. Irrigation with isopropyl alcohol will not cause swelling.

✗ Do not attempt to remove a large or hard object with bayonet or similar forceps. The bony canal will slowly close the forceps as they are advanced, and the object will be pushed farther into the canal. Alligator forceps are designed for use in the canal, but even they will push a large, hard foreign body farther into the ear.

Discussion

The external ear canal narrows at the junction of the cartilaginous segment and the bony segment, and then at the isthmus of the bony segment. Most foreign bodies are found at these two narrow loci. The cross-section of the canal is elliptic; therefore the physician can usually find an opening around a circular foreign object in which to place an instrument or for water to get behind when irrigating.

Some physicians do not recommend the use of a Waterpik for irrigation, because the high-pressure water jet has the potential for rupturing the tympanic membrane.

When the foreign body within the ear canal is a cyanoacrylate adhesive (Super Glue, Dermabond),

it can be removed more easily after 48 hours when desquamation occurs. If the glue adheres to the tympanic membrane, an ENT referral may be most prudent.

On telephone consultation, patients can be instructed to use cooking or baby oil, or ethyl or isopropyl alcohol, instilled into the ear canal, to kill an insect at home. It can then be removed at a subsequent office visit.

Complications of foreign body removal from the ear canal include trauma to the skin of the canal, canal hematoma, otitis externa, tympanic membrane perforation, or ossicular dislocations and, rarely, facial nerve palsy.

Suggested Readings

Antonelli PJ, Ahmadi A, Prevatt A: Insecticidal activity of common reagents for insect foreign bodies of the ear, *Laryngoscope* 111:15–20, 2001.

Bressler K, Shelton C: Ear foreign-body removal: a review of 98 consecutive cases, *Laryngoscope* 103:367–370, 1993.

Brown L, Denmark TK, Wittlake WA, et al: Procedural sedation use in the ED: management of pediatric ear and nose foreign bodies, *Am J Emerg Med* 22:310–314, 2004.

Brunskill AJ, Satterthwaite K: Foreign bodies, *Ann Emerg Med* 24:757, 1994.

Heim S, Maughan K: Foreign bodies in the ear, nose, and throat, *Am Fam Physician* 76:1185–1189, 2007.

Leffler S, Cherney P, Tandberg D: Chemical immobilization and killing of intra-aural roaches: an in-vitro comparative study, *Ann Emerg Med* 22:1795–1798, 1993.

McLaughlin R, Ullah R, Heylings D: Comparative prospective study of foreign body removal from external auditory canals of cadavers with right angle hook or cyanoacrylate glue, *Emerg Med J* 19:43–45, 2002.

O'Toole K, Paris PM, Stewart RD, et al: Removing cockroaches from the auditory canal: controlled trial, *N Engl J Med* 312:1197, 1985.

Schulze SL, Kerschner J, Beste D: Pediatric external auditory canal foreign bodies: a review of 698 cases, *Otolaryngol Head Neck Surg* 127:73–78, 2002.

Skinner DW, Chui P: The hazard of button-sized batteries as foreign bodies in the nose and ear, *J Laryngol Otol* 100:1315–1319, 1986.

Foreign Body, Nose

Presentation

Most commonly, a child may admit to his parents that he has inserted something into his nose or someone observed him doing this. Sometimes, however, the history is obscure, and the child presents with local pain; a purulent, unilateral nasal discharge; epistaxis; a nasal voice change; or foul breath. The most commonly encountered nasal foreign bodies are beans, peanuts or other foodstuffs, beads, toy parts, pebbles, paper wads, and eraser tips. Most foreign bodies (FBs) can be seen on direct visualization using a nasal or otoscope speculum. These objects usually lodge on the floor of the nose just below the inferior turbinate or immediately anterior to the middle turbinate.

What To Do:

✓ There are various techniques available for removal of nasal FBs. These include suction, air pressure, ear curettes, curved hooks, alligator forceps, bayonet forceps, balloon catheters, irrigation and glue. The choice will depend of the shape, makeup, and depth of the FB as well as the age and cooperation of the patient.

✓ Before attempting removal techniques in an uncooperative patient, consider use of sedation. Be aware of the higher risk of aspiration of the FB when sedation is used.

✓ Because of the potential for spraying of body fluids from the nose, always practice universal precautions and wear appropriate eye and splash protection.

✓ Before any of the removal procedures, explain in detail what you are about to do to the patient and or parent. Advise that the procedure will be a little uncomfortable, may cause some bleeding and that there is a small risk the FB body could be aspirated. Have advanced airway equipment in the room, including a McGill forceps.

✓ **After initial inspection with a nasal speculum and bright light, suction out any discharge, and insert a small cotton pledget soaked in 4% cocaine or alternatively a 1:1 mixture of phenylephrine (Neo-Synephrine) and tetracaine (Pontocaine), which will shrink the nasal mucosa and provide topical anesthesia.**

✓ Be careful to avoid pushing the FB posteriorly when inserting the pledget. Remove the pledget after 5 to 10 minutes. If you cannot safely insert a pledget, drip or spray the same solution into the nose.

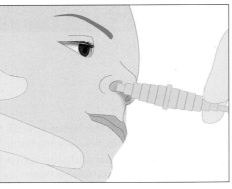

Figure 29-1 Beamsley Blaster technique.

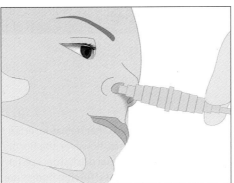

Figure 29-2 Remove foreign bodies with bayonet forceps, right-angle hook, Katz extractor, or alligator forceps.

✓ **After vasoconstriction, some FBs can be blown out of the nose by a cooperative patient or suctioned out, using Frazier tip suction. Further suctioning success may be obtained by placing a piece of soft plastic tubing over the end of the suction tip. Placing water-soluble lubrication on the end of this tubing will also help achieve a better vacuum seal.**

✓ **In infants and children who will not blow their nose on command, a parent may blow a sharp puff of air into the child's mouth while holding the opposite nostril closed.** A tight-fitting Ambu mask over the mouth and a bag-valve device is an alternative means for producing the positive pressure required to force the FB out of the nose.

✓ **Another air pressure technique is to place oxygen tubing, running at 10 to 15 L/min, into the contralateral nostril to the FB (Beamsley Blaster)** (Figure 29-1). This technique, along with the other positive-pressure ones, reduces the risk for forcing the FB posteriorly, thereby reducing the risk of aspiration. These methods may not work as well for FBs that have produced edema or infection.

✓ Alligator forceps may be used to remove cloth, cotton, or paper FBs. Pebbles, beans, and other hard FBs are most easily grasped using bayonet forceps.

✓ **If an object cannot be grasped, it may be rolled out of the nose by using an ear curette or right-angle ear hook to get behind it. After sliding the tool past the FB, twist until it catches the FB and then pull anteriorly. A soft-tipped hook can be made by bending the tip of a metal Calgiswab to a 90-degree angle.**

✓ **A less intrusive approach is to bypass the FB with a lubricated 5-Fogarty biliary balloon probe or small Foley catheter, inflating the balloon with 1 mL of air and gently pulling the catheter and FB out of the nose** (Figure 29-2). A commercially available FB remover, the Katz Extractor (InHealth Technologies, Carpinteria, Calif.), may offer an easier balloon catheter technique, but not necessarily be the least expensive device.

✓ **One can also try the glue technique. After drying the exposed surface of the FB, a drop of cyanoacrylate (Super Glue, Dermabond) can be applied to the cotton end of a regular cotton-tipped applicator, which is then touched to the FB, held there for 1 minute, and used to pull the attached FB out of the nose.**

✓ **Button batteries can cause serious local damage through liquefaction necrosis and should be removed quickly.** Button batteries of all sizes have a distinctive double contour on radiographs; therefore, with a high index of suspicion, radiographs can help assist with an uncertain diagnosis.

✓ **Earring magnets** that become stuck together across the nasal septum must also be removed as soon as possible because of the risk for pressure necrosis leading to septal perforation. Ideally, the septum should be lubricated. Using the balloon catheter technique bilaterally, both magnets should be removed simultaneously to prevent a lone magnet from dropping back into the nasopharynx and being aspirated.

✓ Bleeding, which will often occur during FB removal, can usually be stopped by reinsertion of a cotton pledget soaked in the topical solution used prior to the procedure.

✓ **Small, particulate material may be irrigated from the nasal cavity by insertion of an irrigation syringe into one nostril while the patient sits up, leans forward, and repeats "eng" as you irrigate. The "eng" sound will close the back of the throat during irrigation. Slowly flush the debris out the opposite nostril** (Figure 29-3).

✓ After FB removal, inspect the nasal cavity again, checking for additional objects. Always look in the other nostril, and it may be wise to check the ears.

✓ If a foreign body cannot be located, but is suspected, or if attempts to remove a visible FB have failed, an ear-nose-throat (ENT) consultation is warranted.

What Not To Do:

✗ Do not inspect the nasal cavity by opening the nasal speculum in the horizontal plane. The speculum should be opened in the vertical plane and not pressed against the nasal septum.

✗ Do not ignore unilateral nasal discharge in a child. It must be assumed to be caused by the presence of a FB until proven otherwise.

✗ Do not push a FB down the back of a patient's throat by attempting to remove a large, solid, smooth FB with alligator or bayonet forceps. It may be aspirated into the trachea.

✗ Do not attempt to remove a FB from the nose without first using a topical anesthetic and vasoconstrictor.

✗ Do not leave a button battery in the nose or magnets across the nasal tissue. These objects can cause quick tissue necrosis and must be removed as soon as possible. If you suspect a button battery in the nose but cannot find it, consider a radiograph for confirmation.

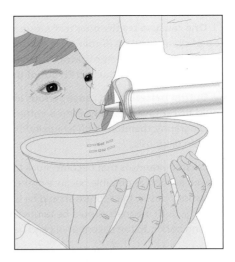

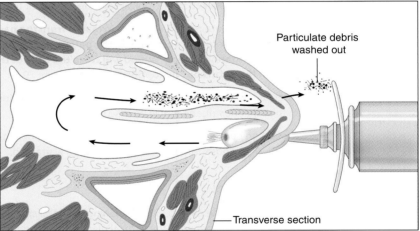

Figure 29-3 Nasal irrigation.

Discussion

The symptoms produced by a nasal FB will vary with its size, composition, location, and the length of time it has been present. Most nasal foreign bodies can be removed easily and safely by emergency clinicians. There is generally no need for emergent intervention. There is time available to provide procedural sedation, if necessary, as well as to assemble all of the supplies and instruments necessary to help ensure the success of this procedure. Because nasal FBs have different sizes, shapes, and locations within the nares, the emergency clinician should be familiar with several removal techniques.

The mucous membrane lining the nasal cavity allows the tactical advantages of vasoconstriction and topical anesthesia. The patient who has unsuccessfully attempted to blow an FB out of his nose may be successful after instillation of an anesthetic vasoconstrictive solution.

Discussion continued

If a patient has swallowed a foreign body that was pushed back into the nasopharynx, this is usually harmless, and the patient and parents can be reassured (see Chapter 72). If the object has been aspirated into the tracheobronchial tree, it may produce coughing and wheezing, and bronchoscopy under anesthesia is required for retrieval.

Animate foreign bodies (myiasis) of the nose are common in warm tropical climates and are associated with poor hygiene. The most common of all infestations is the fly maggot. These maggots can cause varying degrees of inflammatory reaction, including local tissue destruction, fetid discharge, and pain. The symptoms tend to be bilateral. Inspection after suctioning may reveal constant motion and masses of different worms. These worms are firmly attached and difficult to extract. An ENT consultation is required.

Suggested Readings

Backlin SA: Positive-pressure technique for nasal foreign body retrieval in children, *Ann Emerg Med* 25:554–555, 1995.

Brown L, Denmark TK, Wittlake WA, et al: Procedural sedation use in the ED: management of pediatric ear and nose foreign bodies, *Am J Emerg Med* 22:310–314, 2004.

Heim S, Maughan K: Foreign bodies in the ear, nose, and throat, *Am Fam Physician* 76:1185–1189, 2007.

Lin VY, Daniel SJ, Papsin BC: Button batteries in the ear, nose, and upper aerodigestive tract, *Int J Pediatr Otorhinolaryngol* 68:473–479, 2004.

Navitsky RC, Beamsley A, McLaughlin S: Nasal positive-pressure technique for nasal foreign body removal in children, *Am J Emerg Med* 20:103–104, 2002.

Ngo A, Ng KC, Sim TP: Otorhinolaryngeal foreign bodies in children presenting to the emergency department, *Singapore Med J* 46:172–178, 2005.

Noorily AD, Noorily SH, Otto RA: Cocaine, lidocaine, tetracaine: which is best for topical nasal anesthesia? *Anesth Analg* 81:724–727, 1995.

Foreign Body, Throat

Presentation

The patient is usually convinced that there is a foreign body (FB) stuck in his throat, because he recently swallowed something, such as a fish or chicken bone, and can still feel a "sensation" in the throat, especially (perhaps painfully) when swallowing. He may be able to localize the FB sensation to precisely above the thyroid cartilage (which implies an FB in the hypopharynx that may be visible), or he may only vaguely localize the FB sensation to the suprasternal notch (which could imply an FB anywhere in the esophagus).

Those with dentures, especially full dentures, are more likely to swallow a bone because of reduced sensitivity and inability to chew properly. Fish bones, which are usually long, are commonly caught in the oropharynx, particularly at the region of the tonsils and the tonsillar pillars. At these regions, fish bones can usually be grasped and extracted, as long as they can be visualized.

An FB lodged in the tracheobronchial tree usually stimulates coughing and wheezing. Obstruction of the esophagus produces drooling and causes the patient to spit up whatever fluid is swallowed. Any infant who refuses to eat or who has trouble handling buccal secretions should be evaluated for an FB.

What To Do:

✓ FBs in the throat can lead to partial or complete airway obstruction. If complete or near-complete obstruction is present, immediate intervention with direct visualization using a laryngoscope and removal with an instrument, such as a McGill forceps, is indicated.

✓ If the patient can cough and verbalize and is not in significant distress, but appears to have a partial airway obstruction, it is better to place him in the most comfortable position, provide supplemental oxygen, and call in a multidisciplinary team, including an ear-nose-throat (ENT) specialist and anesthesiologist, to perform removal in the operating room.

✓ If the patient has no evidence of airway obstruction, but only the sensation of an FB in the throat, establish exactly what was swallowed, when, and the progression of symptoms. Patients can accurately tell if an FB is on the right or left side.

✓ Examine the anterior neck for tenderness, masses, or subcutaneous emphysema (suggests perforation). Percuss and ascultate the chest. An FB sensation in the throat can be produced by a pneumothorax, pneumomediastinum, or esophageal disease, all of which may show up on a chest radiograph.

✅ **Inspect the hypopharynx using a good light or headlamp mirror and tongue depressor, paying special attention to the base of the tongue, tonsils, and vallecula, where foreign bodies are likely to lodge.** Place the tongue depressor at the middle third of the tongue and press firmly downward to give good exposure without making the patient gag. You can also maximize visibility and exposure, without making the patient gag, by holding the tongue out (use a washcloth or 4 × 4-inch gauze for traction), taking care not to lacerate the frenulum of the tongue on the lower incisors, and then instruct the patient to raise his soft palate by "panting like a dog."

✅ This may be accomplished without topical anesthesia, but **if the patient tends to gag, the soft palate and posterior pharynx can be anesthetized by spraying with Cetacaine, Hurricane, or 10% lidocaine, or by having the patient gargle with lidocaine (viscous Xylocaine) diluted 1:1 with water.** Some patients may continue to gag even with the topical anesthesia.

✅ **If the object can be seen directly, carefully grasp and remove it with bayonet or curved forceps** (Figure 30-1). Objects at the base of the tongue or in the hypopharynx may require a mirror or indirect laryngoscope for visualization. Small fish bones are frequently difficult to see. They may be overlooked entirely except for their tips, or they may only appear to be threads of mucus. Fiberoptic nasopharyngoscopy, usually performed by an ENT specialist, is preferred, when available.

✅ **If the symptoms are mild and a foreign body cannot be visualized, test the patient's ability to swallow, first using a small cup of water and then a small piece of soft bread. If the patient can swallow liquids and solids, they may be safely discharged.** They should be instructed to seek follow-up care as soon as possible if the pain worsens, fever develops, or if breathing or swallowing is difficult. They should be seen by an ENT specialist or return to the ED or clinic if they are not better in 2 days.

✅ If the pain or FB sensation is moderate to severe, or if there is bleeding or fever, and the FB cannot be visualized, **CT scanning is the test of choice to diagnose FBs that may not be easily seen on plain radiography.**

✅ **If an FB is discovered on CT, but cannot be visualized on physical examination, obtain an ENT consultation.** Consider an ENT consultation even if the CT is negative and you are still very suspicious of an FB, because CT scanning is associated with a small percentage of false-negative examinations.

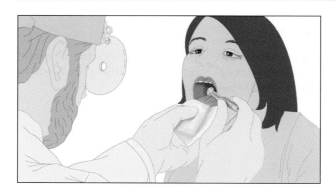

Figure 30-1 Carefully grasp and remove any foreign body that can be seen in the throat.

✅ **If the ENT evaluation of the hypopharynx is negative and the pain is persistent, (especially pain localized to the suprasternal notch), consider that the FB may be in the esophagus and consult a gastroenterologist.**

✅ **An impacted button battery represents a true emergency and requires rapid removal, because leaking alkali produces liquefactive necrosis.** Button batteries of all sizes have a distinctive double contour on radiography.

✅ A tablet composed of irritating medicine, if swallowed without adequate liquid, may stick to the mucosa of the pharynx or esophagus and cause an irritating ulcer with a foreign body sensation.

✅ When coughing or wheezing suggests aspiration of an FB into the tracheobronchial tree, a chest radiograph with expiratory views should be obtained. If these are negative, a chest CT scan should be performed. If a foreign body is found in the pulmonary tree, a pulmonary specialist consultation should be obtained.

✅ **If CT studies are normal, careful inspection does not reveal an FB, and the patient is afebrile with only mild discomfort, he may be sent home. Reassure him that a scratch on the mucosa can produce a sensation that the FB is still there. Also inform him that if the symptoms worsen or fail to resolve in 2 days, he may need further endoscopic studies to look for a hidden problem.**

What Not To Do:

❌ Do not assume that a foreign body is absent just because the pain disappears after a local anesthetic is applied.

❌ Do not order plain radiographs or a barium swallow to evaluate suspected fish bone impactions. The results are unreliable or misleading, and with barium, subsequent examinations of a coated esophagus are made more difficult.

❌ Do not attempt to remove a strand of mucus that mimics the appearance of a delicate fish bone; when you grab it and it behaves like a thread of mucus, it *is* a thread of mucus.

❌ Do not reassure the patient that the presence of a foreign body has been ruled out if it has not been completely ruled out. Explain that although you think there is a low probability that a foreign body exists, careful follow-up needs to be obtained if symptoms do not resolve.

❌ Do not overlook the possibility of preexisting pathologic conditions discovered incidentally during swallowing.

❌ Do not attempt to remove a foreign body from the throat blindly by using a finger or instrument, because the object may be pushed farther down into the airway and obstruct it or may cause damage to surrounding structures.

Discussion

Most of these patients have a sharp pricking-pain sensation on swallowing, but no specific sign or symptom will consistently rule in or rule out a retained bone.

During swallowing, as the base of the tongue pushes a bolus of food posteriorly, any sharp object hidden in that bolus may become embedded in the tonsil, the tonsillar pillar, the pharyngeal wall, or the tongue base itself. Symptomatic patients are convinced that they have a bone stuck in the throat, although in most patients no bone is found and the symptoms resolve spontaneously. In two studies, approximately 25% of the patients with symptoms of an embedded fish bone had no demonstrable pathologic findings, and their symptoms resolved in 48 hours. Only 20% actually had an embedded fish bone, and most of these were easily identified and removed on the initial visit.

All patients who complain of a foreign body in the throat should be taken seriously. Even relatively smooth or rounded objects that remain impacted in the esophagus have the potential to cause serious problems. A fish bone can perforate the esophagus in only a few days, and chicken bones carry even greater risk for serious injuries, such as a neck abscess, mediastinitis, and an esophageal carotid artery fistula.

The sensation of a lump in the throat, unrelated to swallowing food or drink, may be globus hystericus, which is related to cricopharyngeal spasm and anxiety. The initial workup is the same as that for any foreign body sensation in the throat.

Suggested Readings

D'Agostino J: Pediatric airway nightmares, *Emerg Med Clin N Am* 28:119–126, 2010.

Digoy P: Diagnosis and management of upper aerodigestive tract foreign bodies, *Otolaryngol Clin N Am* 41:485–496, 2008.

Haliloglu M, Ciftci AO, Oto A, et al: CT virtual bronchoscopy in the evaluation of children with suspected foreign body aspiration, *Eur J Rad* 48:188–192, 2003.

Heim S, Maughan K: Foreign bodies in the ear, nose, and throat, *Am Fam Physician* 76:1185–1189, 2007.

Lue AJ, Fang WD, Manolidis S: Use of plain radiography and computed tomography to identify fish bone foreign bodies, *Otolaryngol Head Neck* 123:435–438, 2000.

Laryngotracheobronchitis

(Croup)

Presentation

A child, most often between the ages of 3 months and 3 years (peak incidence 1 to 2 years, but can be seen up to 6 years), arrives with a characteristic "barking" cough that sounds very much like a trained seal. There is usually a prodrome of low-grade fever and symptoms of a mild upper respiratory infection. The barking cough tends to occur at night, with symptoms worsening on the second night.

The parents are usually alarmed by the sound of the cough, but the child is usually in no distress and appears nontoxic. The throat is clear and normal in appearance, and there may be varying degrees of stridor (predominately inspiratory) or retractions of the accessory chest muscles. Wheezes may be present on chest auscultation.

What To Do:

✅ **Perform a complete examination, with attention directed to the child's throat.** Although now rare in children, acute epiglottitis should be eliminated as a possibility by noting a healthy-appearing supraglottic region with absence of high fever, sudden onset, drooling, and laryngeal tenderness. At times, a normal-appearing epiglottis can be seen (Figure 31-1). There should also be no worsening of the child's condition when lying supine.

✅ Make the child as comfortable as possible, and avoid agitating the child with unnecessary procedures and examinations.

✅ **When available, monitor O_2 saturation with pulse oximetry or CO_2 level with capnometry.** Humidified air or cool-mist therapy may be used, but neither has been proven to be effective.

✅ Humidified oxygen should be administered to any patient with O_2 saturation less than 95%.

✅ **When the patient is showing any signs of distress, it is most appropriate to give a combination of nebulized racemic epinephrine and corticosteroid. Administer racemic epinephrine (Vaponefrin), 2.25% solution diluted in 3 mL of normal saline nebulized q4-6h (0.25 mL for infants younger than 6 months and weighing less than 20 kg; 0.5 mL for a child older than 6 months and weighing more than 20 kg). If no racemic epinephrine is available or if an inexpensive alternative is desired, 0.1 to 0.3 mL (0.01 mL/kg) of regular epinephrine (L-epinephrine) 1:1000 may be substituted for a racemic epinephrine and diluted in 3 mL of normal saline for nebulization.**

✅ An adjunct to treatment with epinephrine is the use of a continuous 70/30 helium and oxygen mixture (heliox) administered through a facemask.

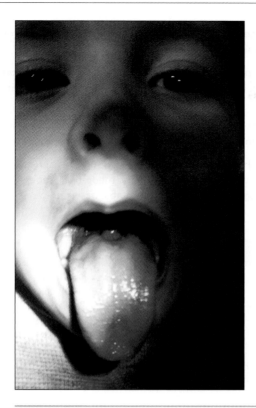

Figure 31-1 A normal-appearing epiglottis.

✓ **Give dexamethasone (Decadron) elixir, 0.5 mg/5 mL, 0.6 mg/kg PO once (maximum dose 10 mg). If the patient is vomiting or unable or unwilling to take dexamethasone PO, it can be given IM as an injectable suspension, 8 mg/mL, or even nebulized in 3 mL of normal saline.**

✓ Observe the patient for signs of improvement or worsening over a period of 2 to 3 hours.

✓ **In general, admit all children with a toxic appearance, inability to keep down fluids with unreliable parents, or with no improvement with epinephrine administration or if worsening occurs at 2 to 3 hours following initial epinephrine administration.**

✓ For the mildest cases of croup, it is reasonable to treat with supportive measures alone. Adding one dose of dexamethasone to prevent worsening of symptoms later is also a justifiable addition. For moderate cases, and certainly for more severe cases, adding racemic or L-epinephrine is required to bring about the most rapid and effective relief.

What Not To Do:

✗ Do not routinely obtain soft tissue neck radiographs. These should be reserved for atypical presentations when more severe disease (i.e., epiglottitis or abscess) or a foreign body is suspected. In croup, an anteroposterior soft tissue neck radiograph may show subglottic narrowing, which is called the steeple or pencil-point sign.

(X) Do not separate the child with croup from the parents unless unavoidable. Any separation may increase anxiety and make breathing more difficult.

(X) Do not routinely obtain blood work. The resultant pain and agitation will do more to worsen symptoms than is justified by the small potential for any useful information that might be obtained.

(X) Do not prescribe antibiotics. This is a viral illness, and unless there is an alternative source of bacterial infection, antibiotic use will be ineffective and is inappropriate.

(X) Do not discharge the patient prior to at least 2 hours of observation after racemic epinephrine has been administered. Although the theoretical rebound phenomenon has been discredited, patients might return to an unacceptable baseline.

Discussion

Laryngotracheobronchitis, or viral croup, is the most common infectious cause of acute upper airway obstruction in children. Most cases occur in the late fall and early spring. Parainfluenza viruses cause most cases of croup. Other responsible viruses include influenza A and B, adenovirus, respiratory syncytial virus, and rhinovirus. The viral infection leads to inflammation of the nasopharynx and subglottic area of the upper airway.

Stridor in children with croup occurs from the mucosal and submucosal edema of this subglottic portion of the airway, which is the narrowest portion of a child's upper airway.

Not all children with stridor have croup. Excluding other causes, especially foreign body aspirations or ingestions, is crucial.

In contrast with viral croup, a nonseasonal allergic variant, known as spasmodic croup, may occur. This disorder typically has an abrupt onset, with no preceding upper respiratory infection and no fever. Spasmodic croup usually resolves quickly with exposure to humidified air, only to recur for the next few days.

When high fever, toxicity, and worsening respiratory distress develop after several days of crouplike illness, consider the possibility of the more serious but uncommon diagnosis of bacterial tracheitis.

Suggested Readings

Everard M: Acute bronchiolitis and croup, *Pediatr Clin North Am* 56:119–133, 2009.

Geelhoed GC: Sixteen years of croup in a western Australian teaching hospital: effects of routine steroid treatment, *Ann Emerg Med* 28:621–626, 1996.

Geelhoed GC, Macdonald WBG: Oral dexamethasone in the treatment of croup, *Pediatr Pulmonol* 20:362–368, 1995.

Johnson DW, Jacobson S, Edney PC, et al: A comparison of nebulized budesonide, intramuscular dexamethasone, and placebo for moderately severe croup, *N Engl J Med* 339:498–503, 1998.

Klassen TP, Craig WR, Moher D, et al: Nebulized budesonide and oral dexamethasone for treatment of croup, *JAMA* 279:1629–1632, 1998.

Klassen TP, Watters LK, Feldman ME, et al: The efficacy of nebulized budesonide in dexamethasone-treated outpatients with croup, *Pediatrics* 97:463–466, 1996.

Kunkel NC, Baker MD: Use of racemic epinephrine, dexamethasone, and mist in the outpatient management of croup, *Pediatr Emerg Care* 12:156–159, 1996.

Luria JW, Gonzalez-del Rey, Digiulio GA, et al: Effectiveness of oral or nebulized dexamethasone for children with mild croup, *Arch Pediatr Adolesc Med* 155:1340–1345, 2001.

McDonogh AJ: The use of steroids and nebulized adrenaline in the treatment of viral croup over a seven-year period at a district hospital, *Anaesth Intens Care* 22:175–178, 1994.

Neto GM, Kentab O, Klassen TP, et al: A randomized controlled trial of mist in the acute treatment of moderate croup, *Acad Emerg Med* 9:873–879, 2002.

Prendergast M, Jones JS, Hartman D: Racemic epinephrine in the treatment of laryngotracheitis: can we identify children for outpatient therapy? *Am J Emerg Med* 12:613–616, 1994.

Rittichier KK, Ledwith CA: Outpatient treatment of moderate croup with dexamethasone: intramuscular versus oral dosing, *Pediatrics* 106:1344–1348, 2000.

Rizos JD, DiGravio BE, Sehl MJ, et al: The disposition of children with croup treated with racemic epinephrine and dexamethasone in the emergency department, *J Emerg Med* 16:535–539, 1998.

Rowe BH: Corticosteroid treatment for acute croup, *Ann Emerg Med* 40:353–355, 2002.

Sobol SE, Zapata S: Epiglottitis and croup, *Otolaryngol Clin North Am* 41:551–566, 2008.

Weber JE, Chudnosfsky CR, Younger JG, et al: A randomized comparison of helium-oxygen mixture (heliox) and racemic epinephrine for the treatment of moderate to severe croup, *Pediatrics* 107:E96, 2001.

Mononucleosis

(Glandular Fever)

Presentation

The patient is usually an adolescent or a young adult between the ages of 15 and 25 who complains of several days of fever, malaise, lassitude, myalgias, and anorexia, culminating in a severe sore throat. The physical examination is remarkable for generalized lymphadenopathy, including the anterior and posterior cervical chains, and huge tonsils, perhaps meeting in the midline and covered with a dirty-looking exudate. There may also be palatal petechiae and swelling, periorbital edema (an early finding), splenomegaly (often not evident clinically), hepatomegaly, and, less commonly, a diffuse maculopapular rash or jaundice (more common in patients who are older than 40 years of age).

What To Do:

✓ **Perform a complete physical examination, looking for signs of other ailments and the rare complications of airway obstruction, encephalitis, hemolytic anemia, thrombocytopenic purpura, myocarditis, pericarditis, hepatitis, and rupture of the spleen.**

✓ **Send blood samples to be tested. Obtain a differential white cell count (looking for atypical lymphocytes) and a heterophil or monospot test.** Either of these tests, along with the generalized lymphadenopathy, will help confirm the diagnosis of mononucleosis. Atypical lymphocytes are less specific, because they are present in several viral infections.

✓ **Culture the throat or obtain a rapid *Streptococcus* test.** Patients with mononucleosis harbor group A *Streptococcus* and require penicillin with approximately the same frequency as anyone else with a sore throat.

✓ **When the diagnosis has been confirmed, warn the patient that the period of convalescence for mononucleosis is longer than that for most other viral illnesses (typically 2 to 4 weeks, occasionally more) and that he should seek attention if he experiences lightheadedness, abdominal or shoulder pain, or any other sign of the rare complications mentioned earlier.**

✓ **Symptomatic treatment is the mainstay of care. This includes adequate hydration, analgesics, antipyretics, and adequate rest. Bed rest should not be enforced, and the patient's energy level should guide activity.**

✓ **These patients should be withdrawn from contact or collision sports or any strenuous athletic activity for 4 weeks after the onset of symptoms.**

✅ Patients should be warned that, in a few cases, fatigue, myalgias, and an excessive need for sleep may persist for several months.

✅ Corticosteroids, acyclovir, and antihistamines are not recommended for routine treatment. If there is impending airway obstruction caused by tonsillar swelling, hospitalization is necessary, along with IV fluids, humidified air, and corticosteroids.

✅ **Dexamethasone, in doses up to 10 mg, has been used to treat impending airway obstruction caused by markedly enlarged "kissing tonsils."**

✅ Arrange for medical follow-up.

What Not To Do:

❌ Do not routinely begin therapy with penicillin for the pharyngitis, and certainly do not use ampicillin. In a patient with mononucleosis, ampicillin will produce an uncomfortable maculopapular rash (in 95% to 100% of cases), which incidentally does not imply that the patient is allergic to ampicillin.

❌ Do not routinely evaluate the degree of splenomegaly with ultrasonography to determine when an athlete may return to contact sports. There is little evidence to support its routine use.

❌ Do not unnecessarily frighten the patient about possible splenic rupture. If the spleen is clinically enlarged, he should avoid contact sports, but spontaneous ruptures are rare, usually occurring within 3 weeks of onset of symptoms, with an incidence of 0.1% to 0.5% (spontaneous or after mild trauma).

Discussion

Infectious mononucleosis is caused by Epstein-Barr virus (EBV). EBV is a tumorigenic herpes virus that is ubiquitous in the adult population. EBV establishes a harmless lifelong infection in almost everyone worldwide and rarely causes disease unless the host–virus balance is upset. After an acute infection, a patient can shed and transmit virus through saliva for up to 3 months, and persistent virus shedding has been reported for up to 18 months. The incubation period for infectious mononucleosis is 4 to 8 weeks. In most cases, primary infection occurs subclinically during childhood, often spread between family members by salivary contact. It is commonly assumed that those who remain uninfected throughout childhood generally become infected as adolescents through kissing (thus it is called the kissing disease). It is when the primary infection is delayed until adolescence or beyond that clinical illness is caused by an intense immunopathologic reaction. Similar

mononucleosis-like illnesses can be caused by other infectious agents, including cytomegalovirus, streptococcal infection, adenovirus, and *Toxoplasma gondii*. Infectious mononucleosis should be suspected in patients who are 10 to 30 years of age who present with sore throat, fever, and lymphadenopathy.

Atypical lymphocytosis of at least 20%, or atypical lymphocytosis of at least 10% plus lymphocytosis of at least 50%, strongly supports the diagnosis, as does a positive heterophil antibody test. False-negative results of monospot tests are relatively common early in the course of infection. Patients with negative results may have another infection, such as the examples given earlier. Although reasonably specific, positive tests are also seen in other conditions, including human immunodeficiency virus (HIV), lymphoma, systemic lupus, rubella, parvovirus, and other viral infections.

(continued)

Discussion continued

Mild thrombocytopenia, elevations of hepatocellular enzymes, microscopic hematuria, and proteinuria are often present but self-limiting abnormalities.

Although there are some cases of prolonged fatigue after infectious mononucleosis, there is no convincing evidence that EBV infection or recurrence of EBV infection is linked to a chronic fatigue syndrome. For previously healthy adolescents and young adults, infectious mononucleosis is a self-limited illness. Many have symptoms for less than 1 week, and most have returned to their usual state of health within a month.

Because concern for splenic rupture is the major consideration in limiting athletes from returning to strenuous sports, interestingly, more than half of the cases of splenic rupture related to infectious mononucleosis had no clearly notable previous trauma.

Suggested Readings

Auwaeter PG: Infectious mononucleosis: return to play, *Clin Sports Med* 23:485–497, 2004.

Bass MH: Periorbital edema as the initial sign of infectious mononucleosis, *J Pediatr* 45:204–205, 1954.

Ebell MH: Epstein-Barr virus infectious mononucleosis, *Am Fam Physician* 70:1279–1287, 2004.

Ellen Rimsza ME, Kirk GM: Common medical problems of the college student, *Pediatr Clin North Am* 52:9–24, 2005.

Macsween KF, Crawford DH: Epstein-Barr virus—recent advances, *Lancet Infect Dis* 3:131–140, 2003.

Mandell GL, Bennett JE, Dolin R, editors: *Mandell, Douglas, and Bennett's principles and practice of infectious diseases*, ed 7, Philadelphia, 2009, Churchill Livingstone.

Nasal Fracture

(Broken Nose)

Presentation

After a direct blow to the nose from a fight, fall, sports injury, or motor vehicle crash, the patient usually arrives at the ED or clinic concerned that his nose is broken. There is usually minimal continued hemorrhage. There may be tender ecchymotic swelling over the nasal bones or the anterior maxillary spine, and inspection and palpation may or may not disclose a nasal deformity. Alcohol consumption is an important contributing factor in many cases.

What To Do:

✓ To help determine the nature and extent of the injury, obtain a history of the mechanism of injury. A direct frontal blow can cause fractured bones to telescope posteriorly. A laterally directed injury can cause a depression on the side of the impact, often with a corresponding outward displacement on the opposite side of the nose.

✓ Additional history should include information regarding previous surgeries and injuries, as well as a subjective assessment of baseline nasal function and appearance.

✓ Examine the patient for any associated injuries (e.g., blow-out fractures, zygoma fractures, mandible fractures, and eye injuries). A general screening exam should include special attention to the cervical spine.

✓ A deformity of the nose usually will be evident when a nasal fracture has occurred. Edema and ecchymosis of the nose and periorbital structures ordinarily will be present. **Palpation of the nasal structures should be done to elicit crepitus, indentation, or irregularity of the nasal bone. Bony crepitus and nasal segment mobility are both diagnostic for nasal fracture.**

✓ If a facial or mandibular fracture is suspected, assessment with a CT scan is indicated. Uncommon findings, such as a cerebrospinal fluid leak posing as clear rhinorrhea, subcutaneous emphysema, mental status changes, new malocclusion, or limited extraocular movement, also require CT evaluation and subspecialty consultation.

✓ **An internal nasal examination should be conducted with good lighting, suction, and vasoconstriction with topical anesthesia. A nasal speculum and a headlamp will improve visualization.** Clots should be removed with Frazier tip suction and cotton-tipped applicators. With swelling and/or continued bleeding, instill cotton pledgets soaked in 4% cocaine or, alternatively, 2% tetracaine (Pontocaine) or 4% lidocaine (Xylocaine) mixed 1:1 with 1% phenylephrine (Neo-Synephrine) or oxymetazoline (Afrin).

✓ After removing these pledgets, **inspect for nasal airway patency, ongoing epistaxis, septal deformities, and, most important, septal hematomas, which may appear as slightly white or purple areas of fluctuance lying on one or both sides of the nasal septum.** Bimanual palpation of the septum with cotton-tipped applicators helps to differentiate hematoma, which tends to be more compressible from tissue edema. Areas of increased mobility are suggestive of septal fracture. If bleeding continues, treat this epistaxis as described in Chapter 27.

✓ When an uncomplicated nasal fracture is suspected, plain radiography rarely is indicated. In fact, because of poor sensitivity and specificity, plain radiographs may serve only to confuse the clinical picture.

✓ **Explain to the patient that for minor injuries, radiographic examinations are not routinely used. They expose him to unnecessary radiation and usually are not helpful because all therapeutic decisions are made on the basis of the physical examination.** If there is a fracture, but it is stable and in a good position clinically, the nose need not be reset. Conversely, a broken and displaced cartilage may obstruct breathing and require operation but may never show up on the film.

✓ **Patients with suspected or possible nondisplaced fractures and no nasal deformity should be sent home with analgesics, cold packs, and instructions to keep the head elevated and avoid contact sports and related activities for 6 weeks.** When nasal deformity cannot be visualized or palpated because of marked swelling, have the patient seen in follow-up within 3 to 5 days when the swelling has subsided.

✓ **Patients with suspected displaced fractures, nasal deformity, or both should be referred for otolaryngologic or plastic surgery consultation to discuss immediate or delayed reduction. Patients can be instructed that reduction is more accurate after the swelling subsides and that there is no greater difficulty if it is done between the 5th and 10th day after the injury.**

✓ **Septal hematomas should be drained immediately** to prevent septal necrosis and the development of a saddle-nose deformity. If improperly managed, a septal hematoma may still result in this disastrous outcome; therefore otolaryngologic consultation is advisable.

✓ **A minor isolated fracture of the anterior nasal spine** (in the columella of the nose) does not necessitate restriction of activities. Such fractures hurt only when the patient smiles.

✓ **A laceration over a nasal fracture should probably be closed with antibiotic prophylaxis, such as cephalexin (Keflex), 500 mg qid, or cefadroxil (Duricef), 500 mg bid for 3 to 5 days.**

✓ Physical abuse should be considered in children and women and should be appropriately ruled out and managed.

What Not To Do:

✗ Do not focus solely on the obviously traumatized nose. Consider cervical spine injury as well as other facial injuries and other remote trauma.

✗ Do not automatically obtain radiographs of every injured nose. Patients may expect this because it used to be standard practice (and they are still regularly obtained), but routine films have turned out to be mostly useless.

Ⓧ When a deformity is apparent, do not assume that a normal radiographic examination means that there is no fracture. Radiographs can often be inaccurate in determining the presence and nature of a nasal fracture. Rely on the clinical assessment. If there is swelling, arrange for reexamination in 3 to 5 days when the swelling has subsided, and then look for subtle deformities.

Ⓧ Do not pack an injured nose that does not continue to bleed. Packing is generally unnecessary and will only add to the patient's discomfort.

Discussion

The nose is easily exposed to trauma, because it is the most prominent and anterior feature of the face. The nose is supported by cartilage, anteriorly and inferiorly, and by bone, posteriorly and superiorly. Although most of the nasal structures are cartilaginous, the nasal bones usually are fractured in an injury.

Fights and sports injuries account for most nasal fractures in adults, followed by falls and vehicle crashes.

The two most common indications for reducing a nasal fracture are an unacceptable appearance and the patient's inability to breathe through the nose. Regardless of radiographic findings, if neither breathing nor cosmesis is a concern, it is not necessary to reduce the fracture.

Nasal fractures are uncommon in young children, because their noses are composed of mostly pliable cartilage. For this reason, radiographic examination has even less accuracy than in an adult.

It should be noted, however, that with significant trauma to the face, children may develop devastating growth retardation of the nose and midface. Refer all young children with posttraumatic nasal asymmetry, bony crepitus, epistaxis, periorbital ecchymosis, significant edema, or overlying skin lacerations to an otolaryngologist for reexamination within 2 to 4 days. Because of faster rates of bone healing, realignment in children should ideally be performed within 4 days of injury.

Suspect septal hematoma when a patient's nasal airway is completely occluded. Within 48 to 72 hours, a hematoma can compromise the blood supply to the cartilage and cause irreversible damage.

Suggested Readings

Altreuter RW: Facial form and function: film versus physical examination, *Ann Emerg Med* 15:240–244, 1986.

Kucik CJ, Clenney T, Phelan J: Management of acute nasal fractures, *Am Fam Physician* 70:1315–1320, 2004.

Li S, Papsin B, Brown DH: Value of nasal radiographs in nasal trauma management, *J Otolaryngol* 25:162–164, 1996.

Otitis Externa (Swimmer's Ear), Acute

Presentation

In acute otitis externa (AOE), the patient complains of ear pain, which is always uncomfortable and sometimes unbearable, often accompanied by drainage and a blocked sensation, decreased hearing, and sometimes by fever. When the condition is mild or chronic, there may be itching rather than pain. Pulling on the auricle or pushing on the tragus of the ear classically causes increased pain (Figure 34-1). The tissue lining of the canal may be swollen, and, in severe cases, the swelling can extend into the soft tissue surrounding the ear. Tender erythematous swelling or an underlying furuncle may be present, and it may be pointing or draining.

The canal may be erythematous and dry, or it may be covered with fuzzy cotton-like grayish or black fungal plaques (wet newspaper appearance). Most often, the canal lining is moist and covered with purulent drainage and debris, and cerumen is characteristically absent. The canal may be so swollen that it is difficult or impossible to view the tympanic membrane (TM), which, when visible, often looks dull.

A pruritic vesiculopapular eruption in the canal is most consistent with an allergic reaction to a topical agent (often neomycin) (see Chapter 160).

What To Do:

✓ Determine if the patient has had tympanostomy tubes or a history of chronic suppurative otitis media with recurrent ear drainage; if so, he will probably have an open TM.

✓ **Meticulous and repeated clearing of the canal is the cornerstone of treatment.** Irrigation can be very effective in cleaning out the canal, using a 1:1 dilution of 3% hydrogen peroxide (if the TM is intact). Other cleaning methods include suction, cotton swabs, and ear curettes.

✓ **Inspect the ear for the presence of a foreign body.**

✓ **Incise and drain any furuncle that is pointing or fluctuant.**

✓ **If the ear canal is too narrow to allow medication to flow freely, insert a wick. The best wick is the Pope ear wick (Merocel Corporation, Mystic, Conn.),** which is about 1 × 10 mm of compressed cellulose; it is thin enough to slip into an occluded canal but expands when wet. If this wick is not available, try using alligator forceps to insert a 1-cm strip of ¼-inch plain gauze or a twisted wisp of cotton that may be obtained from a cotton ball or the end of a cotton-tipped applicator. (This method is more painful.) Advance the wick cautiously to avoid damaging the middle-ear structures or puncturing the TM. **After the wick is inserted, water must be kept out**

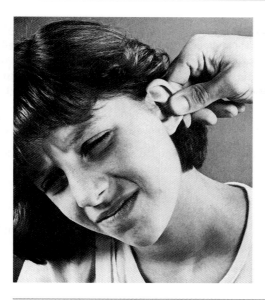

Figure 34-1 Pulling on the ear causes increased pain.

of the ear, and the patient must be instructed to use soft wax earplugs while showering. Wicks may be replaced every 1 to 3 days if the symptoms persist.

✓ **Studies have shown no difference in cure rate between topical antibiotics, topical antiseptics and topical antibiotic/steroid preparations, but that these agents are significantly superior to placebo.**

✓ Acidifying solutions, such as acetic acid, work by lowering canal pH, thus inhibiting fungal and bacterial growth. The addition of a steroid to the antimicrobial or acidifying solution has been shown to decrease time to symptom relief. A typical acidifying solution is 2% acetic acid. (Add 2 parts of 5% acetic acid [or household vinegar] to 3 parts water and you will render 2% acetic acid.) *Pseudomonas aeruginosa* and *Staphylococcus* are the most common bacteria responsible for AOE.

✓ **There are several antibiotic choices, but ciprofloxacin and ofloxacin have the advantage of good bacterial coverage, bid dosing, and ability to use if the TM is perforated. Suggestions are ciprofloxacin-hydrocortisone (Cipro HC Otic) otic suspension, 10 mL, 3 drops in ear(s) bid × 7 days, or ofloxacin (Floxin Otic), 10 mL, 0.3%, 5 drops in ear(s) bid × 7 days. If the TM is intact, other choices are gentamycin (Garamycin) or tobramycin (Tobrex) ophthalmic solution 0.3%, 5 mL, 4 to 6 drops in ear(s) qid × 7 days.**

✓ Fungal infections cause about 10% of AOE. Patients usually complain more of itching than pain, and edema of the canal is often milder than in bacterial infection. Fungal filaments can sometimes be seen, and *Candida* typically reveals sebaceous-like material in the canal. Topical antifungals, such as acetic acid and aluminum acetate (Domeboro Otic), 60 mL, 4 to 6 drops in ear(s) q2-3h × 7 days; acetic acid (VoSol Otic) 15%, 30 mL, 5 drops in ear(s) tid to qid (VoSol HC Otic adds hydrocortisone 1% [only generic is available]); or clotrimazole (Lotrimin) 10 mL, 1% solution, 4 to 6 drops in ear(s) bid × 7 days, may be prescribed. **Acetic acid preparations should not be used if an open TM is known or suspected to be present because of theoretical ototoxicity.**

⊘ **For moderate to severe pain and soft tissue swelling or other signs of cellulitis, prescribe an appropriate analgesic. Systemic antibiotics are indicated in patients with diabetes mellitus, immunodeficiency, history of radiation to the ear, or when infection has spread beyond the external ear canal, or if the canal cannot be adequately cleared to allow the topical agent to work. Systemic antibiotics include levofloxacin (Levaquin), 500 mg qd × 10 days, or ciprofloxacin (Cipro) 500 mg bid × 10 days.**

⊘ Provide follow-up in 2 to 3 days to remove a wick and any remaining debris from the ear canal.

⊘ When administering ear drops without a wick, instruct the patient to lie on her side for 20 minutes after instilling, to maximize medication exposure.

What Not To Do:

⊗ Do not routinely culture ear drainage. This should be reserved for severe cases or where there is persistent or refractory infection.

⊗ Do not use oral antibiotics to treat simple otitis externa without evidence of cellulitis or concurrent otitis media.

⊗ Do not use topical antibiotics for prophylaxis. Long-term use of any topical antibiotics can lead to a fungal superinfection.

⊗ Do not instill medication without first cleansing the ear canal, unless restricted because of pain and/or swelling.

⊗ Do not expect medicine to enter a canal that is swollen shut without using a wick.

⊗ Do not use eardrops containing neomycin, which sometimes causes severe allergic contact dermatitis.

⊗ Do not miss the case of malignant (necrotizing) external otitis in the elderly diabetic patient who presents with exquisitely painful otorrhea. These patients require otolaryngologic consultation, special diagnostic evaluation, and prolonged administration of an oral quinolone.

Discussion

Acute otitis externa has a seasonal occurrence, being more frequently encountered in the summer months, when the climate and contaminated swimming water will most likely precipitate a fungal or *Pseudomonas aeruginosa* bacterial infection. *P. aeruginosa* is the most common bacterium involved in this infection, with *Staphylococcus* species being the next most common pathogen. Fungi are only responsible for approximately 2% of cases but may well be more prominent in cases of persistent or chronic infection. Various dermatoses, diabetes, aggressive ear cleaning with cotton-tipped swabs, previous external ear infections, and furunculosis also predispose patients to developing otitis externa.

The healthy ear canal is coated with cerumen and sloughed epithelium. Cerumen is water repellent and acidic and contains a number of antimicrobial substances. Repeated washing or cleaning can remove this defensive coating. Moisture retained in the ear canal is readily absorbed by the stratum corneum. The skin becomes macerated and edematous, and the accumulation of debris may block gland ducts, preventing further production of the protective cerumen. Finally, endogenous or

Discussion continued

exogenous organisms invade the damaged canal epithelium and cause the infection.

In most cases of uncomplicated acute otitis externa, topical antibiotics are the first-line treatment choice. There is no evidence that systemic antibiotics alone or combined with topical preparations improve treatment outcome compared with topical antibiotics alone, and they may contribute to the development of bacterial resistance. When a perforation exists or a patent tympanostomy tube is present, quinolone drops offer superior safety and efficacy. It should be realized, however, that the risk for ototoxicity is negligible when using aminoglycoside combination drops or acetic acid drops when the TM is intact, and that these preparations are consistently effective and less expensive first-line treatments. Clearly, systemic antibiotics are indicated to treat the more serious manifestations of the disease, such as periauricular cellulitis or necrotizing otitis externa.

Malignant or necrotizing external otitis is a potentially life-threatening condition that occurs primarily in elderly diabetic patients and immunocompromised individuals. *P. aeruginosa* is isolated from the aural drainage in more than 90% of cases. The pathophysiology is incompletely understood, although irrigation for cerumen impaction has been reported as a potential iatrogenic factor.

The typical patient presents with severe headache or ear pain, swelling, and drainage. Granulation tissue on the floor of the ear canal may be present. The TM is almost always intact. Disease progression is associated with osteomyelitis of the skull base and temporomandibular joint. Cranial nerve palsies generally indicate advancing infection. Paralysis of the facial nerve is most common. Patients are usually afebrile with normal white blood cell (WBC) and differential counts. The erythrocyte sedimentation rate (ESR) is usually markedly increased. CT scans are ideal to assess for bone erosion. In a prospective study, presence of bone erosion and soft tissue abnormalities in the infratemporal fossa were most helpful in making the diagnosis of malignant external otitis. There is no role for topical antibiotics, even quinolones, in the treatment of this disease. Instillation of antipseudomonal topical agents only increases the difficulty of isolating the pathogenic organism from the ear canal. Systemic antipseudomonal antibiotics are the primary therapy for malignant external otitis. The availability of oral agents has eliminated the need for hospitalization in all but the most recalcitrant cases. Ciprofloxacin (Cipro), 750 mg orally bid, seems to be the antibiotic of choice. Despite the rapid relief of symptoms (pain and otorrhea), prolonged treatment for 6 to 8 weeks is still recommended, as indicated for osteomyelitis. Early consultation should be obtained if there is any suspicion of this condition in a susceptible patient with a draining ear.

The ear is innervated by the fifth, seventh, ninth, and tenth cranial nerves and the second and third cervical nerves. Because of this rich nerve supply, the skin is extremely sensitive. Otalgia may arise directly from the seventh cranial nerve (geniculate ganglion), ninth cranial nerve (tympanic branch), external ear, mastoid air cells, mouth, teeth, or esophagus. Ear pain can result from sinusitis, trigeminal neuralgia, and temporomandibular joint dysfunction or may be referred from disorders of the pharynx and larynx. A mild pain referred to the ear may be felt as itching, may cause the patient to scratch the ear canal, and may present as external otitis.

It is important to consider the possibility of malignancy in the evaluation of a patient with otalgia and apparently refractory otitis externa. When the source of ear pain is not readily apparent, the patient should be referred for a more complete otolaryngologic investigation.

Suggested Readings

Cummings C, editor: *Otolaryngology: head and neck surgery*, ed 4, St Louis, 2005, Mosby.

Hannley MT, Denneny JC, Holzer SS: Use of ototopical antibiotics in treating 3 common ear diseases, *Otolaryngol Head Neck Surg* 122:934–940, 2000.

Kaushik V, Malik T, Saeed SR: Interventions for acute otitis externa, *Cochrane Database Syst Rev* (1):CD004740, 2010.

Rosenfeld RM, Brown L, Cannon CR, et al: Clinical practice guideline: acute otitis externa, *Otolaryngol Head Neck Surg* 134(Suppl 4):S4–S23, 2006.

Rosenfeld RM, Singer M, Wasserman JM, Stinnett SS: Systematic review of topical antimicrobial therapy for acute otitis externa, *Otolaryngol Head Neck Surg* 134(Suppl 4):S24–S48, 2006.

Rubin Grandis JR, Branstetter BF 4th, Yu VL: The changing face of malignant (necrotizing) external otitis: clinical, radiological, and anatomic correlations, *Lancet Infect Dis* 4:34–39, 2004.

Ruben RJ: Efficacy of ofloxacin and other otic preparations for otitis externa, *Pediatr Infect Dis J* 20:108–110, 2001.

van Balen FA, Zuithoff BP, Verheij TJ: Clinical efficacy of three common treatments in acute otitis externa in primary care: randomized controlled trial, *Br Med J* 327:1201–1205, 2003.

van Balen FA, Smit WM, Zuithoff NP, Verheij TJ: Clinical efficacy of three common treatments in acute otitis externa in primary care: randomised controlled trial, *BMJ* 327:1201–1205, 2003.

Wong DLH, Rutka JA: Do aminoglycoside otic preparations cause ototoxicity in the presence of tympanic membrane perforations? *Otolaryngol Head Neck Surg* 116:404–410, 1994.

Wooltorton E: Ototoxic effects from gentamicin ear drops, *Can Med Assoc J* 167:56, 2002.

Otitis Media, Acute

Presentation

In acute otitis media (AOM), adults and older children will complain of ear pain. There may or may not be accompanying symptoms of upper respiratory tract infection. In the younger child or infant, parents may report irritability, decreased appetite, and sleeplessness, with or without fever or pulling at the ears. The real diagnosis comes not from symptoms or history but from tympanic membrane (TM) findings (Figures 35-1 and 35-2). The TM may show marked redness, but contrary to what many clinicians were taught during training, erythema of the TM is the least specific finding for AOM.

Expanding middle-ear effusion volume and intense inflammation produce the key TM findings that are essential for an AOM diagnosis. These findings point to fullness or a bulging TM, with decreased clarity of the bony landmarks and decreased mobility on pneumatic otoscopy. A normal TM snaps briskly like a sail filling with air from a sudden breeze. With fluid behind the TM, there will be either sluggish or no movement at all. A diagnosis of AOM also can be established if the TM has perforated and acute purulent otorrhea is present that is not attributable to otitis externa (see Chapter 34).

Note that increased vascularity or erythema is not sufficient to diagnose AOM but does strengthen the diagnosis by providing the identification of possible TM inflammation. Keep in mind that a child's vigorous crying is a common cause of an erythematous TM that otherwise has normal findings. Therefore, under these circumstances, avoid diagnosing AOM if erythema of the TM is the only finding suggesting AOM.

What To Do:

✓ Investigate for any other underlying illness. When clinical evidence of AOM is obscure or absent, consider other sources of ear pain, such as dental or oral disease, temporomandibular joint dysfunction, or disorders of the mastoid, pharynx, or larynx.

✓ There are many antibiotics available for the treatment of AOM. **Amoxicillin remains the treatment of choice** according to the guidelines of the American Academy of Pediatrics, based on efficacy, palatability, side-effect profile, and cost. **High-dose amoxicillin at 80 mg/kg/day dosed bid provides better coverage of resistant organisms than standard 40 mg/kg/day dosing. Amoxicillin should not be used if**

(1) There has been treatment failure with amoxicillin in the past 30 days.

(2) Concurrent purulent conjunctivitis is present (usually caused by *Haemophilus influenzae*).

(3) The patients are already on chronic suppressive therapy with amoxicillin.

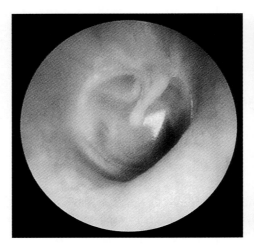 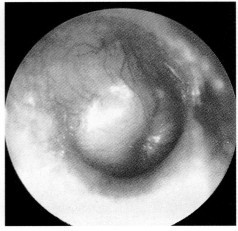

Figure 35-1 Normal right tympanic membrane and middle ear. (From Meniscus Educational Institute: *Otitis media: management strategies for the 21st century*. Bala Cynwyd, Pa, 1998.)

Figure 35-2 Bulging right tympanic membrane in acute otitis media. (From Meniscus Educational Institute: *Otitis media: management strategies for the 21st century*. Bala Cynwyd, Pa, 1998.)

✅ **For those patients in whom an alternative to amoxicillin is needed and there is no penicillin allergy, choices include amoxicillin-clavulanate (Augmentin) 90 mg/kg/day dosed bid (maximum dose 3 g/day), Cefpodoxime 10 mg/kg dosed once daily (maximum dose 800 mg/day), or Cefuroxime 30 mg/kg/day dosed bid (maximum dose 1 g/day).**

✅ **For patients allergic to penicillin, the best choice is erythromycin plus sulfisoxazole (Pediazole) 75 mg/kg/day of the erythromycin component dosed qid (maximum dose 2 g erythromycin component).** Azithromycin and trimethoprim-sulfamethoxazole have significant problems with resistance.

✅ **Studies suggest that 10 days of oral therapy for AOM is more effective than shorter courses in children less than 2 years of age. After 2 years of age, consideration may be given to shorter courses of 5 to 7 days.**

✅ **Ceftriaxone (Rocephin) can be used in a dose of 50 mg/kg IM once daily for 1 to 3 days when compliance problems are anticipated.** A three-dose regimen of IM ceftriaxone may be more efficacious than a single dose for patients with nonresponsive AOM.

✅ **When there is reliable follow-up and the parents are responsible, mild cases of AOM may be treated initially with analgesics alone, adding antimicrobials as an option if symptoms persist or worsen. All children younger than 6 months and all those with moderate to severe ear pain and fever greater than 39° C in the past 24 hours, bilateral disease or otorrhea, should be treated immediately.**

✅ **Parents can be very satisfied with a wait-and-see approach, in which an antibiotic is prescribed, but the parents are asked to wait 72 hours before filling it.** They are to have the prescription filled only if their child still has substantial ear pain or fever at that point or if he is not starting to get better. Provide follow-up by telephone or office visit within 3 days to reassess.

✓ **Acute draining OM** (by either spontaneous perforation or tympanostomy tube) usually is caused by standard AOM pathogens. The usual systemic antibiotics are, in most cases, successful at curing the otitis and stopping the drainage. **In children with no symptoms other than the drainage, ofloxacin (Floxin Otic), 5 mL 0.3%, 5 drops in ear(s) bid × 7 to 10 days, has been shown to produce clinical success in more than 75% of cases, without oral antibiotics.** Topical agents alone, however, are not recommended for children whose draining AOM is accompanied by fever or otalgia. Aminoglycoside topical agents should not be used because of the potential for ototoxicity.

✓ **Provide pain and fever control with acetaminophen or ibuprofen elixir. Additional pain relief may be obtained using antipyrine, benzocaine, oxyquinoline, and glycerin (Auralgan Otic) drops if perforation or tympanostomy tubes are not present.**

✓ Advise parents that pacifier use, exposure to tobacco smoke, and bottle feeding an infant in a reclining rather than an upright position all increase the risk for AOM. Daycare with more than five attendees has been shown to be the most powerful risk factor for frequent AOM. Children who have one or more parents or siblings who experienced frequent AOM or who had pressure-equalizing tubes also will often have frequent AOM or need pressure-equalizing tubes.

✓ **Recommend a 10-day follow-up examination for all patients younger than 2 years of age, in those cases in which the parents do not believe that the infection has resolved or the child's symptoms persist, and when there is a family history of recurrent otitis or the accuracy of the parental observations may be in doubt.**

✓ Because otitis media is much less common in adults, these patients should also have follow-up in 2 weeks, with possible otolaryngologic consultation.

✓ Middle-ear effusion will often persist after resolution of acute infection. Persistence of this effusion without symptoms does not indicate need for further antibiotics.

What Not To Do:

✗ Do not overlook underlying illnesses, such as meningitis.

✗ Do not prescribe antihistamines or decongestants. These drugs do not decrease the incidence or hasten the resolution of AOM. The American Academy of Pediatrics recommends that over-the-counter cough and cold medications should not be given to children younger than 2 years of age because of the risk of life-threatening side effects.

Discussion

AOM is primarily a disease of children younger than 3 years of age, although AOM is not totally unexpected up to age 5. Age-related factors that directly cause AOM are the result of immature anatomy and immature immune systems coupled with excessive exposure to pathogens. The main reasons for AOM are not bacterial, although bacteria are the final ingredients. Bacterial AOM pathogens merely take advantage of the main cause of

AOM (i.e., dysfunction of the middle-ear–flushing mechanism, the eustachian tube). Eustachian tubes are dysfunctional to some degree in every young child but gradually become fully functional by age 5.

Most AOM is caused by a viral infection, and most patients do well regardless of the antibiotic chosen. Some 50% to 80% of cases of AOM will

(continued)

Discussion continued

spontaneously clear without antibiotics. (Older children with infrequent AOM are more likely to experience spontaneous clearing, whereas more severe AOM or AOM occurring soon after a previous episode is less likely to clear spontaneously.) Because AOM usually occurs secondary to acute viral infections (respiratory syncytial virus, influenza, and rhinovirus), rapid initiation of antibiotic treatment may result in eradication or reduction of the susceptible organisms in both the middle-ear fluid and the nasopharynx, permitting the overgrowth of the nasopharyngeal flora organisms that are not susceptible to the drug. Because the predisposing condition (the viral infection causing ciliary and mucosal damage, plus overproduction of secretions)

may still be present, a new infection of the middle ear may then take place with the newly selected resistant pathogen. Despite the increase in antimicrobial resistance of community-acquired *Streptococcus pneumoniae, Haemophilus influenzae,* and *Moraxella catarrhalis* and the plethora of alternative antibiotics available, amoxicillin remains the drug of choice in the treatment of uncomplicated AOM.

Bullous myringitis is the result of acute bacterial infection of the tympanic membrane, producing intraepithelial fluid collections. These patients present with bullae on the TM and can have severe pain. They respond well to anesthetic otic drops (Auralgan), oral antibiotics, corticosteroids, and analgesia.

Suggested Readings

American Academy of Pediatrics Subcommittee on the Management of Otitis Media: Diagnosis and management of acute otitis media, *Pediatrics* 113:1451–1465, 2004.

Arguedas A, Emparanza P, Schwartz RH, et al: A randomized, multicenter, double blind, double dummy trial of single dose azithromycin versus high dose amoxicillin for treatment of uncomplicated acute otitis media, *Pediatr Infect Dis J* 24:153–161, 2005.

Bell LM: The new clinical practice guidelines for acute otitis media: an editorial, *Ann Emerg Med* 45:514–516, 2005.

Cohen R, Levy C, Boucherat M, et al: Five vs. ten days of antibiotic therapy for acute otitis media in young children, *Pediatr Infect Dis J* 19:458–463, 2000.

Culpepper L, Froom J: Routine antimicrobial treatment of acute otitis media: is it necessary? (editorial), *JAMA* 278:1643–1645, 1997.

Del Mar C, Glaszion P, Hayem M: Are antimicrobials indicated as initial treatment for children with acute otitis media? A meta-analysis, *BMJ* 314:1526–1529, 1997.

Eskin B: Evidence-based emergency medicine/systemic review abstract. Should children with otitis media be treated with antibiotics? *Ann Emerg Med* 44:537–539, 2004.

Froom J, Culpepper L, Jacobs M, et al: Antimicrobials for acute otitis media? A review for the international primary care network, *BMJ* 315:98–102, 1997.

Garbutt J, St. Geme JW, May A, et al: Developing community-specific recommendations for first-line treatment of acute otitis media: is high-dose amoxicillin necessary? *Pediatrics* 114:342–347, 2004.

Klein J, Pelton S: *Acute otitis media in children: treatment [UpToDate* website]. Available at http://www.uptodate.com.

Kozyrskyj AL, Hildes-Ripstein E, Longstaffe S, et al: Treatment of acute otitis media with a shortened course of antibiotics, *JAMA* 279:1736–1742, 1998.

Le Saux N, Gaboury I, Baird M, et al: A randomized, double-blind, placebo-controlled noninferiority trial of amoxicillin for clinically diagnosed acute otitis media in children 6 months to 5 years of age, *CMAJ* 172:335–341, 2005.

Marchetti F, Ranfani L, Nibali SC, et al: Delayed prescription may reduce the use of antibiotics for acute otitis media, *Arch Pediatr Adolesc Med* 159:679–684, 2005.

McCormick DP, Chonmaitree T, Pittman C, et al: Nonsevere acute otitis media: a clinical trial comparing outcomes of watchful waiting versus immediate antibiotic treatment, *Pediatrics* 115:1455–1465, 2005.

Niemela M, Uhari M, Jounio-Ervasti K, et al: Lack of specific symptomatology in children with acute otitis media, *Pediatr Infect Dis J* 13:765–768, 1994.

Paradise JL: Managing otitis media: a time for change [editorial], *Pediatrics* 96:712–715, 1995.

Pelton SI: Otoscopy for the diagnosis of otitis media, *Pediatr Infect Dis J* 17:540–543, 1998.

Rosenfeld RM, Vertrees JE, Carr J, et al: Clinical efficacy of antimicrobial drugs for acute otitis media: meta-analysis of 5400 children from thirty-three randomized trials, *J Pediatr* 124:355–367, 1994.

Use of codeine- and dextromethorphan-containing cough remedies in children: American Academy of Pediatrics. (A statement of reaffirmation for this policy was published on February 1, 2007). Committee on Drugs, *Pediatrics* 99:918–920, 1997.

Otitis Media with Effusion; Serous (Secretory) Otitis Media (Glue Ear)

Presentation

After an upper respiratory tract infection, an episode of acute otitis media (AOM), an airplane flight, or during a bout of allergies, an adult may complain of a feeling of fullness in the ears, an inability to equalize middle-ear pressure, decreased hearing, and a clicking, popping, or crackling sound, especially when he moves his head. There is little pain or tenderness. Otitis media with effusion (OME) is usually asymptomatic in children, except for tugging at the ears or signs of decreased hearing (lack of attention, talking too loud, sitting nearer to the television set). When viewed through the otoscope, the tympanic membrane (TM) appears retracted, with bony landmarks that are clearly visible and that are associated with a dull to normal light reflex with minimal if any injection. The best test to diagnose OME is pneumatic otoscopy, showing poor motion of the TM on insufflation. An air-fluid level or bubbles through the eardrum may be visible (Figure 36-1). There may be a lack of translucency, with a yellow or grayish effusion (Figure 36-2). Hearing may be decreased, and the Rinne test may show decreased air conduction (i.e., a tuning fork is heard no better through air than through bone).

It should be emphasized that there is no pain, fever or inflammation, or bulging of the TM, as one might expect to see in AOM (see Chapter 35).

What To Do:

✓ **In children without underlying developmental delay, preexisting hearing or vision problems, or other prior speech or language issues, OME can be observed for 3 months from the time of symptom onset or diagnosis without specific workup or treatment.** If the OME lasts longer than 3 months or the child has preexisting problems, as outlined earlier, a hearing evaluation should be obtained.

✓ **Adults with OME may request symptomatic relief of the nasal congestion or middle-ear symptoms. Over-the-counter vasoconstrictor nose sprays, such as phenylephrine (Neo-Synephrine) or oxymetazoline 0.05% (Afrin), may be recommended.**

✓ **Also, fluticasone (Flonase) topical corticosteroid spray may be prescribed (two sprays per nostril daily).** However, in studies of children, neither vasoconstrictor sprays nor corticosteroids have been shown to lead to long-term resolution of OME.

✓ **Autoinflation has been shown to afford some improvement without side effects in audiometry at 1 month.** To perform this, instruct the patient to insufflate his middle ear through the eustachian tube by closing his mouth, pinching his nose shut, and blowing until his ears "pop."

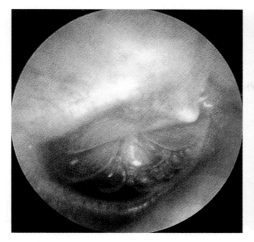

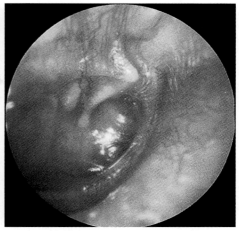

Figure 36-1 Air-fluid level and bubbles visible through right retracted, translucent tympanic membrane in otitis media with effusion. (From Meniscus Educational Institute: *Otitis media: management strategies for the 21st century.* Bala Cynwyd, Pa, 1998.)

Figure 36-2 Severely retracted, opaque right tympanic membrane in otitis media with effusion. (From Meniscus Educational Institute: *Otitis media: management strategies for the 21st century.* Bala Cynwyd, Pa, 1998.)

⊘ **A course of antibiotics may improve clearance of OME. Use the same antibiotics as for AOM. Do not prescribe more than one course.**

⊘ Instruct the patient to seek follow-up with a primary care doctor or ear-nose-throat (ENT) specialist if the condition does not improve within 1 week.

⊘ Parents of children should be informed that bottle feeding, feeding a supine child, attending daycare, and living in a home in which people smoke increases the prevalence of OME.

What Not To Do:

✗ Do not allow the patient to become habituated to vasoconstrictor sprays. After a few days of use, the sprays become ineffective, and the nasal mucosa develops a rebound swelling known as rhinitis medicamentosa, when the medicine is withdrawn.

✗ Do not use oral antihistamines or decongestants. They have been shown not to be effective in the treatment of OME.

✗ Do not use oral or topical corticosteroids for the treatment of children with OME. There may be significant side effects with use of these medications in children. The American Academy of Pediatrics guidelines recommend against their use.

✗ Do not miss a nasopharyngeal mass, which should be considered in all patients with unilateral OME.

Discussion

Among children who have had an episode of AOM, as many as 45% have persistent effusion after 1 month. OME is defined as fluid in the middle ear without signs or symptoms of ear infection. Approximately 90% of cases of OME resolve spontaneously within 6 months. There is significant controversy regarding the routine treatment of this condition.

Most episodes resolve spontaneously within 1 to 2 months. The treatments described here are directed mainly at reestablishing normal function of the eustachian tube. It is unclear if any of these recommended treatments alter the natural course of this disease; therefore symptomatic relief should guide the clinician toward the most effective management for each individual patient.

Fluid in the middle ear is more common in children because of frequent viral upper respiratory tract infections and an underdeveloped eustachian tube.

The highest incidence of OME occurs in children younger than 2 years, and the incidence decreases dramatically in those older than 6 years. Children are also more prone to bacterial superinfection of the fluid in the middle ear. When accompanied by fever and pain, this condition merits treatment with analgesics and antibiotics.

When the diagnosis of OME is uncertain, the patient should be referred for tympanometry or acoustic reflectometry. Children with persistent OME, who do not have the aforementioned risk factors, should be examined at 3- to 6-month intervals until the effusion clears or hearing abnormalities are discovered. Tympanostomy tube insertion is now recommended if there is hearing loss of 40 dB or greater persisting for 4 to 6 months. Repeated bouts of OME in an adult, especially if unilateral, should raise suspicion regarding a tumor obstructing the eustachian tube.

Suggested Readings

American Academy of Family Physicians: American Academy of Otolarygology—Head and Neck Surgery; American Academy of Pediatrics Subcommittee on Otitis Media with Effusion: Otitis media with effusion, *Pediatrics* 113: 1412–1429, 2004.

Csortan E, Jones J, Haan M, et al: Efficacy of pseudoephedrine for the prevention of barotrauma during air travel, *Ann Emerg Med* 23:1324–1327, 1994.

Griffin GH, Flynn C, Bailey RE: Schultz JK: Antihistamines and/or decongestants for otitis media with effusion (OME) in children, *Cochrane Database Syst Rev*(4):CD003423, Oct 18, 2006.

Harrison CJ: The laws of acute otitis media, *Prim Care* 30:109–135, 2003.

Jones JS, Sheffield W, White LJ, et al: A double-blind comparison between oral pseudoephedrine and topical oxymetazoline in the prevention of barotraumas during air travel, *Am J Emerg Med* 16:262–264, 1998.

Klein J, Pelton S: Otitis media with effusion (serious otitis media) in children. [*UptoDate* website]. Available at http://www.uptodate.com. Accessed November 2010.

McCracken GH: Diagnosis and management of acute otitis media in the urgent care setting. *Ann Emerg Med* 39:413–421, 2002.

Onusko E, Tympanometry: *Am Fam Physician* 70:1713–1720, 2004.

Reidpath DD, Glasziou PP, Del Mar C: Systematic review of autoinflation for treatment of glue ear in children, *BMJ* 318:1177, 1999.

Rosenfeld RM, Post JC: Meta-analysis of antibiotics for the treatment of otitis media with effusion, *Otolaryngol Head Neck Surg* 106:378–386, 1992.

Williams RL, Chalmers TC, Strange KC, et al: Use of antibiotics in preventing recurrent acute otitis media and in treating otitis media with effusion. A meta-analytic attempt to resolve the brouhaha, *JAMA* 270:1344–1351, 1993.

Perforated Tympanic Membrane

(Ruptured Eardrum)

Presentation

The patient experiences ear pain after barotrauma, such as a blow or slap on the ear, an exploding firecracker, a fall while water skiing or during a deep water dive, or after direct trauma inflicted with a stick or other sharp object, such as a paper clip or cerumen curette. Hemorrhage is often noticed within the external canal, and the patient will experience the acute onset of pain (which tends to subside quickly) and some partial hearing loss. Tinnitus or transient vertigo may also be present. Otoscopic examination reveals a defect in the tympanic membrane (TM) that may or may not be accompanied by disruption of the ossicles (Figure 37-1). The presence of blood may make assessment difficult.

What To Do:

✓ When necessary, clear any debris from the canal, using gentle suction.

✓ **Determine if this is just an abrasion of the wall of the ear canal or if an actual TM perforation is present. If so, note its size and location.**

✓ Test for nystagmus and gross hearing loss.

✓ **With a true TM perforation, place a protective cotton plug inside the ear canal, and instruct the patient to keep the canal dry by using soft wax earplugs while showering. He should also avoid submerging his head under water until the perforation is completely healed.**

✓ Prescribe an appropriate analgesic, such as ibuprofen (Motrin), naproxen (Anaprox), or acetaminophen with hydrocodone (Lorcet) or with oxycodone (Percocet).

✓ **Prescribe the ototopical antibiotic ofloxacin (Floxin Otic) 5 mL, 3 to 5 drops in ear bid × 3 to 5 days, only if the lacerated TM and middle ear were contaminated with lake water, seawater, or a dirty object, such as a tree branch.** Systemic antibiotics may be added in cases in which contamination is severe.

✓ **Ensure that the patient gets early follow-up with an otolaryngologist. This is especially important with sharp, penetrating trauma in the posterior superior quadrant of the TM, where disruption of the ossicles is most likely to occur. The patient should be seen regularly until the TM is well healed.**

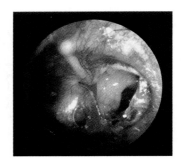

Figure 37-1 Small traumatic perforation of the tympanic membrane.

What Not To Do:

(X) Do not suction or attempt to clear blood or debris close to the TM, if the canal is filled with clotted blood or if damage to the ossicles has occurred; vigorous suctioning may further traumatize these structures.

(X) Do not attempt to remove a foreign body you think may have penetrated the middle-ear space. Consult an ear-nose-throat (ENT) specialist in these cases.

(X) Do not instill any fluid other than Floxin Otic into the external canal or allow the patient to get water into his ear. Water in the middle ear is painful and irritating and may introduce bacteria. Wax earplugs or a cotton plug covered with petroleum jelly will allow the patient to shower more safely.

Discussion

Small uncomplicated perforations usually heal without sequelae over a period of days to weeks. Small defects (less than 2 mm) will heal spontaneously almost 100% of the time, but larger defects or marginal defects may not heal and would then require either myringoplasty or tympanoplastic procedures. When there is nystagmus, vertigo, profound hearing loss, or disruption of the ossicles, early otolaryngologic consultation is advisable.

If healing has not taken place after 8 weeks or if there is persistent hearing loss after healing, then surgical repair may be indicated.

Suggested Readings

Amadasun JEO: An observational study of the management of traumatic tympanic membrane perforations, *J Laryngol Otol* 116:181–184, 2002.

Evans AK, Handler SD: Evaluation and management of middle ear trauma. [*UpToDate* website]. Available at http://www.uptodate.com. Accessed November 2010.

Fagan P, Patel N: A hole in the drum. An overview of tympanic membrane perforations, *Aust Fam Physician* 31:707–710, 2002.

Isaacson JE, Vora NM: Differential diagnosis and treatment of hearing loss, *Am Fam Physician* 68:1125–1132, 2003.

Segal S: Inner ear damage in children due to noise exposure from toy cap pistols and firecrackers: a retrospective review of 53 cases, *Noise Health* 5:13–18, 2003.

Pharyngitis

(Sore Throat)

Presentation

The patient with bacterial pharyngitis complains of a rapid onset of throat pain worsened by swallowing. There is usually sudden onset of the following: fever; pharyngeal erythema; edematous uvula; palatine petechiae; purulent, patchy yellow, gray, or white exudate; tender anterior cervical adenopathy; headache; and absence of a cough. Children who are younger than 3 years of age more often have coryza and are less likely to present with exudative pharyngitis. Viral infections are typically accompanied by conjunctivitis, nasal congestion, hoarseness, cough, aphthous ulcers on the soft palate, and myalgias. Children with viral pharyngitis can present with mouth breathing, vomiting, abdominal pain, and diarrhea. It is helpful to differentiate pain on swallowing (odynophagia) from difficulty swallowing (dysphagia); the latter is more likely to be caused by obstruction or abnormal muscular movement.

What To Do:

✓ Obtain important historical information, including onset, duration, and progression of symptoms as well as the presence of associated fever, cough, respiratory difficulty, or swollen lymph nodes.

✓ First, examine the ears, nose, and mouth, which are, after all, connected to the pharynx and often contain clues to the diagnosis. The pharynx should be evaluated for erythema, hypertrophy, foreign body, exudates, and petechiae (using a tongue blade). It is also important to assess the patient for fever, rash, cervical adenopathy, and coryza. Also, listen for the presence of a heart murmur and evaluate the patient for hepatosplenomegaly.

✓ **Patients usually fall into three clinical categories: those who appear to have *Streptococcus* pharyngitis, those who clearly have a viral illness, and those with symptoms of both. Scoring systems have been developed that can aid in decision making.**

✓ There are other uncommon causes of pharyngitis that should be kept in mind, such as primary human immunodeficiency virus (HIV) infection, diphtheria, as well as noninfectious causes, such as gastroesophageal reflux, postnasal drip, thyroiditis, allergies, and foreign bodies.

✓ **The Centor scoring system has been validated for adults and places people into high-, moderate-, and low-risk groups (for *Streptococcus* pharyngitis), based on four criteria: tonsillar exudates, tender anterior cervical lymphadenopathy, absence of a cough, and history of fever. High-risk patients have three or four positive criteria. Low-risk patients have zero or one positive criterion.**

✅ **The McIsaac scoring system has been validated in both children and adults and uses seven factors: fever, absence of a cough, tender anterior cervical adenopathy, tonsillar swelling or exudates, age younger than 15 years, each of which scores 1 point. Age 15 to 45 years scores 0 points. Age over 45 scores –1 point. High-risk patients have a score of 4 or 5 points. Low-risk patients have a score of 0 or –1 point.**

✅ **Patients in the low-risk category, in either scoring system, should be neither treated nor tested. Patients in the high-risk category may be treated empirically with antibiotics or tested and then treated if positive. Patients with moderate risk should be tested and only treated if positive for group A *Streptococcus* (GAS) infection.**

✅ **Testing can be done with the rapid streptococcal test or with a throat culture.** The throat culture will take at least 1 day to get results. According to some studies, the practice of treating high-risk patients without testing leads to significant overprescribing of antibiotics. **Doing a culture or rapid streptococcal test on all moderate- to high-risk adult patients leads to the most appropriate use of antibiotics.**

✅ **Children should be handled differently than adults when it comes to testing for GAS.** Children have a higher risk of rheumatic fever and are much more likely to transmit GAS to others. Therefore, if rapid strep testing is used at the initial test and it is negative, a follow-up streptococcal culture is recommended. For this reason, **initial testing with a throat culture may be the most cost effective practice in children.**

✅ **When antibiotics are indicated, the first choice is penicillin V potassium (Pen-Vee K), 500 mg bid × 10 days, or oral solution 50 mg/kg/day divided bid × 10 days.** If there is concern about compliance, give the penicillin IM, using penicillin G benzathine (Bicillin L-A), 1.2 million units IM × 1, or for the pediatric patient less than 27 kg, give 25,000 units/kg IM × 1.

✅ In the penicillin-allergic patient, prescribe erythromycin base, 333 mg tid × 10 days or erythromycin ethyl succinate (EES) suspension 40 mg/kg/day divided bid × 10 days.

✅ **Cephalosporins can also be used, such as cefadroxil (Duricef), 500 mg bid × 10 days, or suspension 30 mg/kg/day divided bid × 10 days.** Refractory cases may be treated with clindamycin 300 mg qid × 10 days or, for pediatric patients, 30 mg/kg/day divided qid × 10 days.

✅ If mononucleosis is suspected, draw a test for atypical lymphocytes, and perform a heterophil antibody (monospot) test to confirm the diagnosis (see Chapter 32).

✅ **Relieve pain with acetaminophen or ibuprofen given on a regular basis rather than on an "as needed" basis.** Warm saline gargles, and gargles or lozenges containing phenol as a mucosal anesthetic (e.g., Chloraseptic, Cepastat), may be soothing. Tessalon Perles may be bitten, with the anesthetic liquid held in the back of the throat and then swallowed. Gargling a 1:1 mixture of diphenhydramine and kaolin-pectin suspension can also provide temporary relief of throat pain.

✅ **For severe pain, in patients without contraindications, one dose of dexamethasone, 10 mg (0.6 mg/kg) IM or PO, or prednisone, 60 mg PO (in adults), has been used in conjunction with antibiotics and can provide a more rapid onset of pain relief. Narcotics can be considered for patients with severe pain.**

What Not To Do:

(X) Do not prescribe an antibiotic to patients with a clear viral infection (low-risk Centor or McIsaac scores). Treatment of viral pharyngitis with antibiotics is a major source of antibiotic resistance.

(X) Do not miss scarlet fever, which is associated with group A beta-hemolytic *Streptococcus* (GABHS) pharyngitis and usually presents as a punctate, erythematous, blanchable, sandpaper-like exanthema. The rash is found in the neck, groin, and axilla and is accentuated in body folds and creases (the Pastia lines). The tongue may be bright red with a white coating (strawberry tongue).

(X) Do not overlook acute epiglottic or supraglottic inflammation. In children, this presents as a sudden, severe pharyngitis, with a guttural rather than hoarse voice (because it hurts to speak), drooling (because it hurts to swallow), and respiratory distress (because swelling narrows the airway). Adults usually have a more gradual onset over several days and are not as prone to a sudden airway occlusion, unless they present later in the progression of the swelling and are already experiencing some respiratory distress.

(X) Do not prescribe ciprofloxacin, tetracycline, doxycycline, and sulfamethoxazole/trimethoprim for acute pharyngitis. These drugs are considered to be ineffective.

(X) Do not give ampicillin to a patient with mononucleosis. Although the resulting rash helps make the diagnosis, it does not imply ampicillin allergy and can be uncomfortable.

(X) Do not overlook peritonsillar abscesses, which often require hospitalization and IV penicillin, incision and drainage, or needle aspiration. Peritonsillar abscesses or cellulitis causes the tonsillar pillar to bulge toward the midline. Patients typically have a toxic appearance and may present with a "hot potato voice." With an abscess, there is a very tender, fluctuant, peritonsillar mass and asymmetric deviation of the uvula. Intraoral ultrasound examination or CT examination are diagnostic tests that can provide an accurate diagnosis if the clinical picture is unclear.

(X) Do not overlook gonococcal pharyngitis in sexually active patients at risk. This can produce a clinical syndrome with fever, severe sore throat, dysuria, and characteristic greenish exudates that require special culture on Thayer-Martin medium or testing with a nucleic acid probe. This requires special treatment (see Chapter 83).

(X) Do not overlook Kawasaki disease. A malady that most often affects children younger than 5 years of age, it has characteristic signs and symptoms that include sore throat, fever, bilateral nonpurulent conjunctivitis, anterior cervical node enlargement, erythematous oral mucosa, and an inflamed pharynx with a strawberry tongue. Within 3 days of the onset of fever, the patient will develop cracked red lips, a generalized erythematous rash with edema and erythema of the hands and feet, and periungual desquamation followed by peeling of the palms.

(X) Do not overlook diphtheria. This acute upper respiratory tract infection is characterized by a sore throat, low-grade fever, and an adherent grayish membrane with surrounding inflammation of the tonsils, pharynx, and nasal passages with a serosanguineous nasal discharge.

Discussion

Members of the general public know to see a doctor for a sore throat, but the actual benefit of this visit is unclear. Rheumatic fever is exceedingly rare in the United States and other developed countries (annual incidence less than one case per 100,000). Only 15% to 30% of cases in children and 5% to 15% of cases in adults are culture-positive GABHS pharyngitis. Poststreptococcal glomerulonephritis is usually a self-limiting illness and is not prevented with antibiotic treatment.

On the other hand, penicillin and other antibiotic therapies do prevent the rare development of acute rheumatic fever and may sometimes reduce symptoms or shorten the course of a sore throat. Antibiotics probably inhibit the infection from progressing into tonsillitis, peritonsillar and retropharyngeal abscesses, adenitis, and pneumonia.

Group A streptococcal infection cannot be diagnosed reliably based on clinical signs and symptoms. Typically, 25% of throat cultures grow group A *Streptococcus,* and 50% of those represent carriers who do not raise antistreptococcal antibodies and risk rheumatic fever.

Rapid streptococcal screens are less sensitive than cultures, but because of improvements in rapid streptococcal antigen tests, throat culture can be reserved for patients whose symptoms do not improve over time or who do not respond to antibiotics.

Clinical prediction rules have been developed that use several key elements of the history and physical examination to predict the probability of strep throat. Using a clinical prediction rule gives a clinician a rational basis for assigning a patient to a low-risk category (requires neither testing nor treatment), a high-risk category (empiric antibiotic may be indicated), or a moderate-risk category (may require further diagnostic testing). One of the best validated scoring systems is a simple four-item clinical prediction rule developed by Centor. The Centor score has been validated in three distinct adult populations. McIsaac modified the Centor score and validated it prospectively in a mixed population of adults and children. There is controversy surrounding these and other similar clinical prediction rules. Therefore clinical judgment and monitoring of the most recent literature on the subject are still advised when deciding whether or not to test or treat with antibiotics.

Suggested Readings

Adam D, Scholz H, Helmerking M: Short-course antibiotic treatment of 4782 culture-proven cases of group A streptococcal tonsillopharyngitis and incidence of poststreptococcal sequelae, *J Infect Dis* 182:509–516, 2000.

Bisno A, Lichtenberger P: Evaluation of acute pharyngitis in adults. [*UpToDate* website]. Available at http://www.uptodate.com. Accessed November 2010.

Bisno AL, Garnet SP, Kaplan EL: Diagnosis of strep throat in adults: are clinical criteria really good enough? *Clin Infect Dis* 35:126–129, 2002.

Bisno AL, Gerber MA, Gwaltney JM, et al: Diagnosis and management of group A streptococcal pharyngitis: a practice guideline, *Clin Infect Dis* 25:574–583, 1997.

Bulloch B, Kabani A, Tenenbein M: Oral dexamethasone for the treatment of pain in children with acute pharyngitis: a randomized, double-blind, placebo-controlled trial, *Ann Emerg Med* 41:601–608, 2003.

Casey JR, Pichichero ME: Meta-analysis of cephalosporins versus penicillin for treatment for group A streptococcal tonsillopharyngitis in adults, *Clin Infect Dis* 38:1526–1534, 2004.

Cohen R, Reinert P, de la Rocque F, et al: Comparison of two dosages of azithromycin for three days versus penicillin V for ten days in acute group A streptococcal tonsillopharyngitis, *Pediatr Infect Dis J* 21:297–303, 2002.

Coonan KM, Kaplan EL: in vitro susceptibility of recent North American group A streptococcal isolates to eleven oral antibiotics, *Pediatr Infect Dis J* 13:630–635, 1994.

Cooper RJ, Hoffman JR, Bartlett JG, et al: Principles of appropriate antibiotic use for acute pharyngitis in adults: background, *Ann Emerg Med* 37:711–719, 2001.

DiMatteo LA, Lowenstein SR, Brinhall B: The relationship between the clinical features of pharyngitis and the sensitivity of a rapid antigen test: evidence of spectrum bias, *Ann Emerg Med* 38:648–652, 2001.

Ebell MH, Smith MA, Barry HC, et al: Does this patient have strep throat? *JAMA* 284:2912–2918, 2000.

Hall MC, Kieke B, Gonzales R, et al: Spectrum bias of a rapid antigen detection test for group A beta-hemolytic streptococcal pharyngitis in a pediatric population, *Pediatrics* 114:182–186, 2004.

Huovinen P, Lahhtonen R, Ziegler T, et al: Pharyngitis in adults: the presence and coexistence of viruses and bacterial organisms, *Ann Intern Med* 110:612–616, 1989.

Marvez-Valls EG, Stuckey A, Ernst AA: A randomized clinical trial of oral versus intramuscular delivery of steroids in acute exudative pharyngitis, *Acad Emerg Med* 9:9–14, 2002.

Mayes T, Pichichero ME: Are follow-up throat cultures necessary when rapid antigen detection tests are negative for group A streptococcus? *Clin Pediatr* 40:191–195, 2001.

McIsaac WJ: The validity of a sore throat score in family practice, *CMAJ* 163:811–815, 2000.

McIsaac WJ, Kellner JD, Aufricht P, et al: Empirical validation of guidelines for the management of pharyngitis in children and adults, *JAMA* 291:1587–1595, 2004.

Neuner JM, Hamel MB, Phillips RS, et al: Diagnosis and management of adults with pharyngitis, *Ann Intern Med* 139:113–122, 2003.

O'Brien JF, Meade JL, Falk JL: Dexamethasone as adjuvant therapy for severe acute pharyngitis, *Ann Emerg Med* 22:212–214, 1993.

Pichichero ME: Group A streptococcal tonsillopharyngitis: cost-effective diagnosis and treatment, *Ann Emerg Med* 25:390–403, 1995. editorial 404–406.

Vincent MT, Celestin N, Hussain N: Pharyngitis. *Am Fam Physician* 69:1465–1470, 2004.

Webb KH, Needham CA, Kurtz SR: Use of a high-sensitivity rapid strep test without culture confirmation of negative results, *J Fam Pract* 49:34–38, 2000.

Yeh B, Eskin B: Evidence-based emergency medicine/systematic review abstract. Should sore throats be treated with antibiotics? *Ann Emerg Med* 45:82–84, 2005.

Rhinitis, Acute

(Runny Nose)

CHAPTER 39

Presentation

In allergic rhinitis, patients typically complain of rhinorrhea ("runny nose"), nasal congestion, sneezing, nasal itching, and "itchy eyes." There may be a problem with sleep disturbance (from nasal congestion), malaise, fatigue, irritability, and neurocognitive deficits.

Typically, patients with allergic rhinitis have clear discharge, swollen turbinates, and bluish or pale mucosa. There may be "allergic shiners"—infraorbital darkening thought to be caused by chronic venous pooling—or an "allergic salute" in children who rub their noses upward because of nasal discomfort, sometimes producing a persistent horizontal crease across the nose. Mild bilateral conjunctivitis with nonpurulent discharge is strongly suggestive of an allergic cause when it is accompanied by pruritus. The patient with a "summer cold" lasting a full month is likely to have allergic rhinitis.

Precipitating factors may be known or may be elicited from the patient. Common allergens include airborne dust-mite fecal particles, cockroach residues, animal danders (especially cats and dogs), molds, and pollens (hence the origin of the term *hay fever*). Vasomotor (idiopathic) rhinitis may occur in response to environmental conditions, such as changes in temperature or relative humidity, odors (e.g., perfume or cleaning materials), passive tobacco smoke, alcohol, sexual arousal, or emotional factors.

Drug-induced rhinitis may be caused by oral medications, including angiotensin-converting enzyme (ACE) inhibitors, beta-blockers, various antihypertensive agents, chlorpromazine, aspirin, other nonsteroidal anti-inflammatory drugs (NSAIDs), and oral contraceptives as well as topical α-adrenergic decongestant sprays that have been used for more than 5 to 7 days (rhinitis medicamentosa). Repeated use of intranasal cocaine and methamphetamines may also result in rebound congestion and, on occasion, septal erosion and perforation.

In viral rhinitis, patients generally complain of an annoying, persistent mucoid nasal discharge accompanied by nasal and facial congestion, along with a constellation of viral symptoms, including low-grade fever, myalgias, and sore throat. These patients generally seek care, because they feel miserable, cannot sleep, and want relief. They often believe that antibiotics are needed to cure their problem.

On physical examination, there is only nasal mucous membrane congestion, which may appear erythematous, along with cloudy nasal secretions, which may become somewhat yellow and thick after several days. Resolution occurs within 10 days to 2 weeks.

Always keep in mind that young children may place intranasal foreign bodies in their noses (e.g., beads or beans), leading to foul-smelling, purulent, unilateral nasal discharge (see Chapter 29).

What To Do:

Allergic Rhinitis

✓ Determine which specific symptoms are most bothersome to the patient (e.g., nasal congestion, pruritus, rhinorrhea, sneezing), the pattern of the symptoms (e.g., intermittent, seasonal, perennial), any precipitating factors in the home or occupational environment, the response to previous medications, and any coexisting conditions.

✓ Use a hand-held otoscope or headlamp with nasal speculum to view the anterior nasal airway. (A topical decongestant improves visualization of the nasal cavity.)

✓ **Educate the patient about avoidance of any known inciting factors.** In particular, patients who are allergic to house dust mites should use allergen-impermeable encasings on the bed and pillows. For patients with seasonal allergies, pollen exposure can be reduced by having them keep windows closed, using an air conditioner, and limiting the amount of time spent outdoors.

✓ **Intranasal corticosteroids are the most effective medication class for treatment of allergic rhinitis and should be used as a single first-line agent; although, it should be kept in mind that these are generally expensive items.** These preparations are generally not associated with significant systemic side effects in adults. **Prescribe fluticasone (Flonase) nasal spray (which has been shown to be beneficial even when used on an as-needed basis) for adults and children older than 12 years of age, 2 sprays (50 µg/spray) in each nostril qd, or 1 spray in each nostril bid. Other options include flunisolide (Nasalide)** nasal spray, 2 sprays in each nostril bid (may increase to tid to qid), or, for children 6 to 14 years old, 1 spray in each nostril tid or 2 sprays each nostril bid; **mometasone furoate (Nasonex)** for adults and children older than 12 years of age, 2 sprays in each nostril qd; and **budesonide (Rhinocort Aqua)** nasal spray for adults and children older than 6 years of age, 1 spray in each nostril qam.

✓ Patients should be instructed to direct sprays away from the nasal septum to avoid irritation and not to tilt the head back when spraying, to avoid having the drug run out of the nasal cavity and into the throat.

✓ **Antihistamines are a second-line agent in allergic rhinitis treatment** but have less effect on nasal congestion. **Prescribe a nonsedating second-generation antihistamine, such as fexofenadine (Allegra), 180 mg qd (for children 6 to 11 years old, 30 mg bid); desloratadine (Clarinex), 5 mg qd; loratadine (Claritin), 10 mg qd, or syrup, 10 mg/10 mL (for children 2 to 5 years old, 5 mg qd; for children 6 to 11 years old, 10 mg qd); cetirizine (Zyrtec), 5 to 10 mg qd, or syrup, 5 mg/5 mL (for children 2 to 5 years old, ½ to 1 tsp [2 to 2.5 mg] qd; for children 6 to 11 years old, 1 to 2 tsp [5 to 10 mg] qd).**

✓ **An alternative to oral antihistamines is the intranasal antihistamine azelastine (Astelin Nasal Spray) for adults and children older than 12 years of age, 2 sprays per nostril bid.** Side effects many include a bitter taste in the mouth and sedation.

✓ **Topical decongestant nasal sprays and oral decongestants can effectively reduce nasal congestion for both allergic and nonallergic forms of rhinitis, but they can cause side effects** (especially the oral forms) of insomnia, nervousness, loss of appetite, and urinary retention in males. They should be used with caution or not at all in patients with arrhythmias, hypertension, or hyperthyroidism. **Prescribe pseudoephedrine (Sudafed), 60 mg q6h; time-released version, 120 mg bid, or syrup, 3 mg/mL (for children 2 to 5 years old, 5 to 30 mg q4-6h; for children 6 to 12 years old, 30 mg q4-6h or 4 mg/kg/day divided q6h [1 mg/kg/dose]).**

✓ **Two effective nasal decongestant sprays are oxymetazoline (Afrin) 0.05%, 2 sprays per nostril bid (or, for pediatric patients, 0.025%, 1 to 2 sprays per nostril bid), and phenylephrine (Neo-Synephrine Nasal) 0.025%, 0.05%, or 1%, 1 to 2 sprays per nostril q3-4h (or, for pediatric patients older than 2 years, 0.125% or 0.25%). Use must be limited to 3 to 5 days to avoid rebound nasal congestion (rhinitis medicamentosa).**

✓ The same cautions and contraindications exist for nasal decongestants as for the oral medications. Because of the use of pseudoephedrine in the illegal manufacture of amphetamine drugs, it now must be purchased behind the counter.

✓ **Other products that have some efficacy in allergic rhinitis are cromolyn sodium, a mast cell stabilizer, and montelukast (Singulair), a leukotriene receptor antagonist, for adults, 10 mg qhs (for children 2 to 5 years old, 4 mg chewable tab qhs; for children 6 to 14 years old, 5 mg chewable tab qhs).**

✓ In addition, ipratropium bromide (Atrovent Nasal Spray) 0.06%, two sprays per nostril tid to qid have been shown to help but works best in vasomotor (idiopathic) rhinitis.

Viral Rhinitis

✓ Determine which specific symptoms are most bothersome to the patient (e.g., nasal congestion, rhinorrhea, scratchy throat, general aches, fever, or cough).

✓ Perform a general examination, including a careful nasal examination, to exclude any associated diseases, such as rhinosinusitis, otitis media, bacterial pharyngitis, and asthmatic bronchitis.

✓ **For nasal congestion, prescribe oral or topical decongestants, as you would for allergic rhinitis (described earlier). For rhinorrhea, you can prescribe ipratropium bromide (Atrovent Nasal Spray) 0.06%, 2 sprays per nostril tid to qid.**

✓ Although antihistamines are effective for treatment of rhinitis related to allergy, they are much less effective for rhinitis related to the common cold. The side effects often outweigh the benefit and thus are not recommended.

✓ **Nasal saline irrigation has been shown to have some efficacy in the relief of viral rhinitis. This can easily be accomplished with a commercially available neti pot.**

✓ **Provide symptomatic relief for associated symptoms (e.g., acetaminophen [Tylenol] or ibuprofen [Motrin] for fever, general aches, and scratchy throat, or albuterol [Ventolin] metered-dose inhaler for cough).**

✓ **Warm facial compresses, steam inhalation, warm tea, and chicken soup are all comforting, and chicken soup may possibly be therapeutic.**

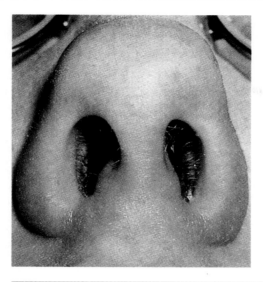

Figure 39-1 Example of nasal vestibulitis. (Adapted from Park YW, Littlejohn R, Eley J: Diagnosis at a glance. *Emerg Med* 5:9, 2002.)

When **pain, redness and tender swelling around the nostrils** occur **because of nose picking or excessive rubbing or blowing of the nose (nasal vestibulitis)** (Figure 39-1), treat with an antistaphylococcal antibiotic ointment—mupirocin (Bactroban) 2%, apply tid × 2 weeks—and recommend warm compresses. Patients with diabetes, immune deficiency, or progressive infection should be placed on a systemic antistaphylococcal antibiotic to avoid potential spread to the cavernous sinus.

What Not To Do:

Do not prescribe sedating antihistamines for symptoms of hay fever.

Do not prescribe antihistamines or nasal steroids for the common cold.

Do not obtain imaging studies of the sinuses unless the criteria for bacterial rhinosinusitis are met (symptoms lasting more than 7 days and including facial or dental pain or tenderness along with purulent nasal drainage).

Do not prescribe antibiotics for cold symptoms. Antibiotics should only be considered if symptoms persist for more than 7 days and are accompanied by signs of rhinosinusitis (see Chapter 40).

Do not bother recommending the use of zinc lozenges. Despite numerous randomized trials, the evidence for their effectiveness in reducing the duration of common cold symptoms is still lacking.

Discussion

Rhinitis is an inflammation of the nasal mucous membranes. Allergic rhinitis triggers a systemic increase in inflammation. Within minutes of allergen exposure, immune cells release histamine, proteases, cysteinyl leukotrienes, prostaglandins, and cytokines. Systemic circulation of inflammatory cells permits their infiltration into other tissues where chemoattractant and adhesion molecules already exist. Consequently, allergic rhinitis is linked to comorbid conditions: asthma, chronic hyperplastic eosinophilic sinusitis, nasal polyposis, and serous otitis media. Effective therapy should ideally be directed at the underlying inflammation and its systemic manifestations. It should improve the rhinitis and the comorbid conditions.

Antihistamines relieve early symptoms, but they do not significantly influence the proinflammatory loop. Oral corticosteroids provide the systemic anti-inflammatory effect needed, but their toxicity precludes extended routine use. Intranasal corticosteroids effectively target the local inflammatory processes of rhinitis, but they only reduce the local inflammatory cells within the nares. Leukotriene modifiers have both systemic anti-inflammatory effects and an acceptable safety profile.

Immunotherapy (allergy shots) is the only treatment that produces long-term relief of symptoms. Patients should be considered candidates for these treatments, based on the severity of their symptoms and the failure or unacceptability of the other treatment modalities.

Nasal polyps are benign inflammatory growths that arise from the inflamed mucosa lining the paranasal sinuses. They are frequently associated with sinus disease. Unilateral nasal polyps should raise consideration of a possible neoplasm.

Suggested Readings

Borish L: Allergic rhinitis: systemic inflammation and implications for management, *J Allergy Clin Immunol* 112: 1021–1031, 2003.

Dykewicz MS: Rhinitis and sinusitis, *J Allergy Clin Immunol* 111:S520–S529, 2003.

Diamond L, Dockhorn RJ, Grossman J, et al: A dose-response study of the efficacy and safety of ipratropium bromide nasal spray in the treatment of the common cold, *J Allergy Clin Immunol* 95:1139–1146, 1995.

Fletcher R: An overview of rhinitis. [*UpToDate* website]. Available at http://www.uptodate.com. Accessed November 2010.

Friedman N, Sexton D: The common cold in adults: treatment and prevention. [*UpToDate* website]. Available at http://www.uptodate.com. Accessed November 2010.

Jackson JL, Peterson C, Lesho E: A meta-analysis of zinc salts lozenges and the common cold, *Arch Intern Med* 157:2373–2376, 1997.

Linder JA, Singer DE: Desire for antibiotics and antibiotic prescribing for adults with upper respiratory tract infections, *J Gen Intern Med* 18:795–801, 2003.

Macknin ML, Piedmonte M, Calendine C, et al: Zinc gluconate lozenges for treating the common cold in children, *JAMA* 279:1962–1967, 1998.

Mainous AG, Hueston WJ, Clark JR: Antibiotics and upper respiratory infection: do some folks think there is a cure for the common cold? *J Fam Pract* 42:357–361, 1996.

Prasad AS, Fitzgerald JT, Bao B, et al: Duration of symptoms and plasma cytokine levels in patients with the common cold treated with zinc acetate: a randomized double-blind, placebo-controlled trial, *Ann Emerg Med* 38:245–252, 2001.

Rosenwasser LJ: Treatment of allergic rhinitis, *Am J Med* 113(Suppl 9A):17S–24S, 2002.

Rhinosinusitis

(Sinusitis)

Presentation

After a viral infection or with chronic allergies, the patient may complain of a dull facial pain, which is usually unilateral, gradually increases over a couple of days, is exacerbated by sudden motion of the head or bending over with the head dependent, may radiate to the upper molar teeth (through the maxillary antrum), and may increase with eye movement (through the ethmoid sinuses). Often, there is a sensation of facial congestion and stuffiness. The child with sinusitis often has a cough, rhinorrhea, and fetid breath. The patient's voice may have a resonance similar to that of an individual with a "stopped up" nose, and she may complain of a foul taste in her mouth or reduced sense of smell. Stuffy ears and impaired hearing are common because of associated otitis media with effusion and eustachian tube dysfunction. A colored nasal discharge is a particularly sensitive finding. Fever is present in only half of all patients with acute infection and is usually low grade. A high fever and severe headache usually indicate a serious complication, such as meningitis or another diagnosis altogether. Transillumination of sinuses in the acute care setting is usually unrewarding, but tenderness may be elicited on gentle percussion or firm palpation over the maxillary or frontal sinuses or between the eyes (ethmoid sinuses). Swelling and erythema may exist. Pus may be visible draining below the nasal turbinates (most often in the middle meatus) with a purulent yellow-green or chronic infection, sometimes with a foul-smelling discharge from the nose or running down the posterior pharynx.

What To Do:

✓ Rule out other possible causes of facial pain or headache through the patient's history and physical examination (palpate the scalp muscles, temporal arteries, temporomandibular joints, eyes, and teeth). Consider the diagnosis of viral or allergic rhinitis (see Chapter 39).

✓ **Shrink swollen nasal mucosa (and thereby provide symptomatic relief of nasal obstruction) with 1% phenylephrine (Neo-Synephrine) or 0.05% oxymetazoline (Afrin) nose drops.** Instill 2 drops in each nostril, allow the patient to lie supine for 2 minutes, and then repeat the process. (Repeating the process allows the first applications to open the anterior nose so that the second dose gets farther back.) Have the patient repeat this process every 4 hours but for no more than 3 to 5 days (to avoid rhinitis medicamentosa).

✓ Examine the nose for purulent drainage before and, when practical, after shrinking the nasal mucosa with a topical vasoconstrictor.

✓ **Unless contraindicated by age, hypertension, benign prostatic hypertrophy, or underlying cardiac disease, prescribe systemic sympathomimetic decongestants such as pseudoephedrine (Sudafed), 60 mg q6h.**

✅ **Antibiotics should be limited to patients who have symptoms lasting 7 or more days, with unilateral maxillary pain or tenderness of the face or teeth accompanied by purulent nasal secretions or to those patients who present initially with more severe symptoms.**

✅ **Prescribe amoxicillin (Amoxil), 1 g tid × 10 days, 90 mg/kg/day divided bid or tid (suspension 125, 200, 250, and 400 mg/5mL).** Studies have shown that the newer broad-spectrum antibiotics are no better than the older, less expensive narrow-spectrum ones.

✅ **If the patient has taken antibiotics within the past month or the prevalence of drug-resistant *Streptococcus pneumoniae* is greater than approximately 30% in the community, prescribe amoxicillin clavulanate (Augmentin XR), 2000/125 mg bid (prescribed as 2 tabs 1000/62.5 mg bid), or extra strength pediatric suspension, 90 mg amoxicillin component/kg/day divided bid × 10 days.**

✅ The best choice in penicillin-allergic patients is either trimethoprim-sulfamethoxazole (Bactrim) 1 PO bid × 7 days or azithromycin (Zithromax) 500 mg PO day 1 then 250 mg PO qd days 2 to 5.

✅ **The more expensive respiratory fluoroquinolones should be considered in adults only if penicillin-resistant *S. pneumoniae* is a major concern or for treatment failures.**

✅ **Most cases of acute rhinosinusitis are viral in origin,** and the clinical differentiation of viral from bacterial causes is difficult. Therefore, **when a patient presents early in the course of his illness, unnecessary treatment with antibiotics can often be avoided by not starting a patient on antibiotics initially but, instead, writing a backup prescription that can be filled if symptoms persist for a total of 7 days.**

✅ **Provide pain relief** (e.g., ibuprofen, naproxen, acetaminophen, oxycodone, hydrocodone) when necessary.

✅ **If allergic rhinitis is suspected** (see Chapter 39), **a second-generation antihistamine is a logical addition to therapy, or an intranasal steroid may be helpful,** but it may be difficult to distinguish viral from allergic sinus symptoms.

✅ **For symptomatic relief, recommend that the patient try hot facial compresses and hot water vapor inhalation using a simple teakettle, a hot shower, a steam vaporizer, or a home facial sauna device. Hot soups or teas can also be comforting. Plain saline nasal sprays and irrigations have been shown to lessen symptoms as well.**

✅ Arrange for follow-up within 1 to 7 days, depending on the severity of the initial findings. Specialist evaluation is appropriate when sinusitis is refractory to treatment or is recurrent.

✅ Give the patient an explanation of the rationale for management and inform him about the signs and symptoms of worsening that should prompt him to seek immediate medical attention.

What Not To Do:

❌ Do not ignore signs of orbital cellulitis (swelling, erythema, decreased extraocular movements, and possible proptosis). These patients require consultation and hospital admission for IV antibiotic therapy.

❌ Do not ignore the toxic patient who has marked swelling, high fever, severe pain, profuse drainage, or other signs and symptoms of a serious infection. (See the potential complications described later.) These patients require immediate consultation and intervention.

(X) Do not order routine radiograph or CT examinations. Reserve them for difficult diagnoses and treatment failures.

(X) Do not prescribe first-generation antihistamines, which are sedating and can make mucous secretions dry and thick and can interfere with necessary drainage.

(X) Do not allow the patient to use decongestant nose drops for more than 3 to 5 days; this will prevent the nasal mucosa from becoming habituated to topical sympathomimetic medication. If she uses the drops for more than 5 days, the patient may suffer rebound nasal congestion (rhinitis medicamentosa) when use of the drops is discontinued; resolution of this condition requires time, topical steroids, and reeducation.

(X) Do not prescribe long-term topical or systemic sympathomimetic decongestants to a patient who suffers from increased intraocular pressure, hypertension, ischemic heart disease, tachycardia, or difficulty initiating urination, all of which may be exacerbated.

(X) Do not prescribe antibiotics to patients with mild symptoms who do not have persistent maxillary facial or dental pain or tenderness or who do not have purulent nasal drainage. These patients are unlikely to have bacterial rhinosinusitis, regardless of duration of illness.

Discussion

The term *rhinosinusitis* is considered to be more accurate than sinusitis, because sinusitis is, in most instances, a continuum and eventual consequence of rhinitis (see Chapter 39). Acute sinusitis is defined as inflammation of the sinuses for less than 4 weeks.

Sinusitis is the most common health care complaint in the United States. The paranasal sinuses drain through tiny ostia under the nasal turbinates. Occlusion of these ostia allows secretions and pressure differences to build up, resulting in the pressure and pain of acute sinusitis and the air-fluid levels sometimes visible on radiographs. Early mild cases do not require treatment with antibiotics. However, congested sinuses can become a site for bacterial superinfection.

Most cases of rhinosinusitis begin with ostial obstruction caused by mucosal swelling associated with viral upper respiratory tract infection. Other causes include allergic rhinitis; barotraumas caused by flying, swimming, or diving; nasal polyps and tumors; and foreign bodies, including nasogastric and endotracheal tubes placed in hospitalized patients. Abscessed teeth can also be the source of maxillary sinusitis. If there is tenderness on percussion of the bicuspids or molars, arrange for dental consultation.

A CT scan of the sinuses is the study of choice for evaluating sinusitis but is needed urgently only with complicated cases or treatment failures. Radiologic studies performed within days of the onset of symptoms may lead to an incorrect conclusion that bacterial infection is present. Up to 40% of sinus radiographs and more than 80% of CT scans may be abnormal in viral sinusitis if obtained within 7 days of the onset of illness.

Most patients can receive initial treatment on the basis of the history and physical examination alone. Anyone who has moderate to severe unilateral facial or dental pain or purulent nasal discharge persisting for more than 7 days, with or without fever, should probably be treated empirically for acute bacterial rhinosinusitis. Be aware that most cases of milder acute bacterial rhinosinusitis will resolve without the need to prescribe antibiotics, and complications of untreated bacterial disease are rare.

Many patients have been conditioned by the advertising of over-the-counter antihistamines for "sinus" problems (usually meaning "allergic rhinitis") and may relate a history of "sinuses," which on closer questioning turns out to be uncomplicated rhinitis.

Suggested Readings

Clement PAR, Bluestone CD, Gordts F, et al: Management of rhinosinusitis in children, *Arch Otolaryngol Head Neck Surg* 124:31–124, 1998.

Dykewicz MS: Rhinitis and sinusitis, *J Allergy Clin Immunol* 111:S520–S529, 2003.

Garbutt JM, Goldstein M, Gellman E, et al: A randomized, placebo-controlled trial of antimicrobial treatment for children with clinically diagnosed acute sinusitis, *Pediatrics* 107:619–625, 2001.

Gwaltney J: Acute community-acquired sinusitis, *Clin Infect Dis* 23:1209–1223, 1996.

Hickner JM, Bartlett JG, Besser RE: Principles of appropriate antibiotic use for acute rhinosinusitis in adults: background, *Ann Emerg Med* 37:703–710, 2001.

Hwang, P, Getz, A: Acute rhinosinusitis. [*UptoDate* website]. Available at www.uptodate.com. Accessed November 2010.

Low DE, Desrosiers M, McSherry J, et al: A practical guide for the diagnosis and treatment of acute sinusitis, *CMAJ* 156(Suppl 6):S1–S14, 1997.

Piccirillo JF, Mager DE, Frisse ME, et al: Impact of first-line vs second-line antibiotics for the treatment of acute uncomplicated sinusitis, *JAMA* 286:1849–1856, 2001.

Rosenfeld RM, Andes D, Bhattacharyya N, et al: Clinical practice guidelines: adult sinusitis, *Otolaryngol Head Neck Surg* 137:S1–S31, 2007.

Slavin RG: Nasal polyps and sinusitis, *JAMA* 278:1849–1854, 1997.

Tang A, Frazee B: Antibiotic treatment for acute maxillary sinusitis, *Ann Emerg Med* 42:705–708, 2003.

Van Buchem FL, Knottnerus JA, Schrijnemaekers VJ: Primary-care-based randomized placebo-controlled trial of antibiotic treatment in acute maxillary sinusitis, *Lancet* 349:683–687, 1997.

Williams JW, Simel DL: Does this patient have sinusitis? Diagnosing acute sinusitis by history and physical examination, *J Am Med Assoc* 270:1242–1246, 1993.

PART 4

Oral and Dental Emergencies

■ Philip Buttaravoli ■ Daniel Wolfson

CHAPTER

Aphthous Ulcer

(Canker Sore)

41

Presentation

The patient complains of a painful lesion in her mouth and may be worried about having herpes. Lesions are painful and may interfere with eating, speaking, or swallowing. Minor oral trauma from dental appliances, dentures, and orthodontic hardware may be causative, or patients may inadvertently produce traumatic ulcers through biting of the oral mucosa, either accidentally or through unconscious habit.

Simple aphthosis represents the more usual scenario of episodic lesions that are few in number, healing within 1 to 2 weeks, and recurring infrequently. Conversely, complex aphthosis is a more severe phenomenon, presenting as a clinical picture of numerous severe lesions, which are persistent, slow to resolve, and associated with marked pain or disability.

Canker sores can present as one or more flat, even-bordered, round or oval ulcers with a central friable pseudomembranous base surrounded by a bright red halo. They may be seen on nonkeratinized unattached mucosa, such as the buccal or labial mucosa, lingual sulci, soft palate, pharynx, lateral and ventral tongue, or gingiva. Lesions are usually solitary but can be multiple and recurrent without antecedent vesicles or bulla. The pain is usually greater than the size of the lesions would suggest.

Minor aphthae comprise 80% of all aphthae, measure less than 5 to 10 mm in circumference, are usually located on the buccal or labial mucosa, and heal spontaneously in 7 to 10 days without scarring (Figure 41-1). Ten percent of all lesions are major aphthae, which are larger than 10 mm in circumference and are deeper. They may heal over weeks to months and often result in scarring. Major aphthae may also be located posteriorly, on the soft palate, tonsils, and pharynx (Figure 41-2). Major aphthae that last for months and are slow to heal may be associated with human immunodeficiency virus (HIV) infection. The remaining 10% of aphthae are herpetiform aphthae, which are smaller (1 to 3 mm), grouped, or coalescent ulcers that may be present on keratinized mucosa of the dorsal tongue and palate and heal spontaneously over 1 to 4 weeks (Figure 41-3). Herpes simplex virus is not, by definition, found in these lesions.

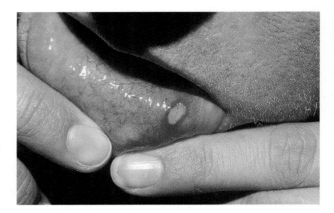

Figure 41-1 Aphthous ulcers. A gray-white oval ulcer with a bright red margin is typical. These lesions are usually quite painful. (From White G, Cox N: *Diseases of the skin*, 2nd ed 2. St Louis, 2006, Mosby.)

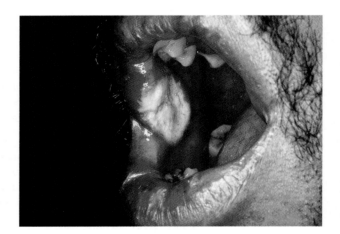

Figure 41-2 Aphthae major in a patient with AIDS. (From Bolognia J, Jorizzo J, Rapini R: *Dermatology.* St Louis, 2003, Mosby.)

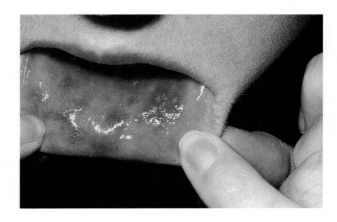

Figure 41-3 Herpetiform mouth ulcers. (From White G, Cox N: *Diseases of the skin*, ed 2. St Louis, 2006, Mosby.)

What To Do:

✅ Through a careful history and physical examination, decide whether the patient is troubled with simple aphthosis or is more likely to have the potentially more serious complex aphthosis.

✅ Attempt to differentiate between the patient's mucosal sores and lesions of herpes simplex (most commonly appearing on the lips and skin outside the mouth) (see Chapter 54).

✅ **For simple aphthosis with minor aphthae, inform the patient that these lesions are benign and usually last 1 to 2 weeks. She should avoid heavily spiced, acidic, or other irritating food and drink, such as pretzels and citrus fruit, and avoid any precipitating factors, such as ill-fitting dentures, a hard-bristled toothbrush, or habitual biting.** Avoidance of sodium lauryl sulfate–containing mouthwash and dentifrices (used for foaming action) may decrease the incidence of aphthous ulcers. Interestingly, the antibacterial, anti-inflammatory chemical triclosan has been demonstrated to prevent the chemotoxicity of sodium lauryl sulfate and reduce aphthous ulcers by 96%. Colgate Total (Colgate-Palmolive, New York, N.Y.) is a commercially available dentifrice containing triclosan.

✅ **If food allergens, such as cereal, fruit, chocolate, nuts, and tomatoes, can be identified as triggering recurrent canker sores, their elimination will reduce or completely relieve symptoms in approximately 90% of cases.**

✅ Recommend acetaminophen (Tylenol) as an analgesic, adding a narcotic as needed.

✅ **Prescribe Triamcinolone 0.1% in orabase (Kenalog in orabase). Apply a thin film to dried ulcers 2 to 4 times daily until healed.**

✅ **Prescribe amlexanox (Aphthasol oral paste) 5%, 5-g tube, to be applied qid (about 0.5 cm to affected area after brushing teeth).** This medication may sting, but it is the first drug to be approved by the U.S. Food and Drug Administration (FDA) for aphthous ulcers in healthy people. This treatment may help canker sores heal only a little faster and could be **reserved for those cases in which pain is severe and sores recur frequently.**

✅ **An alternative treatment that can be used for transient pain relief is a tablet of sucralfate crushed in a small amount of warm water and swirled in the mouth or gargled. Another alternative is tetracycline elixir (or a capsule dissolved in water), not swallowed but applied to the lesions to cauterize them or used as a mouthwash.** This also stings but sometimes can relieve pain after one or more applications.

✅ **Diphenhydramine (Benadryl) elixir mixed 1:1 with kaolin-pectin (Kaopectate), lidocaine (Xylocaine 2% viscous solution), and hydrocortisone (Orabase HCA) applied topically with a cotton-tipped swab can also provide symptomatic relief.** Bioadhesive 2-octyl cyanoacrylate (Dermabond) has been recommended as a topical nonprescription treatment for pain reduction but is cost prohibitive if applied repeatedly.

✅ **For more severe cases, prescribe the topical steroid clobetasol propionate gel (Temovate) 0.05%, 15-g tube. Apply a thin film after drying the area qid until healed. The gel may be mixed with Orabase (OTC) mucosal adherent, although the dilution may affect the strength. Not recommended for patients less 12 years old.**

✅ In very severe cases, try a burst dose of prednisone, 40 to 60 mg qd for 5 days (no tapering required).

Patients with complex aphthosis or with major aphthae can be treated with the same measures as outlined earlier. Approximately 15% of these patients have a systemic disorder in which the oral ulcers are a mucocutaneous marker of the systemic disease. Therefore they should also be referred to a specialist for further evaluation of these possible associated systemic diseases, which may require management with systemic agents to control the aphthae. Such agents include colchicines, thalidomide, dapsone, and cyclosporine. You may also consider vitamin supplementation: zinc lozenges, vitamin C, and vitamin B–complex.

What Not To Do:

Do not give steroids to a patient in whom you suspect there may be an underlying herpes infection.

Do not forget to consider hematologic etiologies if recurrent or slow-healing ulcers are associated with fevers. Check a complete blood count (CBC) with differential to rule out neutropenia or leukemias.

Discussion

Aphthae is a term of ancient origin referring to ulceration of any mucosal surface.

Aphthous stomatitis has been studied for many years by numerous investigators. Although many exacerbating factors have been identified, the cause as yet remains unknown. Lesions can be precipitated by minor trauma (often from a hard-bristled toothbrush), food allergy, stress, genetic predisposition, allergy, medications, nutritional hematinic deficiencies (e.g., iron, folic acid, vitamin B_{12}), systemic illnesses (e.g., inflammatory bowel disease or gluten-sensitive enteropathy [celiac sprue]), or HIV-associated immunosuppression. Recurrent aphthous ulcers may also accompany malignancy or autoimmune disease.

Behçet syndrome is a multisystem inflammatory disorder characterized by recurrent oral ulcers that are clinically indistinguishable from aphthae but are accompanied by genital ulcers, conjunctivitis, retinitis, iritis, leukocytosis, eosinophilia, and increased erythrocyte sedimentation rate. Patients with posterior uveitis (i.e., retinal vasculitis) are at greatest risk for blindness. Patients with Behçet disease usually present with oral aphthae (minor, major, and herpetiform), which may be the only manifestation of disease for an average of 6 to 7 years before the second major manifestation is apparent.

At present, the treatment for both simple and complex aphthosis is only palliative and may not alter the course of the syndrome. Aphthous ulcers may be an immune reaction to damaged mucosa or altered oral bacteria.

Although they are in great pain, patients with simple aphthosis and minor aphthae can be reassured that they do not have a serious problem and that they are not contagious. **Herpangina and hand-foot-and-mouth disease** can produce ulcers resembling aphthous ulcers, but these ulcers are instead part of Coxsackie viral exanthems, usually occurring with fever and in clusters among children.

Suggested Readings

Bruce AJ, Rogers RS: Acute oral ulcers, *Dermatol Clin* 21:1–15, 2003.

Letsinger JA, McCarty MA, Jorizzo JL: Complex aphthosis: a large case series with evaluation algorithm and therapeutic ladder from topicals to thalidomide, *J Am Acad Dermatol* 52:500–508, 2005.

Ship JA: Recurrent aphthous stomatitis: an update, *Oral Surg Oral Med Oral Pathol* 81:141–147, 1996.

Vincent SD, Lilly GE: Clinical, historic and therapeutic features of aphthous stomatitis, *Oral Surg Oral Med Oral Pathol* 74:79–86, 1992.

Zunt SL: Recurrent aphthous stomatitis, *Dermatol Clin* 21:33–39, 2003.

Avulsed Tooth, Dental Subluxation, Dental Luxation

Presentation

After a direct blow to the mouth, the patient, usually a child 7 to 9 years old, may have a permanent tooth that has been completely knocked out of its socket (avulsion) (Figure 42-1). The tooth is intact down to its root, from which hangs the delicate periodontal ligament that used to be attached to alveolar bone. Alternatively, the tooth may have only become loosened within its normal anatomic position (subluxation) or partially displaced laterally, partially extruded from the socket, or intruded into the alveolar ridge (luxation) (Figure 42-2). These disfiguring, hemorrhagic injuries are often dramatic and a frightening experience for the patient, his parents, and other bystanders.

What To Do:

⊘ Reassure everyone that you will be doing everything that can be done to save the patient's tooth (or teeth) and provide comfort.

⊘ Obtain a detailed history that includes the mechanism of injury, conditions that may have led to dental contamination, the length of time that any avulsed tooth has been out of its socket, and how that tooth was stored and handled. **Determine whether there are any missing teeth that cannot be accounted for and also determine if the injured teeth were primary or permanent.**

⊘ **Check to see whether prophylaxis against bacterial endocarditis is required** because of an implanted heart valve, abnormal native valve (leakage/blockage), congenital heart defect (ventricular septal defect [VSD], atrial septal defect [ASD], patent ductus arteriosus [PDA], complex anomaly), significant mitral valve prolapse, pacemaker, or Dacron or Teflon vascular graft or patch over cardiac defect.

⊘ Examination should include evaluation of surrounding soft tissue for lacerations (see Chapter 51), with special attention to possible embedded foreign bodies (e.g., chipped teeth). Grasp the injured teeth between your gloved fingers to see if a tooth or an entire segment of teeth (e.g., alveolar ridge fractures) is mobile.

⊘ Check for malocclusion and other signs of mandibular fracture as well as any other associated injuries that might be overlooked with the distracting oral trauma.

⊘ **Radiographs need only be obtained if a mandibular or alveolar fracture is suspected, if a dental fragment is missing in the soft tissues of the mouth, or if a tooth may have been intruded down into its socket, is no longer visible, and appears to be missing.**

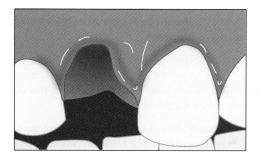

Figure 42-1 The site of an avulsed tooth. (Adapted from Honsik KA: Emergency treatment of dentoalveolar trauma. *Physician Sports Med* 32:23-29, 2004.)

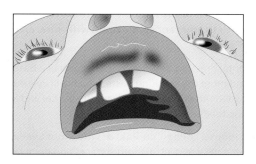

Figure 42-2 A partially extruded and laterally displaced tooth (luxation). (From Honsik KA: Emergency treatment of dentoalveolar trauma. *Physician Sports Med* 32:23-29, 2004.)

✅ **If a tooth is lost and cannot be accounted for, order a chest radiograph to rule out bronchial aspiration.**

✅ **The best way to preserve a tooth that has been knocked out (avulsed) is to put it back in its socket as quickly as possible.** Do not delay replanting a tooth because you are waiting for radiograph results, unless you suspect an alveolar ridge fracture. Keep in mind that more accurate dental films can be done at the time of dental follow-up.

✅ **Primary tooth: A primary tooth that has been avulsed should not be reimplanted. The risk of injury to the developing permanent tooth is high.**

✅ **If the permanent tooth is only partially avulsed and is just protruding farther out of its socket than normal or is angulated, simply push it back in, using firm pressure until it sits in its proper position.** If the tooth is very sensitive and painful to touch, quickly provide analgesia, using an appropriate oral nerve block (see Appendix D). To ensure that the tooth is firmly reseated, have the patient bite down hard on a piece of gauze.

✅ **In the field, fully extruded permanent teeth may be stored under the tongue or in the buccal vestibule between the gums and the teeth. If the patient is unconscious, the tooth can be stored in cold milk or saline solution—or, if nothing else is available, water—until a better preservation solution is available.** A child's permanent tooth might be preserved, if necessary, in the parent's mouth.

✅ **Place the tooth in protective solution as soon as possible after patient arrival,** even before obtaining additional history. Use commercially available protective solutions, such as Hank balanced salt solution or Save-A-Tooth kit. *Note:* Contact-lens solution is not an appropriate storage medium.

✓ If the tooth is contaminated, *hold it by the crown only* and irrigate it with normal saline. *Do not rub or scrub the root surface.*

✓ Replacing a tooth into its socket can be facilitated by first anesthetizing the tooth socket with a dental block (see Appendix D). **After the socket is numb, irrigate the socket and gently suction out any remaining debris or blood. Once the socket is prepared in this manner, replace the tooth back into the socket.**

✓ If the permanent tooth has been out of its socket for less than 15 minutes, **take it by the crown, drop it in a tooth-preservation solution (see earlier), and gently flush the socket with the same solution or normal saline. Then reimplant the tooth firmly, first checking its proper orientation. Instruct the patient to bite down hard on a piece of gauze to help stabilize the tooth. Most of the time the tooth will remain stable in the socket. If necessary, secure the tooth to adjacent stable teeth with wire, arch bars, or a temporary periodontal pack (Coe-Pak).**

✓ Coe-Pak is a periodontal dressing that comes in the form of a base and a catalyst. Mix together the two parts and mold the resulting paste, which will eventually set semihard, over the gingival line and between the dried teeth on both the buccal and lingual sides but not over the occlusive surface of the teeth.

✓ **If a temporary periodontal splint (Coe-Pak) or wire is not available** to stabilize loose teeth, spread soft wax over palatal and labial tooth surfaces and neighboring teeth as a temporary splint. If this item is not available, there is a case report showing the use of a pliable metal nasal bridge from a respirator mask to stabilize the replanted tooth. This splint is molded to the outer surface of the teeth and then glued to the reimplanted tooth and the stabilizing adjacent teeth using 2-octyl cyanoacrylate (2-OCA; Dermabond and others) (Figure 42-3).

✓ **Put the patient on a soft diet, prescribe penicillin V potassium, 500 mg (12.5 mg/kg for pediatric patients) qid for 2 weeks,** and schedule a dental appointment as soon as possible. Instruct the patient to brush all but the splinted teeth. Some endorse chlorhexidine mouth rinse in addition to brushing.

✓ If the permanent tooth has been out of its socket for 15 minutes to 2 hours, **first soak it in the previously mentioned protective solution for 30 minutes to replenish nutrients before reimplanting. Local anesthesia will probably be needed before the tooth can be reimplanted as described earlier** (see Appendix D).

✓ If the permanent tooth has been out of its socket for longer than 2 hours, **the periodontal ligament is dead and should be removed, along with the pulp.** Soak the tooth for 30 minutes in 5% sodium hypochlorite (Clorox) and 5 minutes each in saturated citric acid, 1% stannous fluoride, and 5% doxycycline before reimplanting. The dead tooth should ankylose into the alveolar bone of the socket as with a dental implant.

✓ Even when the tooth has been out less than 2 hours, if the patient is between 6 and 10 years of age, **soak the tooth for 5 minutes in 5% doxycycline to kill bacteria that could enter the immature apex and form an abscess.**

✓ If all this cannot be done right away, **simply keep the tooth soaking in the preservation solution until a dentist can get to it. The solution should preserve the tooth safely for up to 4 days.**

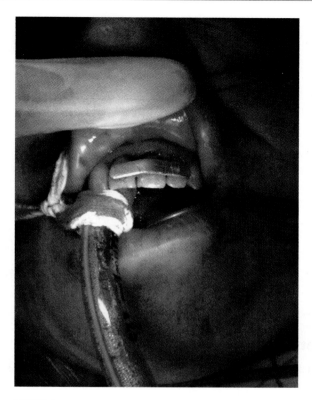

Figure 42-3 Pliable metal nasal bridge of respirator mask bonded to teeth using 2-OCA for reimplantation and stabilization of avulsed left upper central incisor (tooth 9). (Adapted from Rosenberg H, Rosenberg H, Hickey M: Emergency management of a traumatic tooth avulsion. *Ann Emerg Med* 57:375-377, 2011.)

✓ **When consulting a dentist or an oral surgeon, the use of a dental map will help in communicating the exact tooth/teeth involved** (Figure 42-4).

✓ **Provide antibiotic prophylaxis to all patients with even minor dental trauma (e.g., subluxation) if they are at risk for bacterial endocarditis.**

✓ Consider the possibility of domestic or child abuse as the source of the trauma; if suspected, notify the appropriate authorities.

✓ Add tetanus prophylaxis to the treatment protocol if required (see Appendix H).

✓ Inform the patient or his parents that any trauma to the teeth can lead to the death of a tooth or infection or root absorption and the eventual loss of the tooth. Also let them know that they will require dental referral for possible repositioning, more durable splinting, possible root canal therapy, and long-term follow-up. **Root canal therapy will definitely be required on all permanent teeth that have been completely avulsed.**

✓ **Prescribe appropriate pain medication, such as oxycodone and acetaminophen (Percocet)** 5 mg/325 mg, 1 to 2 tablets q4-6h prn for pain; for children 6 to 12 years old, ¼ to ½ tablet of 2.5 mg/325 mg q6h prn for pain, or for children 12 to 18 years old, ½ to 1 tablet of 2.5 mg/325 mg q6h prn for pain. Have the patient try acetaminophen or a nonsteroidal anti-inflammatory drug (NSAID) alone first to see if a narcotic is necessary. May use oxycodone oral solution 5 mg/5 mL concentration. Give 0.05 to 0.15 mg/kg PO q4-6h prn.

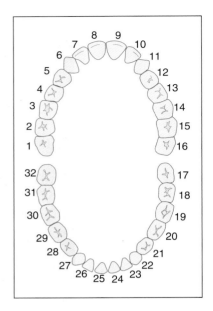

Figure 42-4 Dental map.

What Not To Do:

(X) Do not allow an avulsed tooth to dry out. The total length of dry storage time has the greatest negative impact on the success or failure of dental reimplantation.

(X) Do not touch a viable root with fingers, forceps, gauze, or anything else, and do not try to scrub or clean it. The periodontal ligament will be injured and unable to revascularize the reimplanted tooth. Only hold an avulsed tooth by its crown.

(X) Do not overlook fractures of teeth and alveolar ridges.

(X) Do not substitute the calcium hydroxide composition (Dycal) used for covering fractured teeth for the temporary periodontal pack (Coe-Pak) used to stabilize luxated teeth. They are different products.

(X) Do not reimplant an avulsed tooth if there is a complicated crown fracture, a fractured root, or an alveolar ridge fracture.

(X) Do not replace primary deciduous or baby teeth, although this has been done under very special circumstances. Reimplanted primary teeth heal by ankylosis; they literally fuse to the bone, which can lead to cosmetic deformity because the area of ankylosis will not grow at the same rate as the rest of the dentofacial complex. Ankylosis can also interfere with eruption of the permanent tooth.

(X) Do not confuse an avulsed adult tooth with a child's deciduous tooth, which would fall out soon anyway. Normal developmental shedding of primary decidual teeth is preceded by absorption of the root. If such a tooth is brought in by mistake, there is no root to reimplant and little or no empty socket; instead, a new permanent tooth may be visible or palpable underneath.

(X) Do not release a patient with an unsplinted tooth that is so loose that it is in danger of falling out and being aspirated.

Discussion

Accidents at home, at school, or in a motor vehicle, as well as altercations and contact sports, lead to injuries of the teeth. The maxillary central incisors are the teeth most commonly affected. When teeth are avulsed, the prognosis is best when teeth are reimplanted within 5 minutes of avulsion; yet, such optimal treatment is not always possible.

Before commercially available reconstitution solutions (e.g., Hank balanced salt solution, 320 mOsm, pH 7.2), the best treatment that could be offered the avulsed tooth was rapid reimplantation. Without a preservation solution, the chances of successful reimplantation decline approximately one percentage point every minute the tooth is absent from the oral cavity.

In mature teeth (those more than 10 years old), the pulp will not survive avulsion, even if the periodontal ligament does. At the 1-week follow-up visit with the dentist, the necrotic pulp will be removed (root canal) to prevent a chronic inflammatory reaction from interfering with the healing of the periodontal ligament.

The primary goal of rapid reimplantation is to preserve the periodontal ligament, not the tooth. With survival of the periodontal ligament, the tooth is more likely to function for a longer period of time, with less resorption of the root and reduced ankylosis.

Almost half of teeth with luxation injuries become necrotic after 3 years. The correct and timely management of these cases can increase the success of treatment.

Successful reimplantation of avulsed anterior permanent teeth can delay or negate the need for prosthetic or complex and expensive restorative procedures. Several studies have shown that teeth can function for 20 years or more after reimplantation. A number of cases have been reported in which reimplanted teeth have been functional for 20 to 40 years with a normal periodontium.

Suggested Readings

Cho S, Cheng AC: Replantation of an avulsed incisor after prolonged dry storage: a case report, *J Can Dent Assoc* 68:297–300, 2002.

Douglass AB: Common dental emergencies, *Am Fam Physician* 67:511–516, 2003.

Krasner P: Modern treatment of avulsed teeth by emergency physicians, *Am J Emerg Med* 12:241–246, 1994.

Martins WD, Westphalen VPD, Westphalen FH: Tooth replantation after traumatic avulsion: a 27-year follow up, *Den Traumatol* 20:101–105, 2004.

Rosenberg H, Rosenberg H, Hickey M: Emergency management of a traumatic tooth avulsion, *Ann Emerg Med* 57:375–377, 2011.

Zamon EL, Kenny DJ: Replantation of avulsed primary incisors: a risk–benefit assessment, *J Can Dent Assoc* 67:386, 2001.

Bleeding after Dental Surgery

Presentation

The patient who had an extraction or other dental surgery performed earlier in the day now has excessive bleeding at the site and is unable to visit the dentist. The patient may also be using aspirin, Coumadin, Plavix, or other anticoagulant medications.

What To Do:

✓ Ask the patient what procedure was done and estimate how much bleeding has occurred. Inquire about ingestion of antiplatelet drugs (aspirin, Coumadin, Plavix, or Pradaxa), underlying coagulopathies, and previous experiences with unusual bleeding.

✓ **Using suction and saline irrigation, clear any packing and blood from the bleeding site.**

✓ **Roll a 2 × 2–inch gauze pad, insert it over the bleeding site, and have the patient apply constant pressure on it (biting down usually suffices) for 30 to 45 minutes.**

✓ **If the site is still bleeding after 30 to 45 minutes of gauze pressure, infiltrate the extraction area and inject a local anesthetic and vasoconstrictor, such as 2% lidocaine with 1:100,000 or 1:200,000 epinephrine, into the socket and surrounding gingiva until the tissue blanches.** Again, have the patient bite on a gauze pad for 45 minutes. The anesthetic allows the patient to bite down harder, and the epinephrine helps restrict the bleeding.

✓ **If this injection does not stop the bleeding, pack the bleeding site with Gelfoam, Surgicel, or gauze soaked in topical thrombin. Then place the gauze pad on top, and apply pressure again. Alternatively, HemCon dental gauze (HemCon Medical Technologies, Portland, Ore.) can be applied. Place the HemCon dental dressing into the extraction wound. The dressing is most effective when in contact with blood from the wound, which wets the dressing. The top of the dressing should be flush with the gingival margin. Place sterile gauze over the HemCon dental dressing, and have the patient bite down, applying gentle pressure for 1 to 2 minutes. Visualize the site to confirm proper placement of the dressing, and replace the gauze on top. The HemCon dressing dissolves in 48 hours to 7 days and does not need to be removed. The patient may irrigate the wound site at 7 days to ensure removal of any residual material.**

✓ **Another approach** to the bleeding is to saturate the gauze sponge with tranexamic acid (Cyklokapron) injectable solution, 100 mg/mL at a dose of 25 mg/kg (which can be swallowed), and have the patient bite down hard for another 30 to 45 minutes.

✅ An arterial bleeder resistant to all the aforementioned treatments may require ligation with a figure-eight stitch.

✅ Assess any possible large blood loss by obtaining orthostatic vital signs.

✅ **When the bleeding stops, remove the overlying gauze and instruct the patient to leave the site alone for a day and see her dentist for follow-up.**

What Not To Do:

❌ Do not routinely obtain laboratory clotting studies or hematocrit levels, unless there is reason to suspect a bleeding disorder such as hemophilia A or von Willebrand disease, over-medication with warfarin (Coumadin), or severe blood loss.

❌ Do not allow a patient to intermittently remove the gauze. It is the constant, prolonged pressure that is most likely to provide successful hemostasis.

Discussion

Serious hemorrhage is rare even in the presence of a bleeding diathesis or anticoagulant therapy. Most patients are merely annoyed by the continued bleeding and often only need to stop dabbing the area and apply constant pressure to get the bleeding to stop.

Occasionally this problem can be handled with telephone consultation alone. Some say a moistened tea bag, which contains the hemostatic effects of tannic acid, works even better than a gauze pad when constant pressure is applied.

Suggested Readings

Federici AB: Clinical diagnosis of von Willebrand disease, *Haemophilia* 10:169–176, 2004.

Gazda H, Grabowska A: Topical treatment of oral bleeding in children with clotting disturbances (in Polish), *Wiad Lek* 46:111–115, 1993.

Petersen JK, Krogsgaard J, Nielsen KM, et al: A comparison between 2 absorbable hemostatic agents: gelatin sponge (Spongostan) and oxidized regenerated cellulose (Surgicel), *Int J Oral Surg* 13:406–410, 1984.

Senghore N, Harris M: The effect of tranexamic acid (Cyclokapron) on blood loss after third molar extraction under a day case general anaesthetic, *Br Dent J* 186:634–636, 1999.

Songra AK, Darbar UR: Post-extraction bleeding—an aid to diagnosis? *Aust Dent J* 43:242–243, 1998.

Waly NG: Local antifibrinolytic treatment with tranexamic acid in hemophilic children undergoing dental extractions, *Egypt Dent J* 41:961–968, 1995.

Zanon E, Martinelli F, Bacci C, et al: Safety of dental extraction among consecutive patients on oral anticoagulant treatment managed using a specific dental management protocol, *Blood Coagul Fibrinolysis* 14:27–30, 2003.

Burning Mouth Syndrome, Burning Tongue

(Glossodynia)

Presentation

The patient is very uncomfortable because of a painful sensation of the tongue or mouth. The pain is variably described as a burning, tingling, hot, scalded, or numb sensation, the magnitude of which is similar to a toothache. The sensation occurs most commonly on the anterior two thirds and tip of the tongue but may include the upper alveolar region, palate, lips, and lower alveolar region. Burning mouth syndrome (BMS) affects women seven times more frequently than men. It particularly affects the middle-aged and elderly population (mean age 60 years) and has not been reported in children.

There may be xerostomia (dry mouth) (Figure 44-1), dental disease or dentures, geographic tongue (Figure 44-2), smooth tongue (Figure 44-3), candidiasis (see Chapter 53), or no visible explanation for the pain.

What To Do:

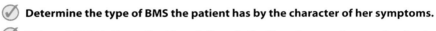 Determine the type of BMS the patient has by the character of her symptoms.

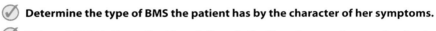 **In type 1 (35%), the patient has daily pain that is not present on awakening but progresses throughout the day and is most severe during the evening hours.** This type of pain is usually not associated with psychiatric disorders.

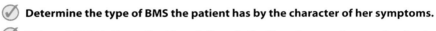 **In type 2 (55%), the patient awakens with a constant daily pain. This type of pain is associated with psychiatric conditions, especially chronic anxiety.**

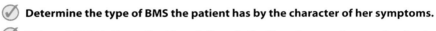 **In type 3 (10%), the patient has intermittent pain with symptom-free intervals. The pain occurs in unusual sites, such as the buccal mucosa, floor of the mouth, and throat. This type of pain is associated with allergies to food additives or flavorings.**

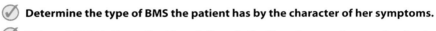 Try to determine if the patient's pain is associated with systemic, local, psychiatric or psychological, or idiopathic factors.

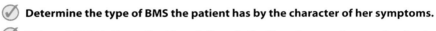 **The most common associations include psychiatric or psychological disorders, xerostomia, nutritional deficiencies, allergic contact stomatitis, denture-related factors, parafunctional behavior (e.g., bruxism and tongue thrusting), candidiasis, diabetes mellitus, and drug-related BMS. There may be more than one cause.**

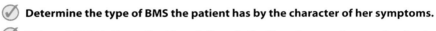 A history should include the duration of pain, its character, its pattern, and the site of involvement. Ask about depression, anxiety, and fear of cancer. Are there any exacerbating factors, such as food, mouthwash, mints, lip cosmetics, or smoking? Is there a relationship of the pain to denture use, dental work, tongue thrusting, bruxism, or jaw clenching? Look into medication use that has xerostomic potential.

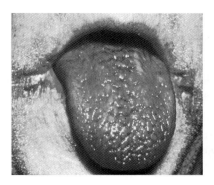

Figure 44-1 Xerostomia. (From Drage LA, Rogers RS: Burning mouth syndrome. *Dermatol Clin* 21:135-145, 2003.)

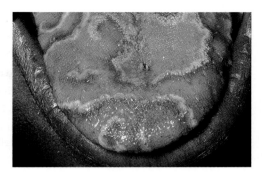

Figure 44-2 Geographic tongue. (From Bolognia J, Jorizzo J, Rapini R: *Dermatology*. St Louis, 2003, Mosby.)

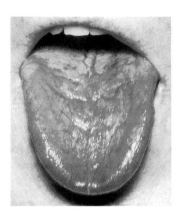

Figure 44-3 Smooth tongue. (From Drage LA, Rogers RS: Burning mouth syndrome. *Dermatol Clin* 21:135-147, 2003.)

✓ A general physical examination should be performed with emphasis on a thorough oral evaluation, and, when appropriate, reassurance that cancer is not present. Look for erythema, ulcers, glossitis, atrophy, candidiasis, dentures, geographic tongue, lichen planus, and xerostomia.

✓ When a psychiatric disorder is suspected, referral for psychiatric evaluation, medication, and psychotherapy evaluation may play a role in alleviating the symptoms. Antidepressants and anxiolytics with less anticholinergic impact (hence, less xerostomia) are preferred. Serotonin reuptake inhibitors may be a good choice in this setting. Medical management may also include tricyclic antidepressants (amitriptyline 10 to 150 mg per day), benzodiazepines (clonazepam 0.25 to 2 mg per day), or anticonvulsants (gabapentin 300 to 1800 mg per day).

✓ Reassurance that cancer is not present should be stated clearly and repeatedly.

✓ Potential dental problems require evaluation of any dental work, dentures, and parafunctional behavior (e.g., bruxism) by a specialist. Avoidance of irritants, removal of dentures at night, treatment of dentures with anticandidal agents, and a review of dental hygiene should occur.

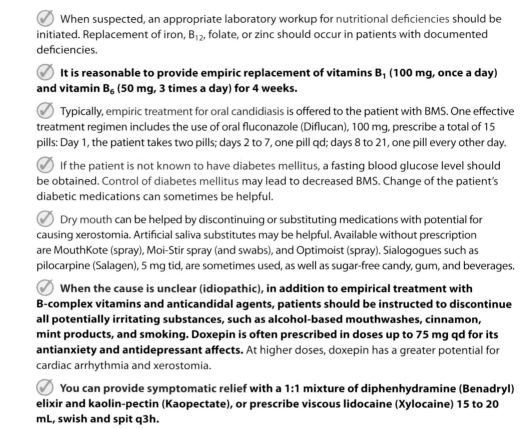

When suspected, an appropriate laboratory workup for nutritional deficiencies should be initiated. Replacement of iron, B_{12}, folate, or zinc should occur in patients with documented deficiencies.

It is reasonable to provide empiric replacement of vitamins B_1 (100 mg, once a day) and vitamin B_6 (50 mg, 3 times a day) for 4 weeks.

Typically, empiric treatment for oral candidiasis is offered to the patient with BMS. One effective treatment regimen includes the use of oral fluconazole (Diflucan), 100 mg, prescribe a total of 15 pills: Day 1, the patient takes two pills; days 2 to 7, one pill qd; days 8 to 21, one pill every other day.

If the patient is not known to have diabetes mellitus, a fasting blood glucose level should be obtained. Control of diabetes mellitus may lead to decreased BMS. Change of the patient's diabetic medications can sometimes be helpful.

Dry mouth can be helped by discontinuing or substituting medications with potential for causing xerostomia. Artificial saliva substitutes may be helpful. Available without prescription are MouthKote (spray), Moi-Stir spray (and swabs), and Optimoist (spray). Sialogogues such as pilocarpine (Salagen), 5 mg tid, are sometimes used, as well as sugar-free candy, gum, and beverages.

When the cause is unclear (idiopathic), in addition to empirical treatment with B-complex vitamins and anticandidal agents, patients should be instructed to discontinue all potentially irritating substances, such as alcohol-based mouthwashes, cinnamon, mint products, and smoking. Doxepin is often prescribed in doses up to 75 mg qd for its antianxiety and antidepressant affects. At higher doses, doxepin has a greater potential for cardiac arrhythmia and xerostomia.

You can provide symptomatic relief with a 1:1 mixture of diphenhydramine (Benadryl) elixir and kaolin-pectin (Kaopectate), or prescribe viscous lidocaine (Xylocaine) 15 to 20 mL, swish and spit q3h.

If the onset is recent, an alternative approach is to have the patient rinse with a topical anesthetic mouth rinse for 3 minutes and then apply capsaicin gel (0.025%) for 3 minutes. This is repeated morning and evening for 6 weeks. (This works best in neuropathic pain of recent onset.)

If the cause is uncertain and persists, refer the patient for a comprehensive medical evaluation.

What Not To Do:

Do not assume that the patient has a purely psychiatric cause for her pain until all other potential causes have been considered and appropriate consultations have been made.

Discussion

Burning mouth syndrome is the occurrence of oral pain in a patient with a normal oral mucosal examination.

Psychiatric disease is a common underlying factor in patients with BMS. At least one third of patients may have an underlying psychiatric diagnosis, most commonly depression or anxiety disorders. A phobic concern regarding cancer is also prominent in 20% of patients. Remember that depression and psychological disturbance are common in chronic pain populations and may be secondary to the chronic pain, rather than the cause of BMS. In addition, many

Discussion continued

of the medications that are used to treat psychiatric disease can cause xerostomia and exacerbate BMS.

Dry mouth is a frequent complaint among BMS patients. Drug-related xerostomia is common and can occur with many medications, including tricyclic antidepressants, benzodiazepines, monoamine oxidase inhibitors, antihypertensives, and antihistamines. Connective tissue diseases, such as Sjögren syndrome, or sicca syndrome, can cause xerostomia, as can a history of local irradiation or diabetes mellitus. Even stress and anxiety can lead to a dry mouth.

Because of rapid cell turnover and trauma, the oral cavity is especially sensitive to nutritional deficiencies and may be the first indicator of such a problem. Iron-deficiency anemia, pernicious anemia (an autoimmune B_{12} deficiency), zinc deficiency, and B-complex vitamin deficiency have all been reported to cause BMS.

Flavoring or food additives have been implicated as possible allergens in BMS. Cinnamon aldehyde (cinnamon), sorbic acid, tartrazine, benzoic acid, propylene glycol, menthol, and peppermint have all been identified as potential causes of mouth pain.

Denture-related pain is usually caused by faulty design, irritation, or parafunctional behavior. Candidiasis can also contribute to denture-related pain. Most BMS patients with dentures or significant dental work benefit from referral for a formal dental consultation to assess dental work, dentures, occlusion, and the need for modification or replacement.

Candidiasis is reported as a causative factor in 6% to 30% of patients with BMS. The mucosal alterations typically seen with candidiasis (thrush) may be minimal or absent. Candidal overgrowth occurs with xerostomia, corticosteroid treatment, antibiotic treatment, denture use, and diabetes mellitus. Empiric treatment for oral candidiasis is often prescribed to patients with BMS.

Approximately 5% of BMS patients have diabetes mellitus. BMS is the second most common oral complaint after xerostomia in a study of diabetic patients. Improved control of their diabetes mellitus may lead to improvement or cure of BMS.

The angiotensin-converting enzyme inhibitors enalapril, captopril, and lisinopril can cause scalded mouth or BMS. There is often improvement with reduction or discontinuation of the medication.

Although they are often regarded as asymptomatic variants of normal, multiple studies have shown geographic, fissured, or scalloped tongues more frequently in patients with tongue pain. When these patients complain of pain, technically they do not fit under the rubric of BMS but can be treated as such and should be reassured about their possibly increased fear of cancer.

Identification of correctable causes of BMS should be emphasized, and psychiatric causes should not be invoked without thorough evaluation of the patient. Such a thoughtful and structured evaluation has been associated with improvement in approximately 70% of these patients.

Suggested Readings

Drage LA, Rogers RS: Burning mouth syndrome, *Dermatol Clin* 21:135–145, 2003.

Grushka M, Epstein J, Gorsky M: Burning mouth syndrome, *Am Fam Physician* 65:615–621, 2002.

Vickers R: *Burning mouth/tongue syndrome (glossodynia/glossopyrosis)* Available at www.painmanagement.usyd.edu.au/html/orofacial_burning_mouth.htm.

Dental Pain, Periapical Abscess

(Tooth Abscess)

Presentation

The patient complains of severe, constant facial or dental pain, often associated with facial swelling, regional lymphadenopathy, and cellulitis, and may be accompanied by signs of systemic toxicity. The pain may be gnawing or throbbing or sharp and shooting. Dental caries may or may not be apparent. Percussion of the offending tooth causes increased pain (Figure 45-1). The severe toothache may be exacerbated by thermal changes, especially cold drinks. On the other hand, hot and cold sensitivity may no longer be present because of necrosis of the pulp. A fluctuant abscess may be palpated in the buccal or palatal gingiva, but usually extending toward the buccal side and to the gingival–buccal reflection.

See normal anatomy (Figure 45-2) with subsequent development of periapical abscess and cellulitis (Figure 45-3).

What To Do:

⊘ **The quickest way to control dental pain is with a dental block. See Appendix D for inferior alveolar or apical nerve block.** Use of bupivacaine (Marcaine) as the anesthetic agent will give prolonged pain relief.

⊘ **Adequate pain medication should be administered and prescribed for continued pain relief until dental follow-up can be arranged.** Nonsteroidal anti-inflammatory drugs (NSAIDs) are excellent for dental pain and often suffice or can be administered in combination with narcotic pain medications for synergistic analgesia if necessary. Provide a small prescription for 15 tabs of acetaminophen with hydrocodone or oxycodone (Vicodin or Percocet) to help manage the patient's pain until he can follow up with a dentist.

⊘ Antibiotics are not necessary to treat apical abscesses unless concurrent cellulitis is present.

⊘ **When cellulitis and facial swelling are present, depending on the level of toxicity, the patient initially should be treated with either parenteral or oral penicillin. A 10-day course of penicillin VK, 500 mg qid, should be prescribed in adults or 50 mg/kg/day divided into three doses in children. Erythromycin or clindamycin may be substituted if the patient is allergic to penicillin.**

⊘ If a fluctuant gingival abscess cavity is present (Figure 45-4), **perform incision and drainage at the most dependent location.** Provide local anesthesia with 1% lidocaine (Xylocaine) with epinephrine. With gingival swelling and fluctuance, incision and drainage can often be accomplished by sliding a No. 15 scalpel blade between the tooth and gingiva.

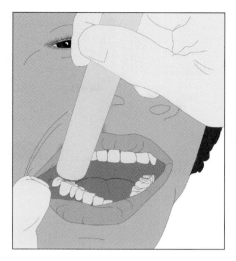

Figure 45-1 Percussion of tooth with tongue blade.

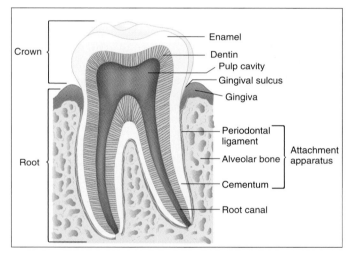

Figure 45-2 Normal tooth anatomy. (From Marx JA, Hockberger RS, Walls RM, et al: *Rosen's emergency medicine concepts and clinical practice*, ed 7. Philadelphia, 2010, Mosby.)

Instruct the patient to apply warm compresses to the affected area and seek follow-up care from a dentist within 24 hours. Definitive therapy is root canal treatment or extraction.

When drug-seeking behavior is suspected, limit narcotic prescriptions, and assist the patient by ensuring that early dental consultation is obtained.

What Not To Do:

Do not obtain radiographs for an uncomplicated abscess.

Do not insert an obstructing pack (i.e., cotton soaked with oil of cloves) into a tooth cavity when an abscess or cellulitis is present.

Do not prescribe aspirin if it is possible that a tooth will need to be extracted.

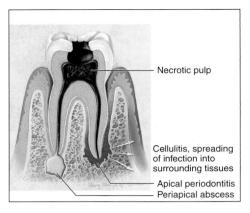

Necrotic pulp

Cellulitis, spreading
of infection into
surrounding tissues

Apical periodontitis

Periapical abscess

Figure 45-3 Apical periodontitis, periapical abscess, and cellulitis.
(From Douglass AB, Douglass JM: Common dental emergencies. *Am Fam Physician* 67:511-513, 2003.)

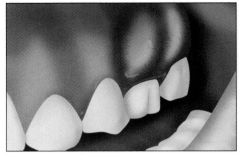

Figure 45-4 Abscess adjacent to primary tooth.

Discussion

A periapical abscess originates in the dental pulp, usually secondary to dental caries that erode the protective layers of the tooth (enamel, dentin) and allow bacteria to invade the pulp, producing a pulpitis. A severely inflamed pulp (pulpitis) will eventually necrose, causing apical periodontitis, which is inflammation around the apex of the tooth. Apical abscess is a localized, purulent form of apical periodontitis. Cellulitis may follow apical periodontitis or abscess if the infection spreads into the surrounding tissues (see Figure 45-4). This is the most common dental abscess in children.

Dental pain may be referred to the ear, temple, eye, neck, or other teeth. Conversely, what appears to be dental pain may, in fact, be caused by overlying maxillary sinusitis or otitis.

Diabetes, immune deficiency diseases, and valvular heart disease increase the risk for complications from bacteremia. Local extension of infection can lead to retropharyngeal abscess, Ludwig cellulitis, cavernous sinus thrombosis, osteomyelitis, mediastinitis, and pulmonary abscess, which are all serious complications requiring immediate consultation with an appropriate specialist.

An acute periodontal (as opposed to periapical) abscess, involves the supporting structures of the teeth (periodontal ligaments, alveolar bone), and causes localized, painful, fluctuant swelling of the gingiva, either between the teeth or laterally, and is associated with vital teeth that are not usually sensitive to percussion. This condition is found in patients with chronic periodontal disease and is the most common dental abscess in adults. It may also occur in patients (including children) who have a foreign object lodged in the gingiva. The involved tooth may be tender to percussion and show increased mobility. Treatment consists of local infiltrative anesthesia and drainage by subgingival curettage. In severe cases or cases in which there is fever, prescribe doxycycline, 100 mg bid for 10 days. Also, instruct the patient to rinse his mouth with warm salt water and consult a dentist for further treatment. Severe periodontitis in a young patient should raise the possibility of an underlying immune disorder.

Suggested Reading

Douglass AB: Common dental emergencies, *Am Fam Physician* 67:511–516, 2003.

Dental Pain, Pericoronitis

Presentation

The patient is between the ages of 17 and 25 and seeks help because of painful swelling and infection around an erupting or impacted third molar (wisdom tooth). There may be a bad taste caused by pus oozing from the area. The pain may be mild but is usually quite intense and may radiate to the external neck, the throat, the ear, or the oral floor. Occasionally, there is trismus (the inability to open the jaws more than a few millimeters) or pain on biting. The site appears red and swollen, with a flap that may reveal a partial tooth eruption beneath it. There may be purulent drainage when the flap is pulled open. There should be no pain on percussion of the tooth.

Even with relatively minor enlargement of the operculum (flap), the third molar region of the mandible can be very painful (Figure 46-1). Cervical lymphadenopathy, fever, and malaise may be present in the more advanced cases.

What To Do:

✓ **Irrigate with a weak (2%) hydrogen peroxide solution. Purulent material can be released by placing the catheter tip of the irrigating syringe under the tissue flap overlying the impacted molar. A syringe with an Angiocath catheter will work well to accomplish this.**

✓ **Prescribe oral analgesics for comfort.**

✓ **When the problem is no longer localized and there is evidence of cellulitis, prescribe penicillin to be taken over the next 10 days (penicillin V potassium, 500 mg qid). Use erythromycin, azithromycin, or clindamycin in penicillin-allergic individuals. Cefuroxime axetil is also effective in the treatment of acute dental infections.**

✓ Instruct the patient regarding the importance of cleansing away any food particles that collect beneath the gingival flap. This can be accomplished simply by using a soft toothbrush or by using water-jet irrigation. Have the patient rinse and swish with a hot, salty mouthwash after meals and at least four times per day.

✓ **A follow-up visit with a dentist should be arranged** so that the resolution of the acute infection can be observed and so that the patient can be evaluated to see if symptomatic treatment can suffice until eruption is complete or if surgical therapy to remove the gum flap or underlying tooth is necessary.

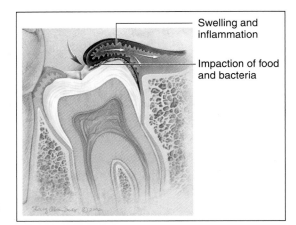

Swelling and inflammation

Impaction of food and bacteria

Figure 46-1 Mild pericoronitis. (From Douglass AB, Douglass JM: Common dental emergencies. *Am Fam Physician* 67:511-516, 2003.)

What Not To Do:

Ⓧ Do not undertake any major blunt dissection while draining pus. This could spread a superficial infection into the deep spaces of the head and neck or follow a deep abscess posteriorly into the carotid sheath.

Discussion

Pericoronitis is a special type of acute periodontal abscess that occurs when gingival tissue (gum flap, or operculum) overlies a partially erupted or impacted tooth (usually a third molar, also known as a wisdom tooth). Recurring acute symptoms are usually initiated by trauma inflicted by the opposing tooth or by impaction of food or debris under the flap of tissue that partially covers the erupting tooth.

When dental referral is not readily available, one procedure that can relieve the pain is surgical removal of the operculum. Inject local anesthetic, such as lidocaine (Xylocaine) 1% with epinephrine, directly into the overlying tissue, and then cut it away using the outline of the tooth as a guide for the incision. Sutures are not required.

Suggested Reading

Sasaki I, Morihana T, Kaneko A, et al: Clinical evaluation of cefuroxime axetil in acute dental infections (in Japanese), *Jpn J Antibiot* 43:2035–2068, 1990.

Dental Pain, Postextraction Alveolar Osteitis

(Dry Socket)

Presentation

The patient develops severe, dull, throbbing pain 2 to 4 days after a tooth extraction. The pain is often excruciating, may radiate to the ear, and is not relieved by oral analgesics. There may be associated foul taste and odor (halitosis). The extraction blood clot is absent from the tooth socket, the bony walls of which are denuded and exquisitely sensitive to even gentle probing.

If untreated, the pain may last for 10 to 40 days.

What To Do:

✓ **Treatment is optimized by first administering an anesthetic nerve block with a long-acting local anesthetic, such as bupivacaine (Marcaine) 0.5% (see Appendix D).**

✓ **Irrigate the socket with warm normal saline solution or with 0.12% warmed chlorhexidine, and remove all retained debris.**

✓ Pack the socket with ¼-inch iodoform gauze soaked in oil of cloves (eugenol).

✓ **An alternative to packing with iodoform gauze is to fill the socket with zinc oxide or, when available, commercial dry socket dressing material (Alvogyl).** It has been reported that immediate pain relief can be obtained by mixing this paste with one crushed aspirin and 2 drops of eugenol. This mixture can be inserted with the wooden end of a cotton-tipped applicator. Placing a moistened, folded gauze pad over the site will prevent this material from coming out. Have the patient keep it covered for a few hours.

✓ **Have the patient take 4000 mg/day of vitamin C. This has been associated with rapid recovery from dry socket in one study.**

✓ **Prescribe oxycodone (Percocet, Tylox) and nonsteroidal anti-inflammatory drugs (NSAIDs) for additional pain relief.**

✓ Refer the patient back to her dentist for follow-up. The gauze packing should be removed and replaced every 24 hours until symptoms subside. Advise the patient that the dry socket paste will dissolve over the next few days and likely need to be replaced by the dentist at least one more time in most cases.

What Not To Do:

✖ Do not try to create a new clot by stirring up bleeding. Scraping the socket can implant bacteria in the alveolar bone, setting the stage for osteomyelitis.

Discussion

Dry socket results from a pathologic process combining loss of the healing blood clot with a localized inflammation (alveolar osteitis). Fibrinolysis produced by bacterial activity may contribute to the production of the dry socket.

It most commonly occurs with difficult extractions of the mandibular molars, especially third retained molars. This condition may be promoted by smoking, spitting, or drinking through a straw—

activities that create negative pressure in the oral cavity. Thirty percent of women taking **oral contraceptives** experience dry sockets after their surgery. (The best time for them to have their wisdom teeth removed is during the last week of their menstrual cycle—days 23 through 28.)

Intractable pain usually responds to a nerve block with long-acting local anesthetics.

Suggested Readings

Carvalho P, Mariano R, Okamoto T: Treatment of fibrinolytic alveolitis with rifamycin B diethylamide associated with Gelfoam: a histological study, *Braz Dent J* 8:3–8, 1997.

Halberstein RA, Abrahnsohn GM: Clinical management and control of alveolalgia ("dry socket") with vitamin C, *Am J Dent* 16:152–154, 2003.

Torres-Lagares D, Serrera-Figallo MA, Romero-Ruíz MM, et al: Update on dry socket: a review of the literature (in Spanish), *Med Oral Patol Oral Cir Bucal* 10:81–85, 77–81, 2005.

Turner PS: A clinical study of "dry socket", *Int J Oral Surg* 11:226–231, 1982.

Dental Pain, Pulpitis

Presentation

The patient develops an acute toothache with sharp, throbbing pain that is often worse with recumbent position. The patient may or may not be aware that he has a cavity in the affected tooth. Initially, the pain is decreased by heat application and increased by cold application, but as the condition progresses, heat application worsens the pain, whereas application of ice dramatically relieves it. (The patient might come to the emergency department with his own cup of ice and may not allow examination unless ice can be kept on the tooth.) Oral examination may reveal dental cavities (caries) or an extensive tooth restoration, without facial or gingival swelling.

What To Do:

✓ **Administer a strong analgesic, such as oxycodone in combination with acetaminophen (Percocet, Tylox), and prescribe additional medication, including nonsteroidal anti-inflammatory drugs (NSAIDs), for home use. Severe pain may necessitate a nerve block with a long-acting local anesthetic, such as bupivacaine (Marcaine) 0.5% (see Appendix D).**

✓ If a cavity is present, insert a small cotton pledget soaked in oil of cloves (eugenol). The cotton should fill the cavity loosely without rising above the opening (where it would strike the opposing tooth). An alternative to eugenol is a pearl of benzonatate (Tessalon Perles), opened so that the contents can soak the small cotton pledget. Alternatively, benzonatate pearls can be prescribed, and the patient can bite them for repeated topical anesthesia.

✓ **Refer the patient to a dentist for definitive therapy (removal of caries, removal of pulp, or removal of the tooth) within 12 hours.**

What Not To Do:

✗ Do not prescribe antibiotics if there are no signs of cellulitis or visible abscess formation.

✗ Do not pack a tooth cavity tightly with eugenol-soaked cotton. If an abscess develops, this cavity may serve as a route for drainage.

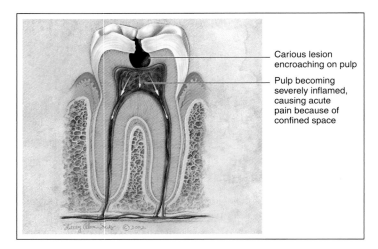

Carious lesion
encroaching on pulp

Pulp becoming
severely inflamed,
causing acute
pain because of
confined space

Figure 48-1 Irreversible pulpitis. (From Douglass AB, Douglass JM: Common dental emergencies. *Am Fam Physician* 67:511-516, 2003.)

Discussion

Dental decay presents visually as opaque white areas of enamel with gray undertones or, in more advanced cases, as brownish, discolored cavitations. Caries are initially asymptomatic. Pain does not occur until the decay impinges on the pulp and an inflammatory process develops. **Reversible pulpitis** is mild inflammation of the tooth pulp caused by caries encroaching on the pulp. Pain is triggered by hot, cold, and sweet stimuli; lasts for a few seconds; and resolves spontaneously. Treatment involves removal of the carious tissue and replacement with a dental restoration or filling.

As the patient's condition progresses from reversible pulpitis to **irreversible pulpitis** (Figure 48-1) and pulpal necrosis, he experiences excruciating pain caused by fluid and gaseous pressure within a closed space. Heat increases the pressure and pain, whereas cold reduces it. The pain is persistent and is often poorly localized.

Intractable pain usually responds to nerve block techniques with injection of long-acting local anesthetics.

If a patient refuses a nerve block or a nerve block fails to relieve the pain, consider the possibility that the patient is seeking drugs. At the same time, remember that some people have extreme phobias about dental injections. When in doubt, err on the side of compassion.

The only way to definitively treat the discomfort of irreversible pulpitis is root canal treatment (removal of the pulp and filling of the empty pulp chamber and canal) or extraction of the tooth. The urgency of referral to a dentist should be determined by the patient's level of discomfort, but examination should not be delayed for more than a few days. Patients should be warned to return if they develop signs of cellulitis, such as facial swelling, fever, and malaise.

Suggested Reading

Douglass AB, Douglas JM: Common dental emergencies, *Am Fam Physician* 67:511–516, 2003.

Dental Trauma

(Fracture, Subluxation, and Displacement)

Presentation

After a direct blow to the mouth in an accidental fall, motor vehicle collision, sports activity, or fight, a portion of a patient's tooth (most often one of the maxillary incisors) may be broken off, or a tooth may be loosened to a variable degree.

Ellis class I dental fractures (Figure 49-1) involve only enamel and are a problem only if they have left a sharp edge, which can be filed down with an emery board. Ellis class II fractures (Figure 49-2) expose yellow dentin, which is sensitive to temperature, percussion, and forced air; can become infected; and should be covered. Ellis class III fractures (Figure 49-3) expose pulp that is pink, may bleed, and usually hurt.

A tooth that is either impacted inward or partially avulsed outward is recognizable, because its occlusal surface is out of alignment compared with adjacent teeth. There is also usually some hemorrhaging at the gingival margin. If several teeth move together, suspect a fracture of the alveolar ridge. Figure 49-4 shows normal dental anatomy.

What To Do:

✓ Assess the patient for any associated injuries, such as facial or mandibular fractures. Pay special attention to the temporomandibular joints. Clean and irrigate the mouth to expose all injuries. Touch injured teeth with a tongue depressor, or grasp them between gloved fingers to see if they are loose, sensitive, painful, or bleeding.

✓ **Consider possible locations of any tooth fragments.** Broken tooth fragments may be embedded in the soft tissue, swallowed, or aspirated. Intraoral wounds should be explored for retained dental fragments. **Ultrasonography can be used to detect foreign bodies that may be deeply imbedded and difficult to palpate. A chest radiograph examination can disclose tooth fragments that have been aspirated into the bronchial tree.**

✓ When there is an open wound, provide tetanus prophylaxis as indicated.

✓ For uncomplicated **Ellis class I fractures,** the patient can be instructed to file the rough edges with an emery board and then to see a dentist for reshaping and polishing the broken tooth or, for larger fractures, providing composite fillings to replace the broken portion.

✓ For sensitive **Ellis class II fractures** exposing dentin, **cover the exposed surface with a calcium hydroxide composition (Dycal), zinc oxide, tooth varnish (copal ether varnish), cyanoacrylate (Dermabond), a strip of Stomahesive, or clear nail polish to decrease sensitivity.** Younger patients have less dentin; therefore the pulp is closer to the enamel

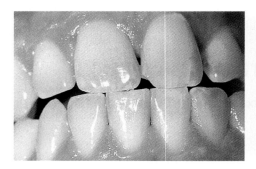

Figure 49-1 Ellis class I dental fracture. (From Knoop KJ, Stack LB, Storrow AB: *Atlas of emergency medicine.* New York, 2002, McGraw-Hill.)

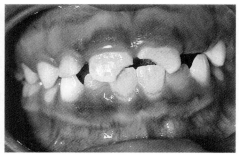

Figure 49-2 Ellis class II dental fracture. (From Knoop KJ, Stack LB, Storrow AB: *Atlas of emergency medicine.* New York, 2002, McGraw-Hill.)

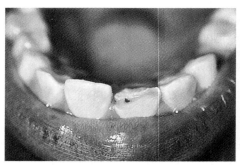

Figure 49-3 Ellis class III dental fracture. (From Knoop KJ, Stack LB, Storrow AB: *Atlas of emergency medicine.* New York, 2002, McGraw-Hill.)

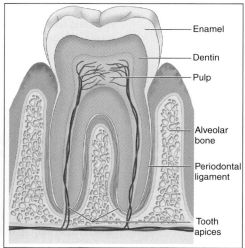

Figure 49-4 Anatomy of the tooth.

and is at greater risk for injury and infection. Treat these patients aggressively. **Provide pain medications,** instruct the patient to avoid hot and cold food or drink, and arrange for follow-up with a dentist the next day. Children should be referred the same day if possible.

Patients with **Ellis class III fractures** exposing pulp **should be seen by a dentist immediately (ideally within 3 hours). The tooth should be cleaned, then calcium hydroxide or moist cotton covered with foil be used as a temporary covering. Alternatively, medical-grade cyanoacrylate (Dermabond) can be placed on the exposed pulp to decrease the risk for infection and reduce the pain of an exposed nerve. Provide analgesics as needed.**

Prescribe penicillin (Pen-Vee K), 500 mg qid × 10 days. Use erythromycin or azithromycin in penicillin-allergic individuals. Root canal will have to be performed to avoid dental extraction.

✓ **Minimally subluxed (loosened) teeth** may require no emergency treatment other than a soft diet for 1 to 2 weeks and dental follow-up. **Very loose teeth** should be pressed back into their sockets (see Chapter 42) and wired or covered with a temporary periodontal splint (Coe-Pak) for stability for up to 48 hours. The patient should be scheduled for dental follow-up, definitive fixation, and a possible root canal. These patients should be placed on a soft food or liquid diet to prevent further tooth motion. Antibiotic prophylaxis with penicillin should be provided (Pen-Vee K), 500 mg qid for 5 to 10 days.

✓ **Intruded primary teeth and permanent teeth** of young patients can be left alone and allowed to re-erupt. Intruded teeth of adolescents and older patients are usually repositioned by an oral surgeon.

✓ **An extruded primary or permanent tooth** can be readily returned to its original position by applying firm pressure with your fingers. Both intrusive and extrusive injuries require early dental follow-up and antibiotic prophylaxis, such as penicillin V potassium, 500 mg qid × 10 days (see Chapter 42).

✓ **Inform patients that any trauma to teeth can disrupt the blood supply to a tooth and lead to the eventual need for root canal.**

What Not To Do:

✗ Do not fail to consider or recognize domestic abuse and/or child abuse.

✗ Do not overlook associated injuries of the alveolar ridge, mandible, facial bones, or neck.

✗ Do not use bone wax on complicated crown fractures with exposure of the pulp. It can cause inflammatory reactions.

Discussion

Accurately describing the dental anatomy can be very helpful when communicating with your dental consultant. The adult mouth consists of 32 teeth, named from midline to lateral. There is a set of central incisors and lateral incisors, a set of canines (or cuspids), two sets of premolars (or bicuspids), and three sets of permanent molars (first, second, and third molars). The third molars are referred to as "wisdom" teeth.

Each tooth is assigned a number starting with the right maxillary third molar as number 1, ending with the left maxillary third molar as number 16. The number 17 is assigned to the left mandibular third molar and the number 32 to the right mandibular third molar (Figure 49-5).

Dentists generally no longer use the Ellis system for classifying dental fractures. These fractures can simply be described as being an uncomplicated "enamel fracture" or a fracture with "exposed dentin"

or a complicated crown fracture that involves the pulp of the tooth. Exposure of dentin leads to variable sequelae, depending on the age of the patient. Because it is composed of microtubules, dentin can serve as a conduit for pathogenic microorganisms.

In children, the exposed dentin in an Ellis class II fracture lies nearer the neurovascular pulp and is more likely to lead to a pulp infection. Therefore, **in patients younger than 12 years of age**, this injury requires a dressing such as a calcium hydroxide composition (Dycal). Mix a drop of resin and catalyst over the fracture, and, although unnecessary, if you wish, cover it with dry aluminum foil. When in doubt, consult a dentist. If these fractures are covered quickly, pulpal contamination can be prevented, and subsequent root canal may be avoided.

(continued)

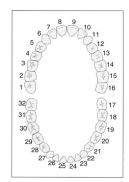

Figure 49-5 Dental map.

Discussion continued

In older patients with Ellis class II fractures, the previously mentioned treatment may be applied; however, treatment, including administration of analgesics, avoidance of hot and cold foods, and follow-up with a dentist within 24 hours, is quite adequate.

If a temporary periodontal splint (Coe-Pak) or wire is not available to stabilize loose teeth, spread soft wax over palatal and labial tooth surfaces and neighboring teeth as a temporary splint (see Chapter 42 for additional techniques).

Root fractures are clinically difficult to diagnose; patients may notice abnormal mobility and sensitivity to percussion of the tooth.

Suggested Reading

Hile LM, Linklater DR: Use of 2-octyl cyanoacrylate for the repair of a fractured molar tooth, *Ann Emerg Med* 47:424–426, 2006.

Gingivitis and Acute Necrotizing Ulcerative Gingivitis

(Trench Mouth)

Presentation

With mild gingivitis, the patient's gums bleed easily and become red and swollen with increased sensitivity. As symptoms worsen, the gums begin to recede and take on a beefy red, inflamed color.

Further progression leads to the most severe periodontal infection, trench mouth, or acute necrotizing ulcerative gingivitis (ANUG). The patient complains of generalized severe pain of the gums, often with a foul taste or fetid odor. The gingiva will appear edematous and red, with a grayish necrotic membrane between the teeth. The gums bleed spontaneously or on gentle touch, and there is loss of gingival tissue, especially the interdental papillae. The teeth will eventually become loose, and the patient may become febrile and show signs of systemic infection with generalized weakness.

What To Do:

✓ **For the more severe forms of gingivitis, prescribe (in order of preference) tetracycline, penicillin V potassium, or erythromycin, 250 to 500 mg qid for 10 days. Do not use tetracycline in children younger than 8 years of age, because it may cause permanent discoloration of the teeth.**

✓ **For milder cases, instruct the patient to rinse with warm saline every 1 to 2 hours, floss, and gently brush with sodium bicarbonate toothpaste.** The use of a power toothbrush with rotating/oscillating motion is better than a manual brush.

✓ **In all cases, have the patient rinse his mouth with an antiseptic solution: Use chlorhexidine 0.12% oral rinse (PerioGard), 15 mL (1 tablespoon), swished in the mouth for 30 seconds, and spit out qid. Half-strength hydrogen peroxide may also be used as a mouth rinse.**

✓ For comfort, prescribe viscous lidocaine (Xylocaine) 2%. Rinse and spit 1 tbsp q6-8h.

✓ A narcotic analgesic (hydrocodone [Vicodin]) may sometimes be required.

✓ **For definitive care and the prevention of periodontal disease, refer the patient for dental follow-up. The dentist will remove any dead gum tissue (débridement) to promote healing and help reduce pain. In severe cases, periodontal surgery may be required to restore gum tissue.**

✓ **Nonsteroidal anti-inflammatory drugs (NSAIDs) have been shown to speed the resolution of inflammation** when teeth are being cleaned and scaled to remove plaque. With appropriate treatment, patients usually respond dramatically in 48 to 72 hours.

What Not To Do:

(X) Do not obtain radiographs or diagnostic blood work. Gingivitis is a clinical diagnosis, and special testing is required only if the patient is very ill or not responding to initial therapy or when a more serious underlying disease is suspected.

Discussion

Gingivitis and trench mouth are infections of the gum tissue. The most common type of gingivitis involves the marginal gingiva and is brought on by the accumulation of microbial plaques in persons with inadequate oral hygiene. Eventually, the gingiva separates from the tooth, pockets develop, the periodontal ligaments break down, and, along with alveolar bone destruction, the teeth loosen and eventually fall out.

Acute necrotizing ulcerative gingivitis is also known as trench mouth or Vincent *angina*. This condition is usually seen in those patients who practice very poor oral hygiene, those who are under stress, those who smoke, and sometimes those who have immune deficiencies. The term *trench mouth* was coined in World War I, when ANUG was common among trench-bound soldiers.

ANUG is different from simple gingivitis in that it is an acute infection of the gingiva, with organisms such as *Prevotella intermedia,* alpha-hemolytic streptococci, *Actinomyces* species, or any number of different oral spirochetes. Systemic diseases that may simulate the appearance of ANUG include infectious mononucleosis, leukemia, aplastic anemia, and agranulocytosis.

Treatment of trench mouth is generally highly effective, and complete healing often occurs in a few weeks. Healing may take longer if the patient's immune system is compromised, such as by HIV/AIDS.

Lacerations of the Mouth

Presentation

Because of the rich vascularity of the soft tissues of the mouth, impact injuries often lead to dramatic hemorrhages that bring patients with relatively trivial lacerations to the ED and other healthcare facilities. Blunt trauma to the face can cause secondary lacerations of the lips, frenulum, buccal mucosa, gingiva, and tongue. Active bleeding has usually stopped by the time a patient with a minor laceration has reached the clinic or ED.

What To Do:

✓ Provide appropriate tetanus prophylaxis (see Appendix H), and check for associated injuries, such as loose teeth and mandibular or facial fractures. Crushed ice wrapped in clean gauze and held inside the cheek may help limit swelling, bleeding, and discomfort.

✓ If dental fractures or avulsions are present, explore wounds thoroughly with your gloved finger, looking for a dental fragment within the wound. **In deep wounds or whenever there is the question of a retained foreign body, obtain radiographs or perform ultrasonography (using a 6.5-MHz endocavity transducer) to rule it in or out.** Ideally, all missing teeth or dental fragments should be accounted for (see Chapter 42).

✓ **When only small lacerations (less than 2 cm) are present and only minimal gaping of the wound occurs, reassurance and simple aftercare are all that is required.** Inform the patient that the wound will become somewhat uncomfortable and covered with pus over the next 48 hours, and **instruct him to rinse with lukewarm water or half-strength hydrogen peroxide for several days after meals and every 1 to 2 hours while awake. Patients may rinse with chlorhexidine 0.12% oral rinse, swished in mouth for 30 seconds and spit out four times daily.**

✓ **If there is continued bleeding or the wound edges fall between chewing surfaces, or if the wound edges gape significantly (especially on the edge of the tongue), or there is a flap or deformity when the underlying musculature contracts, the wound should be anesthetized using lidocaine with epinephrine, cleansed thoroughly with saline, and loosely approximated using a 5-0 or 6-0 absorbable suture.**

✓ **Most tongue lacerations heal well without suturing. The decision of whether or not to repair tongue lacerations depends on the estimated risk of compromised function after healing.** Lacerations that should be considered for repair **include large lacerations (greater than 1 cm in length) that extend into or pass through the muscular layers of the tongue, deep lacerations on the lateral border of the tongue, gaping lacerations or those with large flaps, or lacerations that may cause dysfunction if healed improperly (anterior split tongue). **Tongue lacerations that do not need repair include those less than 1 cm in length, nongaping lacerations, or lacerations assessed to be clinically minor.**

 ✓ Consider using procedural sedation and analgesia when suturing children who cannot cooperate (see Appendix E).

✓ A traction stitch or special rubber-tipped clamp can be very helpful when attempting to suture the tongue of a small child or an intoxicated adult (Figure 51-1). The same aftercare as described earlier applies here as well.

✓ **When the exterior surface of the lip is lacerated, any separation of the underlying musculature must be repaired with buried absorbable sutures.**

✓ **To avoid an unsightly scar when the lip heals, precise skin approximation is very important. First, approximate the vermilion border, making this the key suture** (Figure 51-2). Fine nonabsorbable suture material (e.g., 6-0 nylon or Prolene) is most appropriate for the skin surfaces of the lip, whereas a fine absorbable suture (e.g., 6-0 Dexon or Vicryl) is quite acceptable for use on the mucosa and vermilion.

✓ Although in most cases antibiotics are not indicated, for deep lacerations of the mucosa or lip or **for any sutured laceration in the mouth, it is reasonable to prescribe prophylactic penicillin (penicillin V potassium, 500 mg tid for 3 to 4 days) to prevent deep tissue infections.** (Erythromycin or azithromycin may be substituted in penicillin-allergic individuals.)

✓ Recommend acetaminophen or ibuprofen for pain.

✓ **Instruct patient to return in 48 hours for a wound reevaluation.**

✓ Recommend that the patient consume only cool liquids and soft foods beginning 4 hours after the repair.

What Not To Do:

✗ Do not bother to repair a simple laceration or avulsion of the frenulum of the upper lip. It will heal quite nicely on its own (Figure 51-3).

✗ Do not use nonabsorbable suture material on the tongue, gingiva, or buccal mucosa. There is no advantage, and suture removal on a small child will be an unpleasant struggle at best.

✗ Do not overlook domestic abuse or child abuse.

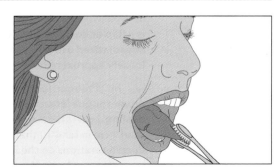

Figure 51-1 Proper use of a rubber-tipped clamp.

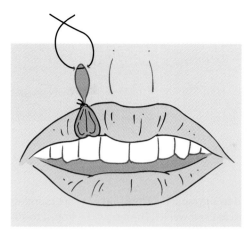

Figure 51-2 In the repair of lip lacerations, the first stitch should be placed at the vermilion-cutaneous border to obtain proper alignment. (From Grabb WC, Kleinert HE: *Techniques in surgery: facial and hand injuries.* Somerville, NJ, 1980, Ethicon, Inc.)

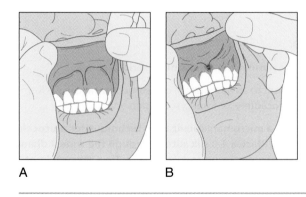

A   B

Figure 51-3 Simple laceration or avulsion of the frenulum of the upper lip. **A,** Normal frenulum. **B,** Lacerated frenulum.

Discussion

Imprecise repair of the vermilion border will lead to a "step-off" or puckering that is unsightly and difficult to repair later.

Fortunately, the tongue and oral mucosa usually heal with few complicating infections, and there is a low risk for subsequent tissue necrosis.

Suggested Reading

Grabb WC, Kleinert HE: *Techniques in surgery: facial and hand injuries*, Somerville, NJ, 1980, Ethicon, Inc.

Mucocele

(Mucous Cyst)

Presentation

A patient may be alarmed by the rapid development of a soft, rounded, nontender, fluctuant cyst, most often found inside the lower lip. The cyst varies from 2 to 10 mm in diameter. The surface is made up of pearly or translucent mucosa. It is relatively painless or asymptomatic (Figure 52-1). The patient may be aware of previous recent or remote trauma to the lip, or he may have a habit of biting his lip.

What To Do:

✓ **Reassure the patient that this is not a serious tumor.**

✓ Refer the patient to an appropriate oral surgeon who can perform laser ablation cryosurgery, electrocautery, or total cyst excision.

✓ **Alternatively, a micromarsupialization technique for mucoceles in pediatric patients has been reported. Place a 4-0 silk suture through the widest diameter of the dome of the lesion without engaging the underlying tissue. Tie a surgical knot, and leave the suture in place for 7 days, allowing a new epithelial-lined duct to form and providing egress of saliva from the obstructed minor salivary gland. The recurrence rate after this procedure was approximately 14% in pediatric patients.**

What Not To Do:

✗ Do not use the micromarsupialization technique on mucoceles that are larger than 1 cm in diameter.

✗ Do not simply unroof these lesions. They will typically recur.

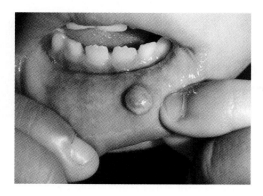

Figure 52-1 Traumatic mucous cyst. (Copyright © Vilma Pineda, DDS, Dermatlas; http://www.dermatlas.org.)

Discussion

This cyst, which is of minor salivary gland origin, is caused by traumatic rupture of the mucous gland duct, with extravasation of sialomucin into the submucosa. It usually occurs inside the lower lip but may also occur under the tongue or in the buccal mucosa. These traumatic mucus-retention cysts rupture easily, releasing sticky, straw-colored fluid. Most mucoceles occur in young individuals, with 70% of individuals being younger than 20 years.

Suggested Reading

Witman PM, Rogers RS: Pediatric oral medicine, *Dermatol Clin* 21:157–170, 2003.

Oral Candidiasis

(Thrush or Yeast Infection)

Presentation

An infant (who often has a concurrent diaper rash) has white patches in his mouth, or an older patient (who usually has poor oral hygiene, diabetes, a hematologic malignancy, an immunodeficiency, or who is on antibiotic, cytotoxic, or steroid therapy) may have few complaints or complains of a sore mouth and sensitivity to foods that are spicy or acidic. On physical examination, painless white patches are found in the mouth and on the tongue. The patches wipe off easily with a swab, leaving an erythematous base that may bleed. There also may be intense, dark red inflammation throughout the oral cavity.

What To Do:

✅ If there is any doubt about the cause, confirm the diagnosis by smearing, Gram staining, and examining the exudate under a microscope for large, gram-positive pseudohyphae and spores. Mycologic confirmation can be achieved rapidly by 10% potassium hydroxide (KOH preparation) or normal saline microscopic examination. A fungal culture may also confirm the diagnosis but is usually unnecessary and does not distinguish between colonization and true infection.

✅ **Mild cases in infants may be watched without treatment. For topical treatment, prescribe an oral suspension of nystatin (Mycostatin), 100,000 U/mL; place 1 mL in each cheek for infants and 4 to 6 mL in each cheek for children and adults.** Instruct the patient to gargle and swish the liquid in his mouth as long as possible before swallowing, 4 times a day, for at least 2 days beyond resolution of symptoms. Nystatin is also available in pastilles (lozenges) of 200,000 U; one or two pastilles can be dissolved in the mouth 4 to 5 times daily. Alternatively, for children younger than 3 years old, prescribe clotrimazole (Mycelex) in 10-mg troches to be dissolved slowly in the mouth 5 times a day for 7 to 14 days. The best time to administer medication is between meals, because this allows longer contact time. Nystatin suspension is the least expensive option, more palatable, and possibly more effective. When treating patients with diabetes, remember that nystatin suspension has a high sugar content.

✅ **For adults who do not have acquired immunodeficiency syndrome (AIDS), fluconazole (Diflucan), 100 mg qd for 14 days, may be a better regimen. Sometimes a single 200-mg oral dose is effective, but the longer course decreases the risk for recurrence. An acceptable compromise is to give 200 mg qd on day 1, followed by 100 mg qd for four more days.** Itraconazole (Sporanox) suspension (10 mg/mL), 100 to 200 mg daily for 7 days, is as effective as fluconazole.

✅ In patients with AIDS, give fluconazole, 200 mg on day 1, then 100 mg qd for 14 days or until improvement.

⊘ **Have** patients with removable dental appliances or dentures **soak them overnight in a nystatin suspension to prevent reinfection with these contaminated objects.**

⊘ **Look elsewhere for _Candida_ infection** (e.g., esophagitis, intertrigo, vaginitis, diaper rash), and treat these conditions appropriately.

⊘ For healthy newborns or infants, reassure the parents about the benign origin and course of this minor superficial yeast infection.

What Not To Do:

⊗ Do not overlook diarrhea, rashes (other than diaper rash), failure to thrive, hepatosplenomegaly, or repeated infections that may suggest an underlying immunodeficiency. Beyond infancy, be especially vigilant for those patients who have no apparent underlying cause for thrush (e.g., antibiotics, steroids).

Discussion

Oropharyngeal candidiasis or thrush is a local infection commonly found in young infants, older individuals with poor oral hygiene or dentures, diabetics, or patients treated with antibiotics, steroids, chemotherapy, or radiation therapy. Thrush can also be found in those with a hematologic malignancy or immunodeficiency, such as human immunodeficiency virus (HIV)/AIDS.

In the healthy newborn, thrush is a self-limited infection, but it usually should be treated to avoid feeding problems. The neonate acquires the yeast from the mother at the time of delivery. Most often, thrush will appear at about 1 week of age; the incidence peaks around the fourth week of life. Infants who fail to respond to treatment with nystatin oral suspension can be given nystatin or clotrimazole vaginal suppositories placed in a split pacifier, which will provide a more prolonged topical application.

In adults, oral candidiasis is found in a variety of acute and chronic forms. The pseudomembranous form is the most common and appears as white plaques on the buccal mucosa, palate, tongue, or the oropharynx. The atrophic form does not have plaques, is more common in adults with dentures, and is known as denture stomatitis. This form of oral candidiasis presents with localized erythema and erosions with minimal white exudate, which may be caused by candidal colonies beneath dentures. It is severalfold more frequent in women than in men. Thrush may also present simply as a beefy red tongue.

Thrush may be the first sign of HIV infection; its appearance in advanced HIV indicates poor prognosis. Maintenance prophylaxis may be required in patients with AIDS who have several recurrences of symptomatic oral candidiasis. After an initial 200-mg dose, fluconazole can be continued at 100 mg qd or given intermittently (200 mg weekly). A recurrence rate of 10% to 20% can be anticipated with intermittent prophylaxis.

Suggested Reading

Vazquez JA, Sobel JD: Mucosal candidiasis, _Infect Dis Clin North Am_ 16:793–820, 2002.

Oral Herpes Simplex

(Cold Sore, Fever Blister)

Presentation

Patients have swelling, burning, or soreness at the vermilion border of the lips followed by the appearance of clusters of small painful vesicles on an erythematous base (Figure 54-1). The vesicles then rupture to produce red, irregular ulcerations with swollen borders and crusting, which eventually heal without leaving a scar. These lesions can also occur on the hard palate or gingiva. Episodes may recur after exposure to sunlight or emotional or physical stress. The initial episode is usually the worst, with generalized malaise, low-grade fever, tender cervical adenopathy, and occasional exudative pharyngitis lasting 2 to 3 weeks. Recurrences are milder and shorter, with a prodrome of itching or burning at the lesion site. The painful ulcers that eventually form last 7 to 10 days.

What To Do:

✓ When there is any doubt about the diagnosis, scrape the base of a vesicle (warn the patient that this hurts), smear it on a slide, stain it with Wright or Giemsa solution, and examine it for multinucleate giant cells (look for nuclear molding). This is called a *Tzanck preparation* and establishes the diagnosis of herpes. Alternatively, a swab can be sent for viral cultures, which may take days to grow. When performing a culture, the ulcer base should be swabbed vigorously, because herpes simplex virus (HSV) is an intracellular infection and adequate cell sampling is required.

✓ **For minor symptoms,** docosanol (Abreva), a topical cream available without a prescription, started within 12 hours of prodromal symptoms, decreases time to healing by about half a day.

✓ **For moderate-to-severe symptoms, prescribe penciclovir 1% cream (Denavir), 1.5 g. Have the patient apply it every 2 waking hours for 4 days.** This treatment has been shown to hasten the resolution of lesions and pain in immunocompetent adults who have recurrent herpes simplex labialis, regardless of whether it is applied early or late in the course of the eruption. Started within 1 hour of papule appearance and applied every 2 hours while awake, it will decrease healing time by about 1 day.

✓ **An alternative treatment is oral acyclovir (Zovirax), 400 mg 5 times per day for 7 days.** This therapy reduces viral shedding, appearance of new lesions, and severity of pain and has been shown to decrease time to healing by 1 day. **A much more convenient regimen with the same efficacy is a 1-day course of valacyclovir (Valtrex),** to begin with the first symptoms of herpes labialis, 2 g q12h (2 doses). A much more costly regimen of famciclovir (Famvir), 500 mg bid for 7 days, can shorten the duration of symptoms by 2 days.

✓ **Treat recurrences early, if possible during the prodrome or at the first sign of the first skin lesion.**

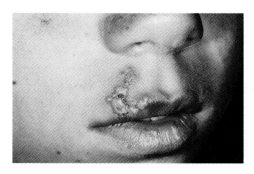

Figure 54-1 Herpes simplex labialis. (From Bolognia J, Jorizzo J, Rapini R: *Dermatology.* St Louis, 2003, Mosby.)

✓ **For comforting topical treatment,** an equal mixture of kaolin-pectin (Kaopectate) and diphenhydramine (Benadryl) elixir can coat and dry the area and reduce pain. By adding an equal part of lidocaine (Xylocaine) 2% viscous solution, a mouthwash is created that can be swished in the mouth and then expectorated (do every 3 to 4 hours). **Topical lip salves (Orabase, Zilactin, or Aphthasol) and application of cold compresses will also relieve the pain.**

✓ **Prescribe nonsteroidal anti-inflammatory drugs (NSAIDs) or even narcotics and mild sedation for the most severe pain.**

✓ Instruct the patient to keep lesions clean and to avoid touching them, which will prevent spreading the virus to the eyes, unaffected skin, and other people. Instruct the patient about the benefits of thorough hand washing. The patient should avoid kissing and other close contact while lesions are apparent.

✓ Inform the patient that oral herpes need not be related to genital herpes, that the vesicles and pain should resolve over about 2 weeks (barring superinfection), that they are infectious during this period (and perhaps at other times as well), and that the herpes simplex virus, residing in sensory ganglia, can be expected to cause recurrences from time to time (especially during periods of illness or stress). If the patient has more than six outbreaks a year, his primary care physician should consider prescribing acyclovir prophylactically.

What Not To Do:

✗ Do not prescribe topical acyclovir or corticosteroids. They are ineffective. Do not use topical anesthetics on keratinized skin. They are effective only on oral mucosa and lip vermilion.

Discussion

In most cases, **herpes labialis** is caused by herpes simplex virus type 1 (HSV-1). Primary herpes usually appears as **gingivostomatitis** (Figure 54-2), pharyngitis, or a combination of the two, whereas recurrent infections usually occur as intraoral or labial ulcers.

Primary infection is acquired mainly by direct person-to-person contact, such as kissing, wrestling, sexual intercourse, and inadvertent touching of lesions. Healthcare workers are at particular risk for **finger or hand infections** (whitlows). Primary infection tends to be a disease of childhood or young adulthood; is more severe than recurring episodes; is preceded by a temperature of up to 105° F, sore throat, and headache; and is followed by red, swollen gums that bleed easily.

(continued)

Discussion continued

This gingivostomatitis may need to be differentiated from herpangina, acute necrotizing ulcerative gingivitis, Stevens-Johnson syndrome, Behçet syndrome, and hand-foot-and-mouth disease. Herpangina is caused by Coxsackievirus group A and involves the posterior pharynx. The 1- to 4-mm intraoral vesicles do not extend beyond the soft palate and tonsillar pillars. Acute necrotizing ulcerative gingivitis, also known as *Vincent angina* or *trench mouth,* is bacterial in origin, causes characteristic blunting of the interdental gingival papillae, and responds rapidly to treatment with penicillin. Stevens-Johnson syndrome is a severe form of erythema multiforme. In this syndrome, there are characteristic lip lesions, the gingiva is only rarely affected, and there may be bull's-eye skin lesions on the hands and feet. Behçet syndrome is thought to be an autoimmune response and is associated with genital ulcers and inflammatory ocular lesions. Hand-foot-and-mouth disease is also caused by Coxsackievirus group A and is associated with concurrent lesions of the palms and soles. Fifteen percent of these cases present with oral ulceration only, making differentiation from herpes difficult, but tender cervical adenopathy is uncommon in hand-foot-and-mouth disease. Recurrent aphthous stomatitis (RAS) (see Chapter 41) is usually located on the loose mucosal surfaces of lips or buccal mucosa of the cheeks.

Recurrent HSV infection most commonly occurs on the cutaneous lip and vermilion (herpes simplex labialis). Primary infection, unlike recurrent HSV, affects both the keratinized surfaces of the oral mucosa (such as the hard palate and gingiva, where the mucosa is tightly adherent to underlying bone) and the nonkeratinized mucosal surfaces.

Secondary recurrences of cold sores are due to reactivation of latent infection in the trigeminal ganglion. Possible causes of HSV-1 reactivation include stress, fever, menstruation, gastrointestinal disturbance, infection, fatigue, and exposure to cold or sunlight.

Home remedies for cold sores include application of ether, lecithin, lysine, and vitamin E. Because herpes is a self-limiting affliction, all of these therapies work, but in controlled studies, none has outperformed placebos (which also do very well).

Among **immunocompetent patients,** HSV infections are usually self limiting, and reactivation is rapidly controlled by the host's immune system. **In the immunocompromised person,** however, the reactivated virus might continue to replicate, forming large, slowly expanding, long-lasting ulcerative lesions. More important, potentially fatal herpetic encephalitis or disseminated HSV infection is possible.

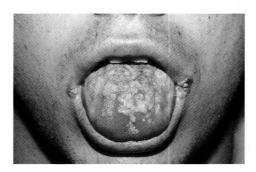

Figure 54-2 Acute herpes simplex gingivostomatitis in a young adult. (From White G, Cox N: *Diseases of the skin,* ed 2. St Louis, 2006, Mosby.)

Suggested Readings

Bruce AJ, Rogers RS: Acute oral ulcers, *Dermatol Clin* 21:1–15, 2003.

Chilukuri S, Rosen T: Management of acyclovir-resistant herpes simplex virus, *Dermatol Clin* 21:311–320, 2003.

Raborn GW, Dip MS, McGaw WT, et al: Treatment of herpes labialis with acyclovir, *Am J Med* 85(Suppl 2A):39–42, 1988.

Spruance SL, Rea TL, Thoming C, et al: Penciclovir cream for the treatment of herpes simplex labialis: a randomized, multicenter, double-blind, placebo-controlled trial, *JAMA* 277:1374–1379, 1997.

Orthodontic Complications

Presentation

Someone wearing braces on his teeth was struck on the mouth, or his orthodontic appliances broke spontaneously, puncturing, hooking, or otherwise entrapping some oral mucosa. There may be pain, blood, lacerations, a confusing tangle of wires and elastic bands, and panic on the part of the patient and family. Other problems involve food, candy, or chewing gum becoming stuck and causing gingival infection.

What To Do:

⊘ Irrigate and cleanse the mouth so that the nature of the problem can be clearly visualized.

⊘ **Inject local anesthetic (e.g., lidocaine [Xylocaine] 1% with epinephrine) into entrapped or punctured mucosa to ease the patient's discomfort and allow necessary manipulation.**

⊘ **Release mucosa from hooklike attachments** by pushing the lip against the teeth and moving it (usually upward) to unhook it. You may have to use a closed hemostat to manipulate the mucosa off of the bent wire or hooked piece of metal.

⊘ **Bend any exposed sharp wire end so that it points toward the teeth rather than toward sensitive lips and gums.** Use a hemostat to grasp the wire. If a brace wire has popped out of the bands around the molars, and the grooves (that the wire fits in) are visible, just slide the wire back in place.

⊘ **When a sharp wire cannot be moved, cover the point with any soft wax, orthodontic wax, cotton, or sugarless chewing gum.**

⊘ A loose band or bracket can generally be left in place until the patient is seen by the orthodontist. If a bracket or wire becomes excessively loose, it can usually be removed with judicious tinkering. If a wire must be cut and small wire cutters are unavailable, try repeatedly bending the appliance until the metal fatigues and breaks.

⊘ Treat gingival infections with frequent warm saline rinses and, if severe, with penicillin or erythromycin, 250 to 500 mg qid for 10 days (see Chapter 50).

⊘ With any continued discomfort, recommend over-the-counter (OTC) analgesics.

⊘ **Arrange for early orthodontic follow-up and definitive repair. Dental fractures or loosened or avulsed teeth require follow-up by a general dentist** (see Chapters 42 and 49).

What Not To Do:

(X) If at all possible, do not cut a protruding wire. It will only create another sharp edge.

(X) Do not administer antibiotics for minor oral abrasions, punctures, or small lacerations.

Discussion

Broken or disturbed appliances are likely to occur from time to time during orthodontic treatment. Fortunately, after orthodontic trauma, the tongue and oral mucosa usually heal with few complicating infections and little tissue necrosis.

Perlèche

(Angular Cheilitis)

Presentation

The patient complains of inflammation and soreness of the skin and contiguous labial mucous membranes at the angles of the mouth (Figure 56-1). On examination, there is erythema, fissuring, and maceration of the oral commissures. In severe cases, the splits can bleed when the mouth is opened, and shallow ulcers or a crust may form.

What To Do:

✓ Attempt to identify a precipitating cause, and advise corrective action when possible.

✓ **Prescribe topical antifungal cream, such as ketoconazole 2% (Nizoral), econazole 1% (Spectazole), or ciclopirox olamine 0.77% (Loprox) applied bid, followed in a few hours by a corticosteroid in a nongreasy base, such as triamcinolone 0.1% (Kenalog) cream 15 g. Discontinue the steroids when the inflammation subsides in favor of a protective lip balm, such as ChapStick.**

✓ It is critical that the oral commissure be kept dry to decrease the chances of reinfection. Continue the antifungal cream for a few weeks for greatest effectiveness.

✓ Treat any associated oral candidiasis with an appropriate oral antimycotic (see Chapter 53).

What Not To Do:

✗ Do not use ointments or creams containing neomycin (Neosporin). They are unlikely to be effective and may cause an unnecessary contact dermatitis.

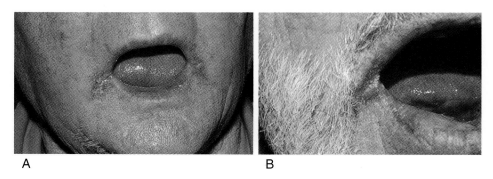

A   B

Figure 56-1 A and **B,** Perlèche. (From White G, Cox N: *Diseases of the skin.* St Louis, 2006, Mosby.)

Discussion

Perlèche is associated with the collection of moisture at the corners of the mouth, which encourages invasion by *Candida albicans*, staphylococci, streptococci, and other organisms. In children, this collection of moisture is often caused by lip-licking, drooling, thumb-sucking, and mouth-breathing. Adults may be troubled by age-related changes in oral architecture commonly seen in edentulous patients and in patients with poorly fitting dentures. The differential diagnosis includes impetigo (see Chapter 172) and herpes simplex (see Chapter 54) infections. Vitamin B_2 or zinc deficiency or iron deficiency anemia can cause perlèche, but this is rare and should not be treated presumptively. The patient should be evaluated for evidence of poor diet or malnutrition (celiac disease). Angular cheilitis can also be a sign of anorexia or bulimia secondary to the associated malnutrition and frequent vomiting. KOH preparation (potassium hydroxide) will confirm a yeast infection. Cheilosis may also be part of a group of symptoms (dysphagia resulting from upper esophageal webs, iron deficiency anemia, burning mouth syndrome with a shiny red tongue resulting from glossitis, along with cheilosis) defining the condition called Plummer-Vinson syndrome.

Suggested Readings

Loo DS: Cutaneous fungal infections in the elderly, *Dermatol Clin* 22:33–50, 2004.

Martin ES, Elewski BE: Cutaneous fungal infections in the elderly, *Clin Geriatr Med* 18:59–75, 2002.

Sialolithiasis

(Salivary Duct Stones)

Presentation

Patients of any age may develop salivary duct stones, although they are more common in men of age 30 to 60 years and less common in children. Most salivary stones occur in the Wharton duct from the submandibular gland. The patient is alarmed by the rapid swelling that suddenly appears beneath his jaw while he is eating. The swelling may be painful but is not hot or red and usually subsides within 2 hours. This swelling may only be intermittent and may not occur with every meal. Infection can occur and will be accompanied by increased pain, exquisite tenderness, erythema, and fever. Under these circumstances, pus can sometimes be expressed from the opening of the duct when the gland is pressed (Figure 57-1).

What To Do:

✓ Conservative care is the mainstay of treatment for salivary duct stones. Patients should be advised to stay well hydrated, to apply warm compresses frequently while gently massaging the gland or "milking" the duct, and to suck on lemon drops or other hard tart candy (sialogogues, which promote ductal secretions) throughout the day as frequently as tolerated.

✓ If possible, discontinue anticholinergic medications that may inhibit ductal secretions, such as diphenhydramine or amitriptyline.

✓ Control pain with nonsteroidal anti-inflammatory drugs (NSAIDs), or add narcotics if necessary.

✓ **Bimanually palpate the course of the salivary duct, feeling for stones.** For the submandibular gland, palpate the floor of the mouth anterior to this gland in order to find a stone in the Wharton duct. For the parotid gland, palpate the buccal mucosa around the orifice to the Stensen duct and along the line from the earlobe to the jawline (see Figure 57-1).

✓ **When a small superficial stone can be felt, anesthetize the tissue beneath the duct and its orifice with a small amount of lidocaine 1% with epinephrine. If available, a punctum dilator can be used to widen the orifice of the blocked duct. Milk the gland and duct with your fingers to express the stone or stones.**

✓ **If the stone cannot be palpated, try to locate it through radiographic examination.** The imaging modality of choice for the evaluation of salivary stones is high-resolution non-contrast CT scanning. Fine cuts must be requested so that the stones are not missed. CT scans have a 10-fold greater sensitivity in detecting stones than do plain films and also provide

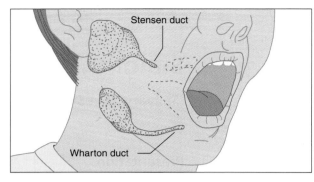

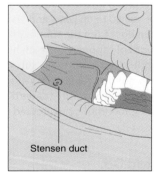

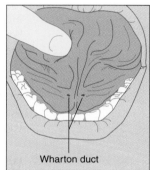

Figure 57-1 Most salivary duct stones occur in the Wharton duct.

the sensitivity to diagnose other pathology, such as a glandular mass. Standard radiographs may identify radiopaque stones with a sensitivity of 80% to 95% for submandibular stones, which tend to be larger, but only 60% for parotid stones, which tend to be smaller or not radiopaque. Dental radiographs shot at right angles to the floor of the mouth are much more likely to demonstrate small stones in the Wharton duct than standard radiograph studies. Ultrasonography is another good imaging option, identifying greater than 90% of stones that are 2 mm in diameter or larger, and it is better than sialography for describing the periglandular structures and is less invasive.

When a stone cannot be demonstrated or manually expressed, the patient should be referred for contrast sialography or surgical removal of the stone. Often, sialography, ultrasonography, CT scanning, or MRI will show whether an obstruction is due to stenosis, a stone, or a tumor.

If the patient has pain, swelling, erythema, and purulent discharge expressed from the gland and, possibly, systemic symptoms (fever/chills/tachycardia), suspect an associated infection, sialadenitis. Initiate treatment with amoxicillin/clavulanate (Augmentin), 875/125 mg bid, or clindamycin (Cleocin), 450 mg q6h, for 10 days after obtaining cultures. For the more severe infections (e.g., when there is fever, tachycardia, severe swelling, and pain), consider hospitalization for administration of IV antibiotics.

What Not To Do:

Ⓧ Do not attempt to dilate a salivary duct if the patient has a suspected case of mumps. Acute, persistent pain and swelling of the parotid gland along with inflammation of the papilla of the Stensen duct, fever, lymphocytosis, hyperamylasemia, and malaise should raise suspicion for mumps or other viruses that may cause sialadenitis.

Ⓧ Do not obtain sialography with acute infection. Injection of dye into an acutely inflamed gland may push the infection outside the gland capsule and into the surrounding soft tissues.

Discussion

Sialolithiasis is the most common disorder of the salivary glands and may range from tiny particles to stones that are several centimeters in length. Salivary duct stones are generally composed of calcium phosphate and hydroxyapatite. Uric acid stones may form in patients with gout. Although the majority, approximately 92%, form in the Wharton duct (which arises from the medial surface of the submandibular glands) in the floor of the mouth, approximately 6% to 20% occur in the Stensen duct (which arises from the anterior border of the parotid gland) in the cheek, and 1% to 2% occur in the sublingual ducts. The exact cause of stone formation is unclear but it is felt to be secondary to secretion of saliva rich in calcium in the setting of partial obstruction of the duct caused by local inflammation or ductal injury, with consequent promotion of stone formation. Dehydration, anticholinergic medications and trauma may also contribute to the formation of salivary duct stones. Depending on the location and the size of the stone,

the presenting symptoms vary. Although most salivary stones are asymptomatic or cause minimal discomfort, larger stones may interfere with the flow of saliva and may cause pain and swelling. **As a rule, the onset of swelling is sudden and associated with salivation during a meal.**

The differential diagnosis for sialolithiasis includes other disease processes that may affect the salivary gland: infections, inflammatory conditions, and neoplastic and nonneoplastic masses.

If left untreated, salivary stones can result in chronic sialadenitis and glandular atrophy. Conservative treatment may consist of oral analgesics and antibiotics. Surgical management may include salivary lithotripsy, basket retrieval, and sialendoscopy.

The presence of dry eyes and dry mouth with arthralgia or arthritis may suggest the diagnosis of Sjögren syndrome as the cause of chronic sialadenitis.

Suggested Reading

Knight J: Diagnosis and treatment of sialolithiasis, *Ir Med J* 97:314–315, 2004.

Temporomandibular Disorder

(TMD, TMJ Syndrome)

Presentation

Patients usually complain of poorly localized facial pain or headache that does not appear to conform to a strict anatomic distribution. The pain is generally dull and unilateral, centered in the temple above and behind the eye, and in and around the ear. The pain may be associated with mastication and passive movement of the mandible, instability of the temporomandibular joint (TMJ), crepitus, or clicking with movement of the jaw. It is often described as an earache.

Other less obvious symptoms include radiation of pain down the carotid sheath, tinnitus, dizziness, decreased hearing, itching, sinus symptoms, a foreign body sensation in the external ear canal, and trigeminal, occipital, and glossopharyngeal neuralgias.

Patients may have been previously diagnosed as suffering from migraine headaches, sinusitis, or recurrent external otitis. Predisposing factors include malocclusion, trauma, recent extensive dental work, or a habit of grinding the teeth (bruxism), all of which put unusual stress on the TMJ.

Clinical signs include tenderness of the chewing muscles, the ear canal, or the joint itself; restricted opening of the jaw or lateral deviation on opening; and a normal neurologic examination.

What To Do:

✓ The patient should be asked about TMJ pain with jaw motion, such as chewing or yawning. Determine if there is a history of jaw trauma or involvement of other joints (which may be indicative of an underlying rheumatologic disorder).

✓ Examine the head thoroughly for other causes of the pain, including assessment of visual acuity, examination of the cranial nerves, and palpation of the scalp muscles and the temporal arteries.

✓ The TMJ examination should focus on the joint and the muscles of mastication, with careful attention to whether palpation can reproduce the patient's pain. While your fingers are firmly palpating the preauricular area, ask the patient to repeatedly open and close her mouth. This maneuver will be painful if the TMJ is the source of her pain. Intraoral palpation of the pterygoid muscles allows evaluation of spasm and tenderness of the muscle. The mandible can be distracted laterally by the patient to assess for pain during range of motion of the TMJ. Crepitus or a "click" may be heard or palpated with movement of the mandible. One should note, however, that given the prevalence of TMJ crepitance, the presence of these findings does not necessarily implicate the TMJ as the cause of the patient's symptoms.

✅ Muscular trigger points that reproduce or intensify the patient's pain on firm palpation indicate a myofascial origin that may benefit from a trigger point injection (see Chapter 123). Look for signs of bruxism, such as ground-down teeth, and percuss the teeth to possibly elicit dental pain as the source of the patient's discomfort.

✅ If the patient has a headache, perform a complete neurologic examination, including funduscopy. If the temporal artery is tender, swollen, or inflamed, send blood to be tested for an erythrocyte sedimentation rate (see Chapters 6 and 9).

✅ Complete evaluation of TMJ disorders, in addition to a thorough physical examination, includes panoramic or plain radiographs and can include MRI studies. These **imaging studies can be deferred until it is clear that symptoms are not resolving after 3 to 4 weeks of conservative therapy.**

✅ **If the pain is severe and clearly isolated to the joint, try an injection into the TMJ, just anterior to the tragus, with 1 to 2 mL of plain lidocaine 1% (Xylocaine) or bupivacaine 0.5% (Marcaine). If symptoms have been prolonged, you can combine this with 10 mg (0.25 mL) of methylprednisolone (Depo-Medrol)** (Figure 58-1). **If this helps, the diagnosis may have been made, and if a steroid was given, long-term relief may have been provided.**

✅ Explain to the patient the pathophysiology of the syndrome, including how many different symptoms may be produced by inflammation at one joint, how TMJ pain is not necessarily related to arthritis at other joints, and how common it is (some estimates are as high as 20% of the population).

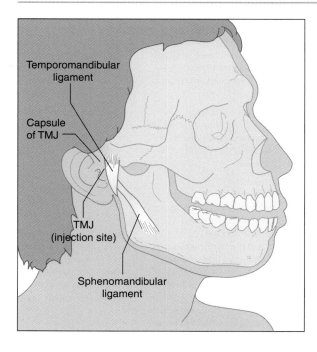

Figure 58-1 Proper temporomandibular joint (TMJ) injection site.

✅ **Prescribe anti-inflammatory analgesics (e.g., ibuprofen, naproxen), a soft diet, application of heat, and muscle relaxants (e.g., metaxalone [Skelaxin]) if necessary for muscle spasm. Application of ice can also be comforting.**

✅ **Have the patient avoid extreme jaw movements, such as yawning, yelling, and singing as well as chewing (especially gum or ice).**

✅ If the symptoms do not clear after 2 to 4 weeks, refer the patient for follow-up with a dentist or an otolaryngologist who has some interest in and experience with TMJ problems. Long-term treatments include orthodontic correction, physical therapy, and, sometimes, psychotherapy and treatment with antidepressants. Surgical intervention should be a last resort. Earlier follow-up should be provided if symptoms dramatically worsen or change.

What Not To Do:

❌ Do not rule out TMJ arthritis simply because the joint is not tender on examination. This syndrome typically fluctuates, and the diagnosis often is made based on the history alone.

❌ Do not omit examining the TMJ in the workup of any headache or earache.

❌ Do not administer narcotics unless there is going to be early follow-up.

Discussion

Painful disorders of the temporomandibular joint involve the trigeminal nerve. Other areas innervated by the trigeminal nerve help explain referred pain from the TMJ. Included are the dura mater, orbit, paranasal sinuses, tympanic membrane, and oral cavity and teeth, which help explain headaches, eye pain, sinus pressure, otalgia, and dental pain, respectively.

The muscles of mastication are abductors (jaw opening) and adductors (jaw closing) muscles. The temporalis, masseter, and medial pterygoids are adductors, whereas the lateral pterygoids are the primary abductors of the jaw.

The relative causative roles of abnormal joint anatomy, inadequate dentition, unsatisfactory occlusion, bruxism, dysfunction of the masticatory muscles, and emotional disorders remain controversial. To stress the role played by muscles, it has been suggested that the term *myofascial pain dysfunction syndrome* is more accurate than the term *TMJ arthritis*. Both these terms, as well as TMJ syndrome, are now considered to be outdated. The term *temporomandibular joint disorder* (TMD) is an umbrella term that combines a true disorder of the TMJ with involvement of the muscles of mastication.

There is also much debate as to the indications for and the efficacy of treatment modalities aimed at these presumed causes. At the least, irreversible treatments such as surgery should be replaced by more conservative therapy. The use of bite blocks for bruxism was based on outdated information and may serve only to alter normal dental occlusion, with deleterious effects.

Perhaps everyone suffers pain in the TMJ occasionally, and only a few require treatment or modification of lifestyle to reduce symptoms. In the emergency department or urgent care clinic, the diagnosis of TMJ pain is often suspected but seldom made definitively. It can be gratifying, however, to see patients with a myriad of seemingly unrelated symptoms respond dramatically after only conservative measures and advice are offered.

It is worth noting that a study of approximately 450 patients with TMJ pain demonstrated otalgia to be the presenting complaint in 48%. In this study, the TMD (and hence otalgia) was successfully managed with conservative therapies, such as heat, massage, patient education, occlusal splints, and pain control.

Suggested Readings

Guralnick W, Kaban LB, Merrill RG: Temporomandibular joint afflictions, *N Engl J Med* 299:123–128, 1978.

Seedorf H, Jüde HD: Otalgia as a result of certain temporomandibular joint disorders. [Article in German] *Laryngorhinootologie* 85:327–332, 2006.

Shah RK, Blevins NH: Otalgia, *Otolaryngol Clin North Am* 36:1137–1151, 2003.

Temporomandibular Joint Dislocation

(Jaw Dislocation)

Presentation

The patient's jaw is "out" and will not close, usually after yawning, taking a large bite of food, or perhaps after laughing, having a dental extraction, or suffering a jaw injury, such as a punch or kick to the mandible, or having a dystonic drug reaction. Such patients have difficulty enunciating clearly. Although they usually have only mild to moderate discomfort, they may have severe pain anterior to the ear. A depression can be seen or felt in the preauricular area, and the jaw may appear to be protruding forward (underbite). If only one side is dislocated, the mandible appears tilted and lies lower on the affected side.

What To Do:

⊘ If there was no trauma (and especially if the patient's jaw is dislocated often), attempt reduction immediately before muscle spasm around the joint makes the reduction more difficult. If there is any possibility of an associated fracture, however, obtain radiographs first. (If available, a panoramic view of the mandible is most accurate.) Excessive pain and tenderness are suggestive of an underlying fracture.

⊘ When the possibility of a fracture has been ruled out, **have the patient sit on a low stool,** with his back and head braced against something firm, either against the wall (facing you) or, as most clinicians prefer, against your body (facing away from you).

⊘ **With gloved hands, wrap your thumbs in gauze, place them on the lower molars, grasp both sides of the mandible, lock your elbows, and, bending from the waist, exert slow, steady pressure downward and posteriorly. The mandible should be at or below the level of your forearm** (Figure 59-1).

⊘ **In a bilateral dislocation, attempt to reduce one side at a time. This helps to reduce the risk for an inadvertent bite to your thumbs. Use of a bite block may also help to prevent being bitten.**

⊘ **Successful reduction is usually evident with the sensation of a palpable "clunk." The teeth will again be able to close easily without malocclusion.**

⊘ If the jaw does not relocate easily or convincingly, it may be necessary to reassess the dislocation with radiographs and to reattempt relocation using IV midazolam to overcome the muscle spasm and 1 to 2 mL of intra-articular 1% lidocaine to overcome the pain. Inject the lidocaine directly into the palpable depression left by the displaced condyle. If you are still unsuccessful, consider using procedural sedation and analgesia, using your institution's standard protocols (see Appendix E).

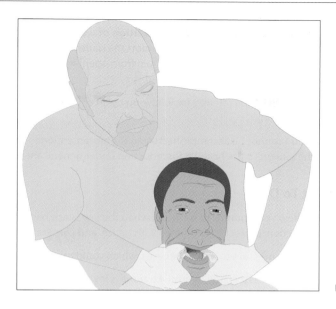

Figure 59-1 Dislocation reduction of the jaw.

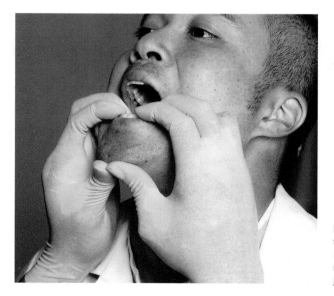

Figure 59-2 The wrist pivot method for temporomandibular joint dislocation reduction. (From Lowery LE, Beeson MS, Lurn KK: The wrist pivot method, a novel technique for temporomandibular joint reduction. *J Emerg Med* 27:167-170, 2004.)

A wrist pivot method for temporomandibular joint (TMJ) reduction **has been described and may be more effective than the traditional techniques described earlier.** While the examiner is facing the patient, who is sitting on a high surface, the mandible is grasped with the clinician's thumbs at the apex of the mentum and fingers on the occlusal surface of the inferior molars (Figure 59-2). Cephalad force is then applied with the thumbs and caudad pressure with the fingers while pivoting at the wrists until the mandible is reduced.

✅ **After the dislocation is reduced, application of a soft cervical collar will reduce the range of motion at the TMJ,** which will comfort the patient. Recommend a soft food diet for several days, and instruct the patient to refrain from opening his or her mouth widely over the next 24 hours. Prescribe analgesics if needed.

✅ All patients should be referred for follow-up by an appropriate specialist (i.e., oral and maxillofacial surgeon).

✅ If reduction cannot be accomplished using the aforementioned techniques, consider admitting the patient to the hospital for reduction under general anesthesia.

What Not To Do:

❌ Do not allow your thumbs to be bitten when the jaw snaps back into position. Maintain firm, steady traction, protect your thumbs with gauze, and consider using a bite block.

❌ Do not apply pressure to oral prostheses, which could cause them to break.

❌ Do not overlook associated injuries if trauma is involved.

❌ Do not try to force the patient's jaw shut.

Discussion

Certain patients with a congenitally shallow mandibular fossa or underdeveloped condyle are predisposed to mandibular dislocation. Most cases of dislocation occur spontaneously without direct trauma.

The mandible usually dislocates anteriorly and subluxes when the jaw is opened wide. Other dislocations imply that a fracture is present and require referral to a surgeon. Dislocation is often a recurring problem (avoided by limiting motion) and is associated with temporomandibular joint dysfunction. If dislocation is not obvious, consider other possible conditions, such as fracture, hemarthrosis, closed lock of the joint meniscus, and myofascial pain.

Suggested Readings

Lowery LE, Beeson MS, Lurn KK: The wrist pivot method: a novel technique for temporomandibular joint reduction, *J Emerg Med* 27:167–170, 2004.

Luyk NH, Larsen PE: The diagnosis and treatment of the dislocated mandible, *Am J Emerg Med* 7:329–335, 1989.

Uvular Edema, Acute

Presentation

The patient complains of a foreign body sensation or a lump or fullness in the throat, possibly associated with a slightly muffled voice and gagging. The patient may be worried after looking in the mirror and seeing a large swelling in his throat. On examination of the throat, the uvula is boggy, swollen, pale, and somewhat translucent and gelatinous appearing (uvular hydrops). If greatly enlarged, the uvula might rest on the tongue and move in and out with respiration. There should be no associated rash or pruritus, soreness, fever, dyspnea, or other areas of edematous involvement, such as the tongue, sublingual region, soft palate, and tonsils.

What To Do:

✓ Because of the known association of uvular edema with hypopharyngeal edema, watch for signs of airway compromise. If the patient complains of respiratory difficulty, breathes with stridor, or has significant voice change or hoarseness, prepare for treatment with IV lines, intubation, and cricothyrotomy equipment at the bedside, and obtain a portable lateral soft tissue neck radiographic examination to rule out epiglottic swelling. Begin medical treatment immediately with signs of impending airway compromise.

✓ If there is no acute respiratory difficulty, ask the patient about precipitating events. **Consider foods, drugs, physical agents, inhalants, insect bites, and, rarely, hereditary angioedema.**

✓ **When fever, sore throat, and pharyngeal injection are present,** swab the throat for a rapid streptococcal screen. If the streptococcal screen is negative, administer an antibiotic effective against *Haemophilus influenzae,* such as clarithromycin (Biaxin), amoxicillin plus clavulanate (Augmentin), or trimethoprim plus sulfamethoxazole (Bactrim). With a positive streptococcal screen, treat acute streptococcal pharyngitis as described in Chapter 38.

✓ If the presentation is confusing, it is reasonable to obtain a complete blood count with a manual differential to demonstrate eosinophilia, which would support the possibility of an allergic reaction, or to demonstrate a high leukocyte count with increased granulocytes and bands, which would support a bacterial infection.

✓ **If there is general pruritus, urticaria, flushing, or facial edema, and an allergic reaction is suspected, the patient should initially receive parenteral H$_1$- and H$_2$-blocking antihistamines, such as hydroxyzine (Vistaril), 50 to 100 mg IM, or diphenhydramine (Benadryl), 25 to 50 mg IV, along with cimetidine (Tagamet), 300 mg IV or PO, or ranitidine (Zantac), 50 mg IV or 150 mg PO or famotidine (Pepcid), 20 mg IV or PO.**

✅ **For more severe cases, give repeated doses of epinephrine, 0.3 mL of 1:1000 SC every 20 minutes for up to three doses. Nebulized isomeric or racemic epinephrine or albuterol is also effective. Topical application of a vasoconstrictor, such as cocaine gel, works very well.**

✅ **Parenteral corticosteroids, such as methylprednisolone (Solu-Medrol), 125 mg IV, are also typically used.**

✅ **When symptoms are mild and there is no clear cause (idiopathic isolated uvular edema), it is reasonable to provide the same treatment as one would give for an allergic reaction, although it is unclear whether or not this will bring about any diminution of the patient's uvular swelling.**

✅ **If the patient is on an angiotensin-converting enzyme (ACE) inhibitor,** such as lisinopril (Prinivil, Zestril), benazepril (Lotensin), captopril (Capoten), cilazapril (Inhibace), enalapril (Vasotec), fosinopril (Monopril), benazepril (Lotensin), moexipril (Univasc), perindopril (Aceon), quinapril (Accupril), ramipril (Altace), or trandolapril (Mavik), **use of that medication should be discontinued, and therapy with an alternative antihypertensive should begin.** The patient will more likely have swelling of the tongue or lips and should be held for several hours of observation. Hospital admission should be considered if the swelling worsens. **Airway compromise can occur rapidly and unpredictably when it is secondary to ACE inhibitor administration, and standard treatments are usually ineffective.** Pronounced edema of the tongue and floor of the mouth are predictors of a need for airway intervention.

✅ Eight patients with acute ACE inhibitor–induced angioedema, in a case series, were successfully treated with a single subcutaneous injection of icatibant. This small series showed complete relief of symptoms at 4.4 hours (standard deviation [SD] 0.8 hours), with the first symptom improvement occurring at a mean time of 50.6 minutes (SD 21 minutes). There were no adverse effects, except erythema occurring at the injection site. The external validity of these impressive results still need to be confirmed in a prospective, randomized, controlled clinical trial.

✅ If the patient has a history of recurrent episodes of edema, and there is a family history of the same, consider ordering tests to determine the C4 complement level or the C1 esterase inhibitor level to screen for hereditary angioedema. In this condition, the edema often involves the uvula and soft palate together. This is a rare condition that also does not respond to standard therapy.

✅ **Uvular decompression may be useful in patients who are resistant to medical therapy or who have rapidly progressing symptoms and in whom there is concern about possible airway compromise.** This procedure consists of grasping the uvula with forceps and either making several lacerations with a sterile needle or snipping the distal centimeter as a partial uvulectomy. **Injecting the uvula with lidocaine 1% (Xylocaine) with epinephrine will provide anesthesia and may be therapeutic.**

✅ **All patients should be observed for an adequate period of time to ensure that there is either improvement or no further increase in the swelling before being sent home.** When discharged, the patient with an allergic or idiopathic cause for their edema should be given a 4- to 5-day supply of H_1 and H_2 blockers and steroids if required.

What Not To Do:

(X) Do not perform a comprehensive and costly laboratory evaluation on every patient. Order only those specific tests that are clearly indicated and will provide results that can be followed up.

(X) Do not obtain lateral soft tissue neck radiographs on patients with acute spontaneous uvular edema who are asymptomatic other than for their foreign body sensation.

Discussion

The uvula (Latin for "little grape") is a small, conical, peduncular process hanging from the middle of the lower border of the soft palate. The soft palate is composed of muscle, connective tissue, and mucous membrane, and the bulk of the uvula consists of glandular tissue with diffuse muscle fibers interspersed throughout. During the acts of deglutition and phonation, the uvula and soft palate are directed upward, thereby walling off the nasal cavity from the pharynx. During swallowing, this prevents ingested substances from entering the nasal cavity.

Most patients who present acutely with isolated angioedema of the uvula have mild symptoms and a benign clinical course with an obscure cause. This idiopathic form of spontaneous swelling of the uvula may or may not be related to other forms of angioedema.

Angioedema, also known as *angioneurotic edema* and *Quincke disease,* is defined as a well-localized edematous condition that may variably involve the deeper skin layers, subcutaneous tissues, and mucosal surfaces of the upper respiratory and gastrointestinal tracts.

Immediate hypersensitivity type I reactions, seen with atopic states and specific allergen sensitivities, are the most common causes of angioedema. These reactions involve the interaction of an allergen with IgE antibodies bound to the surface of basophils or mastocytes. Physical agents, including cold, pressure, light, and vibration, or other processes that increase core temperature may also cause edema through the IgE pathway.

Hereditary angioedema, a genetic disorder of the complement system, is characterized by either an absence or a functional deficiency of C1 esterase inhibitor. This absence or deficiency allows unopposed activation of the first component of complement, with subsequent breakdown of its two substrates, the second (C2) and fourth (C4) components of the complement cascade. This process, in the presence of plasmin, generates a vasoactive kinin-like molecule that causes angioedema. Acquired C1 esterase inhibitor deficiency and other complement consumption states have been described in patients with malignancies and immune complex disorders, including serum sickness and vasculitides.

Other causes of angioedema include certain medications and diagnostic agents (e.g., opiates, D-tubocurarine, curare, radiocontrast materials) that have a direct degranulation effect on mast cells and basophils; substances such as aspirin, nonsteroidal anti-inflammatory drugs (NSAIDs), azo dyes, and benzoates that alter the metabolism of arachidonic acid, thus increasing vascular permeability; and ACE inhibitors, implicated presumably by promoting the production of bradykinin.

The known infectious causes of uvulitis include group A streptococci, *Haemophilus influenzae,* and *Streptococcus pneumoniae.* An associated cellulitis may contiguously involve the uvula and the tonsils, posterior pharynx, or epiglottis.

Suggested Readings

Bas M, Greve J, Stelter K, et al: Therapeutic efficacy of icatibant in angioedema induced by angiotensin-converting enzyme inhibitors: a case series, *Ann Emerg Med* 56:278–282, 2010.

Chiu AG, Newkirk KA, Davidson BJ, et al: Angiotensin-converting enzyme inhibitor-induced angioedema: a multicenter review and an algorithm for airway management, *Ann Otol Rhinol Laryngol* 110:834–840, 2001.

Evans TC, Roberge RJ: Quincke's disease of the uvula, *Am J Emerg Med* 5:211–216, 1987.

Goldberg R, Lawton R, Newton E, et al: Evaluation and management of acute uvular edema, *Ann Emerg Med* 22:251–255, 1993.

Ishoo E, Shah UK, Grillone GA, et al: Predicting airway risk in angioedema: staging system based on presentation, *Otolaryngol Head Neck Surg* 121:263–268, 1999.

Kestler A, Keyes L: Images in clinical medicine. Uvular angioedema (Quincke's disease), *N Engl J Med* 349:867, 2003.

PART 5

Pulmonary and Thoracic Emergencies

■ Philip Buttaravoli   ■ Katherine Walsh

Bronchitis (Chest Cold), Acute

Presentation

The patient's symptoms generally start with 1 to 5 days of fever, malaise, and myalgias that are often indistinguishable from other acute upper respiratory tract infections (URIs). With acute bronchitis, however, this acute phase is followed by a second protracted phase characterized by persistent cough, often accompanied by phlegm production or wheezing. This second phase usually lasts 1 to 3 weeks. The cough may produce hoarseness or may be accompanied by difficult breathing and chest tightness. The patient may be fearful that he is developing pneumonia, wants relief from his symptoms, or wants a prescription for an antibiotic that he believes "cleared up the infection" the last time he had bronchitis.

The patient's vital signs are essentially within normal limits, and he does not appear toxic. If he is producing sputum, it may be clear, white, yellow, brown, or green, and his lung sounds may be clear or reveal rhonchi or wheezes.

What To Do:

✅ Perform a complete history and physical examination; document which of the aforementioned signs and symptoms are present; rule out any other underlying ailment; and note any sign of bacterial superinfection of the ears, sinuses, pharynx, tonsils, epiglottis, bronchi, or lungs, which might require antibiotics or other therapy. In the absence of significant comorbid conditions or asthma, **the primary objective when evaluating patients who have acute cough illness is to exclude pneumonia.**

✅ The absence of abnormal vital signs (heart rate greater than 100 beats/minute, respiratory rate greater than 24 breaths/minute, oral temperature greater than 100.4° F [38° C], hypoxemia), along with the absence of abnormalities on chest examination (focal consolidation, e.g., rales, egophony, fremitus), reduces the likelihood of pneumonia sufficiently to render further diagnostic testing unnecessary.

✅ **Abnormalities in these "pneumonia clinical prediction rules" should prompt the ordering of a chest radiograph.** These rules have limited application in the elderly, because they may present with atypical manifestations of pneumonia (and without vital sign or examination abnormalities). Conversely, during the influenza season, many patients will have fever or tachycardia but not pneumonia.

✅ **The presence or absence of purulent sputum is a poor predictor of bacterial infections.**

✅ In settings where chest radiography is not readily available, **elderly patients who have cough illness or those with clinical findings consistent with pneumonia may be prescribed antibiotics to safeguard against missing a case of pneumonia.**

✅ **Routine antibiotic treatment of acute bronchitis has no consistent effect on either the duration or the severity of illness, and has potential side effects.**

✅ **Patients who have a cough accompanied by the sudden onset of high fever (greater than 101° F), headache, moderate to severe myalgias, and fatigue should be suspected of having influenza in the face of a negative chest radiograph.** Laboratory testing to make the diagnosis is not necessary during an outbreak; otherwise, rapid influenza testing can be performed on a nasopharyngeal specimen. **If it has been less than 48 hours since the onset of symptoms, consider treating with oseltamivir (Tamiflu), 75 mg bid × 5 days (2 mg/kg bid × 5 days in children).** In patients younger than 65 years, who are otherwise healthy and not pregnant, treatment is not necessary but may shorten the duration of illness if initiated promptly. For unvaccinated or high-risk vaccinated patients (elderly, children younger than 2 years old, pregnant women, immunosuppressed patients, or those with underlying lung disease), treatment should be initiated regardless of time from onset of symptoms. Local and national influenza surveillance data should be reviewed to determine appropriate treatment and provide further guidance in choice of antiviral agent.

✅ **Explain the course of the viral illness and the inadvisability of indiscriminate use of antibiotics.** Provide the patient with realistic expectations for the duration of the cough (typically 10 to 14 days) and the ineffectiveness and potential adverse side effects of antibiotics. In addition, inform them that their condition could worsen, because resistant bacteria may be produced. **Let them know that you want to hold antibiotics in reserve in case they develop a true bacterial infection.** Try to avoid using the term *bronchitis,* and instead, refer to their illness as a "chest cold." Positive rapid influenza tests in children can help foster parental acceptance of a management strategy that does not include antibiotics.

✅ Tailor drug treatment to the patient's specific complaint as follows:

- ○ **For fever, headache, and myalgia, prescribe acetaminophen, 650 mg q4h, or ibuprofen, 600 mg q6h (adjust dose for age and weight).**
- ○ **For bronchitis with suspected bronchospasm, treat the cough using inhaled bronchodilators, such as albuterol, two puffs q1-8h prn cough.**

✅ Zinc and vitamin C have been shown to be beneficial in reducing the duration and severity of the common cold when taken within 24 hours of onset of symptoms.

✅ **Recommend comforting regimens, such as using a vaporizer in a dry environment, drinking tea and honey, and eating mother's chicken soup.** There appears to be no evidence in the literature to support the recommendation to drink extra fluids during a respiratory infection. Also, parents of children with an acute cough resulting from URI should be advised that there is almost no meaningful evidence regarding the effectiveness of over-the-counter (OTC) cough preparations, and that the available evidence does not support such treatment.

 Patients with chronic obstructive pulmonary disease (COPD) who have an acute bacterial exacerbation of chronic bronchitis (increased sputum volume or purulence and difficulty breathing) may benefit from antibiotic therapy. For mild to moderate disease, either no treatment or doxycycline or trimethoprim/sulfamethoxazole (TMP/SMX) can be prescribed. For severe disease, amoxicillin/clavulanate (AM/CL), azithromycin, or a respiratory quinolone may be given for a period of 3 to 7 days. If the patient is at risk for *Pseudomonas* (i.e., severe COPD, recent hospitalization, or requiring antibiotics frequently), consider treatment with ciprofloxacin.

 Consider gastroesophageal reflux disease as a possible etiology of new cough, and treat accordingly.

 Arrange for follow-up if symptoms persist or worsen or if new problems develop.

What Not To Do:

 Do not prescribe antibiotics inappropriately. In recent years, patient expectations for antibiotic treatment for URIs have decreased somewhat. It should not be assumed that most patients with a URI want to be treated with antibiotics; when they request one, however, personalize the risks of taking inappropriate antibiotics. Inform them that previous antibiotic use increases their personal risk for carriage of and infection with antibiotic-resistant infections. In addition, antibiotics cause frequent side effects, especially of the gastrointestinal tract.

 Do not obtain sputum for Gram stains and cultures. They have no clinical usefulness in patients with acute bronchitis. Peroxidase released by the leukocytes in sputum causes the color changes.

Discussion

Data from the National Health Interview Survey suggest that 4% to 5% of all adults experience one or more episodes of acute bronchitis each year. Furthermore, more than 90% of acute bronchitis episodes will come to medical attention.

Acute bronchitis is a clinical diagnosis applied to otherwise healthy adults with acute respiratory illness of 1 to 3 weeks' duration. Acute bronchitis usually is distinguished from other acute respiratory infections by the predominance of a cough and the absence of findings suggestive of pneumonia. A **cough lasting longer than 3 weeks** should be considered a "persistent" or "chronic" cough. The diagnostic considerations, under these circumstances, are significantly different from those of acute bronchitis.

The underlying pathophysiology of acute bronchitis is hypersensitivity of the tracheobronchial epithelium and airway receptors (reactive airway disease). Recurrent episodes of "acute bronchitis" may suggest underlying asthma, but a workup for asthma should be reserved for patients with a cough that lasts longer than 3 weeks.

In epidemiologic studies, respiratory viruses seem to cause or serve as a co-pathogen in most cases of acute bronchitis. *Mycoplasma pneumoniae* and *Chlamydia pneumoniae* have been recognized as possible bacterial causes of acute bronchitis. In several studies in which these pathogens were present (as determined by antibody titer or gene amplification), however, treatment with antibiotics appropriate to atypical pathogens did not change the outcome.

(continued)

Discussion continued

Adults with **pertussis** generally present with a persistent cough, with a mean duration of 36 to 48 days. The cough is mostly paroxysmal and often disturbs sleep. Choking or vomiting and whooping can be present, but less commonly than in children or previously unimmunized adults. The diagnosis is made by swabbing the posterior nasopharynx and sending the specimen for polymerase chain reaction (PCR) testing. Antibiotic therapy does not seem to decrease duration of symptoms for pertussis, unless it is initiated within 7 to 10 days of the onset of illness. Macrolide prophylaxis during outbreaks and after intrafamilial contact seems effective, however, and decreases spread of disease.

The societal cost of inappropriate antibiotic use is the rapid emergence of antibiotic resistance among bacterial pathogens and unnecessary prescription expenditures, estimated to be $726 million. On an individual level, a person's risk for carriage and transmission of, and invasive infection with, antibiotic-resistant bacteria is associated strongly with previous antibiotic use. There is ongoing research on using serum levels of **procalcitonin** as a surrogate biomarker of bacterial infection to help guide the need for antibiotic therapy in acute bronchitis. Further research is needed before this is incorporated into standard clinical practice.

Evidence suggests that physicians and patients are more likely to believe that antibiotics are appropriate if purulent secretions are present or if the patient is a smoker, despite significant evidence to the contrary. Patients frequently expect to receive antibiotics for uncomplicated acute bronchitis, and patients or parents who expect antibiotics are more likely to receive them. Communication elements associated with the issuance of antibiotic prescriptions for acute respiratory infections include patient appeals to specific life circumstances (e.g., a pressing social engagement), identification of a previous positive experience with antibiotic use, or the disease being labeled as "acute bronchitis" rather than a "chest cold."

Despite physician concerns about patient expectations, most studies find that satisfaction with care for acute respiratory infections is tied more closely to how much time the physician spent explaining the illness rather than receipt of antibiotics. High patient satisfaction was associated with positive responses to the following statements: "The doctor spent enough time with me"; "the doctor explained the illness to me"; and "the doctor treated me with respect."

Influenza is the most common cause of acute bronchitis, and influenza vaccination is the most effective strategy for preventing influenzal illness. Cough and fever are positive predictors of influenza, whereas severe sore throat is a negative predictor. Prophylactic treatment for high-risk exposed individuals is indicated. Amantadine, rimantadine, zanamivir, and oseltamivir decrease illness duration by approximately 1 day and lead to a half-day quicker return to normal activities. The primary difference between the agents is that the neuraminidase inhibitors are effective against influenza A and B, whereas amantadine and rimantadine are effective only against influenza A, and there is high viral resistance to amantadine. The cost and side effects of these drugs are also significantly different. The relative proportion of cases caused by each type of influenza virus varies from year to year and is determined best through consultation with local public health agencies. Because each of these therapies is effective only if initiated within the first 48 hours (preferably the first 30 hours) of symptom onset, rapid diagnosis is key. During documented influenza outbreaks, the positive predictive value of clinical diagnosis based on clinical judgment is good (correct approximately 70% of the time) and compares favorably with rapid diagnostic tests for influenza (sensitivities of 63% to 81%). Diagnosis of influenza in a non-outbreak period is more difficult, and diagnostic testing should be considered.

The effectiveness of **antitussive therapy** seems to depend on the cause of a cough illness. An acute or early cough caused by colds and other URIs does not seem to respond to dextromethorphan or codeine. Coughs lasting longer than 3 weeks and coughs associated with underlying lung disease seem to respond to these agents.

An herbal extract from the *Pelargonium sidoides* root has been shown to alleviate symptoms of acute bronchitis, including cough and sputum production. In the United States, *P. sidoides* is marketed under the trade name Umcka (4-ounce bottle) 1 tsp, 4 to 5 times per day continued for 48 hours after symptoms subside (Nature's Way, Springville, Utah).

For patients who present with a cough persisting longer than 1 week, pertussis should be considered, as well as bronchial hyperresponsiveness.

Suggested Readings

Aagaard E, Gonzales R: Management of acute bronchitis in healthy adults, *Infect Dis Clin North Am* 18:919–937, 2004.

Agbabiaka TB, Guo R, Ernst E: *Pelargonium sidoides* for acute bronchitis: a systematic review and meta-analysis, *Phytomedicine* 15:378–385, 2008.

Brent S, Saint S, Vittinghoff E, et al: Antibiotics in acute bronchitis: a meta-analysis, *Am J Med* 107:62–67, 1999.

Briel M, Schuetz P, Mueller B: Procalcitonin-guided antibiotic use vs a standard approach for acute respiratory infections in primary care, *Arch Intern Med* 168:2000–2007, 2008.

Clemens CJ, Taylor JA, Almquist JR, et al: Is an antihistamine-decongestant combination effective in temporarily relieving symptoms of the common cold in preschool children? *J Pediatr* 130:463–466, 1997.

Edmonds ML: Antibiotic treatment for acute bronchitis, *Ann Emerg Med* 40:110–112, 2002.

Glezen WP: Clinical practice. Prevention and treatment of seasonal influenza, *N Engl J Med* 359:2579–2585, 2008.

Gonzales R, Barrett PH, Crane LA: Factors associated with antibiotic use for acute bronchitis, *J Gen Intern Med* 13:541–548, 1998.

Gonzales R, Bartlett JG, Besser RE, et al: Principles of appropriate antibiotic use for treatment of uncomplicated acute bronchitis: background, *Ann Intern Med* 134:521–529, 2001.

Gonzales R, Steiner JF, Sande MA: Antibiotic prescribing for adults with colds, upper respiratory infections, and bronchitis by ambulatory care physicians, *JAMA* 278:901–904, 1997.

Guppy MP, Mickan SM, Del Mar CB: "Drink plenty of fluids": a systematic review of evidence for this recommendation in acute respiratory infections, *BMJ* 328:499–500, 2004.

Hamm RM, Hicks RJ, Bemben DA: Antibiotics and respiratory infections: are patients more satisfied when expectations are met? *J Fam Pract* 43:56–62, 1996.

Kaiser L, Wat C, Mills T, et al: Impact of oseltamivir treatment on influenza-related lower respiratory tract complications and hospitalizations, *Arch Intern Med* 163:1667–1672, 2003.

Knutson D, Braun C: Diagnosis and management of acute bronchitis, *Am Fam Physician* 65:2039–2044, 2002.

Linder JA, Singer DE: Desire for antibiotics and antibiotic prescribing for adults with upper respiratory tract infections, *J Gen Intern Med* 18:795–801, 2003.

Linder JA, Sim I: Antibiotic treatment of acute bronchitis in smokers, *J Gen Intern Med* 17:230–234, 2002.

Macfarlane J, Holmes W, Gard P, et al: Providing patient information reduces antibiotic use in acute bronchitis, *BMJ* 324:1–6, 2002.

Paul IM, Yoder KE, Crowell KR, et al: Effect of dextromethorphan, diphenhydramine, and placebo on nocturnal cough and sleep quality for coughing children and their parents, *Pediatrics* 114:e85–e90, 2004.

Rothberg MB, Bellantonio S, Rose DN: Management of influenza in adults older than 65 years of age: cost-effectiveness of rapid testing and antiviral therapy, *Ann Intern Med* 139:321–329, 2003.

Singh M, Das R: Zinc for the common cold, *Cochrane Database Syst Rev* 2:CD001364, 2011.

Smith S, Schroeder K, Fahey T: Over-the-counter medications for acute cough in children and adults in ambulatory settings, *Cochrane Database Syst Rev* 1:CD001831, 2008.

Smucny J, Becker LA, Glazier R: Beta2-agonists for acute bronchitis, *Cochrane Database Syst Rev* 4:CD001726, 2006.

Snow V, Mottur-Pilson C, Gonzales R: Principles of appropriate antibiotic use for treatment of acute bronchitis in adults, *Ann Intern Med* 134:518–520, 2001.

Treanor JJ, Hayden FG, Vrooman PS, et al: Efficacy and safety of the oral neuraminidase inhibitor oseltamivir in treating acute influenza, *JAMA* 283:1016–1024, 2000.

Wilson AA, Crane LA, Barrett PH, et al: Public beliefs and use of antibiotics for acute respiratory illness, *J Gen Intern Med* 14:658–662, 1999.

Zambon M, Hays J, Webster A, et al: Diagnosis of influenza in the community: relationship of clinical diagnosis to confirmed virological, serologic, or molecular detection of influenza, *Arch Intern Med* 161:2116–2122, 2001.

Costochondritis and Musculoskeletal Chest Pain

Presentation

The patient, usually between the ages of 15 and 39, complains of a day or more of steady aching with intermittent stabbing chest pain. The pain may follow an episode of minor trauma, a period of frequent coughing, or unusual physical activity or overuse; may be localized to the left or right of the sternum, without radiation; and may worsen when the patient takes a deep breath, changes position, twists at the torso, pushes or pulls her arms against resistance, or moves her arm or arms overhead. Having the patient arch her back in extension while compressing her thoracic vertebrae with your examining hand may reveal a spinous origin for her pain. She may be concerned about the possibility of a heart attack (though she may not voice her fear), but there is no associated nausea, vomiting, diaphoresis, or dyspnea or any significant cardiac risk factors. The middle anterior costal cartilages (connecting the ribs to the sternum) may be diffusely tender to palpation, without swelling or erythema, and exactly matching the patient's complaint. There may be sites other than the sternal borders, such as the anterior ribs, xyphoid process, or thoracic spine, that are the source of the patient's pain. The rest of the physical examination is normal, along with normal vital signs that include pulse oximetry.

What To Do:

⊘ Obtain a thorough history and perform a complete physical examination. Pay special attention to the specific location and character of the pain (e.g., onset, severity, quality, radiation, duration, and whether or not it is related to strenuous activity, movement, deep breathing, and cough) and associated symptoms (e.g., sensation of a racing heart, palpitations, pallor, syncope or near-syncope, shortness of breath, nausea, vomiting, fever, weight loss, fatigue, diaphoresis, cough, or wheeze). Inquire about any risk factors for pulmonary embolism (e.g., estrogen use, recent surgery, immobilization, history of malignancy, personal or family history of thromboembolic disease) or about a history of preexisting cardiac risk factors (e.g., hypertrophic cardiomyopathy, aortic valvular stenosis, family history of early-onset coronary artery disease, smoking, hypertension, diabetes mellitus, obesity, elevated cholesterol levels, cocaine use). Read the nurse's notes and/or check for critical details the patient may not have repeated to you.

⊘ Look for abnormal vital signs, pleural or pericardial rubs, new murmurs and dysrhythmias, single or paradoxic splitting of the second heart sound, new gallops, unilateral leg swelling, asymmetric pulses, and signs of congestive heart failure, which include rales, peripheral edema, and jugular venous distention. Carefully examine the abdomen using deep palpation under the costal margins, looking for signs of intra-abdominal tenderness.

✓ **At a minimum, obtain a cardiogram, oxygen saturation level, and chest radiograph. If there is some concern for pulmonary embolism (PE), but the patient is low risk, an enzyme-linked immunosorbent assay (ELISA) D-dimer may be obtained to exclude PE.**

✓ If any abnormalities are discovered and there is any suspicion of a pulmonary, cardiac, vascular, or gastrointestinal disorder, begin the appropriate treatment and clinical investigation. **The presence of costochondritis does not exclude the possibility of aortic dissection, myocardial infarction, pericarditis, esophageal or peptic ulcer perforation, pulmonary embolus, pneumomediastinum, pneumothorax, pneumonia, mediastinitis, or pleural effusion. When there is a reasonable possibility for one of these more serious clinical entities to be present, a more complete medical workup is required.**

✓ If there is any suggestion of cardiac, aortic, or serious gastrointestinal or pulmonary disease; if there are complaints of chest tightness or pressure; or if there are significant cardiac risk factors or risk factors for pulmonary embolus, obtain appropriate consultation and strongly consider admission.

✓ **If the ECG and chest radiograph are normal and there is no evidence of other disease (the symptoms are purely musculoskeletal, there are no associated symptoms or significant risk factors, vital signs are normal, and the abnormal physical findings are limited to the chest wall tenderness that mimics their pain), prescribe anti-inflammatory analgesics, have the patient apply heat to ease discomfort, explain the benign nature of the chest wall pain to the patient, and direct the patient to seek follow-up with a primary care practitioner.**

✓ Exquisite tenderness localized over the xiphoid cartilage may represent the rare condition of xiphoidalgia, which may be treated with a course of nonsteroidal anti-inflammatory drugs (NSAIDs) as described earlier. Local injection of a combination of bupivacaine (Marcaine), 0.5% 5 mL mixed with methylprednisolone (Depo-Medrol), 20 to 40 mg, may be helpful in refractory cases or where immediate pain relief clarifies the diagnosis. If this is attempted, extreme caution should be used to not inject posterior to the xiphoid because of the risk of injury to underlying structures.

✓ Instruct all of these patients to return if they experience any fever, palpitations, lightheadedness, shortness of breath, diaphoresis, change in the character of their pain, or radiation of pain to their arm, shoulder, or jaw.

What Not To Do:

✗ Do not rule out myocardial infarction or acute coronary syndrome, especially in the middle-aged or elderly patient, simply because there is tenderness over the costal cartilage, which could represent a coincidental finding, skin hypesthesia, or contiguous inflammation secondary to an infarct.

Discussion

This local inflammatory process is probably related to minor trauma and would not be brought to medical attention so often if it did not occur in the chest, thereby invoking fear of a heart attack. Carefully reassuring the patient and her family is, therefore, most important. This disorder is self-limited, but there may be remissions and exacerbations. The pain usually resolves in weeks to months.

Tietze syndrome is a rare variant that is generally less diffuse and is associated with local swelling. Tumors of the anterior chest wall can also cause these symptoms; if the complaints persist or any swelling progresses, CT or MRI scans should be obtained.

Precordial catch syndrome, or Texidor twinge, is described as a sharp, needle-like pain that is well localized. The pain usually occurs at rest and has a split-second onset, taking the patient by surprise. Typically, the pain lasts only seconds to minutes, with deep breathing making the pain worse. Patients may sit straight up to help relieve the pain. Physical examination is normal, without reproducible pain. These patients are usually young, of light or medium build, and apparently healthy. It can occur once or twice in some people or several times a day for a number of weeks in others. Patients with these symptoms require only reassurance.

Slipping rib syndrome may cause lower chest and upper abdominal pain because of hypermobility at the anterior ends of lower costal cartilages. The diagnosis is made by eliciting tenderness over the costal margin, as well as by performing the "hooking maneuver." This is done by curving your fingers under the costal margin and pulling the ribs forward, thereby eliciting a click that reproduces the patient's pain. Treat with rest and physical therapy.

Chest pain in the pediatric population is most commonly benign, but a careful history and physical examination are critical. If there are any concerning elements in the history (e.g., syncope, dyspnea or pain with exertion, shortness of breath, family history of sudden death), or abnormalities on examination, a workup is indicated. When the history and physical examination reveal a healthy child, routine testing has not been shown to be helpful. An ECG may be useful for providing reassurance, which is the mainstay of therapy in this situation.

In adults, a recent study showed that almost 3% of patients thought to have noncardiac chest pain had an adverse cardiac event (myocardial infarction, coronary artery bypass graft, death) within 30 days. **It is always the medical practitioner's primary responsibility to rule out the worst case scenario. Even when your first impression is that of noncardiac chest pain, if your patient has known coronary artery disease or a history of congestive heart failure, coronary risk factors, weakness, diaphoresis, or chest pain similar to what he may have experienced in a previous acute coronary syndrome event, it may be prudent to pursue a more extensive workup.**

Do not let yourself be led down an incorrect "noncardiac" path by a patient who is downplaying his or her symptoms, acting in a histrionic manner, or has the reputation of being a frequent flyer with similar symptoms. When there are underlying risk factors and symptoms or signs that are not inconsistent with a serious medical disorder of any cause, always play it safe, investigate, consult, and, when necessary, admit.

Suggested Readings

Brown MD: An emergency department guideline for the diagnosis of pulmonary embolism: an outcome study, *Acad Emerg Med* 12:20–25, 2005.

Cava JR, Sayger PL: Chest pain in children and adolescents, *Pediatr Clin North Am* 51:1553–1568, 2004.

Disla E, Rhim HR, Reddy A, et al: Costochondritis: a prospective analysis in an ED setting, *Arch Intern Med* 154:2466–2469, 1994.

Hoogendoorn RJ: Sternal pain: not always harmless, *Ned Tijdschr Geneeskd* 148:2469–2474, 2004.

Miller CD, Lindsell CJ, Khandelwal S: Is the initial diagnostic impression of "noncardiac chest pain" adequate to exclude cardiac disease? *Ann Emerg Med* 44:565–574, 2004.

Perron AD: Chest pain in athletes, *Clin Sports Med* 22:37–50, 2003.

Place R, Vezzetti R: Pediatric and adolescent chest pain, *Pediatr Emerg Med Practice* 4:1–26, 2007.

Proulx A, Zyrd T: Costochrondritis: diagnosis and treatment, *Am Fam Physician* 80:617–620, 2009.

Inhalation Injury

(Smoke Inhalation)

Presentation

The patient was trapped in an enclosed space for some time with toxic gases or fumes (e.g., produced by a fire, a leak, evaporation of a solvent, a chemical reaction, or fermentation of silage) and comes to the emergency department complaining of some combination of coughing, wheezing, shortness of breath, irritated or runny eyes or nose, or skin irritation. More severe symptoms include confusion and narcosis, dizziness, headache, chest pain, nausea, vomiting, and rapidly evolving upper airway obstruction.

Symptoms may develop immediately or after a lag of as much as 1 day. On physical examination, the victim may smell of the agent or be covered with soot or burns. Inflammation of the eyes, nose, mouth, or upper airway may be visible, and pulmonary irritation may be evident as coughing, rhonchi, rales, or wheezing, although these signs may also take up to 1 day to develop.

What To Do:

✓ Separate the victim from the toxic agent by having him remove his clothes, hose himself down, or wash with soap and water.

✓ **Make sure the victim is breathing adequately, and then add oxygen at 15 L/min through a nonrebreather mask with humidification. Oxygen helps treat most inhalation injuries and is essential in treating carbon monoxide (CO) poisoning.**

✓ Mild to moderate carbon monoxide poisoning is common. Patients often present with vague symptoms, such as headache, nausea, vomiting, dizziness, and confusion. The half-life of carboxyhemoglobin (HbCO) with the patient breathing room air is 4 to 6 hours. Breathing 90% to 100% oxygen at 1 atmosphere absolute pressure reduces the HbCO half-life to 60 to 90 minutes. Otherwise asymptomatic patients can be discharged when their CO levels are less than 5%. Hyperbaric oxygen (HBO) can reduce the HbCO half-life to 20 to 30 minutes. Current recommendations for the use of HBO are neurologic compromise (including transient loss of consciousness), metabolic acidosis, ECG evidence of myocardial ischemia or dysrhythmias, HbCO greater than 40%, pregnancy with HbCO greater than 15%, or history of coronary artery disease with HbCO greater than 20%. Early consultation with a hyperbaric center is recommended.

✓ **Bronchodilators can be administered by aerosol inhalation when there is any evidence of bronchospasm.**

✓ The clinical course of inhalation injury is dependent on the agent inhaled and the intensity and duration of exposure. Look for evidence that may clarify the nature of the exposure: Was there a fire? What was burning? What was the estimated length of exposure? Was the patient in an open or a closed space? Was the patient disoriented or unconscious at the scene? What is the status of any other victims? Was there an associated blast?

✓ Determine whether there are significant preexisting conditions, such as smoking, underlying allergies, cardiac or cerebrovascular disease, chronic obstructive pulmonary disease, asthma, or other chronic illness. Patients with underlying pulmonary disease are less able to compensate for inhalation injuries.

✓ What material is on the victim? What does he smell of? What are his current signs and symptoms? Is there soot in the posterior pharynx, singed nasal hair, hoarseness, confusion, tachycardia, tachypnea, use of accessory respiratory muscles, wheezing, rales and rhonchi, or stridor to indicate significant injury to the respiratory tract? Note that the lack of physical findings does not reliably exclude airway injury.

✓ There may be evidence of exposure to a specific toxin that calls for a specific antidote (e.g., muscle fasciculations, small pupils, and wet lungs may imply inhalation of organophosphates, which should be treated with atropine).

✓ **Unless the exposure is insignificant, obtain a chest radiograph, pulse oximetry, and arterial or venous blood gases.** Record the percentage of oxygen being inhaled (Fio_2 approximately 90% at 15 L/min). An increased alveolar-arterial partial pressure of oxygen (Po_2) difference (A-a O_2 gradient) may be the earliest sign of pulmonary injury, but even if the chest radiograph film and arterial blood gases are normal (as they often are), they can serve as a baseline for evaluation of possible later pulmonary problems. An abnormal initial chest radiograph is a poor prognostic factor.

✓ **With significant smoke inhalation, obtain a carboxyhemoglobin level, complete blood count (CBC) and electrolytes, and serial peak flow measurements, if available. With carbon monoxide poisoning, pulse oximetry (Spo_2) is unreliable because of similar light absorption by carboxyhemoglobin and oxyhemoglobin. Carboxyhemoglobin (HbCO) saturation can be directly measured by co-oximetry.** Blood and urine toxicology studies may be obtained to identify coexisting toxicity that may have contributed to the cause of the inhalation injury and also complicate its course.

✓ **Obtain an ECG if there is any loss of consciousness, a history of coronary artery disease, or any complaint of chest pain or palpitations.** Inhalation injuries result in decrease oxygen delivery to the tissues, increasing the risk of cardiac ischemia.

✓ **Consider cyanide toxicity in any patient with smoke inhalation.** Some burning plastics give off cyanide. An anion gap acidosis may be the result of elevated lactate levels secondary to cyanide, carbon monoxide, or hypoxia. A lactate level greater than 8 mmol/L is considered a surrogate marker of elevated cyanide levels and requires treatment. Treatment consists of sodium thiosulfate and/or hydroxocobalamin.

✓ If the patient has difficulty breathing, hoarseness, change in voice, or throat pain—or if he has any abnormality evidenced by the radiography examination, arterial blood gas levels, or physical examination, suggesting acute pulmonary injury—administration of oxygen should be continued, and the patient should be admitted to the hospital or transferred to an appropriate tertiary center. Consider early, elective endotracheal intubation in patients at risk for developing airway compromise, particularly those with hoarseness, difficulty breathing, throat pain, drooling or difficulty swallowing.

✅ **If stridor or other physical evidence of upper airway edema is present or if there is impending respiratory failure, endotracheal intubation should be performed as soon as possible.** Bronchoscopy may be useful in evaluating the extent of injury.

✅ Wheezing and bronchospasm may be allergic reactions and may respond to conventional doses of aerosolized bronchodilators but, if not promptly reversible, are probably signs of pulmonary injury. The elderly (>64 years), the young (<5 years), and persons under the influence of alcohol or other drugs require a lower threshold for admission or transfer.

✅ **After minimal exposure, if no signs or symptoms of inhalation injury develop or if all have resolved in 3 to 4 hours, it may be safe to send the patient home with instructions to return for reevaluation the next day or sooner if any pulmonary signs or symptoms (e.g., stridor, coughing, wheezing, shortness of breath) occur.**

✅ **With minimal to moderate exposure, the patient should be more closely observed for a period of at least 24 hours. Serial arterial blood gas levels, chest radiography, peak expiratory flow rate, airway and lung examination, and bedside spirometry, where available, help detect the evolution of delayed-onset distal airway and pulmonary parenchymal injury.**

What Not To Do:

❌ Do not assume that the patient has not suffered any inhalation injury simply because there are no symptoms or abnormalities evidenced by chest radiography or arterial blood gases in the first few hours after exposure. Some agents produce pulmonary inflammation that develops over 12 to 24 hours.

❌ Do not wait until carboxyhemoglobin levels have been determined before giving 100% oxygen to treat suspected carbon monoxide poisoning. Begin oxygen administration as soon as possible.

❌ Do not insist that the patient breathe room air for a long period before obtaining arterial blood gases. If oxygen administration is helping, its withdrawal is a disservice, and the alveolar-arterial Po_2 gradient can still be estimated while the patient is being given supplemental oxygen.

❌ Do not prescribe corticosteroids unless there is a history of asthma or allergy. Evidence of reduced clearance of lung bacteria and of increased incidence of bacterial pneumonia as a late complication of inhalation injury outweighs any potential anti-inflammatory effects.

❌ Do not prescribe antibiotics unless there is a proven infection.

Discussion

One type of inhalation injury is caused by relatively inert gases, such as carbon dioxide and fuel gases (e.g., methane, ethane, propane, acetylene), which displace air and oxygen, producing asphyxia. Treatment consists of removing the victim from the gas, allowing him to breathe fresh air or oxygen, and attending to any damage (e.g., myocardial infarction, cerebral injury) caused by the period of hypoxia.

A second category of inhalation injury is caused by irritant gases, including ammonia (NH_3), formaldehyde (HCHO), chloramine (NH_2Cl), chlorine (Cl_2), nitrogen

(continued)

Discussion continued

dioxide (NO_2), and phosgene ($COCl_2$). When dissolved in the water lining the respiratory mucosa, irritant gases produce a chemical burn and an inflammatory response. The first three gases listed, which are more soluble in water, tend to produce more upper airway burns, irritating the eyes, nose, and mouth, whereas the latter two gases, being less water soluble, produce more pulmonary injury and respiratory distress. Phosgene can be found is household solvents and can cause delayed severe pulmonary edema, mandating prolonged observation if this agent is suspected. Chlorine is a gas of intermediate solubility and may exert irritant effects widely throughout the respiratory tract. Household bleach contains hypochlorite. Mixing hypochlorite bleach or cleaners with acids, such as hydrochloric acid, sulfuric acid, or phosphoric acid, generates chlorine. Mixing hypochlorite solutions with ammonium hydroxide–containing cleaners generates chloramine.

A third type of inhalation injury is caused by gases that are systemic toxins, such as carbon monoxide (CO), hydrogen cyanide (HCN), and hydrogen sulfide (H_2S). All interfere with the delivery of oxygen for use in cellular energy production and with aromatic and halogenated hydrocarbons, which can result in later liver, kidney, brain, lung, and other organ damage.

A fourth cause of inhalation injury is allergic; inhaled gases, particles, or aerosols produce bronchospasm and edema similar to that caused by asthma or spasmodic croup.

A fifth cause of inhalation injury is direct thermal burns. They are usually limited to the upper airway and produce varying degrees of local edema. Inhalation of steam is far more injurious than heated air. (Steam has approximately 4000 times the heat-carrying capacity of heated air.) Consequently, steam can result in rapidly fatal obstructive glottic edema and lower airway destruction.

The diagnosis of inhalation injury is largely clinical, based on history (disorientation or unconsciousness at the scene, closed space exposure) and physical examination (singed nasal hairs and carbonaceous endobronchial secretions).

In general, treatment of inhalation injury is supportive only. There has been no demonstrated value to prophylactic steroids or antibiotics, but in cases in which the patient is experiencing an exacerbation of underlying COPD or asthma, routine use of steroids is appropriate. Inhaled β-adrenergics can be added if there is bronchospasm. There is promising research evaluating nebulized anticoagulants and N-acetylcysteine for treating inhalation injury.

Because symptoms of acute inhalation injury can be delayed in onset, a key decision that has to be made during the acute evaluation concerns how long to observe a patient for development of more severe respiratory involvement, and whether to admit the patient for hospital treatment. **Current diagnostic tools cannot stratify inhalation injury by severity or accurately predict subsequent clinical course. Again, knowledge of the agent involved and the intensity and duration of exposure is critical.**

Indicators of poor prognosis include a history of altered mental status at the scene, progressive respiratory difficulty, sputum production, rales, burns to the face, hypoxemia, and altered mental status at time of presentation.

■ Although inhalation injuries are often self-limited events, **even mild exposures require early follow-up with clear instructions to the patient** to seek medical care immediately if symptoms worsen. At the follow-up appointments, serial spirometry can assess whether obstructive or restrictive disease is developing.

Suggested Readings

Hall AH, Saiers J, Baud F: Which cyanide antidote? *Crit Rev Toxicol* 39:541–552, 2009.

Miller K, Chang A: Acute inhalation injury, *Emerg Med Clin N Am* 21:533–557, 2003.

Rabinowitz PM, Siegel MD: Acute inhalation injury, *Clin Chest Med* 23:707–715, 2002.

Sheridan R: Specific therapies for inhalation injury, *Crit Care Med* 30(3):718–719, 2002.

Irritant Incapacitant Exposure

(Lacrimators, Riot Control Agents, Tear Gas)

Presentation

The patient may have been sprayed with tear gas (e.g., Mace) during a riot being dispersed by the police, or he may have accidentally sprayed himself with his own can. He complains of burning of the eyes, nose, mouth, and skin; tearing and inability to open his eyes because of the severe stinging; sneezing; coughing; runny nose; and perhaps a metallic taste, with a burning sensation of the tongue, nausea, vomiting, and abdominal pain. These signs and symptoms last 15 to 30 minutes after exposure. Redness and edema may be noted for 1 to 2 days after exposure to these aerosol agents.

What To Do:

✓ Segregate victims so that others are not contaminated. Ideally, this should be done outdoors in the fresh air. Secondary contamination can cause adverse symptoms and injuries in emergency medical personnel, can further contaminate your medical facility, and can potentially lead to costly medical facility closures and evacuations. Medical personnel should don gowns, gloves, and masks before helping victims. (Level C protection with an appropriate air-filtering gas mask approved for riot control agents is adequate.)

✓ **Remove contaminated clothing in a predesignated decontamination area, place the clothing in sealed plastic bags, and then shower with soap and water to remove the irritant incapacitants from the skin.**

✓ **Exposed eyes should be irrigated with copious amounts of tepid water or saline for at least 15 minutes, and contact lenses should be removed. If available, use a Morgan Lens (MorTan, Missoula, Mont.).** Washing the skin with water will remove the residue but will not inactivate it. Removal of contaminated clothing will aid in preventing reexposure. Effects on the eyes and respiratory system generally dissipate within 15 to 30 minutes of cessation of exposure.

✓ **If "pepper spray" (oleoresin capsicum) was the offending agent, some studies suggest that magnesium-aluminum hydroxide suspension (MgAl) (Mylanta), applied to the affected area of skin during the initial 30 minutes, can provide prompt and dramatic relief.** Because MgAl is cheap and readily available and has minimal side effects, it is considered an appropriate early treatment for such dermal exposure.

✓ **If eye pain lasts longer than 15 to 20 minutes, examine the eyes with fluorescein dye, looking for corneal erosions, which may be produced by tear gas or capsicum** (see Chapter 16). **Eye pain from pepper spray is largely dissipated within 1 hour. Topical anesthetics ameliorate the pain, but topical nonsteroidal anti-inflammatory drugs (NSAIDs) do not.**

Patients should be cautioned against rubbing their eyes so that they do not inflict further damage.

✓ Look for signs of, and warn the patient about, allergic reactions to tear gas, including bronchospasm and contact dermatitis. Minor prolonged skin irritation can be treated with hydrocortisone cream 2.5% (1 tube, 30 g), applied bid or qid, or lotion 2.5% (1 bottle, 59 mL), applied bid or qid.

What Not To Do:

✗ Do not rush or allow others to rush to the aid of the patient who has been exposed to tear gas; rushing heedlessly can result in contamination and incapacitation of those attempting to help the patient.

✗ Do not rub the patient's eyes. This may cause mechanical corneal abrasions in addition to the chemical irritation.

Discussion

Irritant incapacitants, also called riot control agents, lacrimators, and tear gases, are currently used by law enforcement agencies and are available to the public for personal protection. These relatively nontoxic agents cause temporary incapacitation by inducing eye pain, lacrimation, and uncontrollable blepharospasm. Exposure to these agents may also result in irritation in the nose and mouth, throat, and airways, causing difficulty breathing and burning sensations in the chest as well as nausea, vomiting, and skin irritation (particularly in moist and warm areas).

Two of the most common riot control agents include chlorobenzylidene malononitrile (CS) (named after its creators, Corson and Stoughton) and oleoresin capsicum (OC), also known as "pepper spray." CS has essentially replaced CN (chloroacetophenone). The U.S. military considers CN obsolete, although it is still common in police agency mixtures and survives as the principal component of Mace.

CS is a white crystalline powder with a pungent pepper-like odor that is immediately detectable. It is used extensively in tear gas. OC is a mixture of compounds obtained by extracting dried, ripe fruit of cayenne peppers. Capsaicin is the principal constituent.

A rinsing solution that may be available in the United States in the future is Diphoterine (Laboratories Prevor, Valmondois, France). Diphoterine is a hypertonic, polyvalent, amphoteric compound developed in France as an eye/skin chemical splash, water-based decontamination solution. In vitro and in vivo, it actively decontaminates approximately 600 chemicals, including acids, alkalis, oxidizing and reducing agents, irritants, lacrimators, solvents, alkylating agents, and radionuclides. Diphoterine and its acid/alkali decontamination residues are not irritating to the eye or skin. Diphoterine is essentially nontoxic. It can prevent eye/skin burns following chemical splashes and results in nearly immediate pain relief. See www.prevor.com and marine suppliers:

R.S. Stern, Inc.
1000 South Highland Avenue
P.O. Box 8872
Baltimore, Md. 21224
or
The Williams & Wells Company
1501 West Blancke Street, Unit B
Linden, N.J. 07036-6219

Although most exposures do not result in life-threatening emergencies, bronchospasm and noncardiogenic pulmonary edema have been seen. Those exposures resulting in respiratory distress should be treated with supplemental oxygen and inhaled bronchodilators.

There is no evidence that a healthy individual will experience long-term health effects from open-air exposures to CS.

Suggested Readings

Blain PG: Tear gases and irritant incapacitants, *Toxicol Rev* 22:103–110, 2003.

Bozeman WP, Dilbero D, Schauben JL: Biologic and chemical weapons of mass destruction, *Emerg Med Clin North Am* 20:975–993, 2002.

Hall AH: Diphoterine for emergent eye/skin chemical splash decontamination: a review, *Vet Hum Toxicol* 44:228–231, 2002.

Horton DK, Burgess P, Rossiter S, et al: Secondary contamination of emergency department personnel from o-chlorobenzylidene malononitrile exposure, 2002, *Ann Emerg Med* 45:655–658, 2005.

Langefeld S: Use of lavage fluid containing diphoterine for irrigation of eyes in first aid emergency treatment, *Ophthalmologe* 199:727–731, 2003.

Lee DC, Ryan JR: Magnesium-aluminum hydroxide suspension for the treatment of dermal capsaicin exposures, *Acad Emerg Med* 10:688–690, 2003.

Merle H: Alkali ocular burns in Martinique. Evaluation of the use of an amphoteric solution as the rinsing product, *Burns* 31:205–211, 2005.

Miller K, Chang A: Acute inhalation injury, *Emerg Med Clin North Am* 21:533–557, 2003.

Zollman TM, Bragg RM, Harrison DA: Clinical effects of oleoresin capsicum (pepper spray) on the human cornea and conjunctiva, *Ophthalmology* 107:2186–2189, 2000.

Rib Fracture and Costochondral Separation

(Broken Rib)

Presentation

A patient with an isolated rib fracture or a minor costochondral separation usually has recently fallen, injuring the side of the chest; been struck by a blunt object; coughed violently; or leaned over a rigid edge. The initial chest pain may subside, but over the next few hours or days the pain increases with movement, interferes with sleep and activity, and becomes severe when the patient coughs or breathes deeply. The patient is often worried about having a broken rib and may have a sensation of bony crepitus or abnormal rib movement. Breath sounds bilaterally should be normal, unless there is substantial splinting or a pneumothorax or hemothorax is present. There is point tenderness over the site of the injury, and occasionally bony crepitus can be felt.

What To Do:

✅ Examine the patient for possible associated injuries, and palpate the abdomen for any signs of a splenic or hepatic injury. What appear to be insignificant mechanisms of injury, such as falling over a chair, hitting the edge of a table, or colliding into a strong ocean wave all have resulted in splenic rupture. **Maintain a high index of suspicion of severe underlying injuries. Consider intra-abdominal injuries in all patients with lower rib fractures and mediastinal injury in those with fractures of the first three ribs. Keep a low threshold for ordering CT scans, especially in the patient with altered mental status or other distracting injuries.**

 ✅ **When there is a history of minor trauma and you do not suspect an intra-abdominal injury, check for rib pain and clinical evidence of fracture by applying indirect stress to the suspected fracture site.** Compress the rib anteroposteriorly if a fracture is suspected at a lateral location. Compress the rib medially if a posterior or anterior fracture is suspected (Figure 65-1). **Pain occurring at the suspected fracture site during application of indirect stress is clinical evidence of a fracture or separation and should be documented on the chart as a "clinical rib fx."** If there is pain with deep inspiration or cough and point tenderness at any position along the rib contours that reproduces this pain, a diagnosis of a clinical rib fracture can also be made. If subcutaneous emphysema is appreciated on examination, the patient is at risk for delayed pneumothorax and should be admitted for observation.

✅ Obtain any history of chronic pulmonary problems or heavy smoking.

✅ **Send the patient for posteroanterior and lateral chest radiographs to rule out a pneumothorax, hemothorax, and pulmonary contusion. Additional oblique rib films for**

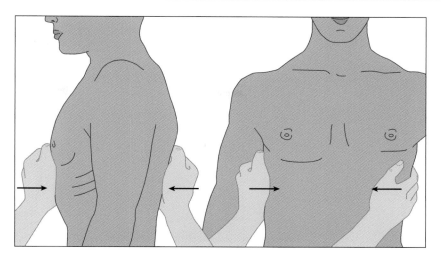

Figure 65-1 Indirect stress test with anteroposterior compression to reveal a lateral rib fracture and lateral-medial compression to reveal an anterior or posterior fracture.

radiologic documentation of a fracture are generally not recommended and rarely add clinical or therapeutic benefit, especially with anterior cartilage injuries. These films may be indicated to document the extent of injury when there is a suspicion of multiple rib fractures, especially in the elderly patient.

Elderly patients with multiple rib fractures have an increased incidence of pneumonia and overall increased mortality and usually require hospital admission with aggressive analgesic management and respiratory care.

If there is no suspicion of a more serious underlying injury, and there is clinical or radiologic evidence of a rib fracture or chondral separation, provide as potent an oral analgesic as needed to control pain. Ibuprofen, naproxen, acetaminophen plus hydrocodone, or acetaminophen plus oxycodone are examples of nonsteroidal anti-inflammatory drugs (NSAIDs) and narcotic preparations that are often most effective when used in combination.

If available, and if the patient is young and healthy, you can place a rib belt on the patient to see if this provides comfort. If there is significant pain relief, you can instruct the patient regarding the intermittent use of this elastic and Velcro belt. Place the bottom of the belt at the inferior tip of the xiphoid process, tightening it around the chest enough to obtain maximum pain relief. The rib belt may be worn almost continuously for the first 1 to 4 days, but it should be removed as comfort allows thereafter (Figure 65-2).

Instruct the patient regarding the importance of deep breathing and coughing (without the rib belt but using a pillow splint) to help prevent pneumonia. Tell him to take enough pain medicine to allow coughing and deep breathing. When available, provide incentive spirometry.

Provide the patient with appropriate documentation for missing work, and refer him for follow-up care in 48 hours. Tell him to expect gradually decreasing discomfort for about

237

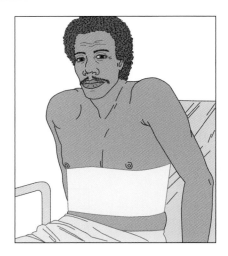

Figure 65-2 Proper placement of elastic and Velcro rib belt.

2 to 4 weeks, but prepare him for an extended period of disability (it will take several weeks to heal and become pain free). **Forbid strenuous activity for approximately 8 weeks.** One study showed that patients with isolated rib fractures returned to work or their usual activities at a mean of 51 days (±39 days).

✅ Severe worsening of chest pain, shortness of breath, fever, or purulent sputum may signal pulmonary complications and should prompt a return visit. A greater incidence of complications can be expected in patients with displaced rib fractures.

✅ **When there is no clinical or radiologic evidence of a fracture, treat the pain as any other contusion would be treated, using an appropriate analgesic.**

What Not To Do:

❌ Do not confuse simple rib fractures with massive blunt trauma to the chest. The evaluation and management are quite different.

❌ Do not overlook child or elder abuse. Rib fractures are uncommon in younger children and are found in 5% to 27% of documented cases of child abuse. Child abuse should be considered in the absence of a plausible history of trauma or conditions of bony fragility, such as osteogenesis imperfecta or rickets.

❌ Do not tape ribs or use continuous strapping. This will lead to hypoventilation and an atelectatic lung that is prone to pneumonia.

❌ Do not assume that there is no fracture just because the radiographs are normal. Rib fractures are often not apparent on radiographs, especially when they occur in the cartilaginous portion of the rib. The patient deserves the disability period and analgesics commensurate with the real injury.

Discussion

Rib fracture pain can be significant, originates at the site of the fractured bone and injured muscle, and is usually reported by patients to be exacerbated by any movement of the chest wall (e.g., with respiration and most certainly with deep breathing and coughing). Although most commonly secondary to trauma, rib fractures may also occur because of repetitive stressors, such as that experienced with coughing or in athletes such as golfers and rowers.

Most isolated fractures and separations cause minimal morbidity or mortality and are treated with immobilization, but ribs are a special problem because patients have to continue breathing. Pain management is crucial. Patients with pain often splint and hypoventilate and thus are predisposed to pneumonia. Outpatient management of isolated rib fractures with oral pain medication is generally adequate.

In the presence of severe pain or multiple rib fractures, consider the use of an intercostal nerve block or injection of the fracture hematoma with 0.5% bupivacaine (Marcaine). Because of the risk for pneumothorax or hemothorax, in most cases, this procedure should be reserved for secondary management when initial treatment has proven inadequate.

Although rib belts are no longer commonly used and their use is even discouraged, they can sometimes provide significant pain relief for young, active patients who are at low risk for pulmonary complications. If used, it may be worn almost continuously for the first 1 to 4 days, but it should be removed as comfort allows thereafter.

Suggested Readings

Bansidhar B, Lagares-Garcia JA, Miller SL: Clinical rib fractures: are follow-up chest x-rays a waste of resources? *Am Surg* 68:449–453, 2002.

Bhavnagri SJ, Mohammed TL: When and how to image a suspected broken rib, *Cleve Clin J Med* 76:309–314, 2009.

Bliss D, Silen M: Pediatric thoracic trauma, *Crit Care Med* 30(Suppl 11):S409–S415, 2002.

Bulger EM, Arneson MA, Mock CN, Jurkovich GH: Rib fractures in the elderly, *Ann Emerg Med* 39:1040–1046, 2002.

Holcomb JB, McMullin NR, Kozar RA, et al: Morbidity from rib fractures increases after age 45, *J Am Coll Med* 196:549–555, 2003.

Holmes JF, Nguyen H, Jacoby RC, et al: Do all patients with left costal margin injuries require radiographic evaluation for intraabdominal injury? *Ann Emerg Med* 46:232–236, 2005.

Kerr-Valentic MA, Arthur M, Mullins RJ, et al: Rib fracture pain and disability: can we do better? *J Trauma* 54: 1058–1064, 2003.

Kieninger AN: Epidural versus intravenous pain control in elderly patients with rib fractures, *Am J Surg* 189:327–330, 2005.

Lazcano A, Dougherty J, Kruger M: Use of rib belts in acute rib fractures, *Am J Emerg Med* 7:97–100, 1989.

Lu MS, Huang YK, Liu YH, et al: Delayed pneumothorax complicating minor rib fracture after chest trauma, *Am J Emerg Med* 26:551–554, 2008.

Quick G: A randomized clinical trial of rib belts for simple fractures, *Am J Emerg Med* 8:277–281, 1990.

Sikka R: Unsuspected internal organ traumatic injuries, *Emerg Med Clin North Am* 22:1067–1080, 2004.

Ullman EA, Donley LP, Brady WJ: Pulmonary trauma, *Emerg Med Clin North Am* 21:291–313, 2003.

PART 6

Gastrointestinal Emergencies

■ Philip Buttaravoli ■ Maj Eisinger

Anal Fissure

Presentation

In most patients, the symptoms are so characteristic that they are nearly diagnostic. Patients complain of severe intense pain with defecation. It can be described as knifelike, cutting, or tearing in character. This pain can persist for hours, with a tight, throbbing quality followed by relative comfort prior to the next bowel movement. Often patients will complain of constipation that predates their anal symptoms. Occasionally, patients have diarrhea or an alternating pattern of constipation and diarrhea.

Bleeding with defecation may occur but is usually slight, only staining the toilet tissue. Mucous discharge may increase perineal moisture and cause itching. Examination of the anus reveals a radial tear or ulceration of the posterior midline 95% of the time (the fissure is anterior in 10% of women but only 1% of men) (Figure 66-1). If the condition becomes chronic, the skin distal to the fissure becomes edematous and enlarged and may form a fibrous skin tag referred to as a "sentinel pile."

What To Do:

✓ Most patients with an anal fissure cannot tolerate a digital rectal examination or anoscopy. Parenteral analgesia may be necessary prior to attempting any examination.

✓ To examine the patient, place him in the left lateral decubitus position with knees bent toward the chest. (Use proper draping to maintain the patient's dignity and to minimize any embarrassment.) Good lighting is essential.

✓ **Gentle retraction of the perianal skin usually allows one to visualize the fissure directly, even in patients with significant spasm.**

✓ **The mainstay of medical treatment for both acute and chronic anal fissures is the avoidance of hard stools.** This can be accomplished with fiber supplementation and stool softeners. **Advise the patient to take methylcellulose (Citrucel), 1 heaping tablespoon in**

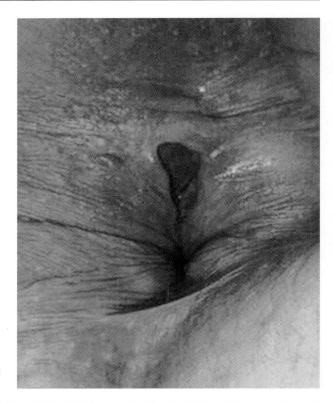

Figure 66-1 With the patient in prone jackknife position, a posterior acute anal fissure is visible once the buttocks are separated. (Courtesy Richard P. Billingham, MD, Seattle, Wash.).

8 oz of water qd to tid, along with docusate sodium (Colace), 50 to 200 mg/day PO, divided in 1 to 4 doses (50, 100, 250 mg capsules). Lubricating glycerin suppositories used bid can also be helpful. All of these products may be purchased over the counter.

To break the cycle of sphincter spasm and tearing of anal mucosa, and thereby promote subsequent healing of the fissure, medical therapy is often necessary. **Prescribe topical nifedipine 0.2%, twice daily for 3 weeks, or diltiazem gel 2%** (these prescriptions often need to be filled at a compounding pharmacy) **with lidocaine HCL 2% gel, maximum dose 4.5 mg/kg, not to exceed 300 mg, to be applied every 12 hours for 8 weeks.**

Topical glyceryl trinitrate 0.2% or nitroglycerin ointment 0.2% (these prescriptions also may need to be filled at a compounding pharmacy) can be substituted for the topical diltiazem and nifedipine, but many patients are unable to tolerate the headaches that frequently occur. Avoid nitroglycerin therapy in patients taking Viagra or other erectile dysfunction medications.

Instruct the patient to use warm, soothing sitz baths after each painful bowel movement.

Prescribe analgesics if needed, but remember that narcotics are constipating.

Botox injection into the sphincter may be considered if the above therapies fail; however, flatus or fecal incontinence is a potential side effect of this. Lateral sphincterotomy is usually successful when medical therapies fail, although complications may occur.

✓ Inform the patient that an acute superficial fissure will take about 4 to 6 weeks to heal. He or she should follow up if symptoms continue. At that point, endoscopy to assess for possible Crohn's disease, and other diagnoses, should be considered.

What Not To Do:

✗ Do not assume that a lesion located outside the anteroposterior midline sagittal plane of the anus is an anal fissure. Lateral location, extension onto the anal verge or above the dentate line, and extension of the base of the ulcer through the internal sphincter are all atypical features. Other possibilities include ulcerative colitis, squamous cell carcinoma, leukemia, tuberculosis, syphilis, herpes, Crohn's disease, sexually transmitted diseases, and trauma from instrumentation and anal intercourse. Appropriate follow-up should be arranged.

✗ Do not confuse a "sentinel pile" with a hemorrhoidal vein.

✗ Do not prescribe 0.2% nitroglycerin ointment for use in patients taking Viagra.

✗ Do not fail to refer an adult patient with rectal bleeding for endoscopy.

Discussion

Anal fissures probably begin by the tearing of the mucosa during defecation. Hard stools are most commonly implicated, but explosive liquid stools can produce the same results. This starts a vicious cycle of pain, causing spasm in the anal sphincter, which results in increased friction during defecation and leads to further tearing and pain.

Currently, ischemia is considered the most likely cause for development of an anal fissure. There is a paucity of anal blood vessels, especially in the posterior midline, and it is thought that anal spasm further reduces blood flow.

After a period of about 4 to 8 weeks, a fissure can be considered chronic. The cycle can be broken with analgesia, stool softening, lubrication, relaxation of spasm, or all four.

Although many acute anal fissures with a fresh skin tear heal spontaneously, some do not. With those that do not, secondary changes develop, with raised edges exposing the white, horizontally oriented fibers of the internal sphincter (chronic fissure). Botulinum toxin, which is a potent inhibitor of acetylcholine release from nerve endings, can be injected into the anal sphincter and can improve healing in patients with chronic fissures. One uncommon adverse effect associated with the drug is flatus incontinence. If the fissure is large, it may become ulcerated and infected, not heal spontaneously, and require surgical excision.

Pruritus ani has multiple causes, although most cases are idiopathic. Infections such as pinworms, *Candida albicans, Tinea cruris,* and erythrasma can cause anal itching. Mechanical trauma from overly vigorous cleansing of the perianal area may also cause pruritus. The latter may be aggravated by diarrhea and the presence of external or prolapsed hemorrhoids or multiple skin tags, which make cleansing more difficult. Another cause of pruritus ani is allergic or contact dermatitis from agents such as soaps, perfumes in toilet tissue, and feminine hygiene sprays, as well as spicy foods, tomatoes, citrus fruits and colas, coffee, and chocolate. Psoriasis, seborrheic dermatitis, atopic eczema, and lichen planus are additional dermatologic sources of itching. Other causes of pruritus ani include chronic anorectal disease, human immunodeficiency virus (HIV)-related infections, diabetes, cancer, and illnesses that produce hyperbilirubinemia. If a specific cause of anal pruritus can be determined, treat it accordingly. If the cause is obscure, the patient can be treated with hydrocortisone cream to reduce itching, scratching, and inflammation, followed by zinc oxide as a barrier cream.

In general, any medications such as antibiotics and laxatives should be discontinued, and the diet should be adjusted as necessary. A bulk-forming

(continued)

Discussion continued

agent can be administered to allow for complete and predictable bowel evacuation, followed by bathing appropriately with warm water and little soap (to reduce chemical irritation). Using a hair dryer will provide gentle drying without further irritation. Moistened rectal wipes can be a reasonable alternative, but wipes containing chemicals such as perfumes, alcohol, or witch hazel should be avoided to reduce any effect of chemical contact dermatitis. Irritation from vigorous cleansing may actually worsen the itch. A systemic antipruritic agent, such

as hydroxyzine (Vistaril), 25 mg orally 3 to 4 times daily, may be prescribed. Follow-up is required.

Proctalgia fugax is a unique entity found mostly in males, causing severe, brief, lancinating episodes of rectal pain lasting seconds to minutes. The pain is excruciating but is spontaneous and unrelated to defecation. The physical examination is completely normal, and treatment primarily consists of reassurance with an explanation of this benign disorder.

Suggested Readings

American Gastroenterological Association: American Gastroenterological Association medical position statement: diagnosis and care of patients with anal fissure, *Gastroenterology* 124:233–234, 2003. Available at http://www.gastro.org/practice/medical-position-statements.

Brenner BE, Simon RR: Anorectal emergencies, *Ann Emerg Med* 12:367–376, 1983.

Brisinda G, Cadeddu F, Brandara F, et al: Randomized clinical trial comparing botulinum toxin injections with 0.2 percent nitroglycerin ointment for chronic anal fissure, *Br J Surg* 94:162–167, 2007.

Ezri T, Susmallian S: Topical nifedipine vs. topical glyceryl trinitrate for treatment of chronic anal fissure, *Dis Colon Rectum* 46:805–808, 2003.

Gopal DV: Diseases of the rectum and anus: a clinical approach to common disorders, *Clin Cornerstone* 4:34–48, 2002.

Herzig DO, Lu KC: Anal fissure, *Surg Clin North Am* 90:33–44, 2010.

Lieberman DA: Common anorectal disorders, *Ann Intern Med* 101:837–846, 1984.

Lund JN, Scholefield JH: A randomized, prospective, double-blind, placebo-controlled trial of glyceryl trinitrate ointment in treatment of anal fissure, *Lancet* 349:11–14, 1997.

Madoff RD, Dykes SL: What's new in colon and rectal surgery, *J Am Coll Surg* 198:98–104, 2004.

Metcalf AM: Anal fissure, *Surg Clin North Am* 82:1291–1297, 2002.

Parellada C: Randomized, prospective trial comparing 0.2 percent isorbide dinitrate ointment with sphincterotomy in treatment of chronic anal fissure: a two year follow-up, *Dis Colon Rectum* 47:437–443, 2004.

Slawson D: Topical nifedipine plus lidocaine gel effective for anal fissures, *Am Fam Physician* 67:1781, 2003.

Zhao X, Pasricha PJ: Botulinum toxin for spastic GI disorders: a systematic review, *Gastrointest Endosc* 57:219–235, 2003.

Constipation, Irritable Bowel Syndrome, and Colic

(Stomach Cramps)

Presentation

Patients with functional constipation will often come in with the complaint of abdominal pain or bloating. Often, it is not until they are asked that they will describe infrequent bowel movements, straining at stooling, incomplete evacuation, hard or small stools, a blockage in the anal region, or the need for digital manipulation to enable defecation.

Patients with irritable bowel syndrome (IBS) will complain of abdominal pain or discomfort, with a change in the form or frequency of defecation. They will have constipation (fewer than three bowel movements per week), diarrhea (more than three bowel movements per day), or alternating constipation and diarrhea. Their pain is relieved by defecation.

At the age of 6 weeks, infants with colic will begin having episodes of inconsolable crying that last more than 3 hours per day for more than 3 days per week and that continue longer than 3 weeks. These infants are well fed and otherwise healthy.

In all of these cases, the patient's discomfort is not accompanied by other symptoms, such as nausea, vomiting, fever, anorexia, or weight loss. Rarely are patients awakened with nocturnal symptoms.

The physical examination is benign, with normal vital signs and no jaundice, tenderness, masses, organomegaly, rectal bleeding, or other abnormalities, and the patient does not appear ill between the episodes of abdominal pain.

What To Do:

✓ Take a thorough history and try to determine the time of onset of symptoms and whether their severity is increasing or decreasing. Ask if there was a similar episode in the past. A careful medication history should be obtained, because many commonly used drugs may cause constipation.

✓ Perform a complete physical examination, including rectal and/or pelvic examination, and a repeat abdominal examination after an interval. The patient's skin is checked for pallor and signs of hypothyroidism (e.g., reduced body hair, skin dryness, fixed edema), and the abdomen is examined for masses, distention, tenderness, and high-pitched bowel sounds. The rectal examination includes careful inspection and palpation for masses, anal fissures, inflammation, and hard stool in the ampulla. Test stool for the presence of occult blood.

✅ **For patients with symptomatic constipation, it is appropriate, but not always necessary, to obtain a complete blood count, biochemical profile, serum calcium, glucose levels, and thyroid-stimulating hormone.**

✅ If the presentation is not clear or there is any concern about significant underlying disease, consider using diagnostic tests, such as urinalysis (to help rule out renal colic or urinary tract infection), an erythrocyte sedimentation rate (a clue to infection or inflammation), abdominal radiographs (to show free peritoneal air, bowel obstruction, or fecal impaction), and ultrasonography (for pyloric stenosis, malrotation and intussusception in children, or gallbladder and pelvic disorders in adults). CT imaging should be used to rule out any suspected intra-abdominal or retroperitoneal catastrophe. Adult patients with a change in bowel habits or hemoccult positive stool should be referred for colonoscopy to assess for malignancy.

✅ **If simple constipation is the problem and there is obstructing stool on rectal examination, disimpact the rectum by pulling out hard stool *(scybala),* and follow with one oil retention enema. This may be very painful and require parenteral analgesia. For dry, obstipated feces, repeated tap-water enemas or phosphate enemas should be administered once or twice daily until clear.**

✅ **Disimpaction by the oral route,** using medication, is noninvasive and more easily accepted by adolescents, who will often be reluctant to receive enemas. If there is no mechanically obstructing fecal impaction, this can also be done for adults. **Magnesium citrate (Citro-Mag), 150 to 300 mL given once or divided doses for those 7 to 12 years old. For pediatric patients younger than 6 years, 2 to 4 mL/kg given once or in divided doses.**

✅ **Disimpaction by means of a combination of the rectal route and the oral route has been shown to be effective.**

✅ Instruct the patient to return if symptoms do not resolve over the next 12 to 24 hours or to return immediately if the pain worsens.

✅ **Instruct the patient to drink plenty of fluids.**

✅ **Instruct the patient that the recommended amount of dietary fiber is 20 to 35 g per day.**

✅ **Suggest adding bulk fiber, 20 to 35 g total fiber intake per day, in the form of bran, psyllium (Metamucil), methylcellulose (Citrucel), or calcium polycarbophil (FiberCon tablets) for prophylaxis.** The last two products are made from synthetic fiber and produce less gas. A high-fiber diet, however, does not benefit all patients with constipation. In general, patients with inadequate fiber intake should be advised (with the help of a dietitian) to increase their intake of natural fiber with fruit and vegetable servings.

✅ **When possible, medications that may be constipating should be discontinued or replaced.** These medications include narcotic analgesics, antacids containing aluminum and calcium, antidepressants, diuretics, nutritional supplements such as iron and calcium, anticonvulsants, antispasmodics, antiparkinson drugs, antihypertensive agents such as calcium channel blockers, and sedatives.

✅ **Laxatives remain the mainstay of treatment for constipation.**

✓ **Osmotic agents with laxative effects include sorbitol solution 70% (30 to 150 mL or 1 to 2 mL/kg as single adult dose) or lactulose (Cephulac, Chronulac) (30 to 150 mL daily, may increase to 60 mL daily if necessary). In recent years, the use of over-the-counter polyethylene glycol 3350 without electrolytes (MiraLax), (17 g [1 heaping tablespoonful] of powder dissolved in 8 oz of water, juice, soda, coffee, or tea once daily, titrated to effect with a maximum of 34 g per day) has become increasingly popular.** It is relatively expensive but generally has fewer side effects. Because it is virtually tasteless, it has led to better compliance with treatment. Polyethylene glycol (e.g., GoLYTELY) is another option, and is supplied in 14-oz and 26-oz containers as a powder to be administered after dissolution of **1 heaping tablespoon in 4 to 8 oz of water, juice, soda, coffee, or tea qd.**

✓ **Additionally, bisacodyl (Dulcolax), 5 to 15 mg as single adult dose, or senna (Senokot), 15 mg once daily, are stimulant laxatives that can be given at bedtime and are available over the counter.** Both sorbitol and senna are less costly than lactulose and have been shown to be at least as efficacious, if not better.

✓ Functional constipation in infants and toddlers is defined as at least 2 weeks of scybalous, pebble-like, hard stools—or firm stools two or fewer times per week—in the absence of structural, endocrine, or metabolic disease.

✓ Constipation in infants and preschool children is usually treated first with sorbitol-containing juices, such as prune, pear, and apple juice; the addition of pureed fruits and vegetables; formula changes; or treatment with a food product with a high sugar content, such as barley malt extract or corn syrup. If, despite these dietary changes, the stool is still hard and painful to evacuate, osmotic laxatives, such as milk of magnesia, 0.5 to 1 mL/kg body weight/day, or polyethylene glycol 3350 without electrolytes (MiraLax), 1 to 1.5 g/kg body weight/day, are easily administered by parents and well-accepted by children. They have a 92% success rate. Glycerin suppositories can be also be effective. Avoid mineral oil in infants, those with neurologic difficulties, and those with gastoesophageal reflux disease (GERD) because of the risk of aspiration pneumonitis. In addition, avoid enemas and stimulant laxatives, such as senna or bisacodyl, in infants.

✓ **If the problem is chronic or recurrent or associated with alternating constipation and diarrhea, consider irritable bowel syndrome (IBS). IBS is characterized by chronic abdominal pain, altered bowel habits, and no organic cause; thus it is a diagnosis of exclusion. The most distinguishing trait of IBS is the presence of discomfort or pain associated with defecation.** The Rome III criteria of 2005 to 2006 include the following criteria for IBS: at least 3 months of symptoms, with onset at least 6 months previously of recurrent abdominal pain or discomfort associated with two or more of the following:

○ Improvement with defecation; and/or

○ Onset associated with change in frequency of stool; and/or

○ Onset associated with a change in form (appearance) of stool.

✓ Warning signs of more serious disease include the following: unintentional or unexpected weight loss; nocturnal symptoms (more common in inflammatory bowel disease, celiac sprue, infection, or cancer); fever, weight loss, and bleeding, which suggest ulcerative colitis infection or cancer; abdominal pain with bloat, anorexia, rectal abscess, and constipation, which could signal Crohn's disease; abdominal pain with iron deficiency and stress fractures, which could be celiac disease or another small-bowel disorder causing malabsorption; and gastrointestinal blood loss (gross or occult), which could be the result of cancer.

✅ If the patient meets the Rome III criteria, if routine testing shows no abnormalities, and if the patient has no warning signs of more serious disease, then you can initiate treatment for IBS and provide follow-up in 3 to 6 weeks (sooner if symptoms change dramatically or the patient's condition deteriorates).

✅ IBS is a chronic condition without known cure. A meticulous dietary history, as it relates to symptoms, can be helpful. Dietary interventions such as a lactose-free diet, restriction of carbohydrates, avoidance of gluten, and avoidance of foods that produce gas may be undertaken.

✅ **For constipation-predominant IBS, you can give synthetic bulk fiber as described earlier.**

✅ **Psychological therapy has been found to have some efficacy in IBS symptom reduction, as noted in the 2009 American College of Gastroenterology Task Force on Irritable Bowel Syndrome, which also provides further guidelines for management of this disorder.**

✅ **The use of pharmacologic agents may also be considered. Antidepressants, such as SSRIs or low-dose TCAs, may be useful in adults with severe, unrelenting symptoms. Antispasmodic drugs, such as dicyclomine (20 mg PO, 4 times daily prn for nongeriatric adult) and hyoscyamine (0.125 to 0.25 mg PO or sublingual tid prn for adult, maximum 1.5 mg/24 h) may provide short-term relief. 5-Hydroxytryptamine (serotonin)-3 (5-HT$_3$) receptor antagonists such as alosetron (Lotronex), for female patients with diarrhea-predominant IBS, were removed from the market because of problems with ischemic colitis and severe constipation, but are now available with tight restrictions. Tegaserod (Zelnorm), a partial 5-HT$_4$ receptor agonist approved for constipation-variant IBS was removed from the market in 2007. Lubiprostone for patients with IBS with constipation has been approved, but there is a lack of controlled studies and long-term safety concerns exist.**

✅ Rifaximin is a nonabsorbable antibiotic that has shown modest benefit in studies with relatively short-term follow-up for those with IBS and bloating.

✅ If there is weight loss, anemia, occult blood in the stool, abdominal distension or mass, or a family history of colon cancer, refer the patient for colonoscopy and gastroenterology consultation.

✅ **For infant colic** (defined as crying for a minimum of 3 hours daily 3 days per week for the previous 3 weeks, without weight loss, vomiting, or diarrhea), **there is no "magic bullet." Use of whey hydrolysate milk is considered likely to be beneficial. Other therapies are of uncertain effectiveness. You may instruct the parents to administer for infants, 2 mL of 24% solution of sucrose in distilled water and for neonates, 0.2 mL of 24% solution, with each episode for a 1- to 2-day trial. If this is not successful, a higher concentration of sucrose may be more effective.** Probiotics *(Lactobacillus reuteri)* have been shown to be beneficial in two randomized trials, with no ill effects observed. However, these are not regulated by the Food and Drug Administration. Homeopathic remedies, simethicone and lactase have no proven benefits.

✅ A product called "Gripe Water," which may include any variety of herbs and herbal oils (such as cardamom, chamomile, cinnamon, clove, dill, fennel, ginger, lemon balm, licorice, peppermint, and yarrow), is available online and in health food stores. It is not entirely without risk. Contaminants and alcohol have been found in some preparations. Parents who choose to use this product should avoid versions made with sugar or alcohol and look for products that were manufactured in the United States.

✓ With breast-feeding mothers, there is a possible therapeutic benefit from eliminating milk products, eggs, wheat, and nuts from the mother's diet.

✓ Some studies suggest that casein hydrolysate formulas (considered hypoallergenic) or replacement of cow's milk formula with a soy-based formula may be beneficial; a trial period of formula substitution can be recommended.

✓ Above all, parents need reassurance that their baby is healthy and that colic is self limited (80% to 90% of infants have symptom resolution by 4 months of age). There are no long-term adverse effects. The potential for child abuse is a real one; parents with crying infants have been known to hurt their babies. Parents should be given reassurance and empathy and have their coping mechanisms addressed; they should be counseled to take breaks from the colicky infant and employ actions to relieve stress. One study concluded that a home-based nursing intervention program reduced both parental stress and overall infant crying time.

What Not To Do:

✗ Do not discharge the patient with significant abdominal pain without 1 to 2 hours of observation and two abdominal examinations. Many abdominal catastrophes may appear improved for short periods, only to worsen in an hour or two.

✗ Do not add fiber supplements without an adequate intake of fluids. Otherwise, they may actually exacerbate symptoms.

✗ Do not settle for a specific benign diagnosis in patients for whom you cannot find a clear cause. Do not fail to refer for colonoscopy.

Discussion

The colon performs several complex functions, which include mixing the ileal effluent, fermenting and salvaging the unabsorbed carbohydrate residues, and desiccating the intraluminal contents to form stool. These functions are regulated by neurotransmitters, intrinsic colonic reflexes, and a plethora of learned and reflex mechanisms that govern stool transport and evacuation, most of which are incompletely understood. Constipation may result from structural, mechanical, metabolic, or functional disorders that affect the colon or anorectum, either directly or indirectly. Because there is a significant interaction between the brain and the gut, it is worth emphasizing that neurologic dysfunction may have profound effects on colon function.

Patients who have had two of the following symptoms for at least 12 months fit the **criteria for functional constipation**: straining, lumpy or hard stools, incomplete bowel evacuation or sensation of anorectal blockage at least a quarter of the time, or less than three bowel movements in a week.

For infants to children 16 years of age, the following constitute functional fecal retention: at least 12 weeks of passage of large-diameter stools at intervals of two per week or fewer and/ or retentive posturing, avoidance of defecation, and use of both pelvic floor and gluteal muscles. Functional constipation is most common in women. Colonic inertia and delayed transit are types of functional constipation caused by decreased muscle activity in the colon. Abnormalities that result in an inability to relax the rectal and anal muscles that allow stool to exit are known as *anorectal dysfunction* or *anismus*.

(continued)

Discussion continued

When constipation becomes chronic and unresponsive to conventional medical and behavioral treatment, it is necessary to rule out organic diseases that can present with constipation. Some of the more common diseases include irritable bowel syndrome, diverticulitis, intestinal obstruction, anal fissure and abdominal tumors. Metabolic causes include uremia, hypokalemia, hyponatremia, hypomagnesemia, hypophosphatemia, and hypercalcemia. Endocrine causes include diabetes mellitus and hypothyroidism. Neuromuscular disorders that lead to constipation include brain tumors, spinal cord compression, multiple sclerosis, Parkinson disease, cerebral palsy, and stroke or other disorders that cause muscle weakness. Acute constipation is more often associated with organic disease than is long-standing constipation. When a particular disorder is suspected, appropriate laboratory studies and colorectal imaging are required.

Flexible sigmoidoscopy and colonoscopy are excellent for identifying lesions that narrow or occlude the bowel. Colonoscopy is the examination of choice in adult patients with constipation who have iron deficiency anemia, a positive guaiac stool test, or a first-degree relative with colon cancer.

In childhood constipation, most difficulties related to defecation are the consequence of painful or psychologically traumatic defecation experiences. In children younger than 1 year of age, the possibility of Hirschsprung disease or cystic fibrosis must be considered. However, in adolescents, constipation is most commonly a consequence of a learned behavior to suppress the urge to defecate. When specifically asked, adolescents readily admit that they do not use the toilet facilities at school. Repeated suppression of the urge to defecate and stool withholding may be contributing factors to the two colorectal disorders associated with constipation: pelvic floor dysfunction and slow-transit constipation.

A reduction in dietary fiber has been associated with a higher prevalence of constipation in children. Illicit substances, particularly opiates such as heroin, OxyContin, and hydrocodone-containing products, are used by approximately 10% of high school seniors nationwide. These substances may cause or exacerbate constipation. Therefore abuse of these substances should be included in the differential diagnosis of the constipated adolescent patient. In addition, constipation is among the most frequently identified concerns in patients who have anorexia nervosa and bulimia. Many patients with eating disorders are distressed by and preoccupied with their infrequent bowel movements.

Occult constipation should be considered in children with recurrent abdominal pain. Because reporting of stool patterns by children is unreliable, rectal examination should be considered in those with recurrent abdominal pain.

IBS is a common condition in adults and adolescents. There is a significant female predominance in those patients who present to physicians with this condition. Patients with IBS view minor illnesses, such as colds and the flu, more seriously and consult physicians more frequently than do patients who do not have IBS.

IBS is a heterogeneous disorder with diverse clinical presentations and multiple pathogenic mechanisms. Its exact pathophysiology remains undefined. The three most important contributing factors seem to be hypersensitivity of the gut, altered motility, and psychosocial dysfunction. Changes in intestinal microflora, including small intestinal bacterial overgrowth, carbohydrate malabsorption, and the development of gluten sensitivity or food specific antibodies are currently being investigated as potential causes. Gastrointestinal infections may act as a triggering factor in a subgroup of patients. Patients with IBS may present with diarrhea, constipation, or a combination of urgency, pain, gas, and bloating. Symptoms are not constant over time. There is temporal fluctuation, with "flare-ups" alternating with periods of relative well-being in most patients. The type of bowel complaint and predominance of specific symptoms may also vary over time.

Patients who are allergic to gliadin (a constituent of rye, barley, and wheat) may present with symptoms that are indistinguishable from IBS. This condition, known as celiac disease, or sprue, can cause a variety of symptoms, including rancid gas, oily or floating stools, bloating, and constipation or diarrhea. Consultation with a gastroenterologist should be obtained prior to starting the patient on a gluten-free diet.

Infant colic can be distressing to parents whose infant is inconsolable during crying episodes. Colic is a diagnosis of exclusion that is made after performing a careful history and physical examination to rule out less common organic causes. Treatment is limited. Feeding changes are sometimes advised. Medications available in the United States have not been proved effective in the

Discussion continued

treatment of colic, and most behavior interventions have not been proved to be clearly more effective than placebo. The cause of infantile colic remains unclear.

Colic attacks usually start when an infant is 7 to 10 days old and increase in frequency for the next 1 to 2 months. They tend to be worse in the late afternoon and evening and subside by the age of 3 months. Colicky infants have attacks of screaming in the evening with associated motor behaviors, such as a flushed face, furrowed brow, and clenched fists. The legs are pulled up to the abdomen, and the infants emit a piercing, high-pitched scream. Crying occurs in prolonged bouts and is unpredictable and spontaneous. It appears to be unrelated to environmental events. The child cannot be soothed, even by feeding. These episodes do not just happen suddenly one night when the infant is 6 to 8 weeks old. In that situation, look for some other acute problem, such as intussusception, corneal abrasion, incarcerated hernia, clothing that may be pinching or pricking, or a digital hair tourniquet. A history of apnea, cyanosis, or struggling to breathe may suggest previously undiagnosed

pulmonary or cardiac conditions. Lethargy, poor skin perfusion, and tachypnea suggest a serious underlying problem. A rectal temperature greater than 100.4° F (38° C) or poor weight gain suggests infection, a gastrointestinal disorder, or nervous system disorder and requires further workup. During the examination, the infant's clothing should be removed to facilitate inspection of the skin, to eliminate any irritation to the skin, and to check for any evidence of trauma or abuse. The examination itself may reassure the parents. Organic causes are found in less than 5% of infants presenting with excessive crying. If the child is not awake and calm for a reasonable period, however, consider hospital admission with a complete diagnostic workup.

Laboratory tests and radiographic examinations usually are unnecessary if the child is gaining weight and has a normal physical examination without worrisome symptoms.

At 1-year follow-up, a group of colicky infants compared with noncolicky infants showed no differences in behavior in nine dimensions assessed by means of the Toddler Temperament Scale.

Suggested Readings

American College of Gastroenterology Task Force on Irritable Bowel Syndrome, Brandt LJ, Chey WD, et al: An evidence-based position statement on the management of irritable bowel syndrome, *Am J Gastroenterol* 104(Suppl 1):S1–S35, 2009.

American College of Gastroenterology Chronic Constipation Task Force: An evidence-based approach to the management of chronic constipation in North America, *Am J Gastroenterol* 100(Suppl 1):S1–S4, 2005.

Arce DA, Ermocilla CA, Costa H: Evaluation of constipation, *Am Fam Physician* 65:2283–2290, 2002.

Chang L: From Rome to Los Angeles—The Rome III Criteria for the Functional GI Disorders, Los Angeles, May 20-25, 2006, Paper presented at Digestive Disorders Week.

Clifford TJ, Campbell K, Speechley KN, et al: Infant colic, *Arch Pediatr Adolesc Med* 156:1183–1188, 2002.

Clifford TJ, Campbell K, Speechley KN, et al: Sequelae of infant colic, *Arch Pediatr Adolesc Med* 156:1123–1128, 2002.

Constipation Guideline Committee of the North American Society for Pediatric Gastroenterology: Hepatology and Nutrition: Evaluation and treatment of constipation in infants and children: recommendations of the North American Society for Pediatric Gastroenterology, Hepatology, and Nutrition, *J Pediatr Gastroenterol Nutr* 43:e1, 2006.

Dalrymple J, Bullock I: Diagnosis and management of irritable bowel syndrome in adults in primary care: summary of NICE guidance, *BMJ* 336:556–558, 2008.

Eidlitz-Markus T, Mimouni M, Zaharia A, et al: Occult constipation: a common cause of recurrent abdominal pain in childhood, *Isr Med Assoc J* 6:677–680, 2004.

Ford AC, Talley NJ, Schoenfeld PS, et al: Efficacy of antidepressants and psychological therapies in irritable bowel syndrome: systematic review and meta-analysis, *Gut* 58:367–378, 2009.

Keefe MR, Lobo ML, Froese-Fretz A: Effectiveness of an intervention for colic, *Clin Pediatr (Phila)* 45:123–133, 2006.

Kilgour T, Wade S: Infantile colic, *Clin Evid* 13:362–372, 2005.

Lehtonen L, Korhonen T, Korvenranta H: Temperament and sleeping patterns in colicky infants during the first year of life, *J Dev Behav Pediatr* 15:416–420, 1994.

Loening-Baucke V: Prevalence, symptoms, and outcome of constipation in infants and toddlers, *J Pediatr* 146: 359–363, 2005.

Pimentel M, Lembo A, Chey WD, et al: Rifaximin therapy for patients with IBS without constipation, *N Engl J Med* 364:22–32, 2011.

Rao S: Constipation: evaluation and treatment, *Gastroenterol Clin North Am* 32:659–683, 2003.

Reijneveld SA, van der Wal MF, Brugman E, et al: Infant crying and abuse, *Lancet* 364:1340–1342, 2004.

Roberts DM, Ostapchuk M, O'Brien JG: Infantile colic, *Am Fam Physician* 70:735–740, 2004.

Savino F, Cordisco L, Tarasco V, et al: *Lactobacillus reuteri* DSM 17938 in infantile colic: a randomized, double-blind, placebo-controlled trial, *Pediatrics* 126:e526–e533, 2010.

Turner TL, Palamountain S: Evaluation and management of colic [*UptoDate* website], 2011. Available at http://www.uptodate.com.

Wald A: Treatment of irritable bowel syndrome [*UpToDate* website], 2011. Available at http://www.uptodate.com.

Wald A: Pathophysiology of irritable bowel syndrome [*UpToDate* website], 2011. Available at http://www.uptodate.com.

Youssef NN, Sanders L, Di Lorenzo C: Adolescent constipation: evaluation and management, *Adolesc Med Clin* 15:37–52, 2004.

Diarrhea

(Acute Gastroenteritis)

Presentation

Complaints may range from acute, copious diarrhea that produces shock to concern because an occasional stool is not well formed. Patients with inflammatory diarrhea usually present with fever, tenesmus (the frequent urge to defecate), abdominal pain, and hemoccult-positive stool. These conditions usually cause a more severe form of diarrhea and require more careful assessment and more aggressive treatment. Noninflammatory diarrhea is usually watery, milder, without significant fever, with only mild abdominal cramping, and without blood or leukocytes in the stool. Nausea and vomiting can occur with both forms of diarrhea.

What To Do:

✅ Ask specifically about the frequency of stools, the volume (much liquid implies a defect in absorption in the small bowel, whereas tenesmus producing little more than mucus implies inflammation of the rectosigmoid wall); the character (color, odor, blood, or mucus); and the consistency (water-like or just loose stool). Ask about travel, medications (including antibiotics), residence, daycare attendance, pregnancy status, immunosuppression, consumption of unpasteurized dairy products or undercooked meat or fish, similar symptoms previously, and nocturnal symptoms (rare with functional disease).

✅ Physical examination should focus on signs of moderate or severe dehydration and signs of systemic toxicity. Extracellular volume can be detected by abnormal vital signs, including fever, tachycardia, and postural changes. **When dehydration is suspected, obtain a urinalysis and weigh pediatric patients.** Any symptoms, fall in blood pressure, or increase in pulse rate of more than 20 beats per minute after standing for a minute suggests hypovolemia. **A urine specific gravity of 1.020 or greater also suggests hypovolemia, and ketones of 2 or greater suggest starvation ketosis.**

✅ Loss of skin turgor and dryness of mucosal membranes are also signs of dehydration. Physical signs in infants and small children may include ill appearance, sunken fontanel, sunken eyes, decreased tears, dry mouth, cool extremities, delayed capillary refill, and a weak cry.

✅ The presence of peritoneal signs or persistent focal tenderness on abdominal examination may suggest an infection with an invasive enteric pathogen or a cause requiring urgent surgical evaluation and management.

✅ **Perform a rectal examination and obtain a sample of stool for occult blood testing and for Wright or Gram staining.** If the rectal ampulla is empty, you can still swab the mucosa and may get an even better specimen for stool culture when required. **Stool cultures for enteropathogens need only be obtained when there is a suspected community** outbreak, involvement of food handlers, special populations (pregnant women, the immunocompromised, the elderly, or those with significant comorbidities who appear ill), temperature greater than 38.5° C, severe or prolonged diarrheal illnesses (generally greater than 1 to 2 weeks in duration), and bloody diarrhea (including Shiga toxin–producing *Escherichia coli*). A spontaneous specimen is also good.

✓ If the patient has been on antibiotics within the past 2 months, test the stool for *Clostridium difficile* toxin.

✓ Severe acute diarrhea warrants immediate medical evaluation and possible hospitalization. The criteria for severe acute diarrhea requiring diagnostic evaluation include volume depletion, fever, six or more stools in 24 hours, an illness lasting longer than 48 hours, significant abdominal pain in individuals older than 50 years of age, and diarrhea in special populations (the elderly, pregnant women, or the immunocompromised) The very young and the very old are at greater risk for developing significant fluid loss, with its attendant complications. In patients with inflammatory bowel disease, it is important to send stool studies to help rule out an infectious process, and differentiate this from an inflammatory bowel disease (IBD) "flare."

✓ If the adult patient is not seriously ill but has a fever higher than 38.5° C (101.3° F), the stool is positive for occult blood, or there are any white blood cells in a 400× field, assume the problem is invasive or inflammatory (e.g., *Campylobacter* organisms, *Salmonella*, *Shigella*, enterohemorrhagic and enteroinvasive *E. coli*, *Entamoeba*, ulcerative colitis, and cytotoxic organisms such as *Clostridium difficile* or *Entamoeba histolytica*). If there is no risk for *C. difficile*, and there is no suspicion for enterohemorrhagic *E. coli*, or fluoroquinolone-resistant *Campylobacter* infection, prescribe ciprofloxacin (Cipro), 500 mg bid for 3 to 5 days, and schedule follow-up.

✓ Because there are reasonable concerns about a possible association between hemolytic-uremic syndrome and antibiotic administration to children, **many authorities believe that children with infectious diarrhea should not be treated empirically;** rather, treatment should be based on culture results. Ask the patient to bring a fresh stool sample in a specimen cup at follow-up if the diarrhea persists, in case it needs to be sent for culture or examined for ova and parasites.

✓ If there are no white blood cells on microscopic examination of the stool or the stool is negative for occult blood, assume the diarrhea results from a virus or toxin.

✓ Afebrile adult patients with limited diarrhea require no diagnostic studies or treatment other than fluid and electrolyte replacement. These patients will not benefit from antibiotics and require follow-up only if they have continued diarrhea, abdominal pain, or fever.

✓ Adult patients who feel sick and appear to be dehydrated will benefit from rapid rehydration with IV 0.9% NaCl or lactated Ringer solution (1 to 2 L over an hour for an adult with normal cardiovascular and renal function). Patients who are not vomiting can often be rehydrated by drinking plenty of fluids, such as diluted fruit juices. To replace lost electrolytes, have them eat foods such as saltine crackers, soups, or broth.

✓ Oral rehydration solutions generally are unnecessary in adults younger than 65 years. When an oral rehydration solution is required, do not use "sports drinks" (e.g., Gatorade), because they contain too much sugar and insufficient salt. If oral rehydration solutions (e.g., Rehydralyte) are unavailable, a less ideal substitute can be prepared by adding one-half teaspoon of table salt and one-half teaspoon of baking soda and 4 tablespoons of sugar to 1 L of purified water.

✓ **Both classes of diarrhea are best treated with absorbent bulk laxatives, such as methylcellulose (Citrucel), using 1 heaping tablespoon in 8 oz water qd to tid.**

✓ **Loperamide (Imodium) often limits symptoms to 1 day. It has antimotility and antisecretory effects and is taken as 4 mg after the first loose stool, followed by 2 mg after each subsequent loose stool to a maximum of 16 mg for 2 days.** Do not use antimotility agents if there is a suspicion for *C. difficile* or concern for enterohemorrhagic *E. coli,* because this may facilitate development of hemolytic uremic syndrome. **Antimotility agents are suggested for symptomatic patients with absent or low-grade fever and nonbloody stools.**

✓ A chewable loperamide-simethicone combination product has been shown to provide faster and more complete relief of acute nonspecific diarrhea and associated gas-related abdominal discomfort than either of its components provided alone. Loperamide may be used in pregnant women but should not be used at all in children with inflammatory diarrhea or who are younger than 2 years old.

✓ **For travelers without signs of invasive or inflammatory diarrhea, give a single dose of ciprofloxacin (Cipro), 500 mg, or norfloxacin (Noroxin), 400 mg PO, to reduce the duration and severity of symptoms.** If symptoms persist or the diarrhea is severe or associated with high fever or bloody stools, prescribe ciprofloxacin, 500 mg bid, or norfloxacin, 400 mg twice daily for 3 days. **Azithromycin (Zithromax), 10 mg per kg daily for 3 days, can be used for children, or 500 mg daily for 1 to 3 days can be used in pregnant women and for other adults with quinolone-resistant *Campylobacter.***

✓ **Probiotics** (*Lactobacillus* preparations [Culturelle Probiotic, Colon Health Probiotic Caps] and yogurt) can also be used; they have efficacy in nonspecific pediatric diarrhea as well as traveler's diarrhea.

✓ **With infants and small children, oral rehydration therapy should be the main treatment. Enteral rehydration by the oral or nasogastric route is as effective as, if not better than, IV rehydration.** Have the parents give an oral rehydration mixture with the goal of replacing the fluid lost. For every 1 cup of diarrhea lost, give a cup of the following recipe:

½ to 1 cup precooked baby rice cereal
2 cups water
¼ tsp salt
Mix the rice cereal, water, and salt together until the mixture thickens but is not too thick to drink. Be sure the ingredients are well mixed. A pinch of the artificial sweetener aspartame (Equal) can be added to make it more palatable. Have the parents give the mixture by spoon often and have them offer the child as much as she will accept (every minute if she will accept it). Instruct the parents that if the child is vomiting, wait 20 minutes and then offer the mixture again in small amounts (½ to 1 tsp) every few minutes. Ondansetron (Zofran ODT) can be used in this situation as an antiemetic. Bananas or other nonsweetened, mashed fruit can help provide potassium.

✓ **Alternatively, one can give commercial rehydration fluids, such as Rehydralyte, Ricelyte, or Pedialyte, which are sold in drugstores.** When parents are sent home with their children, set a specified amount of time that they should continue to try oral rehydration before coming back to see you. Four to 6 hours is a reasonable time period, depending on the age of the child and the degree of dehydration and illness. They should also come back for a recheck if there are more than 10 to 15 stools, minimal urination, or a general worsening of their child's appearance.

✅ **An alternative to voluntary oral rehydration in infants and children who are moderately dehydrated is the use of rapid nasogastric hydration. Patients can be given standard oral rehydration solution down a nasogastric tube of appropriate size administered at a rate of 50 mL/kg of body weight, delivered over 4 hours.**

✅ Infants can become severely dehydrated in short order with viral diarrhea. More severely ill children may benefit from intravenous therapy with normal saline administered at the same rate of 20 to 40 mL/kg over 2 to 4 hours.

✅ **Involve the parents in the decision regarding the method of fluid replacement.**

✅ **During or after diarrhea, children should be given frequent small meals (six or more times a day) and actively encouraged to eat. Nursing infants should continue to breast-feed on demand, and infants and older children should be offered their usual food.** Parents should use well-cooked staple starches that can be easily digested, such as rice, corn, potatoes, or noodles in a soft mashed form. Infants should be given a thick porridge or semiliquid pulp. Milk products and cereals are usually well tolerated.

✅ As soon as an adequate degree of rehydration has been achieved, the diet can be advanced quickly as tolerated, and the usual diet should be started at the earliest opportunity.

✅ All patients with severe dehydration may require large amounts of IV fluids and occasionally must be admitted to the hospital.

What Not To Do:

❌ Do not omit the rectal examination, which may disclose a fecal impaction or rectal abscess.

❌ Do not obtain unnecessary stool cultures. It has been estimated that routine stool cultures are positive in only 2% of patients, and most cases of diarrhea in the United States are self limited and will resolve spontaneously. Follow suggestions for sending stool cultures listed above.

❌ Sending stool samples for ova and parasites is usually only recommended for community or daycare outbreaks, patients with ongoing diarrhea(with or without recent travel), patients who are homosexual men, or if there is bloody diarrhea with a paucity of fecal white blood cells.

❌ Do not stop or reduce breast-feeding when a baby has diarrhea. Infants with diarrhea should be breast-fed as often and for as long as they want.

❌ Do not restrict children or adults from having milk or milk products. Despite the potential for lactose intolerance, clinical evidence of lactase deficiency is uncommon, and most individuals can tolerate nonhuman milk without difficulty.

❌ Do not give or recommend sugary drinks such as Gatorade, sweetened commercial fruit drinks, cola drinks, or apple juice if there is significant dehydration. These may cause an osmotic diarrhea and a net loss of fluid. Clear liquids are also not recommended as a substitute for oral rehydration solutions.

❌ Do not confuse influenza with "stomach flu." Influenza with fever, body aches, cough, and fatigue almost never causes symptoms in the stomach and intestines.

Ⓧ Do not overlook the possibility of acute appendicitis or ischemic bowel disease in those patients with suspicious physical findings or significant risk factors.

Ⓧ Do not have patients use diphenoxylate with atropine (Lomotil). It has central nervous system (CNS) effects that are dangerous if a child accidentally ingests it. It also has unpleasant cholinergic effects.

Ⓧ Do not make the diagnosis of gastroenteritis when the patient is only vomiting. The vomiting may be due to a surgical or nongastrointestinal cause that may possibly be life threatening.

Discussion

Acute infectious gastroenteritis is a common cause of vomiting and diarrhea in the United States. Most patients respond well to symptomatic therapy only. Laboratory testing should be reserved for patients with high fever and bloody or prolonged diarrhea, for the immunocompromised, for suspected cases of antibiotic-associated diarrhea, and for suspected community outbreaks. Empirical antibiotic therapy is generally accepted in adults with fever and hemoccult-positive stool.

Common causes of inflammatory diarrhea include invasive or toxin-producing organisms, such as *Campylobacter jejuni, Clostridium difficile,* enterohemorrhagic and enteroinvasive *E. coli, Shigella* sp., nontyphi *Salmonella* sp., and *Entamoeba histolytica.* Consider pet reptiles, rodents, and dogs as a possible source of *Salmonella* and other forms of infectious diarrhea.

Patients with recent antibiotic exposure who present with diarrhea are at risk for antibiotic-associated diarrhea. Most commonly, these patients are afflicted with *Clostridium difficile* infection, and they should be evaluated specifically for *C. difficile* toxins A and B. Always suspect *C. difficile* as the cause of diarrhea in patients who have been in the hospital for longer than 2 weeks, whatever the reason. Also, inpatients who receive proton pump inhibitors and the elderly are at increased risk for *C. difficile* diarrhea. First-line therapy consists of metronidazole (Flagyl), 500 mg orally 3 times daily for 10 to 14 days, as well as discontinuation of the precipitating antibiotic (if possible).

■ **Viruses** commonly cause diarrhea, but it is rarely severe. Associated symptoms are abrupt onset of nausea and abdominal cramps, followed by vomiting or diarrhea. Fevers occur in approximately 50% of affected individuals. Headache, myalgias, upper respiratory symptoms,

and abdominal pain are common. Stool studies are negative for fecal leukocytes and blood. Common causes include norovirus, rotavirus, and enteric adenovirus. **Other causes of noninflammatory diarrheas** include *Giardia lamblia, Cryptosporidium parvum, Vibrio cholerae,* and enterotoxigenic *E. coli.*

■ **Travelers' diarrhea** usually begins within the first week of travel and usually resolves without consequence after 3 to 5 days. In most cases, however, symptoms are severe enough to force a change of itinerary or result in confinement to bed. In 1% of cases, hospitalization is necessary.

■ High-risk regions include the developing countries of Latin America, Africa, Asia, and parts of the Middle East. Areas of intermediate risk include China, southern Europe, Israel, South Africa, Russia, and several Caribbean islands (especially Haiti and the Dominican Republic).

■ High-risk foods include uncooked vegetables and unpeeled fresh fruit, raw or undercooked meat or seafood (particularly shellfish), and salads. Ice, tap water, and unpasteurized milk carry an increased risk for infection. Safe drinks include bottled carbonated beverages, beer or wine, and boiled or bottled water. Meals eaten in a private home carry reduced risk compared with those eaten in a restaurant. Food from street vendors is particularly risky.

■ **Travelers' diarrhea often cannot be avoided. If these patients are seen by you, they should be treated like any other patient who presents with diarrhea. For patients who are managed in the pretravel period, chemoprophylaxis is generally discouraged. It is most appropriate to prepare the traveler for prompt self-treatment at the first sign of illness using a combination of an antimotility agent (usually loperamide), about 8 doses/person, and an antibiotic (usually a fluoroquinolone),**

(continued)

Discussion continued

6 doses/person, both of which can be obtained prior to departure and carried during travel. Consider azithromycin if the patient is traveling with children or a pregnant adult (see regimen p 255). If symptoms resolve within 24 hours of initiating therapy, no further treatment is necessary. If diarrhea persists after 1 day, treatment should be continued for 1 or 2 more days.

- Rifaximin (Xifaxan) is a nonabsorbed oral antibiotic that has been approved for treatment of travelers' diarrhea, but it is not effective against infections associated with fever or blood in the stool or those caused by *Campylobacter*. It has fewer adverse effects and drug interactions than do systemic antibiotics, but it cannot be taken during pregnancy. For severe diarrhea, the fluoroquinolones or azithromycin remain the preferred antibiotics.

- Acute bloody diarrhea is a frightening symptom that has been associated with *E. coli* 0157:H7 and other Shiga toxin–producing *E. coli* infections, illnesses occasionally complicated by the development of hemolytic-uremic syndrome and death. Suspect this in patients who lack high fever and who have abdominal tenderness and pain with bloody diarrhea. It is recommended that stool samples be cultured for patients with acute bloody diarrhea. Antibiotics and antimotility agents should be avoided in patients with suspected or proven infection with enterohemorrhagic *E. coli*.

- It can be useful if acute care practitioners report any suspected infectious outbreaks to public health departments.

- Patients with prolonged noninflammatory symptom complexes, especially those who have traveled to endemic areas, may benefit from stool evaluation for parasites. For patients with persistent diarrhea (lasting more than 1 week), an empirical trial of metronidazole or nitazoxanide for a protozoal infection is sometimes considered.

- The treatment of diarrhea in immunocompromised patients is essentially the same as that for normal hosts, but such patients may require prolonged courses of antimicrobial therapy and often require subspecialty consultation.

- Noninfectious causes of acute diarrhea include inflammatory bowel disease (most often ulcerative colitis, but diarrhea can also be seen with Crohn disease). Symptoms include diarrhea with mucus, rectal bleeding, and abdominal pain.

- Medications are another noninfectious cause. The most common medications responsible for acute diarrhea are laxatives; antacids containing calcium or magnesium; colchicines; antibiotics; sorbitol gums; and enteral tube feedings, especially if hypertonic. Diarrhea usually resolves after cessation of the medication.

- Other noninfectious causes of diarrhea that need to be considered are pelvic abscess in the area of the rectosigmoid, intestinal ischemia in the elderly, partial small bowel obstruction, obstipation/fecal impaction, or acute appendicitis.

- **Gastroenteritis is probably the most common diagnosis in missed appendicitis cases. Children with acute appendicitis present with a much higher incidence of diarrhea than those in other age groups, but diarrhea can accompany acute appendicitis at any age. Consider using advanced imaging (ultrasonography or if that fails to be diagnostic, CT scan) early in equivocal cases.**

- When inflammatory diarrhea is recurrent, suspect a noninfectious cause such as inflammatory bowel disease.

- In the pregnant patient who has diarrhea and systemic illness, consider listeriosis.

- Ordinary stool cultures only identify *Campylobacter, Shigella, Salmonella, Aeromonas,* and *Yersinia. Aeromonas* and *Yersinia* may be missed on testing unless specifically sought. Testing for other pathogens, such as *Vibrio* sp., enterohemorrhagic *E. coli* 0157:H7, and other Shiga toxin–producing bacteria require special media.

- Routine laboratory tests (complete blood count [CBC], electrolytes, renal function) are generally neither helpful nor indicated in making a diagnosis. These tests may be useful as indicators of severity of disease, especially in the elderly or the very young, but your clinical impression is more important.

- When methylcellulose (Citrucel) is recommended, patients may remind you that they have diarrhea, not constipation. Because these bulk agents absorb water in the gut lumen, however, they can relieve both problems and obviate the rebound constipation often produced by the narcotic and binding agents also used to treat diarrhea.

- Older patients medicated for pain or psychosis can develop a **fecal impaction**, which can also present as diarrhea. **Irritable bowel syndrome, food allergy, lactose intolerance, and parasite infestation** can produce relapsing diarrhea, but the pattern may only become apparent on follow-up.

Suggested Readings

Atherly-John YC, Cunningham SJ, Crain EF, et al: A randomized trial of oral vs intravenous rehydration in a pediatric emergency department, *Arch Ped Adolesc Med* 156:12401243, 2002.

Brown T: Update on emerging infections: news from the Centers for Disease Control and Prevention. Norovirus activity—United States, 2002, *Ann Emerg Med* 42:417–422, 2003.

Chitkara YK: Limited value of routine stool cultures in patients receiving antibiotic therapy? *Am J Clin Pathol* 123:92–95, 2005.

Cohen MB, Mezoff AG, Laney DW, et al: Use of a single solution for oral rehydration and maintenance therapy of infants with diarrhea and mild to moderate dehydration, *Pediatrics* 95:639–645, 1995.

Dial S, Alrasadi K, Manoukian C, et al: Risk of *Clostridium difficile* among hospital inpatients prescribed proton pump inhibitors: cohort and case-control studies, *Can Med Assoc J* 171:33–38, 2004.

Diemert DJ: Prevention and self-treatment of travelers' diarrhea, *Prim Care* 29:843–855, 2002.

Ericsson CD, DuPont HL, Mathewson JJ, et al: Optimal dosing of ofloxacin with loperamide in the treatment of non-dysenteric travelers' diarrhea, *J Travel Med* 8:207–209, 2001.

Feldman M, Friedman L, Brandt L: *Sleisenger and Fordtran's gastrointestinal and liver disease*, ed 9, St Louis, 2010, Elsevier.

Fonseca BK, Holdgate A, Craig JC: Enteral vs intravenous rehydration therapy for children with gastroenteritis, *Arch Pediatr Adolesc Med* 158:483–490, 2004.

Gore JI, Surawicz C: Severe acute diarrhea, *Gastroenterol Clin North Am* 32:1249–1267, 2003.

Grunenberg N: Is gradual introduction of feeding better than immediate normal feeding in children with gastroenteritis? *Arch Dis Child* 88:455–457, 2003.

Kaplan MA, Prior MJ, Ash RR, et al: Loperamide-simethicone vs loperamide alone, simethicone alone, and placebo in the treatment of acute diarrhea with gas-related abdominal discomfort, *Arch Fam Med* 8:243–248, 1999.

Karras DJ, Ong S, Moran GJ, et al: Antibiotic use for emergency department patients with acute diarrhea: prescribing practices, patient expectations, and patient satisfaction, *Ann Emerg Med* 42:835–842, 2003.

Leibovitz E, Janco J, Piglansky L, et al: Oral ciprofloxacin vs intramuscular ceftriaxone as empiric treatment of acute invasive diarrhea in children, *Pediatr Infect Dis J* 19:1060–1067, 2000.

Margolis PA, Litteer T, Hare N, et al: Effects of unrestricted diet on mild infantile diarrhea, *Am J Dis Child* 144:162–164, 1990.

Nager AL, Wang VJ: Comparison of nasogastric and intravenous methods of rehydration in pediatric patients with acute dehydration, *Pediatrics* 109:566–572, 2002.

Phin SJ, McCaskill ME, Browne GJ, Lam LT: Clinical pathway using rapid rehydration for children with gastroenteritis, *J Paed Child Health* 39:343–348, 2003.

Porter SC, Fleisher GR, Kohane IS, et al: The value of parental report for diagnosis and management of dehydration in the emergency department, *Ann Emerg Med* 41:196–205, 2003.

Reid SR, Bonadino WA: Outpatient rapid intravenous rehydration to correct dehydration and resolve vomiting in children with acute gastroenteritis, *Ann Emerg Med* 28:318–323, 1996. editorial 353-354.

Salam I, Katelaris P, Leigh-Smith S, Farthing MJ: Randomized trial of single-dose ciprofloxacin for traveller's diarrhoea, *Lancet* 344:1537–1539, 1994.

Sandhu BK: European Society of Paediatric Gastroenterology, Hepatology and Nutrition Working Group on Acute Diarrhoea: Rationale for early feeding in childhood gastroenteritis, *J Ped Gastroenterol Nutr* 33(Suppl 2):S13–S16, 2001.

Schroeder MS: *Clostridium difficile*–associated diarrhea, *Am Fam Physician* 71:921–928, 2005.

Sigel D, Cohen PT, Neighbor M, et al: Predictive value of stool examination in acute diarrhea, *Arch Pathol Lab Med* 111:715–718, 1987.

Spandorfer PR, Alessandrini EA, Joffe MD, et al: Oral versus intravenous rehydration of moderately dehydrated children, *Pediatrics* 115:295–301, 2005.

Steiner MJ, DeWalt DA, Byerley JS, et al: Is this child dehydrated? *JAMA* 291:2746–2754, 2004.

Steffen R, Collard F, Tornieporth N: Epidemiology, etiology, and impact of traveler's diarrhea in Jamaica, *JAMA* 281:811–817, 1999.

Enterobiasis

(Pinworm, Threadworm, Seatworm)

Presentation

The patient complains of severe perianal and/or vaginal irritation and itching, which is worse at night and may contribute to insomnia or superinfection of the excoriated perianal skin. Children may exhibit only perianal pruritus and nocturnal restlessness. Rarely, more serious disease can result, including weight loss, urinary tract infection, and appendicitis. Often, an entire family is affected.

What To Do:

✓ Examine the anus to rule out other causes of itching, such as rectal prolapse, fecal leakage, hemorrhoids, lice (pediculosis), fungal infections (tinea or candidiasis), or bacterial infections (erythrasma) (see discussion of pruritus ani on p 243).

✓ **Look for pinworms directly (especially if the patient comes in at night) and also by pressing the sticky side of cellophane tape wrapped around a tongue blade (sticky side up) to the perianal skin several times. Remove the tape and place it sticky side down on a glass slide. Examine the tape, under the low power of the microscope, for female worms** (only 5% of infected persons have eggs in their stool) approximately 1 cm long, 0.5 mm in diameter, with pointed tails (Figure 69-1). Adult male pinworms are shorter (2.5 mm in length) and have a blunt tail. (Use shiny rather than "invisible" tape, because the latter's rough surface makes microscopy difficult.) To increase this test's sensitivity to approximately 90%, it should be conducted right after the patient awakens on at least 3 consecutive days.

✓ **If you see pinworms or still suspect them, administer one oral dose of pyrantel pamoate, 11 mg/kg (maximum l g), to all family members. This can be obtained over the counter as Pin-X, Pin-Rid, and Reese's Pinworm Medicine (oral suspension 250 mg/5 mL). This should be repeated in 2 weeks. This treatment has lower efficacy and greater side effects (vomiting, diarrhea, anorexia, and nausea) than the medications available by prescription.**

✓ **Two prescription medications are mebendazole (Vermox), 100-mg chewable tablet once PO (not for children younger than 2 years of age), and albendazole (Albenza), 400 mg in adults or 10 mg/kg in children as a single dose. Both of these prescription medications should be repeated after 2 weeks.** All three of these medications are considered unsafe during pregnancy.

✓ Explain to all concerned that this is not a dangerous infection and should be eradicated from the whole family after one or two treatments. Have the family clean their bedrooms and bedding. Explain that thorough hand washing is important, because pinworms are transmitted by direct anus to mouth spread, by direct contact with dirty linens or clothing, or by dirty hands contaminating food during its preparation or consumption.

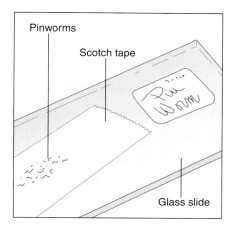

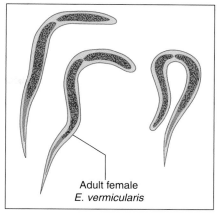

Figure 69-1 Pinworm examples.

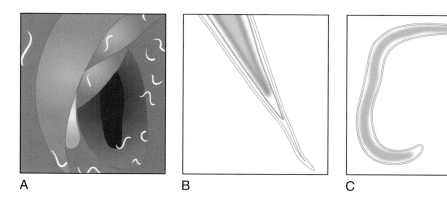

A B C

Figure 69-2 A, Numerous pinworms scattered throughout the colon as seen with colonoscopy. **B,** The adult female worm with a long, pointed tail. **C,** The adult male pinworm is short with a blunt tail. (Adapted from Faruqi S, Ahmed I, Membreno F: Pinworms. *Gastrointest Endosc* 57:566, 2003.)

Discussion

There is evidence of pinworm infection that dates back to Roman-occupied Egypt (30 BC to AD 395). *Enterobius vermicularis* is also the oldest and most common parasite for which we have direct evidence in the New World, with fecal samples positive for pinworm ova from the American Southwest dating back 10,000 years. The pinworm, threadworm, or seatworm is a nematode, or roundworm, with the largest geographic range of any helminth. It is the most prevalent nematode in the United States. Humans are the only known host, and perhaps 10% of the U.S. population may harbor pinworms, especially children.

Adult worms are quite small; the males range in size from 2 to 5 mm, and the females measure 8 to 13 mm (Figure 69-2). The worms live primarily in the cecum of the large intestine, from which the gravid female migrates at night to lay up to 15,000 eggs on the perineum. The eggs can be spread by the fecal–oral route to the original host and new hosts. In this manner, an entire family can become infected. Ingested eggs hatch in the duodenum, and larvae mature during their migration to the large intestine.

(continued)

Discussion continued

Fortunately, most eggs desiccate and die within 72 hours. In the absence of host autoinfection, infestation usually lasts only 4 to 6 weeks. Egg deposition causes perineal, perianal, and vaginal irritation. The patient's constant itching in an attempt to relieve irritation can lead to potentially debilitating sleep disturbance.

Direct visualization of the white-appearing adult worms or microscopic detection of worms or eggs using the "cellophane tape test" confirms the diagnosis.

Pruritus ani has many causes, of which pinworm is just one. Consider diet (coffee, tea, chocolate, citrus), malignancy, anal fistulas, other infections (yeast, sexually transmitted diseases [STDs], *Corynebacterium*), psoriasis, Paget disease, or even incomplete cleansing postdefecation as you evaluate the patient with this complaint.

Suggested Readings

Centers for Disease Control and Prevention: *Enterobiasis (Enterobius vermicularis)*. Available at, http://www.dpd.cdc.gov/DPDx/HTML/Enterobiasis.htm. Accessed November 16, 2011.

Horne PD: First evidence of enterobiasis in ancient Egypt, *J Parasitol* 88:1019–1021, 2002.

Kucik CJ, Martin GL, Sortor BV: Common intestinal parasites, *Am Fam Physician* 69:1161–1168, 2004.

Esophageal Food Bolus Obstruction

(Steakhouse or Café Coronary Syndrome)

Presentation

The patient develops symptoms either immediately after swallowing a large mouthful of food (usually inadequately chewed meat) or as the result of intoxication, wearing dentures, or being too embarrassed to spit out a large piece of gristle. The patient often develops substernal chest pain that may mimic the pain of a myocardial infarction. This discomfort increases with swallowing and is followed by retention of salivary secretions, which, unlike infarction, leads to drooling. The patient usually arrives with a receptacle under his mouth, into which he is repeatedly spitting. At times these secretions will cause paroxysms of coughing, gagging, or choking. Often, the patient can readily tell you where the food has become stuck by pointing to the lower esophagus.

What To Do:

✓ Complete a history and physical examination. If an esophageal perforation is suspected because of severe pain and diaphoresis after swallowing a sharp object, such as a bone, take posteroanterior and lateral radiographs of the neck and chest, looking for subcutaneous emphysema, pneumomediastinum, pneumothorax, and pleural effusion. If these are negative, but a high level of suspicion remains, a contrast study using a low-osmolality iodinated contrast agent (such as Amipaque, Omnipaque, or Hexabrix) should be performed. These agents are much less likely to cause problems if they contaminate the mediastinum or are accidentally aspirated. If a high suspicion for perforation is still present, despite a negative swallowing study, a CT scan may be obtained, which may show air around the mediastinum or esophagus or a mediastinal air–fluid level.

✓ **When there is only mild pain or discomfort and the patient is troubled by drooling and the spitting of saliva, offer to insert a small nasogastric tube to the point of obstruction and attach it to low intermittent suction. This insertion will assist the patient in handling excess secretions and reduce the risk for aspiration.** The patient may prefer to keep spitting to avoid the discomfort of nasogastric tube insertion.

✓ **Provide adequate pain relief, when necessary, with a parenteral analgesic such as hydromorphone (Dilaudid) or fentanyl (Duragesic).**

✓ If the history and physical findings are ambiguous, but there remains a question of esophageal obstruction, give 5 mL of dilute barium PO and obtain radiographs of the chest to locate the foreign body. **When the history and physical findings are classic for a meat impaction in the esophagus, there is no need to perform a barium swallow, which may later obscure the view for a consulting endoscopist.**

✅ **Give 0.5 to 1 mg of glucagon IV to decrease lower esophageal sphincter pressure (infuse slowly to prevent nausea and vomiting). This decrease in pressure will sometimes allow passage of a food bolus.** If there is no response, repeat every 5 to 10 minutes for one to two additional doses. The success rate of this technique is low (only 20% to 40%) and will be of no value in an impaction of the upper two thirds of the esophagus. The side effects of this drug include nausea, vomiting, and hyperglycemia. The hyperglycemia is transient and of no clinical significance and does not require monitoring. Adding diazepam (Valium) to this medication does not improve its effectiveness.

✅ **An alternative IV drug is metoclopramide (Reglan), 10 mg.** Additional modes of therapy include the use of sublingual nitroglycerin or nifedipine to relax the lower esophageal sphincter, but they are not usually as effective as IV glucagon, which itself is of questionable efficacy.

✅ **Another method of passing a lower esophageal meat impaction (of less than 6 hours) into the stomach, if glucagon has failed and there are no signs of esophageal perforation, is to have the patient sit up and drink 100 mL of a carbonated beverage or EZ gas (sodium bicarbonate, citric acid, simethicone), followed by 240 mL of water. EZ gas (also known as Carbex) is sometimes found in the radiology department, if it is not available in the pharmacy.** Another alternative is to use 15 mL of tartaric acid (18.7 g/100 mL), followed by 15 mL of sodium bicarbonate (10 g/100 mL). When these components are combined in the esophagus, **carbon dioxide is produced, which distends the esophagus and, when successful, propels the impacted meat into the stomach. The patient will be able to report when the impaction has been relieved; he will know immediately or the next time he attempts to swallow something. (It should be noted that a complication rate of 3% has been reported using this technique. Reported complications include aspiration and vomiting with an esophageal tear.)**

✅ **If the food does not pass spontaneously, there is no access to a gastroenterologist with an endoscope (flexible esophagoscopy being the treatment of choice),** and the patient is willing, prepare the patient for manual extraction. Start an IV line for drug administration and anesthetize the pharynx with 20% benzocaine (Hurricane) spray, viscous lidocaine 2%, or lidocaine 10% oral spray. Place the patient on his side and slowly administer lorazepam (Ativan), 0.5 to 1 mg intravenously, until the patient is very drowsy but possessing all of his protective reflexes. Take a gastric Ewald lavage tube, cut off the end straight across where there are no side ports, and cut off any sharp edges of the new tip with scissors. Push the Ewald tube through the patient's mouth until the obstruction is reached. Take a large aspiration syringe, have an assistant apply suction to the free end of the Ewald tube, and slowly withdraw it. If suction is maintained, the bolus will come up with the tubing.

✅ **If the clinician does not feel comfortable performing this procedure, the patient is unable to tolerate this procedure, or foreign body removal was unsuccessful, consult with an endoscopist for the earliest possible removal with a flexible fiberoptic esophagoscope. Rigid esophagoscopy performed by an ear-nose-throat (ENT) specialist is an alternative option when flexible esophagoscopy is not available.**

✅ **Be aware that the standard methods for disimpaction outlined above may be ineffective or hazardous in the management of food lodged in a *metallic esophageal stent*.**

✅ When removal of the food bolus has been successful, early medical follow-up should be provided for a comprehensive evaluation of the esophagus.

✓ Patients who have experienced a prolonged obstruction or do not have complete resolution of all their symptoms should be admitted to the hospital for further observation and management.

What Not To Do:

✗ Do not ignore a patient's claims of a foreign body stuck in the esophagus. The patient is usually right.

✗ Do not obtain plain radiograph films for routine food bolus impactions. They are of no value unless a large bone has been ingested.

✗ Do not blindly try to force the food bolus down with the Ewald tube or any other catheter or dilator. This may cause an esophageal tear or perforation. Endoscopists have successfully used an endoscopic push technique, but this has been under direct vision in a controlled manner.

✗ Do not use meat tenderizers or oral enzymes, such as papain, trypsin, or chymotrypsin. This treatment is slow and ineffective and may possibly carry a risk for enzyme-induced esophageal perforation.

✗ Do not discharge a patient prior to removal of the obstruction. The risks of delayed follow-up are too high.

✗ Do not attempt to remove a hard, sharp esophageal foreign body using any of the abovementioned techniques. These techniques very likely will cause an esophageal injury.

✗ Do not give glucagon to patients with pheochromocytoma or insulinoma. It may cause a pheochromocytoma to release catecholamines, or the secondary hyperglycemia may cause an insulinoma to secrete excess insulin and produce hypoglycemia.

✗ Do not use barium-impregnated cotton balls to detect esophageal foreign bodies. If a foreign body is present, they will obscure the view for the endoscopist.

✗ Do not fail to refer a patient in whom a food bolus has passed to an endoscopist, to rule out malignancy and facilitate dilation of any strictures that may be found.

Discussion

Patients who experience a food bolus obstruction of the esophagus are usually older than 60 years of age and often have an underlying structural lesion. Meat impaction occurs most frequently in the distal esophagus. One of the more common lesions is a benign stricture secondary to reflux esophagitis. Another abnormality, the classic Schatzki ring (distal esophageal mucosal ring), especially above a hiatal hernia, may present with the "steakhouse" or "café coronary syndrome," in which obstruction occurs and is relieved spontaneously. Other associated problems include postoperative narrowing, neoplasms, and cervical webs, as well as motility disorders, neurologic disease, and collagen vascular disease. Eosinophilic esophagitis is an increasingly recognized syndrome causing esophageal spasm in response to certain foods (an allergy) with bolus obstruction. It has been described as "asthma of the esophagus."

Meat impacted in the proximal two thirds of the esophagus is unlikely to pass and should be removed as soon as possible. Meat impacted in the lower third frequently does pass spontaneously if given enough time, and the patient can safely wait, under medical observation, up to 12 hours before extraction.

(continued)

Discussion continued

Even if a meat bolus does pass spontaneously, endoscopy must still be done later to assess the almost certain (80% to 90%) chance of an underlying disease. In the great majority of these cases, the underlying disease will be benign.

Flexible endoscopy is the mainstay of esophageal foreign body removal. Reported success rates are high, with few reported complications. Ideally, food impactions should be removed within about 12 hours of presentation. Early removal is recommended because of local pressure-induced ischemia that may occur secondary to the food bolus.

Chicken bones are the foreign bodies that most often cause esophageal perforation in adults.

Suggested Readings

Blair SR, Graeber GM, Cruzzavala JL, et al: Current management of esophageal impactions, *Chest* 104:1205–1209, 1993.

Chae HS, Lee TK, Kim YW, et al: Two cases of steakhouse syndrome associated with nutcracker esophagus, *Dis Esophagus* 15:330–333, 2002.

Kozarek RA, Sanowski RA: Esophageal food impaction: description of a new method for bolus removal, *Dig Dis Sci* 25:100–103, 1980.

Lacy PD, Donnelly MJ, McGrath JP, et al: Acute food bolus impaction: aetiology and management, *Laryngol Otol* 111:1158–1161, 1997.

Lao J, Bostwick HE, Berezin S, et al: Esophageal food impaction in children, *Pediatr Emerg Care* 19:402–407, 2003.

Lee J, Anderson R: Best evidence topic report. Effervescent agents for oesophageal food bolus impaction, *Emerg Med J* 22:123–124, 2005.

Rice BT, Spiegel PK, Dombrowski PJ: Acute esophageal food impaction treated by gas-forming agents, *Radiology* 146:299–301, 1983.

Singer AJ, Konia N: Comparison of topical anesthetics and vasoconstrictors vs lubricants prior to nasogastric intubation: a randomized, controlled trial, *Acad Emerg Med* 6:184–190, 1999.

Tibbling L, Bjorkhoel A, Jansson E, Stenkvist M: Effect of spasmolytic drugs on esophageal foreign bodies, *Dysphagia* 10:126–127, 1995.

Weinstock LB, Shatz BA, Thyssen SE: Esophageal food bolus obstruction: evaluation of extraction and modified push techniques in 75 cases, *Endoscopy* 31:421–425, 1999.

Foreign Body, Rectal

Presentation

Rectal foreign bodies may present with abdominal pain, anorectal pain, obstipation, acute urinary retention, or blood or mucus discharge from the rectum. Such foreign bodies are often difficult to diagnose, because the history may not be offered by the patient unless he or she is directly asked. Sometimes the patient will not volunteer that any object has been inserted or will give outlandish explanations, such as having sat or fallen onto the object. When interviewed privately in a non-judgmental manner, however, the patient will usually give an accurate account of the foreign body.

Rectal foreign bodies most commonly are found when an object, such as a dildo or vibrator, is inserted into the rectum by the patient or a partner for sexual stimulation; it then causes pain or bleeding or becomes irretrievable. Presentation is frequently delayed by embarrassment, or prior attempts on the part of the patient to remove the object.

Rectal foreign bodies also are found with practices such as "body packing," wherein illicit drugs are packed in latex condoms or plastic bags for illegal transport. Rupture of these packets may lead to profound toxicity and death.

Less often, medical instruments, such as enema tips or thermometers, become lodged in the rectum.

What To Do:

✓ Try to determine how long the foreign body has been lodged and if any attempts at removal have been made. Ask specifically about any assault or rape and respond accordingly. Give special consideration to the psychiatric patient.

✓ **The diagnosis of a rectal foreign body can usually be made from the history alone. Perform an abdominal and rectal examination, but defer the rectal examination if the foreign body is suspected to be dangerously sharp.**

✓ If there are signs of peritoneal inflammation (i.e., rebound tenderness or pain with movement) or blood on rectal examination, suspect a perforation of the bowel, start appropriate IV lines, draw blood for laboratory analysis, obtain flat and upright abdominal radiographs to look for free air, notify surgical consultants, and administer IV antibiotics. Surgical consultation should also be obtained in all cases of nonpalpable rectal foreign bodies.

✓ **If there are no signs of perforation, flat and upright abdominal films may still be obtained to help define the location nature, size, and number of foreign objects (as well as to reveal unsuspected free air).**

✓ Those objects that lie in the low or midrectum, up to a level of 10 cm, most often can be removed transanally.

✓ **When there is no suspicion of a bowel perforation, provide procedural sedation to help in the removal of the foreign body (see Appendix E). Perianal nerve blocks with local anesthesia may be helpful for use by those skilled in this procedure.**

✓ Place the patient on his side in the Sims position, or he can lie prone in the knee-chest position. **If anal discomfort persists, instill lidocaine jelly for mucosal anesthesia or locally infiltrate 1% lidocaine with epinephrine into the anal sphincter. In general, a perianal nerve block similar to that used for anorectal surgery works quite well.** Some authors favor using lidocaine (Xylocaine) 1% with epinephrine and bupivacaine 0.5% with epinephrine in a 50:50 mix. A superficial block and then an intersphincteric block circumferentially around the anal verge can be performed. Finally, to ensure the greatest degree of anesthesia, a pudendal nerve block can be performed. The branches of the pudendal nerve that innervate the anal sphincter complex approach the sphincter complex from a posterolateral location. A pudendal nerve block is done by infiltrating the tissues deeply in a fanlike technique approximately 1 cm medial to the ischial tuberosities in the posterolateral location bilaterally. Approximately 2 to 5 mL of the local anesthetic mix is used on each side.

✓ **The method of removal must be individualized, depending on the size, shape, consistency, and fragility of the object. Individual situations demand creative use of standard medical instruments and supplies. Set a time limit for yourself, and let the patient know that if the foreign body cannot be removed within a reasonable length of time (usually 10 to 20 minutes), it will have to be removed in a setting that allows for more potent anesthetics.**

✓ **When the object can be reached by the examining finger and is of a nature that will allow it to be grasped, a lax anal sphincter may allow slow insertion of as much of a gloved hand as possible to grab the object and gradually extricate it. For instance, perforate fruit with the fingertips to obtain a more effective grasp. Having the patient bear down while performing a Valsalva maneuver may help to "deliver" the object. You can also apply suprapubic pressure from above with your free hand.**

✓ **If you are unable to pull out the foreign body by hand,** the following are techniques that can be used to get a purchase on the object and break the vacuum behind it:

○ **Slide a large Foley catheter with a 30-mL balloon past the object, inflate the balloon, and apply traction to the catheter. (This can be used in conjunction with any of the other techniques.)** Two catheters may occasionally be needed, and air should be instilled through the lumen of the catheter to break the vacuum (Figure 71-1). **Alternatively, an endotracheal tube can be passed beyond the foreign body, the cuff inflated, and air gently insufflated down the tube.**

○ **Under direct visualization with an anoscope or a vaginal speculum, attempt to grasp the object with a tenaculum, sponge forceps, Kelly clamp, or tonsil snare** (Figure 71-2). **Brittle objects, especially glass, should be grasped gently, with rubber tubing or gauze covering the metal surfaces of any clamp or forceps.**

✓ **An open object, like a jar or a bottle, can be filled with wet plaster, into which a tongue blade can be inserted like a Popsicle stick. When the plaster hardens, traction can be applied to the tongue blade** (Figure 71-3). **Alternatively, inflation of a Sengstaken-Blakemore tube balloon inside a jar may provide the traction needed to extract the object.**

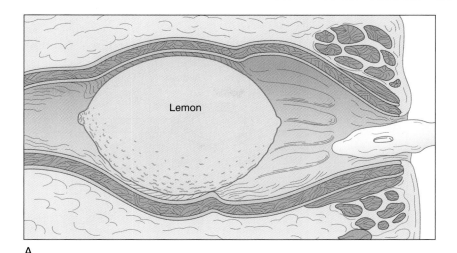

A

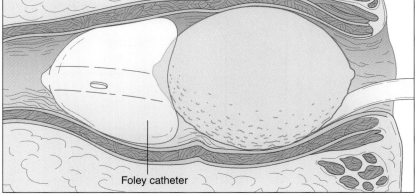

B

Figure 71-1 The Foley catheter technique is used to break a vacuum behind an object.

✓ You may be able to place a screw in some objects, which may allow you to grab them and apply traction. Other objects may have to be cut in sections to be removed.

✓ **Forceps or soup spoons can be used to deliver a round object** (Figure 71-4). **When available, an obstetric vacuum extractor may be even more effective for removing round foreign bodies of compatible size and texture** (Figure 71-5). **Magnets are sometimes useful to help extract metal objects.**

✓ As the object is being removed, the speculum or anoscope should be removed along with it so that the foreign body does not have to fit through these instruments.

✓ With an object that is too high to reach, the patient can be admitted and sedated for removal over the next 6 to 12 hours.

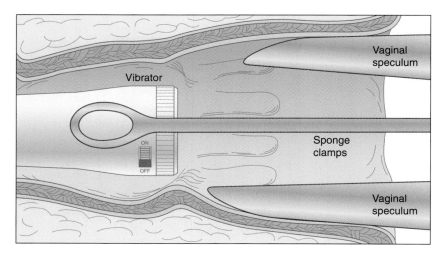

Figure 71-2 Grasp the object with a tenaculum, sponge forceps, Kelly clamp, or tonsil snare.

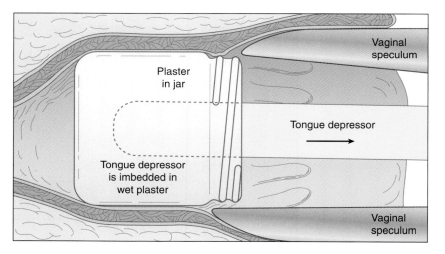

Figure 71-3 Fill jars or bottles with plaster, and insert tongue blade like a Popsicle stick. When plaster hardens, traction can be applied.

When the object cannot be removed because of patient discomfort or sphincter tightness, removal must be accomplished in the operating room under spinal or general anesthesia.

When blood is present in the rectum, when pain is severe or persistent, when there is fever or rectal discharge, or when the object is capable of doing harm to the bowel, proctoscopic evaluation should be performed after removal of the foreign body to rule out rectal injury. Superficial nonbleeding rectal injuries may be left alone. Those that are bleeding or that involve the muscular wall require repair.

When pain persists or there is any lingering suspicion of a bowel perforation, keep the patient for 24 hours of observation and consider performing a water-soluble contrast enema study. If there are any postprocedural problems, surgical consultation is recommended.

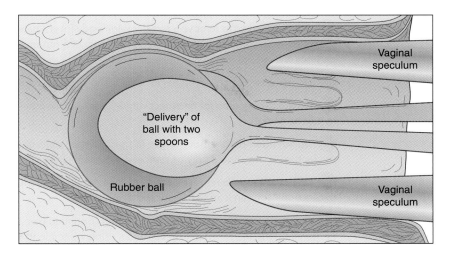

Figure 71-4 Round objects can be removed with forceps or soup spoons.

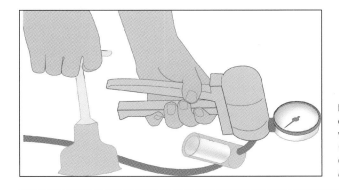

Figure 71-5 Equipment for soft-cup vacuum extraction: cup with traction handle, fluid trap, vacuum gauge, and manual vacuum pump. (Adapted from Putta LV, Spencer JP: Assisted vaginal delivery using the vacuum extractor. *Am Fam Physician* 62:1316-1320, 2000.)

✓ When the foreign body is extracted without difficulty and the potential for bowel injury is minimal, proctoscopic evaluation is probably unnecessary, and the patient can be discharged after a reasonable period of observation.

✓ **Consider recommending sexual or psychological counseling.**

What Not To Do:

✗ Do not pressure the patient into giving you an accurate story. He may be embarrassed, and intimidation will not help. Do not use enemas or cathartics to help speed the removal of these objects. These treatments are not likely to be effective and may actually cause harm.

✗ Do not attempt to remove a rectal foreign body in a patient who is having severe abdominal pain or who has signs of a bowel perforation.

(X) Do not attempt to remove a rectal foreign body from a patient whose rectal pain and spasm are severe and cannot be overcome with the infiltration of local anesthetic. These patients will require regional or general anesthesia.

(X) Do not push the object higher into the colon while attempting to remove it.

(X) Do not blindly grab for an object with a tenaculum or other such device. This can itself lead to a perforation.

(X) Do not attempt to remove fragile or sharp, jagged objects, such as broken glass, through the rectum. These should only be removed under anesthesia in surgery.

(X) Do not attempt to remove packets of illicit drugs with clamps or sharp medical instruments, because spillage can lead to toxicity and death.

(X) Do not send home a patient who is having continued pain. Admit him and observe for peritoneal signs, increased pain, fever, and a rising white blood cell count.

Discussion

Anorectal foreign bodies can be either ingested orally or inserted anally. Although the vast majority are inserted for autoerotic purposes, they may have been placed iatrogenically or as a result of assault or trauma. Ingested objects are rarely a cause of entrapped rectal foreign bodies. Most often, these are bones that become impaled in the anal canal. Iatrogenic foreign bodies include thermometers, enema tips, and catheters. Objects placed as a result of assault, trauma, or eroticism represent a diverse collection, including sex toys; tools; wire hangers and instruments; bottles, cans, and jars; poles, pipes, and tubing; fruits and vegetables; stones; balls; balloons; light bulbs; and flashlights.

Most of these rectal foreign bodies can be removed safely in the emergency department or acute care clinic. Relaxation is essential, and sedation is usually necessary if retrieval is to be successful. Some practitioners quite reasonably forgo radiographs before manipulation if the patient is free of pain and fever and if the object is benign.

Suggested Readings

Couch CH, Tan EGC, Watt AG: Rectal foreign bodies, *Med J Aust* 144:512–515, 1986.

Hellinger MD: Anal trauma and foreign bodies, *Surg Clin North Am* 82:1253–1260, 2002.

Putta LV, Spencer JP: Assisted vaginal delivery using the vacuum extractor, *Am Fam Physician* 62:1316–1320, 2000.

Rodriguez-Hermosa JI, Codina-Cazador A, Ruiz B, et al: Management of foreign bodies in the rectum, *Colorectal Dis* 9:543–548, 2007.

Steele S, Goldberg J: *Rectal foreign bodies* [UptoDate website]. Available at http://www.uptodate.com.

Foreign Body, Swallowed

Presentation

Parents bring in a young child (usually between the ages of 6 months and 6 years) shortly after the child has swallowed a coin, safety pin, or toy. The child may be asymptomatic or have recurrent or transient symptoms of choking, gagging, vomiting, drooling, dysphagia, pain, or a foreign body (FB) sensation. Stridor or dyspnea resulting from tracheal compression may occur in young children. Disturbed or cognitively impaired adults may be brought from mental health facilities to the hospital on repeated occasions, at times accumulating a sizable load of ingested material. Impacted esophageal foreign bodies are more likely to cause the symptoms described, whereas gastric foreign bodies are usually asymptomatic.

What To Do:

Many patients are able to give a clear history of foreign body ingestion; however, young children, psychotic persons, and the cognitively impaired may be unable to give an accurate history.

Ask capable patients about their symptoms and examine them, looking for signs of airway obstruction (e.g., coughing, wheezing), bowel obstruction, or perforation (e.g., vomiting, subcutaneous emphysema, chest pain, melena, abdominal pain, abnormal bowel sounds).

When a foreign body ingestion is suspected, obtain posteroanterior and lateral radiographic views of the throat and chest to at least the midabdomen to determine if indeed anything was ingested or if the FB has become lodged or produced an obstruction. In small children, this should include the area from the nasopharynx to the upper abdomen, which can often be done with a single large radiographic plate. A lateral view will not be necessary if the FB is in the stomach or if it is discovered that no object has actually been swallowed.

A coin located in the proximal esophagus will be oriented in the coronal plane on an anteroposterior projection. Tracheal foreign bodies align in the sagittal plane on a lateral projection (Figure 72-1). Button batteries, which can be hazardous, can be differentiated from a simple coin by their "double ring" appearance on radiographs.

Many foreign bodies are radiolucent; therefore a negative radiograph does not rule out a foreign body.

A foreign body with sharp edges or a blunt FB lodged in the esophagus for more than a day should be removed endoscopically, because it is likely to cause a perforation and is still accessible. Button or disk batteries that are impacted in the esophagus can rapidly

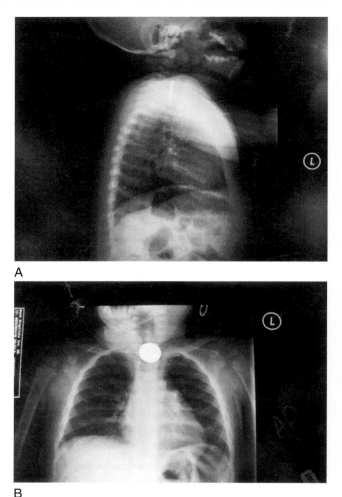

A

B

Figure 72-1 Posteroanterior and lateral combined radiograph views of the chest and neck revealing an upper esophageal coin. (Adapted from Nicholson J: Occult ingestion of foreign body. *Emerg Phys Monthly* April 2005.)

cause tissue necrosis and perforation and therefore must be removed on an emergent basis. Once a button battery has cleared the esophagus, it will usually traverse the remainder of the gastrointestinal tract (GI) without difficulty and would only need to be removed if there were signs and symptoms of gastrointestinal injury, if the battery was larger than 20 mm in diameter, or if it failed to pass the pylorus after 48 hours.

Ⓥ **Many sharp, pointed, and elongated FBs should be removed even if they have passed into the stomach.** Examples include toothpicks, medication blister packs, open safety pins, toothbrushes, plastic bag clips, and elongated nails and wires. FBs longer than 6 cm in children (3 cm in infants) and 10 cm in adults should be removed. Toothpicks are shorter than this, but they are associated with a high incidence of perforation. Plastic bag clips have a propensity to attach to the folds of the small bowel with subsequent small bowel ulceration and the potential for hemorrhage, perforation, and healing with fibrosis and obstruction.

✓ **A child who is brought in immediately after ingesting a coin and is asymptomatic but has a coin impacted in the upper or lower esophagus can initially be fed soft bread with clear fluids and observed for several hours to see if the coin will spontaneously pass into the stomach.** If this is unsuccessful, consult with the parents, along with a pediatric endoscopist, regarding further observation for up to 24 hours as an outpatient or inpatient, or possibly performing endoscopic removal as soon as possible.

✓ **When a coin or other smooth object has been lodged in the upper esophagus of a healthy asymptomatic child for less than 24 hours, and endoscopy is not readily available and the parents are supportive about avoiding general anesthesia, the object can often be removed using a simple Foley catheter technique.** When available, this can be performed under fluoroscopy; although, to avoid this radiation, it can be safely performed as a blind procedure. With the patient mildly sedated (e.g., midazolam [Versed], 0.5 mg/kg per rectum, intranasally or PO, with a half hour allowed for absorption), position the child with the head down (Trendelenburg) and prone to minimize the risk for aspiration. Alternatively, consider ketamine for procedural sedation (see Appendix E). Have a functioning laryngoscope, Magill forceps, and airway equipment at hand. Test the balloon of an 8- to 12-Fr Foley catheter to ensure that it inflates symmetrically. Lubricate the catheter with water-soluble jelly and insert it through the nose into the esophagus to a point distal to the FB. Inflate the balloon with 5 mL of air and apply gentle traction on the catheter until the foreign body reaches the base of the tongue. Terminate the procedure if you encounter any resistance. The patient will reflexively gag, cough, or spit out the foreign body. Immediately deflate the balloon and remove the catheter (Figure 72-2). If a first attempt at removal fails, consult an endoscopist. When removal is successful, repeat the radiograph to be sure that there are no additional coins, and discharge the patient after a brief period of observation.

✓ **Also, when there is parental support, esophageal bougienage is a safe, effective, and inexpensive method to advance coins or smooth objects from the distal esophagus into the stomach without sedation.** After topical anesthesia of the throat, wrap the patient in a bed sheet with arms at the side and have an assistant hold the child upright. Advance a well-lubricated, blunt, round-tipped Hurst-type esophageal dilator through the mouth and esophagus into the stomach, then remove it. Obtain a postprocedure radiograph of the chest and upper abdomen to document the location of the FB. Esophageal bougienage should be limited to witnessed ingestions of a single coin lodged for less than 24 hours with no previous history of esophageal FB, disease, or surgery and no respiratory compromise. Dilator size should be 28 Fr for ages 1 to 2, 32 Fr for ages 2 to 3, 36 Fr for ages 3 to 4, 38 Fr for ages 4 to 5, and 40 Fr for those older than 5 years of age. These two rapid, simple, cost-effective techniques have been shown in the past to be safe and effective. Because of the lack of direct visual control and the potential for injury or aspiration, however, many clinicians forgo these procedures and take advantage of the widespread availability of flexible endoscopy when dealing with esophageal FBs.

✓ **FBs of the esophagus are more difficult to remove when prolonged impaction leads to mucosal edema, swelling, and necrosis.** It is for this reason that Foley catheter manipulation and bougienage are not recommended for coins that have been entrapped for more than 24 hours.

✓ **Children with distal esophageal coins may be safely observed up to 24 hours before an invasive removal procedure, because most will spontaneously pass the coins.**

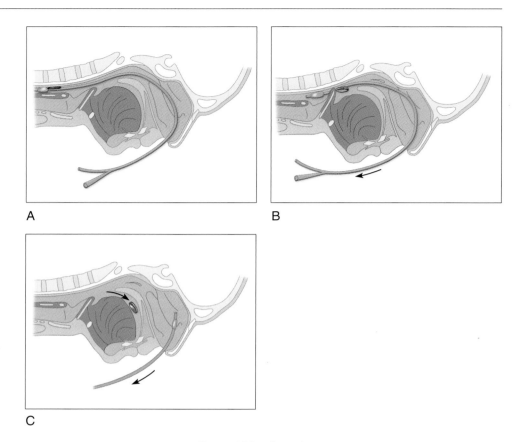

Figure 72-2 Foley catheter technique.

✓ **When an FB has passed into the stomach and there are no symptoms or hazardous circumstances that demand immediate removal, discharge the patient with instructions to return for reevaluation in 3 to 4 days (2 days with button batteries) or sooner if the child develops nausea, vomiting, fever, abdominal pain, rectal pain, or rectal bleeding.**

✓ For potentially hazardous radiopaque objects, repeat radiographs every 3 to 4 days to confirm that passage of the object is necessary. This would not be required for small, smooth objects such as coins.

✓ **All subdiaphragmatic coins seem to pass without incident.** Metal detectors can be used to follow the elimination of metallic FBs without further radiation exposure. Having parents sift through stools is often unproductive. (One missed stool negates days of hard work.) It may be helpful to give a bulk laxative to help decrease the intestinal transit time.

What Not To Do:

✗ Do not use ipecac for FB ingestions. Emesis is effective for emptying the stomach of liquid but not for removing FBs from the esophagus or stomach. It may even result in regurgitation of a gastric disk battery into the esophagus, where it will be much more hazardous.

ⓧ Do not forcefully remove an esophageal FB, especially if it is causing pain. This removal may lead to injury or perforation.

ⓧ Do not worry about the corrosive properties of pennies minted in the United States since 1982, that is, with a high (97.5%) zinc content. Although concerns have been raised in the medical and popular press, they are not associated with more esophageal mucosal injuries than other coins are.

ⓧ Do not automatically assume that an ingested FB should be surgically removed. Most potentially injurious FBs pass through the alimentary tract without mishap. Operate only when the patient is actually being harmed by the swallowed FB or when there is evidence that it is not moving down the alimentary tract.

ⓧ Do not miss additional coins after removing one from the proximal esophagus. Take a repeat radiograph after removal of one coin.

ⓧ Do not routinely refer children with esophageal coins for an additional investigation to look for underlying disease. This is a common occurrence in normal children.

ⓧ Do not ignore the potential hazards of button battery ingestions (see Discussion). Button batteries in the esophagus demand emergent removal.

ⓧ In the patient who presents with food (usually meat) bolus impaction, never use meat tenderizer.

Discussion

Older children and fully conscious, communicative adults may be able to identify the material swallowed and point to the location of the discomfort. Localization of the level of impaction, however, is often not reliable. In many instances, the ingestion goes unrecognized or unreported until the onset of symptoms, which may be remote from the time of ingestion. Young children, the cognitively impaired, or psychiatric patients may present with choking, refusal to eat, vomiting, drooling, wheezing, blood-stained saliva, or respiratory distress.

FB ingestion is most common in children 6 months to 6 years of age, who comprise 75% to 80% of all cases. Coins are the most common FBs in children. Other FBs in children include fish bones, marbles, buttons, button batteries, screws, pins, paper clips, crayons, pen and bottle caps, and small toys. In adults, meat boluses, bones, coins, dentures, fruit pits, and toothpicks are commonly encountered. Ingestion of foreign objects occurs most often in edentulous adults and in individuals with psychiatric conditions, mental retardation, or chemical dependency. Intentional ingestion of various FBs is encountered commonly in prisoners and patients with psychiatric disorders.

Although most coins swallowed by healthy children pass through the gastrointestinal tract without difficulty, patients with previous GI tract surgery or congenital gut malformations are at increased risk for obstruction or perforation. As with coins, most other swallowed FBs in children and adults will traverse the GI tract without difficulty and require no intervention.

The narrowest and least distensible strait in the gastrointestinal tract is usually the cricopharyngeus muscle at the level of the thyroid cartilage. Next narrowest is usually the pylorus, followed by the lower esophageal sphincter and the ileocecal valve. Thus anything that passes the throat will probably pass through the anus as well (although all of these sites are potential locations for FB impaction). In general, FBs below the diaphragm should be left alone.

Complications are related to the type of FB and are more common if it remains entrapped more than 24 hours. These include inconsequential mucosal scratches or abrasions, lacerations, esophageal stricture, esophageal necrosis, retropharyngeal abscess formation, hemorrhage, obstruction, and perforation.

(continued)

Discussion continued

A significant portion of children with esophageal FBs are asymptomatic; therefore any child suspected of ingesting an FB requires radiography to document whether or not it is present, and, if so, where it is located.

Large button batteries (the size of quarters) have become stuck in the esophagus, eroded through the esophageal wall, and produced fatal exsanguination, but the smaller variety and batteries that have passed into the gut have not posed such a danger. A button battery lodged in the esophagus should be considered a true emergency and removed immediately by an endoscopist. A button battery found in the stomach should be allowed to pass spontaneously. Smaller batteries need only weekly radiographic follow-up; the larger ones should be checked every 48 hours. Failure to pass the pylorus within 2 days is an indication for endoscopic removal. The maximum GI transit time for such FBs in children is 5 days.

Any child with respiratory distress should have the coin removed promptly. Time will probably not allow this to be done under ideal conditions in the operating room. Rapid removal using a McIntosh laryngoscope blade to expose the esophageal entrance and then extracting the coin from the esophagus has been described. **Ketamine has been shown to be effective without significant complications in one study that demonstrated its use in the removal of esophageal FBs in pediatric patients. Under critical conditions, combining these two modalities may be quite helpful.**

In adults, esophageal body obstruction is most typically caused by a meat bolus impaction. The upper esophageal sphincter, level of the aortic arch, or the diaphragmatic hiatus are all anatomically narrow and a food bolus may therefore become impacted at any of these sites. Patients with total obstruction, who have inability to pass their secretions, should be treated within 12 hours because of the risk of pulmonary aspiration. A trial of glucagon 1.0 mg IV, administered slowly to avoid nausea and vomiting, may be used in attempt to relax the esophagus. If this is ineffectual, endoscopy allows removal of the impacted food bolus, as well as evaluation of concomitant causative conditions, such as esophageal carcinoma, stricture, achalasia, or eosinophilic esophagitis. Patients who pass a food bolus without endoscopy should be referred for later endoscopy to evaluate for causative conditions.

Suggested Readings

Binder L, Anderson WA: Pediatric gastrointestinal foreign body ingestions, *Ann Emerg Med* 13:112–117, 1984.

Cantu S, Conners GP: Esophageal coins: are pennies different? *Clin Pediatr* 40:677–680, 2001.

Connors GP: A literature-based comparison of three methods of pediatric esophageal coin removal, *Pediatr Emerg Care* 13:154–157, 1997.

Connors GP, Chamberlain JM, Ochsenschlager DW: Symptoms and spontaneous passage of esophageal coins, *Arch Pediatr Adolesc Med* 149:36–39, 1995.

Dokler ML, Bradshaw J, Mollitt DL, et al: Selective management of pediatric esophageal foreign bodies, *Am Surg* 61:132–134, 1995.

Duncan M, Wong RKH: Esophageal emergencies: things that will wake you from a sound sleep, *Gastroenterol Clin North Am* 32:1035–1052, 2003.

Eisen GM, Baron TH, Dominitz JA, et al: Guideline for the management of ingested foreign bodies, *Gastrointest Endosc* 55:802–806, 2002.

Emslander HC, Bonadio W, Klatzo M: Efficacy of esophageal bougienage by emergency physicians in pediatric coin ingestion, *Ann Emerg Med* 27:726–729, 1996.

Ginaldi S: Removal of esophageal foreign bodies using a Foley catheter in adults, *Am J Emerg Med* 3:64–66, 1985.

Gracia C, Frey CF, Bodai BI: Diagnosis and management of ingested foreign bodies: a ten-year experience, *Ann Emerg Med* 13:30–34, 1984.

Hodge D, Tecklinburg F, Fleisher G: Coin ingestion: does every child need a radiograph? *Ann Emerg Med* 14:443–446, 1985.

Hostetler MA, Barnard JA: Removal of esophageal foreign bodies in the pediatric ED: is ketamine an option? *Am J Emerg Med* 20:96–98, 2002.

Mahafza TM: Extracting coins from the upper end of the esophagus using a Magill forceps technique, *Int J Pediatr Otorhinolaryngol* 62:37–39, 2002.

Schunk JE, Harrison M, Corneli HM, et al: Fluoroscopic Foley catheter removal of esophageal foreign bodies in children: experience with 415 episodes, *Pediatrics* 94:709–714, 1994.

Silva RG, Ahluwalia JP: Asymptomatic esophageal perforation after foreign body ingestion, *Gastrointest Endosc* 61:615–619, 2005.

Soprano JV, Fleisher GR, Mandl KD: The spontaneous passage of esophageal coins in children, *Arch Ped Adol Med* 153:1073–1076, 1999.

Triadafilopoulos G: *Ingested foreign bodies and food impactions in adults* [UptoDate website] 2011. Available at http://www.uptodate.com. Accessed March 2012.

Uyemura MC: Foreign body ingestion in children, *Am Fam Physician* 72:287–291, 2005.

Hemorrhoids

(Piles)

Presentation

Patients with external hemorrhoids (Figure 73-1) generally complain of a painful anal lump of sudden onset, which may become intense in severity. It will appear to be purple and is located within the anal canal. It may have been precipitated by straining during defecation, heavy lifting, or pregnancy, but, in most cases, there will be no definite preceding event. The external hemorrhoidal swelling is caused by thrombosis of the venous complex. It is very tender to palpation and usually does not bleed unless there is erosion of the overlying skin.

More commonly, patients with internal hemorrhoids (Figure 73-2) usually seek help because of painless (or nearly painless) bright red bleeding during or after defecation. Patients usually notice intermittent spotting on toilet tissue or blood dripping into the toilet bowl, or both. Blood may be admixed with or streaking the stool. A prolapsed internal hemorrhoid appears as a protrusion of painless, moist red tissue covered with rectal mucosa at the anal verge. Prolapsed internal hemorrhoids may become strangulated and thrombosed, and thus painful. Itching is not a common symptom of hemorrhoids.

What To Do:

✓ If the problem is rectal bleeding, it should be approached as with any other gastrointestinal (GI) bleeding. The amount of bleeding should be quantified with orthostatic vital signs and a hemoglobin and hematocrit. When there is evidence of severe hemorrhage, rapid volume replacement and early surgical consultation should be initiated.

✓ A detailed history will help establish the diagnosis of hemorrhoids. The color and character of anorectal bleeding and any relief the patient may have obtained from reducing a prolapsed hemorrhoid back into the anal canal may lead to the diagnosis.

✓ An adequate physical examination should include careful inspection, palpation, and digital examination. Anoscopy and proctosigmoidoscopy should be performed as soon as possible when there is rectal bleeding. However, evidence of hemorrhoidal bleeding does not exclude other causes of rectal bleeding; therefore a complete colonic evaluation should be done at some point in those who are at a risk, based on family history, or who are at an age for colonic screening evaluation. Young patients in whom hemorrhoids are the obvious source of bleeding may not require more than a digital rectal examination and anoscopy.

✓ **For nonthreatening rectal bleeding from hemorrhoids, the initial management should include a high-fiber diet, stool softeners, and bulk laxatives, and the patient should be instructed to spend less time sitting and straining on the commode.** Patients also should

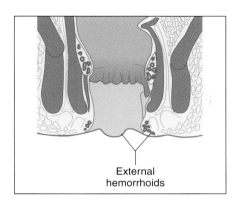

Figure 73-1 External hemorrhoid.

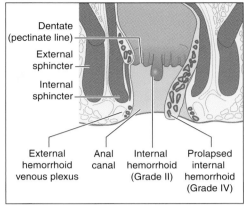

Figure 73-2 Internal hemorrhoid.

be taught not to neglect their first urge to defecate; those who are troubled with constipation should be given an osmotic laxative (see Chapter 67).

✓ Prolapsed or strangulated hemorrhoids warrant surgical consultation and possible hospital admission.

✓ If the problem is mild pain, the rectum should be examined using a topical anesthetic (lidocaine jelly) as a lubricant. First, look for thrombosed external hemorrhoids and prolapsed internal hemorrhoids. Have the patient perform a Valsalva maneuver as you provide traction on the skin of the buttocks to evert the anus. Examine the posterior mucosa for anal fissures. After the topical anesthesia has taken effect, complete the digital rectal examination, looking for evidence of rectal abscesses or other masses. Internal hemorrhoids are usually not palpable unless they have prolapsed.

✓ If topical mucosal anesthetic does not give enough relief to permit examination, follow with subcutaneous injection of 5 to 10 mL of 1% lidocaine with epinephrine or bupivacaine 0.5% with epinephrine for extended pain relief.

✓ **If topical anesthetics on the rectal mucosa help control the pain, provide for more of the same, perhaps also with some added corticosteroid for anti-inflammatory effect (Anusol-HC cream). Suppositories are convenient but may not deliver the medication where it is needed; so, prescribe cream or foam (Proctofoam-HC) applied externally rather than internally.**

✓ **Pain may also be relieved by reducing sphincter spasm. Prescribe topical nifedipine 0.2% or diltiazem gel 2% with lidocaine gel 1.5% to be applied every 12 hours.** Topical glyceryl trinitrate 0.2% or nitroglycerin ointment can be substituted for the diltiazem and nifedipine, but many patients are unable to tolerate the headaches that frequently occur. (These prescriptions often need to be filled at a compounding pharmacy.)

✓ **Instruct the patient to treat lesser pain and itching with witch hazel compresses, a low potency steroid cream, good anal hygiene, and ice packs followed by warm sitz baths or hot compresses. Sitz baths may be the most effective of these therapies;** it consists of a

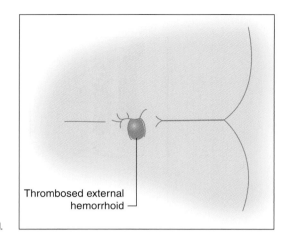

Thrombosed external
hemorrhoid

Figure 73-3 Thrombosed external hemorrhoid.

warm-water (40° C) bath that relieves tissue edema and sphincter spasm. **Zinc oxide paste or petroleum jelly may ease defecation and soothe itching. Prevent constipation by using bulk laxatives (i.e., bran, methylcellulose, polycarbophil)** (see Chapter 67) **and stool softeners (docusate [Colace], 50 to 100 mg qd), and arrange follow-up.** Inform the patient that hemorrhoids may recur and require surgical removal.

✓ Small ulcerated external hemorrhoids usually do not require any treatment for hemostasis. Bulk laxatives and gentle cleansing are generally all that is required. Occasionally, patients present several days after an external hemorrhoid has thrombosed with a small gush of dark blood because of a ruptured pile. This may continue to ooze for a day or two. With or without rupture, if the pain has subsided, all that is required is reassurance and the general measures described previously. Inform the patient that symptoms should resolve in approximately 2 weeks.

✓ **When an acutely thrombosed hemorrhoid is engorged and causing severe pain, and there are no anticipated bleeding problems, the hemorrhoid should be incised to provide pain relief. Consider using procedural sedation** (see Appendix E). Apply an ice pack for 15 minutes; then, using the smallest needle available, inject around it and infiltrate the dome of the mass with a local anesthetic to allow for examination and excision. **As described previously, use lidocaine or bupivacaine with epinephrine. Have an assistant spread the buttocks. The thrombus may be enucleated through an elliptic incision over the anal mucosa. Make the elliptic incision around the clot but not past the cutaneous layer or past the anal verge. Locular clots can be broken up by inserting a straight hemostat into the wound and spreading the tips, thereby allowing the clots to be expressed. Pain relief from this simple surgical technique can be dramatic, but excision is not effective unless the entire thrombosed lesion is completely removed** (Figures 73-3 and 73-4). Apply a compression dressing and tape the buttocks together for 12 hours to minimize bleeding. Occasionally, Gelfoam may be needed to help control oozing. The patient can then begin the nonsurgical treatment described previously. Schedule a follow-up examination in 2 days. Narcotics may be prescribed for a few days but should be switched to nonsteroidal anti-inflammatory drugs (NSAIDs) as soon as the risk of bleeding has lessened so as not to cause constipation.

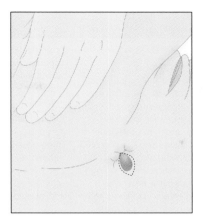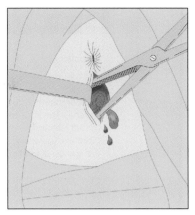

Figure 73-4 Thrombosed hemorrhoid excision.

What Not To Do:

(X) Do not labor to reduce prolapsed hemorrhoids unless they are part of a large rectal prolapse with some strangulation. Everything may prolapse again when the patient stands or strains. Bulky but asymptomatic hemorrhoids should be left alone. Treatment is directed toward symptom control, not appearance, until definitive care is received.

(X) Do not traumatize the patient when doing an examination.

(X) Do not miss infectious, neoplastic, and other anorectal pathologic conditions that can resemble or coexist with hemorrhoids. Consider rectal prolapse, polyps, carcinoma, hypertrophied anal papilla, skin tags, fissure, fistula, and perianal abscess in the differential diagnosis.

(X) Do not excise a thrombosed hemorrhoid when the patient has a bleeding abnormality, is taking an anticoagulant or daily aspirin, or has increased portal venous pressure.

(X) Do not allow patients to use hydrocortisone topical therapy for longer than 7 to 10 days. Prolonged use can lead to mucosal atrophy.

(X) Do not have the patient sit on a doughnut-shaped cushion. This may actually increase venous congestion.

Discussion

The word *hemorrhoid* comes from the Greek *hemo* (blood) plus *rrhoos* (flowing). The word "piles" comes from the Latin *pila*, or ball. As a disease entity, hemorrhoids have been reported to plague the human race since the earliest history of man.

Three quarters of Americans have hemorrhoids at some time in their lives. Predisposing factors include heredity, age, portal hypertension, anal sphincter tone, occupation, low-fiber diet,

(continued)

Discussion continued

obesity, diarrhea, straining to defecate, and pregnancy.

The submucosal tissue within the anal canal is made up of a discontinuous series of vascular cushions that contribute to continence by partially occluding the anus. The three main cushions are found in the left lateral, right anterior, and right posterior positions. These vascular cushions may also protect the anal canal from injury by filling with blood during defecation. The deterioration of supporting tissue to the vascular cushions in the anal canal produces venous distention, erosion, bleeding, and thrombosis. Several theories have been postulated regarding the etiology of hemorrhoids; however, the precise cause is still unknown.

Hemorrhoids are classified according to location and degree of prolapse. The dentate line separates internal from external hemorrhoids. Internal hemorrhoids arise proximal to the dentate line and are covered by mucosa. External hemorrhoids are located distal to the dentate line and are covered by squamous epithelia that contain numerous somatic pain receptors. External skin tags, which represent residual excess skin associated with previous thrombosis of external hemorrhoids, or which can be associated with anal fissures or Crohn disease, are often confused with external hemorrhoids, but they are not hemorrhoids.

There is no widely used classification system for grading external hemorrhoids, but internal hemorrhoids are graded from I to IV. First-degree internal hemorrhoids do not protrude, cannot be palpated by digital examination, and require anoscopy for diagnosis. Second-degree hemorrhoids

protrude with straining or defecation but reduce spontaneously. Third-degree hemorrhoids prolapse with straining or defecation and require manual reduction. Fourth-degree hemorrhoids are irreducibly prolapsed and may strangulate.

External hemorrhoids are usually small, do not itch, and cause pain only when they are acutely thrombosed. Internal hemorrhoids are usually painless, and patients generally present with painless bleeding or a bloody mucoid discharge, often associated with their prolapse, anal soiling, and, occasionally, pruritus.

Elastic banding techniques, which have become one of the most frequently applied methods of treatment of internal hemorrhoids, can be 80% to 90% curative for second-, third-, and fourth-degree lesions. This technique is associated with a low complication rate (<2%). Patients with bleeding diatheses, or both internal and external hemorrhoids, are best treated by means of surgical resection.

The diagnosis of hemorrhoids may cover a variety of minor ailments of the anus that may or may not be related to the hemorrhoidal veins (vascular cushions). Anal and perianal itching can be caused by dermatologic conditions, such as psoriasis, eczema, lichen planus, and allergic dermatitis (see discussion of pruritus ani, p. 243). Infections of the anal and perianal area include herpes simplex, scabies, candidiasis, erythrasma, and pinworms (see Chapter 69). Perianal itching can also be the result of diabetes, leukemia, aplastic anemia, thyroid disease, hyperbilirubinemia, and precancerous and cancerous lesions. Punch biopsy may be indicated when pruritus ani is chronic.

Suggested Readings

Gopal DV: Diseases of the rectum and anus: a clinical approach to common disorders, *Clin Cornerstone* 4:34–48, 2002.

Sardinha TC, Corman ML: Hemorrhoids, *Surg Clin North Am* 82:1153–1167, 2002.

Innocuous Ingestions

Presentation

Frightened parents call or arrive in the ED or clinic with a 2-year-old child who has just swallowed some household product, such as laundry bleach.

What To Do:

✓ Establish exactly what was ingested (have them locate the package or container and have them bring in a sample, if possible), how much was ingested, and how long ago it occurred, as well as any symptoms and treatment so far. It is essential to gather as much information as possible from emergency medical services, bystanders, babysitters, and parents about all of the agents to which the patient might have been exposed.

✓ **If there is any question about the substance, its toxicity, or its treatment, call the regional poison control center** (see Appendix G). **In fact, it is a good policy to call the regional poison center, even if you are completely comfortable managing the case, so that they can record the ingestion for epidemiologic purposes.**

✓ If there is any question of this being a toxic ingestion, follow the instructions of the regional poison center.

✓ Reassure the parents and child, and instruct them to call or return to the ED if there are any problems. Teach parents how to keep all poisons beyond the reach of children and how to call the regional poison center first for any future ingestion(s).

What Not To Do:

✗ Do not totally believe what is told about the nature of the ingestion. Often some of the information immediately available is wrong. Suspect the worst.

✗ Do not depend on product labels to give you accurate information on toxicity. Some lethal poisons carry warnings no more serious than "use as directed" or "for external use only."

✗ Do not follow the instructions on the package regarding what to do if a product is ingested. These are often inaccurate or out of date.

✗ Do not automatically give ipecac for emesis. Follow the recommendation of your regional poison center.

✗ Do not improvise treatment of a patient referred by the regional poison center. He probably has special information and a treatment plan to share, if he has not called already.

Discussion

Fortunately, most products designed to be played with by children are also designed to be nontoxic when ingested. This includes chalk, crayons, ink, paste, paint, and Play-Doh. Many drugs, such as birth control pills and thyroid hormone, are relatively nontoxic, as are most laundry bleaches, the mercury in thermometers, and many plants.

However, some apparently innocuous household products are surprisingly toxic, including camphorated oil, cigarettes, dishwasher soap, oil of wintergreen, and vitamins with iron. Because the ingredients in common products and the treatment of ingestions continue to change, broad statements and lists are not reliable. The best strategy is always to call the regional poison center (see Appendix G).

Suggested Reading

Dantzig PI: A new cutaneous sign of mercury poisoning? *J Am Acad Dermatol* 49:1109–1111, 2003.

Singultus

(Hiccups)

Presentation

Recurring, unpredictable, clonic contractions of the diaphragm produce sharp inhalations. Hiccups are usually precipitated by some combination of laughing, talking, eating, and drinking but may also occur spontaneously. Most cases resolve spontaneously, and patients do not come to a physician's office unless hiccups are prolonged or severe. A bout of hiccups is any episode lasting more than a few minutes. If hiccups last longer than 48 hours, they are considered persistent or protracted. Hiccups lasting longer than 1 month are called intractable.

What To Do:

 ✅ **For a bout of hiccups, stimulate the patient's soft palate by rubbing it with a swab, spoon, catheter tip, or finger, just short of stimulating a gag reflex, and, if necessary, repeat this several times. Alternatively, stimulate the same general area by depositing a tablespoon of granulated sugar at the base of the tongue, in the area of the lingual tonsils, and letting it dissolve.** Such maneuvers (or their placebo effect) may abolish simple cases of hiccups. Other simple measures include having the individual bite on a lemon or inhale a noxious agent (e.g., ammonia). You can also have them perform a Valsalva maneuver, breath hold, or pull their knees up to their chest and lean forward.

✅ With persistent and protracted hiccups, look for an underlying cause and ask about precipitating factors or previous episodes. Drugs that are known to cause hiccups include benzodiazepines, short-acting barbiturates, and dexamethasone. Persistence of hiccups during sleep suggests an organic cause; conversely, if a patient is unable to sleep or if the hiccups stop during sleep and recur promptly on awakening, a psychogenic or idiopathic cause is indicated.

✅ **Perform a complete physical examination.** Look in the ears. (Foreign bodies, such as a hair against the tympanic membrane, can cause hiccups.) Examine the neck (look for thyromegaly and lymphadenopathy), chest, and abdomen, perhaps including an upright chest radiograph, to look for neoplastic, inflammatory, or infectious processes irritating the phrenic nerve or diaphragm. Pericarditis, myocardial infarction, and aberrant cardiac pacemaker electrode placement are potential sources of persistent hiccups, as well as acute and chronic alcohol intoxication and gastroesophageal reflux or other gastrointestinal disorders. Perform a neurologic examination, looking for evidence of partial continuous seizures or brain stem lesions. Early multiple sclerosis is thought to be one of the most frequent neurologic causes of intractable hiccups in young adults.

✅ **Routine laboratory evaluation** may include a complete blood count (CBC) with differential (looking for infection or neoplasm) and a basic metabolic panel. (Hyponatremia, hypokalemia, hypocalcemia, and uremia can cause persistent hiccups.)

✅ **Additional testing** is not limited to, but may include, an ECG, chest CT, and upper endoscopy.

✅ Direct treatment toward the specific illness causing the hiccups, if this is identified.

✅ **If hiccups persist after using simple measures, try chlorpromazine (Thorazine), 25 to 50 mg PO tid or qid.** (The same dose may be given IV or IM.) To avoid or minimize hypotension, consider giving a 500- to 1000-mL bolus of IV normal saline. Chlorpromazine is contraindicated in elderly patients with dementia. Side effects include dystonic reaction, drowsiness, and the risk of tardive dyskinesia. **Alternatively, haloperidol (Haldol), 2 to 5 mg IM, followed by 1 to 4 mg PO tid for 2 days may be equally effective, with less potential for hypotension. Another approach is to use metoclopramide (Reglan), 10 mg PO tid or qid, followed by a maintenance regimen of 10 to 20 mg PO tid to qid for 10 days. Reglan and Haldol are also associated with tardive dyskinesia.**

✅ For intractable hiccups, phenytoin (Dilantin), valproic acid (Depakote), or carbamazepine (Tegretol) can be given in typical anticonvulsant doses. Alternatively, baclofen (a centrally acting muscle relaxant) can be prescribed at 10 to 20 mg 2 to 3 times a day with gabapentin (Neurontin) as an "add-on," if necessary, especially in patients with solid malignancies.

✅ There are some reports of acupuncture or hypnosis being efficacious; these can be tried if the aforementioned are unsuccessful.

✅ **Arrange for follow-up and additional evaluation if the hiccups recur or persist.**

Discussion

The medical term *singultus* apparently originates from the Latin *singult,* which is very descriptive and roughly translates as "the act of catching one's breath while sobbing."

Hiccups result from an involuntary spasmodic contraction of the diaphragm and external intercostal muscles with ensuing quick inspiration. This is followed by a rapid closure of the glottis, which prevents overinflation of the lungs.

Hiccups are mediated by a reflex arch consisting of the afferent and efferent limbs and supraspinal central connection, which are thought to be independent of the respiratory center in the brain stem. The exact cause remains unclear. When there is an organic cause, irritation of the various branches of the vagus nerve are often involved. Despite a

long list of possible causes, in most cases no organic cause can be identified, and a diagnosis of idiopathic chronic hiccups is made.

Although unlikely, there are potentially serious complications, such as dehydration and weight loss, resulting from the inability to tolerate fluids and food.

Patients who experience syncope with the hiccups should be hospitalized and evaluated for possible life-threatening arrhythmias, which have been reported as both the cause and the effect of hiccups.

Hiccups, in general, are a common malady, and fortunately most bouts are usually transient and benign. Persistent or intractable episodes are

Discussion continued

more likely to result from serious pathophysiologic processes that affect a component of the hiccup reflex mechanism.

The common denominator among various hiccup cures for brief episodes seems to be stimulation of the glossopharyngeal nerve, but as for every self-limiting disease, there are always many effective cures.

. . . hold your breath, and if after you have done so for some time the hiccup is no better, then gargle with a little water, and if it still continues, tickle your nose with something and sneeze, and if you sneeze once or twice, even the most violent hiccup is sure to go.

—Eryximachus, the physician to Aristophanes, in
Plato's *Symposium.*

Suggested Readings

Berlin AL, Muhn CY, Billick RC: Hiccups, eructation, and other uncommon prodromal manifestations of herpes zoster, *J Am Acad Dermatol* 49:1121–1124, 2003.

Friedman NL: Hiccups: a treatment review, *Pharmacotherapy* 16:986–995, 1996.

Ge AX, Ryan ME, Giaccone G, et al: Acupuncture treatment for persistent hiccups in patients with cancer, *J Altern Complement Med* 16:811–816, 2010.

Kolodzik PW, Eilers MA: Hiccups (singultus): review and approach to management, *Ann Emerg Med* 20:565–573, 1991.

Launois S, Bizec JL, Whitelaw WA, et al: Hiccup in adults: an overview, *Eur Resp J* 6:563–575, 1993.

Lembo A: *Overview of hiccups. [UpToDate website]*, 2011. Available at http://www.uptodate.com. Accessed March 2012.

Marinella MA: Diagnosis and management of hiccups in the patient with advanced cancer, *J Support Oncol* 7:122–127, 2009.

Nathan MD, Leshner RT, Keller AP: Intractable hiccups (singultus), *Laryngoscope* 90:1612–1618, 1980.

Viera AJ, Sullivan SA: Remedies for prolonged hiccups, *Am Fam Physician* 63:1684–1686, 2001.

Wagner MS, Stapczynski JS: Persistent hiccups, *Ann Emerg Med* 11:24–26, 1982.

Vomiting

(Food Poisoning, Gastroenteritis)

Presentation

The patient seeks medical care 1 to 6 hours after eating because of severe nausea, vomiting, retching, and abdominal cramps that may progress later into diarrhea. He may have relatively minor symptoms or may appear very ill: pale, diaphoretic, tachycardic, orthostatic, perhaps complaining of paresthesias, or feeling as if he is "going to die." Others may have similar symptoms from eating the same food. The physical examination, however, is reassuring. There is minimal abdominal tenderness, localized, if at all, to the epigastrium or to the rectus abdominis muscle (which is strained by the vomiting).

What To Do:

✓ Obtain as much historical information as possible and completely examine the patient. Always consider pregnancy in women of childbearing age who present with vomiting. If there is any suspicion of a more serious underlying disorder (especially in the older patient), perform those tests needed to rule out myocardial infarction, perforated ulcer, aortic aneurysm, or any of the catastrophes that can present in a similar fashion. Always maintain a high index of suspicion for acute appendicitis or other surgical conditions in the patient who presents with abdominal pain and vomiting.

✓ **In the meantime, rapidly infuse 0.9% NaCl or Ringer lactate solution IV and observe the patient, doing repeated vital sign checks and physical examinations. Fluid and electrolyte replenishment is the mainstay of medical treatment.** In adults who have the renal and cardiovascular reserve to handle rapid hydration, 1 to 2 L infused over an hour often provides dramatic improvement of all symptoms.

✓ Older patients require more cautious rehydration and are more likely to require a comprehensive diagnostic workup.

✓ The use of antiemetics for acute gastritis or gastroenteritis is somewhat controversial. With mild symptoms, there is probably no need to add this treatment and incur additional expense as well as risk the potential side effects of some of these drugs. For someone who is actively vomiting, however, these drugs can provide comfort and improve the process of rehydration.

✓ **In adults, ondansetron (Zofran), 4 mg IV is particularly advantageous, because it has minimal side effects. Alternatives include prochlorperazine (Compazine), 10 mg, which can also be given IV, along with diphenhydramine (Benadryl), 12.5 to 25 mg,** to help reduce the incidence of extrapyramidal symptoms (such as dystonic reactions and akathisia). Metoclopramide (Reglan) can also be given (slowly to reduce risk of akathisia) in a dose of 10 mg IV.

✓ **During pregnancy, metoclopramide and ondansetron because they are classified as pregnancy category B drugs.**

✓ **For children who are older than 6 months of age, ondansetron (Zofran), 0.15 mg/kg IV, can be given. Ondansetron (although very expensive under the brand name) can also be given as an oral disintegrating tablet (ODT) (which is reasonably priced as a generic).** Half of a 4-mg tablet (2 mg) is an appropriate dose for an average 2-year-old (weighing 8 to 15 kg). The 4-mg tablet can be given to children weighing 16 to 30 kg, and 8 mg can be given to heavier children. **Alternatively, metoclopramide (Reglan), 0.1 to 0.2 mg/kg IV, can be given.**

✓ **If after 1 to 2 hours the pediatric patient is improving and beginning to tolerate oral fluids and has a benign repeat abdominal examination, discharge him with instructions to advance his diet over the next 24 hours, starting with an oral rehydration solution,** such as the following recipe from the World Health Organization:

- ○ 1 cup of orange juice
- ○ ¾ tsp of table salt
- ○ 1 tsp of baking soda
- ○ 4 tbsp of sugar
- ○ 4 cups of water

✓ He should expect to be eating and feeling well in another 1 or 2 days.

✓ **Children can be rehydrated using the techniques described in Chapter 68.**

✓ If symptoms resolve more slowly, discharge the patient with a single dose of an antiemetic as described earlier.

✓ **Adults with abdominal cramping may be helped with a dose of the antispasmodic dicyclomine (Bentyl), 20 mg qid PO/IM.**

✓ **Patients should always be encouraged to return** for further evaluation and treatment if their symptoms return or if pain continues or worsens.

✓ If hypotension or other significant signs or symptoms persist, if the patient cannot tolerate parenteral rehydration, or if he cannot resume oral intake, he may have to be admitted to the hospital for further evaluation and treatment.

What Not To Do:

✗ Do not presume food poisoning without a good history for it.

✗ Do not overlook pregnancy as a possible cause of vomiting.

✗ Do not assign blame for the cause of any suspected food poisoning. The information available is almost always circumstantial until public health authorities complete their investigation.

✗ Do not skimp on IV fluids. Monitor vital signs and urinary output and generously replace fluid losses.

✗ Do not pursue expensive laboratory investigations for straightforward cases. Diagnostic tests usually are unnecessary in an otherwise healthy patient who is stable and whose history and physical examination are consistent with acute gastroenteritis.

Discussion

- Whenever possible, the cause of vomiting should be ascertained and specific treatment for an underlying cause initiated—particularly when emergent conditions, such as central nervous system (CNS) lesions, myocardial infarction, acute abdomen, bowel obstruction, endocrine/metabolic disorders, are suspected. As mentioned above, always consider pregnancy in women of childbearing age who present with vomiting. Consider bowel obstruction if there is distention and pain on abdominal palpation. Feculent vomiting is concerning for large bowel obstruction. Patients may present with a chief complaint of vomiting and, on exam, have nystagmus; these patients should be evaluated and treated for vertigo. Eating disorders must also be considered. In the diabetic, gastroparesis may be the cause. Frequent use of marijuana may be associated with recurrent vomiting as well. Many prescription drugs may cause nausea and vomiting, **and these will be cured with cessation of the drug;** so, take a good medication history, asking about both prescribed and nonprescribed drugs. **However, in most cases of simple, uncomplicated vomiting with gastroenteritis or foodborne illness, the precise cause need not be determined, and therefore symptomatic treatment is all that is required.**

- Many of the symptoms accompanying any gastroenteritis seem to be related to electrolyte disturbances and dehydration, which can be substantial even in the absence of copious vomiting and diarrhea. Lactated Ringer solution is considered the choice for IV rehydration by many clinicians, because it approximates normal serum electrolytes and can be infused rapidly. Lactated Ringer approximately replaces the electrolytes lost in diarrhea, although normal saline has more of the chloride lost by vomiting. Both work quite well in the acute setting for either diarrhea or vomiting or a combination of the two.

- **Most food items that cause foodborne illness are raw or undercooked foods of animal origin, such as meat, milk, eggs, cheese, fish, or shellfish. A clearly implicated food source may give a clue to the cause: shellfish suggesting** *Vibrio parahaemolyticus;* **rice suggesting** *Bacillus cereus;* **meat or eggs suggesting staphylococci,** *Campylobacter* **organisms, clostridia, salmonellae, shigellae, enteropathic** *Escherichia coli,* **or** *Yersinia* **sp.**

- *Vibrio* bacteria, so named because they are so motile that they appear to vibrate, are most common in states bordering the Gulf of Mexico. These flagellated bacteria inhabit marine environments and can cause gastroenteritis, wound infections, and septicemia. *V. vulnificus* infection more often follows ingestion of raw or undercooked oysters, and *V. parahaemolyticus* infection is more likely to be associated with eating shrimp or crabs. Fever, chills, and headache, in addition to the gastrointestinal symptoms, are common manifestations of this infection. Patients with liver disease, impaired immune systems, and diabetes are at increased risk for fulminant infections.

- *B. cereus* causes an acute emetic syndrome, most commonly within 1 to 6 hours of ingesting fried rice obtained from a Chinese restaurant. *B. cereus* also causes a less common diarrheal syndrome with an onset 8 to 16 hours after ingestion. There is no role for antimicrobial therapy in the treatment of these syndromes.

- **The most common food poisoning** seen in most emergency departments is caused by the heat-stable **toxin of staphylococci,** which is introduced into food from infections in handlers and grows when the food sits warm. Foods that are frequently incriminated in staphylococcal food poisoning include meat and meat products; poultry and egg products; salads, such as egg, tuna, chicken, potato, and macaroni; bakery products, such as cream-filled pastries and cream pies; and milk and dairy products. Foods containing the toxins usually look and taste normal. Sudden onset of nausea, vomiting, abdominal pain, and watery diarrhea usually occurs 30 minutes to 8 hours after eating contaminated food. Because these symptoms are toxin mediated, antibiotics are not indicated.

- **Chemical toxins** have a similar presentation, but the onset of symptoms may be more immediate. Heavy metal poisoning is a rare cause of gastroenteritis and results from gastric irritation caused by copper, zinc, iron, tin, or cadmium. Accidental ingestion of these substances can occur if a person drinks an acidic or carbonated beverage that came into contact with a metal container or metal tubing. Common symptoms include nausea, vomiting, diarrhea, cramps, and, with copper and tin, a metallic taste that usually occurs 5 to 60 minutes after ingestion. For chemical or heavy metal poisoning, consult with a poison control center for advice on appropriate treatment (see Appendix G).

Discussion continued

■ **Other bacterial food poisonings** usually present with onset of symptoms later than 1 to 6 hours after eating, less nausea and vomiting, more cramping and diarrhea, and longer courses. See Chapter 68 for management of these predominantly diarrheal illnesses.

■ **Seafood ingestion syndromes,** such as ciguatera poisoning and scombroid poisoning, can be distinguished from other forms of foodborne illnesses by symptoms such as perioral numbness and reversal of temperature sensation (ciguatera poisoning) or flushing and warmth (scombroid poisoning). Grouper, red snapper, amberjack, sea bass, and barracuda are the most common species of fish implicated in ciguatera poisoning.

■ **Ciguatoxin** is a naturally occurring toxin found in a dinoflagellate *(Gambierdiscus toxicus)* that is consumed by fish. The ciguatoxins become concentrated in these larger fish and are unaffected by normal cooking. Symptoms appear about 5 hours (2 to 30 hours) after eating toxic fish. The first manifestations of poisoning include abdominal pain, nausea, vomiting, painful defecation, and diarrhea. Pruritus and paresthesias, described as uncomfortable tingling sensations, most often develop in the extremities and mouth and, along with a peculiar sensory reversal of hot and cold, are the symptomatic hallmarks of ciguatera poisoning. Pain, paresthesias, pruritus, and weakness may persist for several weeks, and chronic symptoms have been reported. Successful management of these neurologic symptoms with IV mannitol has been described in the past, but a double-blind randomized trial of mannitol therapy in ciguatera fish poisoning did not support single-dose mannitol as standard treatment. Pruritus can be treated with antihistamines, such as hydroxyzine (Atarax, Vistaril), 25 mg 3 to 4 times daily. Treat neuropathic symptoms with gabapentin (Neurontin), 100 mg qd to tid, titrating up to 800 to 1200 mg tid as needed. The patient should be instructed to avoid all fish, alcohol, caffeine, and nuts for 6 months, because these items may precipitate a recurrence of symptoms.

■ **Scombroid** poisoning is caused by improper refrigeration of Scombroidea (bluefin and yellowfin tuna, skipjack, albacore, marlin, and mackerel). Nonscombroid fish, such as mahi-mahi, amberjack, and herring may also produce this syndrome. Bacterial growth and breakdown of the fish flesh result in the production of histamine and the production of a histamine-like toxin, saurine, neither of which are affected by normal cooking temperatures. These fish either may have a bitter, peppery, or metallic taste or may taste perfectly normal. Symptoms consist of a histamine-like reaction that includes flushing, rash, and hot sensations of the skin and mouth, along with headache, anxiety, dizziness, nausea, vomiting, and diarrhea occurring approximately 10 to 30 minutes after ingestion. Antihistamines, such as hydroxyzine (Atarax, Vistaril), 25 mg qd to qid, are effective, along with H_2 blockers, such as ranitidine (Zantac), 150 mg bid, and, in more severe cases, methylprednisolone (Solu-Medrol), 125 mg IV. Symptoms are self-limited, but medications may be required for several days.

■ **When symptoms are severe with large ingestions of either form of fish poisoning,** patients should also be given activated charcoal AD (Superchar), 1 g/kg orally.

■ **Whenever someone suffers any gastrointestinal upset, it is natural, if not instinctive, to implicate the last food eaten. When the index of suspicion for a foodborne illness is high, this information should be reported to the local health department for definitive diagnosis and epidemiologic management.**

Suggested Readings

Apfel CC, Korttila K, Abdalla M, et al: A factorial trial of six interventions for the prevention of postoperative nausea and vomiting, *N Engl J Med* 350:2441–2451, 2004.

American Gastroenterological Association: American Gastroenterological Association medical position statement: nausea and vomiting, *Gastroenterology* 120:261–263, 2001.

Berkovitch M, Mazzota P, Greenberg R, et al: Metoclopramide for nausea and vomiting of pregnancy: a prospective multicenter international study, *Am J Perinatol* 19:311–316, 2002.

Borowitz SM: Are antiemetics helpful in young children suffering from acute viral gastroenteritis? *Arch Dis Child* 90:646–648, 2005.

Büttner M, Walder B, von Elm E, et al: Is low-dose haloperidol a useful antiemetic? *Anesthesiology* 101:1454–1463, 2004.

Parlak I, Atilla R, Cicek M, et al: Rate of metoclopramide infusion affects the severity and incidence of akathisia, *Emerg Med J* 22:621–624, 2005.

Reeves JJ, Shannon MW, Fleisher GR: Ondansetron decreases vomiting associated with acute gastroenteritis: a randomized, controlled trial, *Pediatrics* 109:e62, 2002.

Scorza K, Williams A, Phillips JD, Shaw J: Evaluation of nausea and vomiting, *Am Fam Physician* 76:76–84, 2007.

Schnorf H, Taurarii M, Cundy T: Ciguatera fish poisoning: a double-blind randomized trial of mannitol therapy, *Neurology* 58:873–888, 2002.

Vinson DR: Diphenhydramine in the treatment of akathisia induced by prochlorperazine, *J Emerg Med* 26:265–270, 2004.

PART 7

Urologic Emergencies

■ Philip Buttaravoli   ■ Andrew Bushnell

CHAPTER

77

Blunt Scrotal Trauma

Presentation

Blunt injuries to the scrotum usually occur in patients who are younger than 50 years of age as a result of an athletic injury, a straddle injury, an automobile or industrial accident, or an assault. Patients present with various degrees of pain, ecchymoses, and swelling as well as faintness, nausea, or vomiting (Figure 77-1). The symptoms from minor injuries will gradually resolve on their own after 1 to 2 hours. In the more severe injury of testicular rupture, pain is usually severe, and the scrotal sac may appear full, ecchymotic, and very tender.

What To Do:

✓ Get a clear history of the exact mechanism, the force of the trauma, and the point of maximum impact. Determine if there was any bloody penile discharge or hematuria and whether or not the patient has any preexisting genital disease, such as previous genitourinary surgery, infection, or mass.

✓ Gently examine the external genitalia with the understanding that intense pain may result in a suboptimal examination. If scrotal swelling is not too severe, try to palpate and assess the intrascrotal anatomy.

✓ **When there is minimal pain and tenderness, with normal anatomy, no further evaluation is necessary.**

✓ **There is a high risk for urethral injury in** straddle injuries. **Obtain a urinalysis. If blood is present in the urine (or at the urethral meatus), perform a retrograde urethrogram and obtain urologic consultation.**

✓ After any significant blunt trauma, when pain or swelling prevents demonstration of normal intrascrotal anatomy, **obtain a testicular color Doppler ultrasonograph to help determine the need for urologic consultation and operative intervention.**

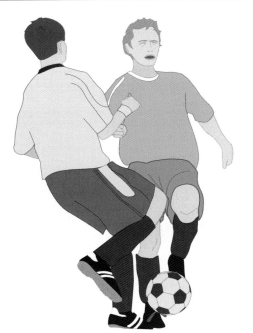

Figure 77-1 Blunt injury to the scrotum.

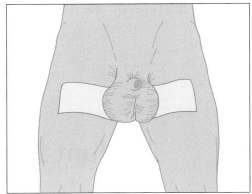

Figure 77-2 Scrotal support.

✔ **Hematomas can involve the testis, epididymis, or scrotal wall. Patients with intratesticular hematomas fare poorly without exploration.** Forty percent of these hematomas result in testicular infection or necrosis, which often requires orchiectomy. **Scrotal exploration is warranted if there is compelling evidence of testicular fracture or rupture on scrotal sonography or physical examination.** It is most appropriate to explore a grossly abnormal scrotum without ultrasonography when the index of suspicion is high. This should occur when there is a clinical hematocele. This may be evidenced by persistent moderate to severe pain, tender ecchymotic fullness of the scrotal sac, and a testicle that feels enlarged and/ or irregular or is difficult to palpate. **The presence of a large hematocele on ultrasonography is another indication for exploration.**

✔ **Small hematoceles, epididymal hematomas, or contusions of the testis generally pose little risk to the patient and do not require surgical exploration.**

✔ **All posttraumatic lesions should be followed to demonstrate sonographic resolution,** because 10% to 15% of testicular tumors first present after an episode of scrotal trauma.

✔ **Simple scrotal lacerations can be closed using Vicryl absorbable suture or tissue adhesive (Dermabond).**

✔ **When emergent urologic intervention is not required, provide analgesia (consider nonsteroidal anti-inflammatory drugs [NSAIDs], bed rest, scrotal support, a cold pack, and urologic follow-up** [Figure 77-2]).

✔ Patients should always be instructed to return immediately if pain increases, becomes severe, or is accompanied by vomiting or lightheadedness.

What Not To Do:

(X) Do not miss testicular torsion, which is associated with minor to moderate blunt trauma approximately 20% of the time. (See symptoms and signs of testicular torsion in Chapter 79.)

(X) Do not miss the rare traumatic testicular dislocation that results in an "empty scrotum." The testis is found superficially beneath the abdominal wall in approximately 80% of such cases. Immediate urology consultation is required.

(X) Do not discharge a patient until he can demonstrate the ability to urinate.

Discussion

Blunt testicular trauma occurs from a direct blow to the testes with impingement against the symphysis pubis or ischial ramus. Trauma can result in contusion, hematoma, fracture, rupture, or, rarely, dislocation of the testis. Testicular rupture is a surgical emergency. More than 80% of ruptured testes can be saved if surgery is performed within 72 hours of injury. Complications of testicular trauma include testicular atrophy, infection, infarction, and infertility, which are much more likely with nonoperative management of serious injuries.

If Doppler studies demonstrate a serious injury, early exploration, evacuation of hematoma, and repair of testicular rupture tend to result in an earlier return to normal activity, with less risk for testicular atrophy, infection, infarction, and infertility.

Sonographic findings in testicular rupture include interruption of the tunica albuginea; contour abnormality; a heterogeneous testis with irregular, poorly defined borders; scrotal wall thickening; and a large hematocele. The sonographic appearance of hematomas varies with time. Acute hematomas appear hyperechoic and subsequently become complex, with cystic components. Color Doppler sonography in posttraumatic patients may reveal focal or diffuse hyperemia of the epididymis, which represents traumatic epididymitis.

Suggested Readings

Bhatt S, Dogra VS: Role of US in testicular and scrotal trauma (review), *Radiographics* 28:1617–1629, 2008.

Chandra RV, Dowling RJ, Ulubasoglu M, Haxhimolla H, Costello AJ: Rational approach to diagnosis and management of blunt scrotal trauma, *Urology* 70:230–234, 2007.

Dogra V, Bhatt S: Acute painful scrotum, *Radiol Clin North Am* 42:349–363, 2004.

Ko S, Ng S, Wan Y, et al: Testicular dislocation: an uncommon and easily overlooked complication of blunt abdominal trauma, *Ann Emerg Med* 43:371–375, 2004.

Rosenstein D, McAninch JW: Urologic emergencies, *Med Clin North Am* 88:495–518, 2004.

Colorful Urine

Presentation

The patient may complain of or be frightened about the color of his urine. Color may be one component of some urinary complaint, or the color may be noted incidentally on urinalysis.

What To Do:

✓ Ask about symptoms of urinary urgency, frequency, and painful urination. Include questions about flank or abdominal pain as well as recent ingestion of any food colorings, over-the-counter (OTC) or prescription medications, or diagnostic dyes. Ascertain the circumstances surrounding the change of urine color: Did the color appear only after the urine contacted the container or the water in the toilet bowl? Did the urine have to sit in the sun for hours before the color appeared?

✓ **Obtain a fresh urine sample for analysis.**

✓ **Persistent foam suggests protein (yellow foam, bilirubin),** which should also show up on a dipstick test.

✓ **With red urine, a positive dipstick for blood implies the presence of red cells, free hemoglobin, or myoglobin,** which can be double-checked by examining the urinary sediment for red cells and the serum for hemoglobinemia. In patients with normal renal function, hemoglobinuria can be distinguished from myoglobinuria by drawing a blood sample, spinning it down, and looking at the serum. **Free hemoglobin produces a pink serum that will test positive with the dipstick. Myoglobin is cleared more efficiently by the kidneys, usually leaving clear serum** that tests negative with the dipstick. Consider sending the urine for microscopic urinalysis to determine the presence of red blood cells.

✓ **If the urine is red and acidic but does not contain hemoglobin, myoglobin, or red blood cells, suspect an indicator dye, such as phenolphthalein (the former laxative in Ex-Lax),** in which case the red should disappear when the urine is alkalinized with a few drops of potassium hydroxide (KOH). **Fourteen percent of individuals who eat beets produce reddish urine** because of the excretion of the pigment betalain. **Blackberries can turn acidic urine red, whereas rhubarb, anthraquinone laxatives, and some diagnostic dyes will redden urine** only when it is alkaline.

✓ **Orange urine may be produced by phenazopyridine (Pyridium) or ethoxazene (Serenium),** both of which are used as urinary tract anesthetics to diminish dysuria. **Rifampin will also turn urine orange, as will carrots, rhubarb, beets, aloe, riboflavin, vitamin A, and vitamin B$_{12}$.**

✅ **Blue or green urine** may be caused by a blue dye, such as methylene blue, a **component in several medications (Trac Tabs, Urised, Uroblue)** used to reduce symptoms of cystitis. **A blue pigment may also be produced by** *Pseudomonas* **infection. Food Dye and Color Blue Number 1 (FD & C Blue No. 1) has been reported to be absorbed from the gastrointestinal (GI) tract in some patients sufficiently to cause the urine to be dark green.**

✅ **In the critically ill patient requiring enteral feeding,** the practice of adding colored dye (including FD & C Blue No. 1) to the tube feeding to quickly detect occult aspiration can also cause urine discoloration.

✅ **Purple urine bag syndrome (PUBS)** is a term that has been used to describe the purple discoloration of the collecting bag and tubing that occurs rarely and is predominantly found in elderly bedridden women with chronic urinary catheterization, alkaline urine, and constipation. No specific cause has been found, and it appears to be a benign condition. PUBS has not been demonstrated to have any implication other than the possibility of a urinary tract infection and has not been proven to change the prognosis of patients.

✅ **Brown or black urine (not resulting from myoglobin or bilirubin) may be caused by l-dopa, melanin, phenacetin, or phenol poisoning as well as anthraquinones mentioned previously.** Metabolites of the antihypertensive methyldopa (Aldomet) may turn black on contact with bleach (which is often present in toilet bowls). **Phenytoin (Dilantin) and the statins (Lipitor, Lescol, Mevacor, Pravachol, and Zocor) are also potential causative agents.** Contamination with povidone-iodine (Betadine) solution or douche can turn urine brown. Melanin and melanogen, found in the urine of patients with melanoma, will darken standing urine from the air-exposed surface downward.

What Not To Do:

❌ Do not allow the patient to alter his urine factitiously. Have someone observe urine collection and inspect the specimen at once.

❌ Do not let a urine dipstick sit too long in the sample (allowing chemical indicators to diffuse out) or hold the dipstick vertically (allowing chemicals to drip from one pad to another and interfere with reagents).

❌ Do not be misled by dye in urine interfering with dipstick indicators. Pyridium can make a dipstick appear falsely positive for bilirubin, while contamination with hypochlorite bleach can cause a false-positive test for hemoglobin. In addition, the urobilinogen dipstick test is not adequate for diagnosing porphyria.

Discussion

Porphyrins or eosin dyes fluoresce under ultraviolet light. Eosin turns urine pink or red but fluoresces green. Automobile radiator antifreeze contains fluorescein, to help locate leaks with ultraviolet light. Because this dye is excreted in the urine, green fluorescence can be a clue to ethylene glycol poisoning.

Suggested Readings

Baran RB, Rowles B: Factors affecting coloration of urine and feces, *J Am Pharm Assoc* 13:139–142 passim, 1973.

Carpenito G, Kurtz I: Green urine in a critically ill patient, *Am J Kidney Dis* 39:E20, 2002.

Vallejo-Manzur F, Mireles-Cabodevila E, Varon J: Purple urine bag syndrome, *Am J Emerg Med* 23:521–524, 2005.

Seak CK, Lin CC, Seak CJ, Hsu TY, Chang CC: A case of black urine and dark skin—cresol poisoning, *Clin Toxicol (Phila)* 48:959–960, 2010.

Su HK, Lee FN, Chen BA, Chen CC: Purple urine bag syndrome, *Emerg Med J* 27:714, 2010.

Epididymitis

Presentation

A male child, adolescent, or adult complains of dull to moderately severe unilateral scrotal pain developing gradually over a period of hours to days and possibly radiating to the ipsilateral lower abdomen or flank. In adult or adolescent males, there may be a history of recent urinary tract infection, urethritis, prostatitis, or prostatectomy (allowing ingress of bacteria), strain from lifting a heavy object, or sexual activity with a full bladder (allowing reflux of urine). Foley catheter drainage, intermittent catheterization, and other forms of urinary tract instrumentation predispose to infection and epididymitis. Drugs, such as amiodarone, also may cause epididymitis (chemical epididymitis), which affects the head of the epididymis only. There may be fever or urinary urgency or frequency. Nausea is unusual.

The epididymis is tender, swollen, warm, and difficult to separate from the firm, nontender testicle. Over time, increasing inflammation can extend up the spermatic cord and fill the entire scrotum, making examinations more difficult, with testicular tenderness, as well as producing frank prostatitis or cystitis. The rectal examination, therefore, may reveal a very tender, boggy prostate.

What To Do:

✓ **The first priority is to rule out the possibility of testicular torsion.** Key details to elicit on initial history include the onset and duration of the symptoms, including any previous such episodes. Testis torsion typically begins suddenly over a matter of minutes with intense pain, whereas epididymitis typically has a more gradual onset over a period of hours to days with more moderate pain. Associated symptoms, such as nausea and vomiting, seem to be more specific for torsion, whereas dysuria, urgency, and frequency point to an infectious or inflammatory cause, such as epididymitis.

✓ The age of the patient may also be helpful in the diagnosis, because testis torsion has a bimodal distribution, with peak incidence in early childhood and preadolescence. The incidence of acute epididymitis increases sharply during adolescence, correlating with increased sexual activity.

✓ The scrotum and its contents should be inspected and palpated. Patients with epididymitis typically appear more comfortable than those with torsion. The position, axis, and lie of the testis should all be documented. A torsed testis is typically enlarged (because of venous congestion) and lies high within the scrotum and may have rotated transversely, giving its axis a more horizontal appearance (Figure 79-1). Conversely, the testis has a normal lie and axis in

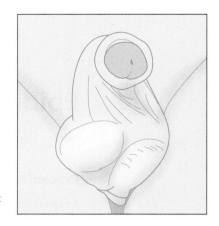

Figure 79-1 The acute scrotum with testicular torsion. Note the horizontal lie and elevated position of the right testis. (Adapted from Rosenstein D, McAninch JW: Urologic emergencies. *Med Clin North Am* 88:495-518, 2004.)

acute epididymitis. After 24 hours, the scrotal appearance of testicular torsion may be identical to that of epididymitis.

✓ Before palpation of the testicles, the cremasteric reflex should be assessed, beginning with the unaffected side. This reflex is elicited by lightly stroking the superomedial aspect of the thigh, causing brisk testicular retraction. **Absence of the cremasteric reflex is highly sensitive for testis torsion.**

✓ The testis and spermatic cord should next be gently palpated. A torsed testis is diffusely tender, whereas in acute epididymitis, the pain may be localized to the head of the epididymis and the superior pole of the testis.

✓ **Laboratory evaluation in acute scrotal pain should include obtaining a midstream urinalysis, Gram stain, and urine culture.** Presence of pyuria or bacteriuria suggests epididymitis but does not confirm the diagnosis or rule out testicular torsion.

✓ **All patients suspected of epididymitis should have an appropriate specimen analyzed for gonococcal and nongonococcal urethritis.** Culture, nucleic acid hybridization tests, and nucleic acid amplification tests (NAATs) are available. Culture and nucleic acid hybridization tests require a urethral swab, whereas NAATs can be performed on a urine sample.

✓ If the clinical diagnosis strongly suggests testis torsion, **there should be no delay in obtaining further testing. Urologic consultation should be obtained immediately to provide expeditious surgical exploration.** Cooling of the affected testicle with an ice pack while awaiting surgery may decrease the ischemic insult. **Manual reduction of a torsed testis can be attempted with or without narcotic analgesia.** Successful detorsion alleviates acute symptoms and may obviate emergent exploration; however, it is not a definitive treatment. Testes usually, but not always, torse in an inward direction. Manual detorsion should proceed with turning the testicle in an outward direction (as in "opening a book") or in the direction that the clinician would supinate his hands when approaching the patient from the feet. With successful detorsion, there will be release and elongation of the cord, followed by a marked diminution in symptoms. If pain increases or the spermatic cord shortens, stop and attempt the maneuver in the reverse direction. As mentioned, successful manual reduction is not a definitive treatment and should soon be followed by elective orchidopexy.

✓ **If the testis has a normal lie, the epididymis is tender, and there is a positive cremasteric reflex, the most likely diagnosis is epididymitis. Testicular torsion is doubtful, and no further workup is indicated.**

✓ **Patients may be treated with narcotic analgesics if needed (nonsteroidal anti-inflammatory drugs [NSAIDs] if not contraindicated) and antibiotics.**

✓ Most pediatric urologists recommend amoxicillin or trimethoprim–sulfamethoxazole for the prepubertal male with epididymitis, even though the urine is usually sterile.

✓ **The sexually active male adolescent to 35-year-old should be treated for a presumed sexually transmitted disease. Prescribe ceftriaxone (Rocephin), 250 mg IM, in the clinic or emergency department, and a prescription for doxycycline (Vibramycin), 100 mg bid for 10 days,** should eradicate *Neisseria gonorrhoeae* and *Chlamydia trachomatis.* An alternative treatment is ofloxacin (Floxin), 300 mg bid for 10 days.

✓ **In men older than 35 years of age who have suspected of epididymitis from enteric organisms, use levofloxacin (Levaquin), 500 mg qd for 10 days, or Ofloxacin, 300 mg bid for 10 days.**

✓ Epididymitis secondary to chronic use of amiodarone responds only to discontinuation or reduction of dosage.

✓ **Arrange for 2 to 3 days of strict bed rest with the scrotum elevated.** The patient should use an athletic supporter when up, soak in warm tub baths, and obtain urologic follow-up within several days. For the first 72 hours, ice compresses may be helpful.

✓ **Always warn patients or parents of the possibility of intermittent torsion and the need to return immediately if severe or worsening pain develops.**

✓ All prepubertal males with confirmed epididymitis should have close follow-up and consideration for referral to a pediatric urologist because of the high incidence of an underlying anatomic abnormality.

✓ **If there is any doubt about the diagnosis because of an atypical history and/or indistinct physical findings, perform an emergent testicular color Doppler ultrasound study. Epididymitis will show a normal or increased blood flow to the testis and epididymis, whereas torsion will show low or no flow.**

✓ **One needs to keep in mind that the testicle may spontaneously detorse before ultrasonography is performed, yielding a normal study or one with postischemic increased flow in a patient still at risk for further episodes of torsion. When the study is nondiagnostic, urologic consultation is required.** Unless you are absolutely certain that your patient does not have testicular torsion, you must insist that the urologist see him as soon as possible.

✓ If the patient is toxic and febrile, have the patient admitted, give antibiotics intravenously, and suspect testicular and/or epididymal abscess.

What Not To Do:

(X) Do not miss testicular torsion. It is far better to have the urologist explore the scrotum and find epididymitis than to delay and lose a testicle to ischemia (which can happen in only 4 to 6 hours). Half of symptomatic males describe previous similar transient episodes of scrotal pain, consistent with intermittent torsion/detorsion. When torsion is strongly suspected, do not delay the management of the case by waiting for the results of ancillary tests.

(X) Do not perform an incomplete manual detorsion of a testicle with a twist greater than or equal to 720 degrees. Partial detorsion may relieve symptoms and improve the examination but not relieve the ischemia. Continue to rotate the testicle one to three turns until the patient is pain free with a normal testicular lie.

(X) Do not overlook the testicular examination in any male with abdominal pain. In some instances of testicular torsion, a gradual onset of testicular and abdominal pain is the primary complaint.

(X) Do not rely on white blood cell counts and urinalysis to help make the diagnosis of acute epididymitis. Although a urinalysis should be performed in all patients with suspected epididymitis, most patients with epididymitis have normal urinalysis.

Discussion

Epididymitis is the most common cause of acute scrotum in adolescent boys and adults. Sexually transmitted *C. trachomatis* and *N. gonorrhoeae* are common pathogens in men younger than 35 years. In prepubertal boys and men older than 35 years of age, the disease is most frequently caused by *Escherichia coli* and *Proteus mirabilis*.

Prehn described the clinical differentiation of scrotal pain associated with epididymitis and acute torsion. Pain is relieved when the testicles are elevated over the symphysis pubis in epididymitis, but the scrotal pain associated with testicular torsion is not lessened with this maneuver **(the Prehn sign). Unfortunately, although a positive sign supports the diagnosis of epididymitis, it in no way excludes the diagnosis of torsion.**

Epididymitis first affects the tail of the epididymis and then spreads to involve its body and head. Orchitis develops in 20% to 40% of cases by direct spread of infection, thereby leading to testicular swelling and tenderness similar to that seen with testicular torsion.

Unlike testicular torsion, torsion of an appendage testis is a self-resolving, benign process and is usually much less painful than epididymitis or testicular torsion, but it is often confused with these two entities. Although appendices can be found on the testicle, epididymis,

or spermatic cord, it is usually the appendix found on the testicle (appendix testis) that is prone to torsion.

The most important aspect of the physical examination is pain and tenderness localized to the region of the appendix testis (usually superior lateral testis). Every attempt should be made to have the patient localize the pain. If only a part of the testis is tender, testicular torsion is doubtful. If the epididymis is not tender, epididymitis is also doubtful. The classic "blue dot sign" of an infarcted appendage may be seen through thin scrotal skin if there is a minimal amount of edema and erythema. These cases are managed conservatively, with attention given to pain management. The pain usually resolves in 2 to 3 days with atrophy of the appendix that may calcify. **The role of sonographic examination in torsion of the testicular appendages is to exclude testicular torsion.**

Testicular torsion causes venous engorgement that results in edema, hemorrhage, and subsequent arterial compromise, which results in testicular ischemia. The extent of testicular ischemia depends on the degree of torsion, which ranges from 180 degrees to 720 degrees or more. **Experimental studies indicate that 720-degree torsion is required to occlude the testicular artery. When torsion is 180 degrees or less, diminished flow is seen.** The testicular salvage rate depends on the

Discussion continued

degree of torsion and the duration of ischemia. A nearly 100% salvage rate exists within the first 6 hours after onset of symptoms, a 70% rate within 6 to 12 hours, and a 20% rate within 12 to 24 hours.

The role of color Doppler and power Doppler sonography in the diagnosis of acute testicular torsion is well established. Torsion may be complete, incomplete, or transient. Cases that show partial or transient torsion present a diagnostic challenge. The ability of color Doppler imaging to diagnose incomplete torsion accurately remains undetermined. The presence of a color or power Doppler signal in a patient with the clinical presentation of torsion does not exclude torsion. **Testicular imaging studies have a 10% to 15% false-negative rate.**

Because of overlapping symptoms, historical findings may be of little use in differentiating epididymitis, testicular torsion, and torsion appendix testis. Physical examination findings are helpful. Patients with testicular torsion are much more likely to have a tender testicle, an abnormal testicular lie, and/or an absent cremasteric reflex when compared with patients with epididymitis. **The presence of the cremasteric reflex is the most valuable clinical finding in ruling out testicular torsion. Color Doppler ultrasonography is extremely helpful in diagnosing the etiology of an acute scrotum, although, at times, diagnostic surgical exploration will be required for making a definitive diagnosis.**

Suggested Readings

Beni-Israel T, Goldman M, Bar Chaim S, Kozer E: Clinical predictors for testicular torsion as seen in the pediatric ED, *Am J Emerg Med* 28:786–789, 2010.

Caldamone AA, Valvo JR, Altebarmakian VK, et al: Acute scrotal swelling in children, *J Pediatr Surg* 19:581–584, 1984.

Centers for Disease Control and Prevention: Sexually transmitted diseases treatment guidelines, 2010. *MMWR Morb Mortal Wkly Rep* 59(No. RR-12):1–110, 2010. Available at http://www.cdc.gov/std/treatment/2010/STD-Treatment-2010-RR5912.pdf. Accessed July 15, 2011.

Kadish H: The tender scrotum, *Clin Pediatr Emerg Med* 3:55–61, 2002.

Kadish HA, Bolte RG: A retrospective review of pediatric patients with epididymitis, testicular torsion, and torsion of testicular appendages, *Pediatrics* 102:73–76, 1998.

Knight PJ, Vassy LE: The diagnosis and treatment of the acute scrotum in children and adolescents, *Ann Surg* 200:664–673, 1984.

Liguori G, Bucci S, Zordani A, et al: Role of US in acute scrotal pain, *World J Urol* 29:639–643, 2011.

Rosenstein D, McAninch JW: Urologic emergencies, *Med Clin North Am* 88:495–518, 2004.

Wan J, Bloom DA: Genitourinary problems in adolescent males, *Adolesc Med* 14:717–731, 2003.

Yang C Jr, Song B, Liu X, et al: Acute scrotum in children: an 18-year retrospective study, *Pediatr Emerg Care* 27:270–274, 2011.

Genital Herpes Simplex

Presentation

The patient may be distraught with severe genital pain, with subsequent outbreak of painful vesicles on the external genitalia that may ulcerate or erode. Alternatively, he may just be concerned about paresthesias and subtle genital lesions. He may want pain relief during a recurrence, or he may be suffering complications, such as superinfection or urinary retention. Often, with primary infection, there are associated systemic symptoms, such as fever, malaise, myalgias, and headache.

Instead of the classic grouped vesicles on an erythematous base, herpes in the genitals usually appears as groupings of 2- to 3-mm ulcers, representing the bases of abraded vesicles (Figures 80-1 to 80-3). Resolving lesions are also less likely to crust on the genitals. Lesions can be tender and should be examined with gloves on, because they shed infectious viral particles. Inguinal lymph nodes may be painful, are usually involved bilaterally, and are not confluent.

What To Do:

✓ If necessary for the diagnosis, perform a Tzanck preparation by scraping the base of the vesicle (this hurts!), spreading the cells on a slide, drying, and staining with Wright or Giemsa stain. The presence of multinucleate giant cells with nuclear molding provides suggestive evidence of herpes infection. This method does not distinguish herpes simplex virus (HSV) from varicella-zoster virus infection. **Confirmation of HSV infection should be obtained by viral culture of a freshly opened lesion or glycoprotein G testing of healing lesions.**

✓ Send a serologic test for syphilis, and culture any cervical or urethral discharge in search of other infections requiring different therapy.

✓ **For the immunocompetent patient, prescribe acyclovir (Zovirax), 400 mg tid for 7 to 10 days. Alternative treatment regimens include famciclovir (Famvir), 250 mg tid for 7 to 10 days, and valacyclovir (Valtrex), 1000 mg bid for 7 to 10 days.**

✓ **For recurrent infections, prescribe any of the following choices: acyclovir, 400 mg tid for 5 days, or 800 mg bid for 5 days or 800 mg tid for 2 days; famciclovir, 125 mg bid or 1000 mg bid for 1 day or 500 mg once, followed by 250 mg bid for 2 days; or valacyclovir, 1000 mg qd for 5 days or 500 mg bid for 3 days.** If there are no contraindications, prescribe adequate anti-inflammatory or narcotic analgesics for pain. Try sitz baths for comfort.

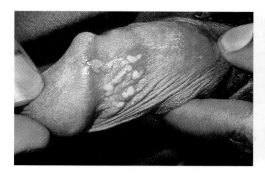

Figure 80-1 Herpes genitalis in a male patient. (Adapted from White GM, Cox NH: *Diseases of the skin*, ed 2. St Louis, 2006, Mosby.)

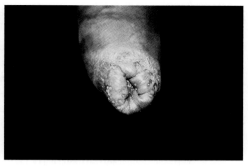

Figure 80-2 Primary genital herpes in a male patient. (Adapted from Bolognia J, Jorizzo J, Rapini R: *Dermatology,* St Louis, 2003, Mosby.)

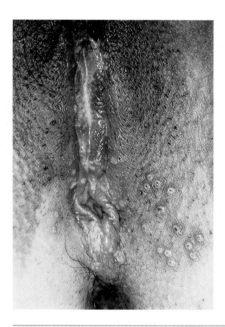

Figure 80-3 Primary genital herpes in a female patient. (Adapted from Bolognia J, Jorizzo J, Rapini R: *Dermatology,* St Louis, 2003, Mosby.)

✓ Warn the patient of the following:

○ Lesions and pain can be expected to last 2 to 3 weeks during the initial attack (usually less in recurrences).

○ Although acyclovir reduces viral shedding, the patient should assume he is contagious whenever there are open lesions (and can potentially transmit the virus at other times as well). Men with HSV infection should be counseled and advised to use barrier contraceptive methods during intercourse.

○ The patient should be careful about touching lesions and washing hands, because other skin can be inoculated.

○ Recurrences can be triggered by any sort of local or systemic stress and will not be helped by topical acyclovir.

○ **Suppressive therapy should be considered for patients who have more than six episodes per year or to reduce transmission in couples where one partner is HSV-2 positive.** This therapy can reduce the frequency of recurrences by 70% to 80%. Prescribe acyclovir, 400 mg bid; famciclovir, 250 mg bid; or valacyclovir, 500 mg to 1 g qd. Because the number of recurrences decreases over time, it is wise to discuss discontinuation of suppressive therapy annually with patients.

What Not To Do:

Ⓧ Do not confuse these lesions with the painless, raised genital ulcer of syphilis or the erosive lesions of Stevens-Johnson syndrome, which will also involve at least one other mucous membrane, such as oral mucosa, pharynx, larynx, lips, or conjunctiva.

Ⓧ Do not delay starting treatment pending culture results. Treatment is more effective if started earlier in the course of the infection.

Discussion

Infection is transmitted by direct contact with infected mucosa or secretions, and the incubation period is 2 to 20 days.

In men, lesions occur on the penile shaft, glans, and prepuce. Men who practice receptive anal intercourse can develop HSV proctitis with pain, tenesmus, and rectal discharge. In women, lesions may be seen on the external or internal genitalia.

Lesions heal over a 3-week period, although latent infection is established in dorsal root ganglia indefinitely and recurrent infection is common. Within 12 months of the initial herpes simplex virus type 2 (HSV-2) episode, 90% of patients have had at least one recurrence, and approximately 40% have had six or more recurrences. Fortunately, recurrences tend to decrease over time. These infections are generally milder in terms of duration, extent of lesions, and pain and may be associated with a prodrome of itching or burning pain.

HSV-2 is the cause of approximately 80% of genital ulcer disease in the United States. Diagnosis of herpes infection can be made largely on clinical grounds with a typical history and physical examination, although typical symptoms and signs are absent in many infected patients. Also, HSV serotyping may influence prognosis, treatment, and counseling, and, therefore, definitive diagnosis should be performed. **Confirmation of HSV infection is best performed by culture of an intact vesicle obtained within 7 days of the initial outbreak or within 2 days of subsequent infections. During active infection, culture sensitivity is approximately 95% from vesicular lesions, whereas it is only 70% from ulcerative lesions and 30% from crusted lesions.**

Type-specific serologic testing for HSV may be useful for diagnosis in patients who have symptomatic disease in the healing stages or in recurrent infections when cultures of lesions are less likely to yield the virus. The Centers for Disease Control and Prevention (CDC) recommends glycoprotein G tests, which have a high sensitivity (80% to 98%) and specificity (>96%). Those tests include POCkit HSV-2 (Diagnology, Research Triangle Park, Durham, N.C.) and HerpeSelect-1 and 2 ELISA and HerpeSelect 1 and 2 Immunoblot (Focus Technologies, Cypress, Calif.).

All the acyclic nucleoside analogue antiviral agents (acyclovir, valacyclovir, famciclovir) are equally effective in the treatment of an acute first episode of genital herpes infection and in the episodic treatment of recurrent herpes. Acyclovir is the least expensive regimen but is less convenient and must be taken more often than valacyclovir and famciclovir.

Counseling is an important part of the management of genital herpes infection. Key points to make when counseling patients should

Discussion continued

include the potential for recurrences and the effectiveness of antiviral medication for the treatment of recurrences. Because HSV infection may initially be asymptomatic, a symptomatic episode does not necessarily mean that the patient's current partner is not monogamous. Patients should be counseled regarding the possibility of transmission during periods of asymptomatic viral shedding and the need to abstain from sexual activity with uninfected partners when lesions or prodromal symptoms are present. They should also be encouraged to use condoms. They should be advised that the risk for HSV transmission to an uninfected partner is not completely eliminated by taking these precautions and that genital ulcer disease increases the risk for transmission of human immunodeficiency virus (HIV).

The diagnosis of genital herpes can be emotionally devastating to a young man or woman who is infected. Although it is advisable for patients to inform future sexual partners about their infection, it is also understandable that discussing this with a future partner can be difficult. It is very important for the physician caring for these patients to provide appropriate psychological as well as medical support.

Currently, there is no role for topical acyclovir in the treatment of genital herpes.

Suggested Readings

Benedetti J, Corel L, Ashley R: Recurrence rates in genital herpes after symptomatic first-episode infection, *Ann Intern Med* 121:847–854, 1994.

Centers for Disease Control and Prevention: Sexually transmitted diseases treatment guidelines, 2010. *MMWR Morb Mortal Wkly Rep* 59(No. RR-12):1–110, 2010. Available at http://www.cdc.gov/std/treatment/2010/STD-Treatment-2010-RR5912.pdf. Accessed July 15, 2011.

Diaz-Mitoma F, Sibbald G, Shafran SD, et al: Oral famciclovir for the recurrent suppression of recurrent genital herpes, *JAMA* 280:887–892, 1998.

Kodner C: Sexually transmitted infections in men, *Prim Care* 30:173–191, 2003.

Merin A, Pachankis JE: The psychological impact of genital herpes stigma (review), *J Health Psychol* 16:80–90, 2011. Epub July 23, 2010.

Rimsza ME: Sexually transmitted infections: new guidelines for an old problem on the college campus, *Pediatr Clin North Am* 52:217–228, 2005.

Warren T, Ebel C: Counseling the patient who has genital herpes or genital human papillomavirus infection, *Infect Dis Clin North Am* 19:459–476, 2005.

Phimosis and Paraphimosis

Presentation

Phimosis is the inability to retract the foreskin over the glans and is usually the result of a contracted preputial opening (Figure 81-1). Patients with phimosis may seek acute medical care when they develop signs and symptoms of infection, such as pain and swelling of the foreskin and a purulent discharge. Pediatric patients with acute phimosis are either fussy or complain of penile pain over hours to days. Children also may develop hematuria or urinary retention because of obstruction or dysuria. On physical examination, the physician discovers a tender foreskin that is not easily retracted.

Paraphimosis occurs when a tight foreskin cannot be re-placed into its normal position after it is retracted behind the glans. The tight ring of preputial skin (phimotic ring), which is caught behind the glans, creates a venous and lymphatic tourniquet that leads to edematous swelling of the foreskin and glans. It usually presents as a swollen tender penis with a large ventral penile-skin bulge and multiple folds just under the glans (Figures 81-2 and 81-3).

What To Do:

✓ **When either of these conditions becomes painful,** provide adequate analgesia with oral or parenteral medication. **A penile nerve block may be required.** Using a 30-g needle, inject 1% lidocaine (Xylocaine) approximately 1 cm distal to the base of the penis, where it exits beneath the pubic arch at the 10-o'clock and 2-o'clock positions of the dorsum of the penis. Use caution not to inject intravascularly. If this does not provide adequate anesthesia, a ring block can be performed around the entire circumference of the base of the penis.

✓ **For paraphimosis, squeeze the glans firmly for at least 10 minutes to reduce the edematous swelling.** Wrap the shaft and swollen glans with a gauze pad followed by a 2-inch elastic bandage to produce constant, gentle compression. **After 10 to 15 minutes, remove the bandage, push the glans proximally, and slide the prepuce back over the glans** (Figure 81-4). An alternative approach for reducing the swelling is to apply an ice-filled surgical glove for 5 minutes.

✓ **If manual reduction fails and the penis does not regain its normal uncircumcised appearance, anesthetize the dorsal foreskin and carefully grasp the foreskin with nonserrated clamps and pull it over the glans penis. If this is unsuccessful, crush the dorsal foreskin with a straight hemostat along the midline and then make a linear incision through this crushed skin track. This incision will relieve the constricting band.** The foreskin is then repositioned over the glans and, when possible, sutured in place.

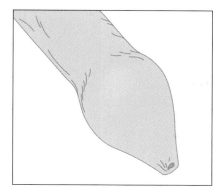

Figure 81-1 Phimosis.

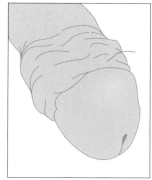

Figure 81-2 Paraphimosis.

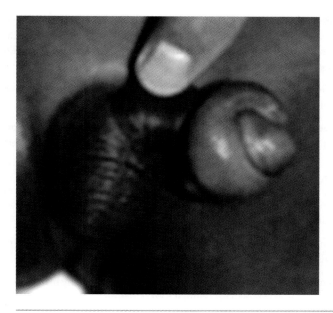

Figure 81-3 Paraphimosis. (Adapted from McGrath N, Howell JM, Davis JE: Pediatric genitourinary emergencies. *Emerg Med Clin North Am* 29:655-666, 2011.)

✅ **If the phimosis patient has secondary urinary obstruction, catheterize the urethra with a small-gauge catheter. If you cannot find the urethral meatus, try using a small nasal speculum or hemostat to widen the opening or anesthetize the dorsal foreskin, and carefully incise the constricting tissue with a vertical incision (dorsal slit) to allow retraction.**

✅ **Treating phimosis usually involves the management of acute infection.** Frequent hot compresses or soaks are needed, along with antibiotics. Topical antibiotics, such as mupirocin (Bactroban), may be adequate when poor hygiene leads to infection in the pediatric patient. Sexually transmitted diseases should be suspected and treated appropriately in adolescents and adults (see Chapter 83). Candidal infections, with their typical white cheesy exudate, are often associated with diabetes mellitus and can be treated with a single dose of fluconazole (Diflucan), 200 mg PO.

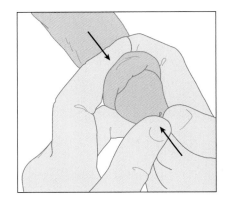

Figure 81-4 Manual reduction of paraphimosis by counter pressure between thumbs and fingers.

✓ **When infection is not a problem, phimosis can be successfully treated with a steroid cream** (0.1% triamcinolone or 0.6% betamethasone), **4 times daily, with a gentle stretch on the foreskin for 2 to 6 weeks. After the phimosis resolves, the foreskin should be retracted daily to prevent recurrence.**

✓ Instruct parents in the technique and importance of proper cleaning of their son's prepuce. Have them place him in a tub of warm water to alleviate dysuria.

✓ **In both paraphimosis and phimosis, follow-up care should be provided. When swelling and inflammation subside, circumcision should be considered.**

What Not To Do:

✗ Do not confuse paraphimosis with, or overlook, a circumferential foreign body (such as a hair or rubber band).

✗ Do not attempt forced retraction when treating phimosis. Forceful retraction causes future adhesions and strictures.

✗ Do not obtain unnecessary studies. Diagnosis is made by history and physical examination, although a radiograph may be useful if a constricting foreign body is suspected.

Discussion

Poor hygiene and chronic inflammation are the usual causes of stenosing fibrosis of the preputial opening. It can be normal for boys up to 5 years of age not to be able to retract the foreskin completely. Repeated inflammation, even through tension on a minimally restrictive aperture from normal erections, may exacerbate the fibrosis and lead to phimosis. Vitamin E cream and topical steroid ointments may help soften a phimotic ring. **When phimosis results in acute urinary retention,** the tip of a hemostat can be inserted into the scarred end of the foreskin and gently opened, allowing the patient to void satisfactorily until urologic consultation can be obtained.

In the case of neglected paraphimosis, arterial occlusion may supervene, and ischemia, skin necrosis, and, eventually, gangrene of the glans develop. One common iatrogenic cause of paraphimosis is negligence in reducing the foreskin after retracting it to clean the glans and insert a Foley catheter.

Suggested Readings

Mackway-Jones K, Teece S: Best evidence topic reports: ice, pins, or sugar to reduce paraphimosis, *Emerg Med J* 21:77–78, 2004.

McGrath N, Howell JM, Davis JE: Pediatric genitourinary emergencies, *Emerg Med Clin North Am* 29:655–666, 2011.

Tanaka S, Brock JW 3rd: Pediatric urologic conditions, including urinary infections, *Med Clin North Am* 95:1–13, 2011.

Wan J, Bloom DA: Genitourinary problems in adolescent males, *Adolesc Med* 14:717–731, viii, 2003.

Prostatitis, Acute Bacterial

Presentation

A man complains of acute onset of malaise, fever, chills, and perineal or low back pain. He also may have dysuria, urinary urgency and frequency, and signs of obstruction to urinary flow, ranging from a weak stream to urinary retention. On gentle examination, the prostate is swollen, hot, and exquisitely tender. The infection may spread from or into the contiguous urogenital tract (epididymis, bladder, urethra) or the bloodstream.

What To Do:

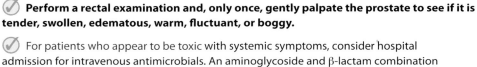 **Perform a rectal examination and, only once, gently palpate the prostate to see if it is tender, swollen, edematous, warm, fluctuant, or boggy.**

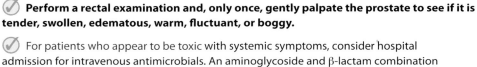 For patients who appear to be toxic with systemic symptoms, consider hospital admission for intravenous antimicrobials. An aminoglycoside and β-lactam combination or a fluoroquinolone may be administered, along with intravenous hydration. Gentamicin (Garamycin), 1 to 1.5 mg/kg IV tid, plus ampicillin (generic), 500 mg IV qid, can be given. Alternatively, give levofloxacin (Levaquin), 750 mg IV qd, or ciprofloxacin, 400 mg IV bid.

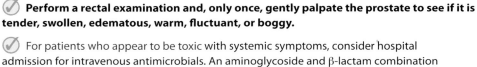 **Evaluate and treat for possible associated urinary retention** (see Chapter 84). In severe cases, a suprapubic catheter may be preferable to a Foley catheter for bladder decompression and urinary drainage, because it avoids trauma to the prostate with resulting pain and hematogenous spread of infection.

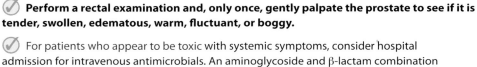 **Culture the urine** to help identify the organism responsible. (This will usually identify the organism involved in acute bacterial prostatitis.) **Test for sexually transmitted diseases,** such as gonorrhea or chlamydia, with a nucleic acid amplification test.

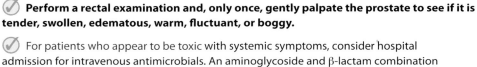 **For the nontoxic patient, empiric therapy should be started. Typical regimens include ciprofloxacin 500 mg PO bid or levofloxacin 500 mg PO qd for 4 to 6 weeks. Alternatively, a less expensive regimen is trimethoprim-sulfamethoxazole PO bid for 4 to 6 weeks. The long duration of treatment is necessary to penetrate deep prostatic tissues.**

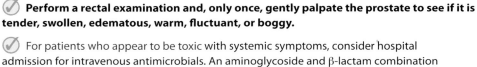 For pain and fever, prescribe nonsteroidal anti-inflammatory drugs (NSAIDs) if there are no contraindications. If the patient needs narcotics, add stool softeners to prevent constipation.

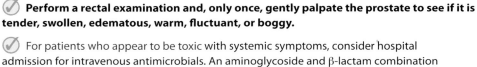 **Arrange for urologic follow-up.**

What Not To Do:

(X) Do not massage or repeatedly palpate the prostate. Rough treatment is unlikely to help drain the infection or produce the responsible organism in the urine but is likely to extend or worsen a bacterial prostatitis or to precipitate bacteremia, urosepsis, or septic shock.

Discussion

Blood in the ejaculate may be a sign of inflammation in the prostate and epididymis or, especially in younger males, may simply be a self-limiting sequela of vigorous sexual activity.

For the treatment of bacterial prostatitis, only trimethoprim and the fluoroquinolones possess both the appropriate bactericidal activity and the ability to diffuse into the prostate. Levofloxacin shows particularly good penetration into prostatic tissue.

The diagnosis of acute prostatitis largely relies on clinical signs and symptoms and a limited number of laboratory findings. Prostate-specific antigen (PSA) levels may be elevated in both acute and chronic bacterial prostatitis. Men who present with an elevated PSA level and findings of prostatitis should be given a course of antibiotics followed by a repeat PSA measurement before any biopsy is performed.

Suggested Readings

David RD, DeBlieux PMC, Press R: Rational antibiotic treatment of outpatient genitourinary infections in a changing environment, *Am J Med* 118(Suppl 7A):7S–13S, 2005.

Hua VN, Schaeffer AJ: Acute and chronic prostatitis, *Med Clin North Am* 88:483–494, 2004.

Krieger JN: Prostatitis revisited: new definitions, new approaches, *Infect Dis Clin North Am* 17:395–409, 2003.

Ramakrishnan K, Salinas RC: Prostatitis: acute and chronic (review), *Prim Care* 37:547–563, viii-ix, 2010.

Sharp VJ, Takacs EB, Powell CR: Prostatitis: diagnosis and treatment (review), *Am Fam Physician* 82:397–406, 2010.

Urethritis

(Drip, Clap)

Presentation

A man complains of dysuria, a burning discomfort along the urethra, pruritus of the urethral meatus, and/or a urethral discharge. A copious, thick yellow-green discharge that stains underwear is characteristic of gonorrhea, whereas a thinner mucopurulent or white scant discharge with milder symptoms is characteristic of *Chlamydia*. These symptoms may be transient.

Urethritis in a woman may be asymptomatic or indistinguishable from cystitis or vaginitis. It may manifest as urinary tract infection (UTI) symptoms with a low concentration of bacteria on urine culture or tenderness localized to the distal periurethral area of the anterior vaginal wall. Female patients may not be able to distinguish urethral discharge from vaginal discharge. In addition to increased vaginal discharge, women who develop cervicitis may have intermenstrual bleeding, especially postcoital spotting or dyspareunia and cervical friability.

What To Do:

✓ Obtain a sexual history that includes number of contacts, gender of contacts, anal/oral practices, and symptoms or illnesses in partners. Determine the color, consistency, and quantity of any discharge as well as any accompanying symptoms, such as genital or abdominal discomfort and dysuria.

✓ Examine the entire genital area for lesions, and check undergarments for discharge staining. Palpate testes and epididymides for any mass or tenderness, or, in the case of a female patient, perform a complete pelvic examination.

✓ Have the male patient milk the ventral surface of his penis to produce any discharge at the urethral meatus. (If discharge is scant, this should be attempted 1 to 2 hours after last voiding.)

✓ **In men, obtain a Gram stain of any urethral discharge, looking for gram-negative diplococci inside white cells, which indicate gonococcal infection. (Their absence does not rule out the possibility.) Urethritis in men is confirmed by any of the following:**

○ The presence of mucopurulent or purulent discharge

○ Five or more white blood cells (WBCs) per oil-immersion field on a Gram stain of urethral secretions

○ Ten or more WBCs per high-power field on microscopic examination of first-void urine

○ Positive leukocyte esterase test on first-void urine

✓ **In female patients, order a urine or blood test to rule out pregnancy.**

✅ **Examine the urine sediment for swimming protozoa, implying infection with** *Trichomonas vaginalis,* **best treated with metronidazole (Flagyl), 2 g PO once or 500 mg bid 7 days.**

✅ **Endocervical swabs from women and urethral swabs or urine specimens from men can be used to detect** *Chlamydia trachomatis* **and** *Neisseria gonorrhoeae* **by using nucleic acid amplification tests (NAATs).** NAATs do not require viable organisms, they are substantially more sensitive than previous tests, and the same specimen can be used to test for both organisms. **When a NAAT is not available or not economical, nucleic acid hybridization assays can be used to detect** *C. trachomatis* **or** *N. gonorrhoeae.* The Gen-Probe PACE 2 (Gen-Probe, San Diego, Calif.) and the Digene Hybrid Capture II (Gen-Probe) assays can detect both organisms in a single specimen. These tests are less sensitive than NAATs.

✅ **Cultures can be performed when transport and storage conditions are conducive to maintaining the viability of** *N. gonorrhoeae* **and** *C. trachomatis,* **especially when an isolate is needed (e.g., sexual abuse or treatment failure) and for monitoring of antimicrobial resistance.** Cultures for *N. gonorrhoeae* have a high sensitivity and specificity and low cost, whereas *C. trachomatis* cell cultures have a relatively low sensitivity at a relatively high cost.

✅ **Order a serologic test for established syphilis.** Further antibiotic treatment is required if the rapid plasma reagin (RPR) or Venereal Disease Research Laboratory (VDRL) test is positive.

✅ **Empirical treatment must be considered in symptomatic patients whose behavior puts them at risk for sexually transmitted infections, those who may be lost to follow-up, and those who have a history of recent exposure to an infected partner, regardless of their symptoms.** Dual treatment of *C. trachomatis* and *N. gonorrhoeae* should be provided when an empirical treatment is instituted.

✅ **Dual treatment is indicated** for the initial management of urethritis or cervicitis unless a sensitive laboratory technology is used to rule out *C. trachomatis* and/or *N. gonorrhoeae.*

✅ **To treat** *N. gonorrhea,* **give ceftriaxone (Rocephin), 250 mg IM × 1, or cefixime (Suprax), 400 mg PO × 1, or cefpodoxime (Vantin), 400 mg PO × 1. To treat** *C. trachomatis,* **give azithromycin (Zithromax), 1 g PO × 1 or doxycycline (Doryx), 100 mg PO bid × 7 days. (Azithromycin provides prophylaxis for syphilis.)** Alternate regimens include levofloxacin, 500 mg PO daily × 7 days, or ofloxacin, 300 mg PO bid × 7 days, or erythromycin base (ERYC), 500 mg PO qid × 7 days, or erythromycin ethylsuccinate (EES), 800 mg PO qid × 7 days.

✅ To treat recurrent and persistent urethritis, give metronidazole (Flagyl), 2 g PO × 1, or tinidazole 2 g PO × 1, plus azithromycin, 1 g PO × 1. **Patients should be instructed to refrain from sexual intercourse until 7 days after therapy is completed.**

✅ **Treat sexual partners** of patients known or suspected to have a sexually transmitted infection with the same antibiotic regimen. (Cultures may be omitted.) These patients should refer all sexual partners within the preceding 60 days for evaluation and treatment; a specific diagnosis may facilitate partner referral. Some physicians feel comfortable providing a prescription for partner therapy, recognizing the limitations on partner referral.

✅ Federal and state reporting regulations should be followed, with subsequent tracking of sexual contacts by state infection control boards.

Patients should be instructed to return if symptoms persist or recur.

 Test-of-cure is not recommended as a routine procedure after therapy for *C. trachomatis* or *N. gonorrhoeae* infection with first-line Centers for Disease Control and Prevention (CDC)– recommended treatment regimens, except after *C. trachomatis* therapy during pregnancy.

 Instruct the patient on the correct use of the condom to prevent reinfection.

What Not To Do:

 Do not perform gram-stain testing for *N. gonorrhoeae* infection among women. The sensitivity of endocervical specimens is lower than that of urethral specimens from men with symptomatic gonorrhea, and adequate specificity requires a skilled microscopist.

 Do not send off a serologic test for syphilis without following up on the results.

Discussion

Common causative organisms for urethritis and cervicitis are *N. gonorrhoeae* and *C. trachomatis*. *Ureaplasma urealyticum*, *Mycoplasma hominis*, *M. genitalium*, and *Trichomonas vaginalis* also are implicated in these clinical conditions. Although they are easily eradicated if treated early, some of these infections have been linked to serious reproductive health consequences; more systemic effects, such as disseminated gonococcal infections and Reiter syndrome; and facilitation of human immunodeficiency virus (HIV) transmission.

N. gonorrhoeae, a gram-negative diplococcus, is a major cause of pelvic inflammatory disease (PID), ectopic pregnancy, and infertility. *C. trachomatis,* an obligate intracellular bacterium, is the most common sexually transmitted bacterial pathogen in the United States and worldwide and is a leading cause of PID. The prevalence of both infections is higher among ethnic minorities and the poor. Age-specific rates are highest among girls and women 15 to 24 years of age and men 20 to 24 years of age. Both *Ureaplasma* and *Mycoplasma* have been isolated in cases of PID and nongonococcal urethritis (NGU). Recent studies have reported serious consequences of trichomoniasis, including increased perinatal mortality and increased HIV transmission. **There is increasing evidence that *T. vaginalis* is a common cause of NGU in men.**

Infections at any one site of the genitourinary tract produce poorly localizing symptoms, particularly in women, which may result in delayed diagnosis or misdiagnosis. Failure to recognize the causal relationship between symptoms of dysuria and sexually transmitted infections by patients and clinicians often results in failure to seek timely diagnosis and treatment. Longer duration and more gradual onset of dysuria may suggest *C. trachomatis* infection, whereas sudden onset of symptoms and hematuria suggests bacterial infection.

Disseminated gonorrhea with arthritis and dermatitis presents with fever, chills, and migratory polyarticular arthritis; a characteristic petechial necrotic pustular or tender papular rash of the distal extremities; and tenosynovitis of extensor tendons of the hands, wrists, or ankle tendons. This represents a more serious infection requiring a more comprehensive evaluation, extended parenteral antibiotic therapy, and hospitalization for all but the mildest cases.

Reiter syndrome is a triad of arthritis, urethritis, and conjunctivitis with associated skin lesions. The pathogenesis is unclear, but *C. trachomatis* has been implicated strongly along with other bacterial organisms. Treatment of Reiter syndrome consists of antimicrobial therapy against *Chlamydia*, NSAIDs, steroid injections of the affected joints, and topical steroids for uveitis.

The Centers for Disease Control and Prevention update treatment recommendations every few years, incorporating changes in antibiotics and sensitivity.

Suggested Readings

Augenbraun M, Bachmann L, Wallace T, et al: Compliance with doxycycline therapy in sexually transmitted disease clinics, *Sex Transm Dis* 25:1–4, 1998.

Bremnor JD, Sadovsky R: Evaluation of dysuria in adults, *Am Fam Physician* 65:1589–1596, 2002.

Brill JR: Diagnosis and treatment of urethritis in men, *Am Fam Physician* 81:873–878, 2010.

Centers for Disease Control and Prevention: Sexually transmittal diseases (STDs): 2010 STD treatment guidelines. Available at http://www.cdc.gov/std/treatment/2010/. Accessed July 15, 2011.

Chen JC: Update on emerging infections: news from the Centers for Disease Control and Prevention, *MMWR Morb Mortal Wkly* 53:197–198, 2004.

Kodner C: Sexually transmitted infections in men, *Prim Care* 30:173–191, 2003.

Simpson T, Oh MK: Urethritis and cervicitis in adolescents, *Adolesc Med Clin* 15:253–271, 2004.

Stamm WE, Hicks CB, Martin DH, et al: Azithromycin for empirical treatment of the nongonococcal urethritis syndrome in men, *J Am Med Assoc* 274:545–549, 1995.

Taylor BD, Haggerty CL: Management of *Chlamydia trachomatis* genital tract infection: screening and treatment challenges, *Infect Drug Resist* 4:19–29, 2011.

Urinary Retention, Acute

Presentation

The patient, usually male, may complain of increasing dull, low-abdominal discomfort or pain and the urge to urinate, without having been able to urinate for many hours. Urinary hesitancy, sensation of incomplete voiding, an interrupted or decreased urinary stream, and straining to void are other typical symptoms of obstruction. Flank pain may accompany obstruction that leads to hydroureter and hydronephrosis.

Elderly and debilitated patients may be asymptomatic or have vague discomfort with urinary frequency but small volumes, overflow, or stress incontinence.

A firm, distended bladder can be palpated between the symphysis pubis and umbilicus. Rectal examination may reveal an enlarged or tender prostate or suspected tumor, although a prostate that is of normal size and consistency by palpation can still be the cause of urethral obstruction.

What To Do:

✅ **In a male patient, distend the urethra with lidocaine jelly 2% in a catheter-tipped syringe (Uroject, Uro-Jet) and try a 16-, 18-, or 20-Fr Foley catheter. When there is minimal distress, leave the lidocaine jelly in place 15 to 20 minutes to obtain good mucosal anesthesia before inserting the catheter** (Figure 84-1).

✅ **When the patient is very uncomfortable,** delay only long enough to provide good aseptic technique, **pass a Foley catheter into the bladder, and collect the urine in a closed collecting system bag.** Reassuring the patient and having him breathe through his mouth may help relax the external sphincter of the bladder and facilitate the passage of the catheter.

✅ **If the problem is negotiating the curve around a large prostate, use a Coudé catheter.**

✅ If the bladder still cannot drain, obtain urologic consultation for instrumentation with stylets, sounds, filiforms, and followers, or consider a percutaneous suprapubic catheterization (but only after it is confirmed that the bladder is distended).

✅ **Check renal and urinary function with urinalysis, a urine culture, and serum blood urea nitrogen (BUN) and creatinine determinations.**

✅ Examine the patient to ascertain the cause of the obstruction. Urinalysis may show hematuria, crystalluria, and/or an elevated pH (>7.5), suggesting the presence of renal calculi. The presence of pyuria, bacteriuria, elevated pH, and/or nitrites suggests infection.

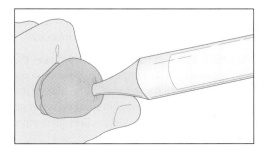

Figure 84-1 Lidocaine jelly administrator.

✓ **Ultrasonography** is useful in determining whether proximal distention is present in the urinary tract. It can also confirm suspected bladder distention, although this can usually be determined clinically from the physical examination, followed by measurement of the urine flow when a bladder catheter is placed.

✓ If there is an infection of the bladder, give antibiotics (see Chapter 85).

✓ **If the volume drained is modest (0.5 to 1.5 L) and the patient is stable and ambulatory, attach the Foley catheter to a leg bag and discharge the patient for urologic follow-up (and probably catheter removal) the next day.**

✓ If the volume drained is small (100 to 200 mL), remove the catheter and search for alternate causes of the abdominal mass and urinary urgency.

✓ **When prostatic enlargement (which is a common cause of bladder outlet obstruction in older men) is suspected, alpha-blocker agents may be helpful, especially in those patients who want to be sent home with a trial without an indwelling urinary catheter. Prescribe alfuzosin (Uroxatral), 10 mg qd taken with food; doxazosin (Cardura XL), 4 mg qd at breakfast; or tamsulosin (Flomax), 0.4 mg qd 30 minutes after eating. These drugs can cause symptomatic hypotension, particularly in patients with ventricular hypertrophy. Giving the first dose at bedtime may help avoid syncope.**

✓ Warn the patient to return if obstructive symptoms recur, and provide early urologic follow-up, ideally within the next 24 to 48 hours.

What Not To Do:

✗ Do not use stylets or sounds unless you have experience instrumenting the urethra; these devices can cause considerable trauma.

✗ Do not remove the catheter right away if the bladder was significantly distended. Bladder tone will take several hours to return, and the bladder may become distended again.

✗ Do not clamp the catheter to slow decompression of the bladder, even if the volume drained is more than 2 L.

✗ Do not use bethanechol (Urecholine) unless it is clear that there is no obstruction, inadequate (parasympathetic) bladder tone is the only cause of the distention, and there is no possibility of gastrointestinal disease.

Ⓧ Do not perform an intravenous pyelogram in patients with compromised renal function. This can cause further renal compromise because of nephrotoxicity.

Ⓧ Do not routinely prescribe prophylactic antibiotics. They lower the incidence of bacteriuria at the expense of selecting out more virulent organisms. Unless the patient is at high risk for the complications of catheter-associated bacteriuria (i.e., renal transplant and granulopenic patients), antibiotic prophylaxis for short-term catheterization is not warranted. A small percentage of low-risk patients with bacteriuria will progress to symptomatic urinary tract infection. However, most will clear spontaneously.

Discussion

Urinary retention is characterized by a urine residual greater than 200 mL after attempted voiding.

Urinary retention may be caused by stones lodged in the urethra or urethral strictures (often from gonorrhea); foreign bodies, including blocked urinary catheters; prostatitis, prostatic carcinoma, or benign prostatic hypertrophy; blood clot, following urologic procedures; and tumor in the bladder.

Any drug with anticholinergic effects or α-adrenergic effects, such as antihistamines, ephedrine sulfate, and phenylpropanolamine, can precipitate urinary retention. Morphine and other narcotics inhibit the voiding reflex and increase the muscle tone of the external sphincter, both of which can contribute to urinary retention. Other drugs that can cause urinary retention are tricyclic antidepressants, detrusor relaxants (e.g., oxybutynin [Ditropan]), and calcium channel blockers.

Neurologic causes include cord lesions, diabetic neuropathy, Parkinson disease, stroke, malignancy that compresses the spinal cord, and multiple sclerosis. Patients with genital herpes or herpes zoster may develop urinary retention from nerve involvement.

Urinary retention has also been reported following vigorous anal intercourse. In addition, anything that causes compression from outside the urinary tract can cause obstruction. Abdominal aneurysms, tumors (primary or metastatic, benign or malignant), pregnancy, ovarian abscess, intra-abdominal abscess (e.g., ruptured appendiceal abscess), and large fecal impactions are some examples of extrinsic lesions that can cause obstruction. The urethral catheterization outlined is the appropriate initial treatment for all these conditions.

Sometimes hematuria develops midway through bladder decompression, probably representing loss of tamponade of vessels that were injured as the bladder distended. This should be watched until the bleeding stops (usually spontaneously) to be sure that there is no great blood loss, no other urologic disease responsible, and no clot obstruction.

Postobstructive diuresis is common, possibly because of increased synthesis of renal prostaglandins. In severe cases, this can lead to electrolyte imbalances and even dehydration. In these severe cases, fluid and electrolyte replacement may be indicated but should be undertaken carefully, because inappropriate replacement can prolong the diuresis.

Suggested Readings

Harmanli OH, Okafor O, Ayaz R, Knee A: Lidocaine jelly and plain aqueous gel for urethral straight catheterization and the Q-tip test: a randomized controlled trial, *Obstet Gynecol* 114:547–550, 2009.

Lucas MG, Stephenson TP, Nargund V: Tamsulosin in the management of patients in acute urinary retention from benign prostatic hyperplasia, *Br J Urol* 95:354–357, 2005.

McNeill SA, Hargreave TB: Members of the Alfaur Study Group: Alfuzosin once daily facilitates return to voiding in patients with acute urinary retention, *J Urol* 171:2316–2320, 2004.

Siderias J, Guadio F, Singer AJ, et al: Comparison of topical anesthetics and lubricants prior to urethral catheterization in males, *Acad Emerg Med* 11:703–706, 2004.

Urinary Tract Infection, Lower (Cystitis), Uncomplicated

Presentation

The patient (usually female) complains of urinary frequency and urgency, internal dysuria, and suprapubic pain or discomfort. The onset of symptoms is generally abrupt, often causing her to seek care within 24 hours. There may have been some antecedent trauma (sexual intercourse) to inoculate the bladder, and there may be blood in the urine (hemorrhagic cystitis). Usually, there is no labial irritation, external dysuria, or vaginal discharge (which would suggest vaginitis or cervicitis), and no fever, chills, nausea, flank pain, or costovertebral angle tenderness (which would suggest an upper urinary tract infection or pyelonephritis).

What To Do:

✅ **Examine a clean-catch urine specimen.** Instruct the patient to wipe the introitus from front to back and begin urinating into the toilet before filling the sample cup. In women of childbearing age, send a urine pregnancy test—this will influence choice of antibiotic and follow-up. Use a dipstick test for leukocyte esterase, send for a urinalysis, or Gram stain a sample of urine. Epithelial cells on the microscopic examination are evidence of contamination from the vagina. The presence of any white blood cells (WBCs) or bacteria in a clean sample confirms the infection. A positive nitrite on dipstick is helpful, but a negative test does not rule out infection, because many bacteria do not produce nitrites. Menses or vaginal discharge makes a clean catch difficult. One technique is to insert a tampon before giving the sample. A better technique is urinary catheterization.

✅ **If the clinical picture is clearly of an uncomplicated lower urinary tract infection (UTI) in a nonpregnant patient and local *Escherichia coli* resistance to trimethoprim-sulfamethoxazole (TMP/SMX) is less than 20%, give trimethoprim, 160 mg, plus sulfamethoxazole, 800 mg (Bactrim DS or Septra DS), one tablet PO bid for 3 days. Otherwise, give fosfomycin (Monurol), 3 g PO × 1, or a 3-day regimen of a quinolone, such as ciprofloxacin (Cipro), 500 mg PO bid, or Cipro XR, 500 mg qd; levofloxacin (Levaquin), 250 mg PO qd; or gatifloxacin (Tequin), 200 to 400 mg PO qd, or nitrofurantoin extended release (Macrobid), 100 mg PO bid × 7 days.** Single-dose treatment with two TMP/SMX DS tablets is also effective in the young healthy female but is associated with a higher early recurrence rate. **In pregnancy, give a 7-day course of nitrofurantoin (Macrodantin), 100 mg PO qid, or nitrofurantoin extended release (Macrobid), 100 mg PO bid.** Cephalosporins (i.e., cephalexin [Keflex], 250 to 500 mg qid × 7 days) are alternatives in pregnancy, but not quinolones (or sulfas 2 weeks before delivery because of the potential increased risk for kernicterus). Trimethoprim is contraindicated during the first trimester because of its antifolate properties.

✓ Instruct the patient to drink plenty of liquids (such as cranberry juice) and remain hydrated, but there is no need to drink excessively.

✓ **If the dysuria is severe, also prescribe phenazopyridine (Pyridium), 200 mg tid for 2 days only, to act as a surface anesthetic in the bladder.** Warn the patient that it will stain her urine (and perhaps clothes) orange.

✓ **Extend antimicrobial therapy to 7 days and obtain cultures when treating a patient who is unreliable, diabetic, symptomatic more than 5 days, older than 50 years of age, or younger than 16 years of age. Also, extend treatment and obtain cultures for all male patients** and for those with an indwelling urinary catheter, renal disease, obstructive urinary tract lesions, recurrent infection, or other significant medical problems. It should be noted that one small double-blind Canadian study of 183 immunocompetent, nondiabetic women aged 65 and older with culture-documented uncomplicated UTI had similarly effective treatment with a 3-day course of ciprofloxacin as they did with a 7-day course (with fewer antibiotic-related side effects).

✓ **If there are no bacteria or few WBCs, no hematuria or suprapubic pain, gradual onset over 7 to 10 days, and a new sexual partner, with a history of vaginal discharge and/or vaginal irritation, the dysuria may be caused by a chlamydial or ureaplasmal urethritis** (see Chapter 83). Perform a pelvic examination and obtain samples for nucleic acid amplification testing, culture, and microscopic examination. Ask the patient about the use of spermicides or douches, which may irritate the periurethral tissue and cause dysuria. Adolescent females who are screened for both *Chlamydia trachomatis* and urinary tract infection have high rates of concurrent disease. Urinary or vaginal symptoms do not differentiate well between these infections. Clinical diagnosis is imprecise, suggesting that **sexually active adolescent females with vaginal or urinary symptoms should be tested for both *C. trachomatis* and UTI.**

✓ **When there is a history of lower UTI symptoms with negative urinalysis, cultures, and workups for sexually transmitted diseases, consider a paraurethral gland infection (sometimes referred to as "female prostatitis")** as the cause of this female urethral syndrome. This is usually associated with tenderness at either side of the distal two thirds of the urethra, adjacent to the urethral meatus (Skene paraurethral glands). During the pelvic examination, press firmly against the posterior and the lateral vaginal walls as a "control" maneuver to demonstrate the lack of pain with firm palpation. Then, bend your examining index finger forward to compress the paraurethral tissue firmly against the flat backside of the pubic bone. An affected patient will have an abrupt pain response, whereas an unaffected patient may only respond with the sensation of having to void. Treat presumed *Chlamydia* with doxycycline, 100 mg bid for an extended 2 to 4 weeks. After an initial treatment failure, older and younger women should be given a quinolone for at least 1 month. Hot sitz baths may provide comfort.

✓ **If there is external dysuria, vaginal discharge, odor, itching, and no frequency or urgency, evaluate for vaginitis** (see Chapter 83) **with a pelvic examination.**

✓ **Arrange for follow-up in 2 days if the symptoms have not completely resolved.** If necessary, urine culture and a longer course of antibiotics can be undertaken.

✓ **Pediatric UTIs** differ from adult UTIs. Pediatric UTIs may indicate a significant genitourinary anomaly; their accurate diagnosis requires invasive collection methods, such as suprapubic aspiration or transurethral catheterization in infants and young children; and accurate diagnosis requires a urine culture rather than relying solely on a simple urinalysis. UTIs in children, especially young children, can manifest as nonspecific symptoms (therefore you must maintain a high index of suspicion). Children, especially those younger than 5 years of age, have increased risk for renal scarring after a single UTI. (Therefore it is important to diagnose quickly and to initiate appropriate broad-spectrum antibiotic therapy.)

✔ Although a midstream, clean-catch void can be a reliable method of urine collection in adults and older children, it is usually impossible for preschool children. For older children, patients and parents should be instructed to cleanse the periurethral area well, spread labia or partially retract the foreskin, and allow the initial urine to be wasted before beginning collection in a sterile container. Having girls sit backward on the toilet may facilitate this.

✔ In small children, transurethral bladder catheterization is the preferred method for obtaining urine by many practitioners and parents.

✔ **The clues to the diagnosis of UTI in children before culture results include urine nitrite, leukocyte esterase, bacteria, or white blood cells. Bacteria on Gram stain are another specific indicator of UTI. The combination of leukocyte esterase, nitrite, and bacteria on microscopy is a sensitive test (sensitivity 99.8%, specificity 70%). The absence of any of these findings on urinalysis and microscopic examination nearly (but not completely) eliminates the diagnosis of UTI.** More than 5 to 10 WBCs per high-powered field on catheter specimen in the presence of a suggestive clinical picture should be presumed to represent a true UTI until proven otherwise by a negative culture.

✔ **For uncomplicated infections in the nontoxic child, prescribe 2 mg of TMP/10 mg of SMX/kg PO qd × 7 days (where local resistance of uropathogens to TMP/SMX is less than 20%); cefixime (Suprax), 8 mg/kg/day divided q12h PO × 7 days; cefprozil (Cefzil), 15 to 30 mg/kg/day divided q12h PO × 7 days; cephalexin (generic), 25 to 100 mg/kg/day divided qid PO × 7 days; or, if the patient is vomiting, ceftriaxone (Rocephin), 50 to 75 mg/kg qd IV or IM.** Because it is difficult to rule out pyelonephritis in febrile infants with UTI, a full 14-day course of antibiotics is indicated.

✔ Arrange follow-up for all children, because a UTI may be the first evidence of underlying urinary tract disease.

What Not To Do:

✘ Do not forget to check for pregnancy.

✘ Do not undertake expensive urine cultures for every lower UTI of recent onset in nonpregnant, normal, healthy women with no history of recent UTI or antibiotic use.

✘ Do not use the single-dose or 3-day regimens for a possible upper UTI or pyelonephritis (see Chapter 86).

✘ Do not rely on gross inspection of the urine sample. Cloudiness is usually caused by crystals, and odors can result from diet or medication.

✘ Do not request a follow-up visit or culture after therapy unless symptoms persist or recur.

Discussion

Lower UTI or cystitis is a superficial bacterial infection of the bladder or urethra. Most of these infections involve *Escherichia coli, Staphylococcus saprophyticus,* or enterococci.

The urine dipstick is a reasonable screening measure that can direct therapy if results are positive. Under the microscope in a clean sediment (free of epithelial cells), one WBC per 400 field suggests significant pyuria, although clinicians accustomed to imperfect samples usually set a threshold of 3 to 5 WBCs per field. In addition, *Trichomonas* organisms may be appreciated swimming in the urinary sediment, indicating a different cause for urinary symptoms or associated vaginitis.

In a straightforward lower UTI, urine culture may be reserved for cases that fail to resolve with single-dose or 3-day therapy. In complicated or doubtful cases or with recurrences, a urine culture before initial treatment may be helpful.

Risk factors for UTI in women include pregnancy, sexual activity, use of diaphragms or spermicides, failure to void postcoitally, and history of previous UTI. Healthy women may be expected to suffer a few episodes of lower UTI in a lifetime without indicating any major structural problem or incurring any long-term medical sequelae, but recurrences at short intervals suggest inadequate treatment or underlying abnormalities.

Young men, however, have longer urethras and far fewer lower UTIs. They probably should be evaluated urologically after just one episode unless they have a risk factor such as an uncircumcised foreskin, HIV infection, or homosexual activity, and they respond successfully to initial treatment. In sexually active men, consider urethritis or prostatitis as the cause. In men who are older than 50 years of age, there is a rapid increase in UTI resulting from prostate hypertrophy, obstruction, and instrumentation.

UTIs among pediatric patients are associated with significantly greater morbidity and long-term sequelae than UTIs among adults, including impaired renal function and end-stage renal disease.

Trimethoprim-sulfamethoxazole has been the standard therapy for UTI; however, *E. coli* is becoming increasingly resistant to this medication. Many experts support using ciprofloxacin as an alternative and, in some cases, as the preferred first-line agent. However, others caution that widespread use of ciprofloxacin will promote increased resistance.

Suggested Readings

Bent S, Nallamothu BK, Simel DL, et al: Does this woman have an acute uncomplicated urinary tract infection? *JAMA* 287:2701–2710, 2002.

Chung A, Arianayagam M, Rashid P: Bacterial cystitis in women (review), *Aust Fam Physician* 39:295–298, 2010.

Gittes RF: Female prostatitis, *Urol Clin North Am* 29:613–616, 2002.

Hoberman A, Wald ER, Hickey RW, et al: Oral versus initial intravenous therapy for urinary tract infections in young febrile children, *Pediatrics* 104:79–86, 1999.

Hooten GK, Stamm WE: Increasing antimicrobial resistance and the management of uncomplicated community-acquired urinary tract infections, *Ann Intern Med* 135:41–50, 2001.

Huppert JS, Biro FM, Mehrabi J, Slap GB: Urinary tract infection and *Chlamydia* infection in adolescent females, *J Pediatr Adolesc Gynecol* 16:133–137, 2003.

Jou WW, Powers RD: Utility of dipstick urinalysis as a guide to management of adults with suspected infection of hematuria, *South Med J* 91:266–269, 1998.

Layton KL: Diagnosis and management of pediatric urinary tract infection, *Clin Fam Pract* 5:367–383, 2003.

McKinnell JA, Stollenwerk NS, Jung CW, Miller LG: Nitrofurantoin compares favorably to recommended agents as empirical treatment of uncomplicated urinary tract infections in a decision and cost analysis, *Mayo Clin Proc* 86:480–488, 2011.

Mehnert-Kay SA: Diagnosis and management of uncomplicated urinary tract infections, *Am Fam Physician* 72:451–456, 2005.

Michael M, Hodson EM, Craig JC, et al: Short compared with standard duration of antibiotic treatment for urinary tract infection: a systematic review of randomised controlled trials, *Arch Dis Child* 87:118–123, 2002.

Raz R, Chazen B, Kennes Y, et al: Empiric use of trimethoprim-sulfamethoxazole (TMP-SMX) in the treatment of women with uncomplicated urinary tract infections, in a geographical area with a high prevalence of TMP-SMX–resistant uropathogens, *Clin Infect Dis* 34:1165–1169, 2002.

Shapiro T, Dalton M, Hammock J, et al: The prevalence of urinary tract infections and sexually transmitted disease in women with symptoms of a simple urinary tract infection stratified by low colony count criteria, *Acad Emerg Med* 12:38–44, 2005.

Stamm WE, Hooton TM: Management of urinary tract infections in adults, *N Engl J Med* 329:1328–1334, 1993.

Valenstein PN, Koepke JA: Unnecessary microscopy in routine urinalysis, *Am J Clin Pathol* 82:444–448, 1984.

Vogel T, Verreault R, Gourdeau M, et al: Optimal duration of antibiotic therapy for uncomplicated urinary tract infection in older women: a double-blind randomized controlled trial, *Can Med Assoc J* 170:469–473, 2004.

Urinary Tract Infection, Upper

(Pyelonephritis)

Presentation

The patient (usually a woman between 18 and 40 years of age) has some combination of urinary frequency, urgency, dysuria, malaise, flank pain, nausea, vomiting, fever (>102° F), and chills that have been progressive over several days.

On physical examination, the patient is febrile and may be ill appearing and tachycardic. There is tenderness elicited by percussing the costovertebral angle over one or both of the kidneys and mild to moderate lateral abdominal and suprapubic tenderness without rebound. The urinalysis may help establish the diagnosis with pyuria, bacteriuria, and possibly tubular casts of white blood cells (WBCs).

What To Do:

✓ Examine the urine using a Gram stain to look for gram-positive cocci (presumably enterococci) or the more usual gram-negative rods, and **send for urinalysis culture and sensitivity** (urine cultures should be obtained before initiation of antibiotic therapy).

✓ Obtain blood cultures before beginning therapy, if blood cultures are thought to be necessary (see Discussion later). Other blood tests that may be helpful include a complete blood count, serum electrolytes, serum creatinine, and blood urea nitrogen (BUN).

✓ **If the patient appears toxic,** with a high fever, high white count, nausea, or vomiting (preventing adequate oral medication and hydration); is immunocompromised (i.e., diabetes mellitus, cancer, sickle cell disease, human immunodeficiency virus (HIV), transplant patients); is pregnant; or shows signs of urinary obstruction or underlying anatomic urinary tract abnormality, she should be admitted to the hospital for IV antibiotics. Other indications for inpatient management include failed outpatient management, progression of uncomplicated UTI, renal failure, suspected urosepsis, age older than 60 years of age, poor social situation, and inadequate access to follow-up. **After cultures are obtained, begin ceftriaxone (Rocephin), 1 g IV, ciprofloxacin (Cipro), 400 mg IV, or levofloxacin (Levaquin), 500 mg IV.**

✓ **For stable, otherwise healthy patients with pyuria of greater than 15 WBCs/hpf, start with a first dose of oral antibiotics in the emergency department or clinic. Prescribe ciprofloxacin 500 mg PO bid or ciprofloxacin extended release (Cipro XR), 1000 mg qd × 7 to 14 days. Alternatively, prescribe levofloxacin (Levaquin), 500 mg qd × 7 to 14 days, gatifloxacin (Tequin), 400 mg qd × 7-14 days, or, if the local resistance of uropathogens to trimethoprim-sulfamethoxazole (TMP/SMX) is less than 20%, TMP/SMX [160/800 mg] (Bactrim DS), one bid × 14 days.**

✔ **Instruct outpatients to return for reevaluation in 24 to 48 hours or sooner if symptoms worsen. Most patients improve on this regimen, but others will require hospital admission if they do not improve in 2 days.**

✔ **All pregnant patients** with pyelonephritis should be hospitalized for at least 24 hours and given IV antibiotics and hydration. Ceftriaxone, 1 g IV, can be started after blood cultures are drawn.

✔ Treatment of pyelonephritis in patients with urinary catheters requires replacement of the catheter as well as the initiation of ampicillin, 1000 mg, plus gentamicin, 1.5 mg IV q8 hours, or levofloxacin (Levaquin), 750 mg IV qd, and hospitalization.

What Not To Do:

✘ Do not forget a pregnancy test in women of childbearing age, and do not give aminoglycosides or fluoroquinolones in pregnancy.

✘ Do not lose the patient to follow-up. Although lower urinary tract infections (UTIs) often resolve without treatment, upper UTIs that are inadequately treated can lead to renal damage or sepsis.

✘ Do not miss a diagnosis of pyelonephritis in the absence of fever when other signs and symptoms are present. An elderly person may have few signs or symptoms other than increased confusion and/or lethargy.

✘ Do not miss an infection above a ureteral stone or obstruction. Cramps, colicky pain, or hematuria with the symptoms listed earlier calls for sonography or unenhanced spiral computed tomography. Antibiotics and hydration alone may not cure an infected obstruction.

Discussion

Most renal parenchymal infections occur secondary to bacterial ascent through the urethra and urinary bladder. In men, prostatitis and prostatic hypertrophy, causing urethral obstruction, predispose to bacteriuria. Hematogenous acute pyelonephritis occurs most often in debilitated chronically ill patients and those receiving immunosuppressive therapy. In more than 80% of cases of acute pyelonephritis, the etiologic agent is *Escherichia coli*. Other etiologic organisms include aerobic gram-negative bacteria, *Staphylococcus saprophyticus*, and enterococci. In elderly patients, *E. coli* is a less common (60%) cause of acute pyelonephritis. The increased use of catheters and instruments among those patients predisposes them to infections with other gram-negative organisms such as *Proteus*, *Klebsiella*, *Serratia*, or *Pseudomonas*.

Patients who have diabetes mellitus tend to have infections caused by *Klebsiella*, *Enterobacter*, *Clostridium*, or *Candida*. They also are at an increased risk for developing emphysematous pyelonephritis and papillary necrosis, leading to shock and renal failure.

Although oral antibiotics are usually sufficient treatment for upper UTIs, there is a significant incidence of renal damage and sepsis as sequelae, mandating good follow-up or admission for IV therapy when necessary. By the same token, lower UTIs can ascend into upper UTIs, or it can be difficult to decide the level of a given UTI, in which case it should be treated as an upper UTI.

In general, the diagnosis of acute pyelonephritis should not be made if flank pain and fever are not present. One should be alert for alternative diagnoses, including pelvic inflammatory disease, lower lobe pneumonia, perforated viscus, the prodrome of herpes zoster, cholecystitis, acute

(continued)

Discussion continued

appendicitis, and diverticulitis. However, up to one third of elderly patients with acute pyelonephritis have no fever; in 20% of elderly patients, the predominant symptoms are gastrointestinal or pulmonary.

Hospitalization is generally recommended for pregnant patients with pyelonephritis because of the risk for serious complications to the mother and fetus; however, outpatient therapy may be appropriate for select patients at less than 24 weeks of gestation.

Because urine culture frequently identifies the responsible organism, it is unclear whether blood cultures alter therapy in the management of pyelonephritis. Therefore some authorities believe that not obtaining blood cultures in immunocompetent, nonpregnant adults with apparently uncomplicated pyelonephritis is within the standard of care. Some say the use of blood cultures should be reserved for patients with an uncertain diagnosis, those who are immunocompromised, and those who are suspected of having hematogenous infection.

Suggested Readings

Chen MY, Zagoria RJ: Can noncontrast helical computed tomography replace intravenous urography for evaluation of patients with acute urinary tract colic, *J Emerg Med* 17:299–303, 1999.

Foxman B: Epidemiology of urinary tract infections: incidence, morbidity, and economic costs, *Dis Mon* 49:53–70, 2003.

Jolley JA, Wing DA: Pyelonephritis in pregnancy: an update on treatment options for optimal outcomes, *Drugs* 70:1643–1655, 2010.

Miller OF, Rineer SK, Reichard SR, et al: Prospective comparison of unenhanced spiral computed tomography and intravenous urogram in the evaluation of acute flank pain, *Urology* 52:982–987, 1998.

Mills AM, Barros S: Are blood cultures necessary in adults with pyelonephritis? *Ann Emerg Med* 46:285–287, 2005.

Mittal P, Wing DA: Urinary tract infections in pregnancy, *Clin Perinatol* 32:749–764, 2005.

Pinson AG, Philbrick JT, Lindbeck GH, et al: ED management of acute pyelonephritis in women: a cohort study, *Am J Emerg Med* 12:271–278, 1994.

Pinson AG, Philbrick JT, Lindbeck GH, et al: Fever in the clinical diagnosis of acute pyelonephritis, *Am J Emerg Med* 15:148–151, 1997.

Ramakrishnan K, Scheid DC: Diagnosis and management of acute pyelonephritis in adults, *Am Fam Physician* 71:933–942, 2005.

Talan DA, Stamm WE, Hooten TM: Comparison of ciprofloxacin (7 days) and trimethoprim-sulfamethoxazole (14 days) for acute uncomplicated pyelonephritis in women: a randomized trial, *JAMA* 283:1583–1590, 2000.

Thanassi M: Utility of urine and blood cultures in pyelonephritis, *Acad Emerg Med* 4:797–800, 1997.

PART 8

Gynecologic Emergencies

■ Philip Buttaravoli ■ Wendy James

Bartholin Abscess

Presentation

A woman complains of vulvar pain (which can become extreme) and swelling that has developed over the past 2 to 3 days, making walking and sitting very uncomfortable. Patients are usually 20 to 30 years old. On physical examination in the lithotomy position, there is a unilateral (occasionally bilateral), tender, fluctuant, mildly erythematous swelling at the 5-o'clock or 7-o'clock position within the posterior labium minus (Figure 87-1).

What To Do:

✅ **If the swelling and pain is mild without fluctuance (bartholinitis) or if the abscess is small, the patient can be placed on antibiotics, such as metronidazole (Flagyl), 500 mg bid × 7 days, or clindamycin (Cleocin), 300 mg qid × 7 days, and instructed to take warm sitz baths. Early follow-up should be provided. If there is any risk for a sexually transmitted disease (STD) that cannot be ruled out with rapid testing, give azithromycin (Zithromax), 1 g orally in a single dose, or oral doxycycline, 100 mg twice a day for 7 days. Also give ciprofloxacin (Cipro), 500 mg orally in a single dose.**

✅ **When the abscess is painful or is enlarged and presents a thin-walled segment, a 0.5- to 1-cm puncture/incision should be made with a No. 15 scalpel blade over the medial bulging mucosal surface of the labia minora and the pus evacuated.** First prepare the mucosal surface with povidone-iodine (Betadine) solution and then thoroughly irrigate with normal saline or sterile water. Anesthetize the overlying tissue with 1% lidocaine (Xylocaine) with epinephrine. A No. 11 blade can be used to make the 5-mm stab incision, about 1.5 cm deep, at or behind the hymenal ring. Hold traction on the cyst with small forceps to prevent collapse of the cyst wall, and maintain visualization of the cavity.

✅ **After drainage, a Word catheter should be inserted through the incision. Insert it to the bottom of the cavity and inflate the tip of the catheter with approximately 1.5 to 3.0 mL of sterile water or saline to hold it in place and prevent premature closure of the**

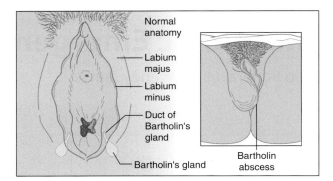

Figure 87-1 Bartholin abscess.

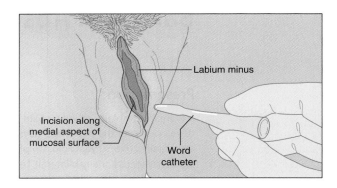

Figure 87-2 Insertion of Word catheter after incision and drainage.

opening (Figure 87-2). If balloon inflation is painful, this may indicate malplacement. Remove and reposition the Word catheter before reinflating. Also reassess the volume of inflation; a smaller amount may hold the catheter in place without maximum inflation. Balloon volumes may be larger; however, 3 mL or less likely will work well. The free end of the catheter may then be tucked up into the vagina.

✓ **After drainage,** use of prophylactic antibiotics is not recommended unless there is significant surrounding cellulitis or signs of systemic illness. One suggestion is Cefixime, 400 mg qd for 7 days, and clindamycin, 300 mg 4 times a day for 7 days. The patient should be instructed to take sitz baths and be provided with mild analgesics for the first day or two. **If there is any risk for an STD, prophylaxis, as noted previously, should be administered.**

✓ **Inform the patient that the catheter should stay in place for 4 to 6 weeks to allow a permanent tract to form (like a pierced ear) and thereby help prevent recurrent abscess formation.**

✓ Arrange for a follow-up examination within 48 hours.

What Not To Do:

(X) Do not make a drainage incision on the outside of the labium.

(X) Do not mistake a nontender Bartholin duct cyst, which does not require immediate treatment, for an inflamed abscess.

(X) Do not mistake a more posterior perirectal abscess for a Bartholin abscess. The perirectal abscess requires a different treatment approach.

(X) Do not miss an underlying malignancy, especially with an older patient with recurrent abscess formation.

(X) Do not use a latex catheter in latex-allergic patients.

Discussion

Bartholin glands are epithelial secretory glands commonly paired within the labia minora at approximately the 5-o'clock and 7-o'clock positions on the posterolateral aspect of the vestibule. Normally pea-sized and draining through a 2.5-cm duct into a fold between the hymenal ring and the labium, obstruction of the gland at the ostium can cause the glands to become cystic and subsequently form abscesses.

Simple incision and drainage without Word catheter placement may be inadequate and lead to a considerable number of recurrences of abscesses. The Word catheter is an inflatable latex balloon on the tip of a 10-Fr, 5-cm, single-barreled catheter designed to retain itself in the abscess cavity for 4 to 6 weeks to help ensure the development of a wide marsupialized opening for continued drainage. It seldom stays in place that long. The size of the incision should be kept less than 1 cm. If the incision is too large when using a Word catheter, the balloon may not be large enough, and this would increase the risk of having it fall out prematurely.

Iodoform or plain ribbon gauze can be inserted into the incised abscess as a substitute. If a wide opening persists, recurrent infections are not likely to occur, but they are common if the stoma closes.

The most common organisms involved in the development of a Bartholin abscess are anaerobic and most commonly include *Bacteroides fragilis* and *Peptostreptococcus*. *Escherichia coli* can also be present. About 10% to 15% of the time, *Neisseria gonorrhoeae* is the causative agent. Bilateral infections are more commonly characteristic of gonorrhea. *Chlamydia trachomatis* is involved less frequently. Often, infections are mixed.

Suggested Readings

Owen JW, Koza J, Shiblee T, et al: Placement of a Word catheter: a resident training model, *Am J Obstet Gynecol* 192:1385–1387, 2005.

Zeger W, Holt K: Gynecologic infections, *Emerg Med Clin North Am* 21:631–648, 2003.

Condylomata Acuminata

(Genital Warts)

Presentation

Patients may complain of perineal itching, burning, pain, and tenderness, although they are commonly asymptomatic, especially with cervical and vaginal involvement. Distinctive fleshy warts can be found on the external genitalia or anus (Figures 88-1 and 88-2). Lesions are pedunculated or broad-based with pink to gray soft excrescences, with multiple papillae arising from a single base. They occur in clusters or individually and can become friable. In addition to the external genitalia (i.e., the penis, vulva, scrotum, perineum, and perianal skin), genital warts can occur on the uterine cervix as well as in and around the vagina, urethra, anus, and mouth.

What To Do:

✅ External warts seldom require biopsy for diagnosis. Biopsy is needed only if the diagnosis is uncertain, the lesions do not respond to standard therapy, the disease worsens during therapy, the patient is immunocompromised, or warts are pigmented, indurated, fixed, and ulcerated. The differential diagnosis of anogenital warts includes molluscum contagiosum (Figures 88-3 and 88-4), verruca vulgaris (common nongenital wart), secondary syphilis (*Condyloma lata,* Figure 88-5), hypertrophic vulvar dystrophies, and vulvar intraepithelial and invasive neoplasias. Consider atypical, pigmented, intravaginal, cervical, and persistent warts for referral for gynecologic evaluation. Recognition of cervical lesions may require colposcopy.

✅ **The primary goal of treating visible genital warts is the removal of symptomatic warts. In most patients, treatment can induce wart-free periods.** Treatment of genital warts should be guided by the number, size, site, and morphology of lesions, as well as the preference of the patient, cost, convenience, available resources, and experience of the healthcare provider. **No definitive evidence suggests that any of the available treatments are superior to the others. Modalities of therapy include physical or chemical destruction, immunologic therapy, or surgical excision.**

✅ **Because of uncertainty regarding the effect of treatment on future transmission and the possibility for spontaneous resolution, an acceptable alternative for some patients is to forgo treatment and await spontaneous resolution.**

✅ Most patients have 10 or less genital warts, with a total wart area of 0.5 to 1.0 cm². These warts respond to most treatment modalities. **Many patients require a course of therapy rather than a single treatment. In general, warts located on moist surfaces and/or in intertriginous areas respond better to topical treatment than do warts on drier surfaces.**

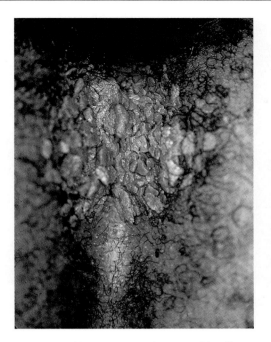

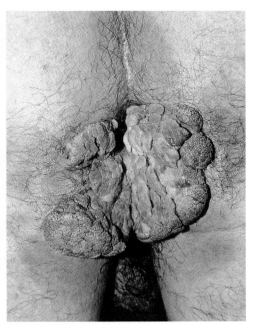

Figure 88-1 Condylomata acuminata on the perineum. (Adapted from Black M, McKay M, Braude P, et al: *Obstetric and gynecologic dermatology,* ed 2. St Louis, 2002, Mosby.)

Figure 88-2 Perianal condyloma acuminatum. (Adapted from White G, Cox N: *Diseases of the skin,* ed 2. St Louis, 2006, Mosby.)

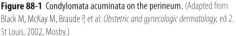

✓ Patients should be warned that persistent hypopigmentation or hyperpigmentation is common with ablative modalities. Rarely, treatment can result in disabling chronic pain syndromes (e.g., vulvodynia or hyperesthesia of the treatment site).

Patient-Applied:

✓ **Prescribe imiquimod (Aldara) cream 5%, 12 single-use packets. Have the nonpregnant patient apply a thin layer of cream once daily to external genital and perianal warts, rubbed in until the cream is no longer visible, with hand washing before and after cream application.** This should be repeated 3 times per week, prior to normal sleeping hours, and left on the skin for 6 to 10 hours before being washed off. This should continue until there is total clearing of the warts or for a maximum of 16 weeks. This cream is very expensive.

✓ **An alternative for self-treatment is to prescribe podofilox 0.5% solution (3.5 mL) or gel 0.5% (3.5 g). Both are moderately expensive. Nonpregnant patients may apply podofilox solution with a cotton swab or podofilox gel with a finger twice daily for 3 days, followed by 4 days of no treatment.** The patient should be careful to avoid the surrounding normal tissue. This cycle may be repeated as necessary for a total of four cycles. Total wart area treated should not exceed 10 cm², and the total volume of podofilox should not exceed 0.5 mL/day. If possible, apply the initial treatment to demonstrate the proper application technique and identify which warts should be treated.

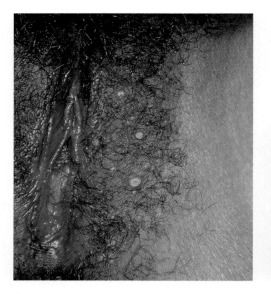

Figure 88-3 Molluscum contagiosum on the labia majora. (Adapted from Black M, McKay M, Braude P, et al: *Obstetric and gynecologic dermatology*, ed 2. St Louis, 2002, Mosby.)

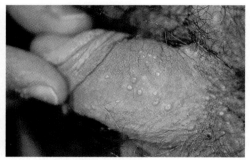

Figure 88-4 Molluscum on the shaft of the penis. (Adapted from White G, Cox N: *Diseases of the skin*, ed 2. St Louis, 2006, Mosby.)

Provider-Administered:

✓ **Apply 25% podophyllin in tincture of benzoin (Podocon-25). Use applicator provided. A small amount should be applied to each wart and allowed to air dry. Leave on briefly for the first treatment to assess for sensitivity, about 30 minutes or so. Thereafter the nonpregnant patient may thoroughly wash off the podophyllin in 1 to 4 hours.** This may be repeated weekly if necessary, but if warts persist after six applications, the patient should be referred for alternative therapy. This is not to be used on mucosal surfaces—never to be applied on cervical or vaginal epithelium.

✓ **Alternatively, apply a small amount of trichloroacetic acid (TCA) or bichloroacetic acid (BCA), 80% to 90%, only to warts and allow it to dry, at which time a white "frosting" develops.** If an excess amount of acid is applied, the treated area can be powdered with baking soda to neutralize unreacted acid. This treatment can be repeated weekly, if necessary. A barrier of petroleum jelly helps protect unaffected surrounding skin, because the solution is highly caustic.

✓ The treatment modality should be changed if a patient has not improved substantially after three provider-administered treatments or if warts have not completely cleared after six treatments.

✓ **Another treatment is the use of 5-fluorouracil epinephrine gel. The gel is injected intralesionally. Inject each lesion once per week for up to 6 weeks.**

✓ **The treatment modality should be changed if the patient has not improved substantially after three provider-administered treatments or if warts have not completely cleared after six treatments.**

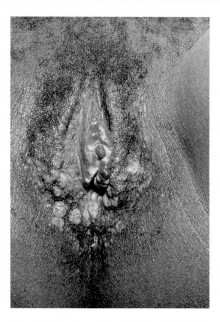

Figure 88-5 Secondary syphilis. (Adapted from White G, Cox N: *Diseases of the skin*, ed 2. St Louis, 2006, Mosby.)

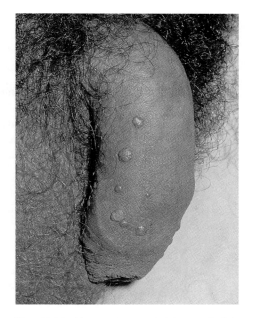

Figure 88-6 Condyloma acuminatum; multiple lesions on the shaft of the penis. (Adapted from White G, Cox N: *Diseases of the skin*, ed 2. St Louis, 2006, Mosby.)

✓ If the patient is pregnant, has severe involvement, or has profuse anal or rectal warts, she should be referred for cryotherapy, ablation with carbon dioxide laser, electrocautery, or surgical excision.

✓ If the patient's male partner also has visible lesions (Figure 88-6), he can be treated using the same regimens. Examination of asymptomatic sex partners is not necessary, but they may benefit from counseling about their potential for future disease.

✓ **Provide patient education and counseling. Inform the patient of the following:**

○ Genital human papillomavirus infection (HPV) is a viral infection that is common among sexually active adults.

○ Infection is almost always sexually transmitted, but the incubation period is variable, and it is often difficult to determine the source of infection. Within ongoing relationships, sex partners usually are infected by the time of the patient's diagnosis, although they may have no symptoms or signs of infection.

○ The natural history of genital warts is generally benign; the types of HPV that usually cause external genital warts are not associated with cancer.

○ Recurrence of genital warts within the first several months after treatment is common and usually indicates recurrence rather than reinfection.

○ The likelihood of transmission to future partners and the duration of infectivity after treatment are unknown. The use of latex condoms may help to prevent the likelihood of further transmission.

○ The value of disclosing a past diagnosis of genital HPV infection to future partners is unclear. Candid discussions about other sexually transmitted diseases (STDs) should be encouraged and attempted whenever possible.

○ After visible genital warts have cleared, a follow-up evaluation is not mandatory but may be helpful. Patients concerned about recurrences should be offered a follow-up evaluation 3 months after treatment.

✓ **Women should be counseled to undergo regular Pap screening, as recommended for women without genital warts. The presence of genital warts is not an indication for a change in the frequency of Pap tests or for cervical colposcopy.**

✓ Counsel both partners about the unpredictable natural history of the disease and the possible increased risk for lower genital tract malignancy (see Discussion). Infected women should have an annual Pap smear.

What Not To Do:

✗ Do not use imiquimod, podofilox, or podophyllin during pregnancy. Safety during pregnancy has not been established for these agents, and there have been a few cases of toxicity reported when large amounts of podophyllin have been used.

✗ Do not mistake "pearly penile papules" for warts (Figure 88-7). These dome-shaped or hairlike projections around the corona of the glans penis are normal variants in up to 10% of men.

✗ **Do not mistake condyloma acuminatum for other lesions. Other lesions include condylomata lata, micropapillumatosis of vulva, molluscum contagiosum, and squamous cell carcinoma. If lesions are not responding to therapy, consider biopsy.**

✗ **Do not advise patients that clearing is a cure; recurrence is the norm.**

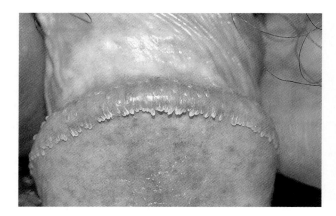

Figure 88-7 Pearly penile papules. (Adapted from White G, Cox N: *Diseases of the skin,* ed 2. St Louis, 2006, Mosby.)

Discussion

Genital warts are a result of infection with HPV. Approximately 35 types of HPV can infect the genital tract. Most HPV infections are asymptomatic, unrecognized, or subclinical. The sexual transmission of HPV is well documented, with the highest prevalence in young, sexually active adolescents and adults. **HPV types 6 and 11 are the most prevalent types associated with condylomata acuminata and are not considered to have the malignant potential of types 16, 18, 31, 33, and 35. The types with malignant potential are found occasionally in visible genital warts and have been associated with external genital squamous intraepithelial neoplasia. Patients who have visible genital warts can be infected simultaneously with multiple HPV types. In addition, HPV frequently coexists with other sexually transmitted diseases.** HPV lesions are difficult to eradicate, with a very high recurrence rate, and there is still no definitive therapy. No evidence indicates that either the presence of genital warts or their treatment is associated with the development of cervical cancer.

Despite current infection with genital warts, patients may still be candidates for the new HPV vaccine. They should be encouraged to seek a specialist's advice.

Imiquimod is a topically active immune enhancer that stimulates production of interferon and other cytokines. Local inflammatory reactions are common with the use of imiquimod; these reactions are usually mild to moderate.

Podofilox, 0.5% solution or gel, an antimitotic drug that destroys warts, is relatively inexpensive, easy to use, safe, and self-applied by patients.

Most patients experience mild to moderate pain or local irritation after treatment.

Podophyllin resin, which contains several compounds, including antimitotic podophyllin lignans, must be allowed to air dry before the treated area comes into contact with clothing, or local irritation caused by spread of the compound to adjacent areas can result.

Both TCA and BCA are caustic agents that destroy warts by chemical coagulation of proteins. TCA solutions have low viscosity, comparable with that of water, and can spread rapidly if applied excessively; thus they also can damage adjacent tissues if not applied sparingly and allowed to dry before the patient sits or stands.

Surgical therapy is a treatment option that has the advantage of usually eliminating warts at a single visit. However, such therapy requires substantial clinical training, additional equipment, and a longer office visit.

Newer therapies, such as topical cidofovir and bacillus Calmette-Guérin (BCG), are under study and show promise.

The goal of present treatments is clearance of visible warts; some evidence exists that treatment reduces infectivity, but there is no evidence that treatment reduces the incidence of genital cancer. Patient-applied therapy, such as imiquimod cream or podofilox, is increasingly recommended. These treatments, used at times in conjunction with surgical excision and/or cryotherapy, are presently the most convenient and effective options.

Biopsy, viral typing, acetowhite staining, and other diagnostic measures are not routinely required.

In patients who fail to respond to therapy or who have extremely large lesions, consider evaluating for an immunosuppressed state, including human immunodeficiency virus (HIV).

Suggested Reading

Kodner CM, Nasraty S: Management of genital warts, *Am Fam Physician* 70:2335–2342, 2004.

Contact Vulvovaginitis

Presentation

Patients complain of severe vulvar itching that may be accompanied by edematous swelling. Occasionally, there will be tenderness, pain, burning, and dysuria severe enough to cause urinary retention. The vulvovaginal area is variably inflamed, erythematous, and edematous. In more severe cases, there may be vesiculation and ulceration; in cases in which there is chronic contact dermatitis, there may be lichenification, scaling, and skin thickening.

What To Do:

✅ **Try to determine if condition is exogenous (from contact) or endogenous (atopic). If an offending agent can be identified, have the patient stop using it. Most reactions are caused by agents that the patient unknowingly applies or uses for hygienic or therapeutic purposes.** Chemically scented douches, soaps, bubble baths, deodorants, perfumes, dyed or scented toilet paper, dyed underwear, scented tampons or pads, and additional feminine hygiene products are the most common causative agents. Neomycin-containing topical medication is another frequent source. Less commonly, plant allergens, such as poison oak or poison ivy, may trigger the reaction. Use of latex condoms and proteins in seminal plasma may also be an inapparent source of contact dermatitis.

✅ If the diagnosis is unclear, rule out an alternative cause of vulvar pruritus, such as pinworms (see Chapter 69) or *Trichomonas* organisms (see Chapter 95). *Candida albicans* may also be the cause of pruritus, but it may present as an overgrowth when contact vulvovaginitis is the primary problem. Atypical herpes simplex virus should also be considered. Atopic or eczematous changes can be causative as well; therefore look at buttock and labial folds.

✅ **When the findings are typical for contact vulvovaginitis, instruct the patient in the use of warm to cool baths twice a day for 5 minutes, and then apply topical steroids as a treatment and to seal in moisture. Trying cool, wet compresses soaked with boric acid or Burow solution (Domeboro) has also been recommended.**

✅ **Prescribe liberal amounts of topical corticosteroids, such as fluocinolone (Synalar cream 0.025%) or triamcinolone (Aristocort A 0.025% cream) bid to qid (dispense 15-g tube). For mild symptoms, hydrocortisone 1% or 2.5% or triamcinolone 0.1% can be used daily for 2 to 4 weeks, then twice per week. For moderate to severe symptoms, clobetasol propionate or betamethasone dipropionate ointment 0.05% can be used nightly for 30 days. One can also try tapering starting with applications twice daily for 2 weeks, then daily for 2 weeks, then on Monday, Wednesday, and Friday for 2 weeks. Finally, the patient** should be reevaluated. In the past, there has been concern about atrophy with steroid use. These potent steroids have been used up to 12 weeks on the vulva without adverse effects.

✓ **In more severe cases, or if topical is increasing the irritation, use triamcinolone intramuscular (IM) 60 mg. This may be used every 6 weeks for up to 3 doses. Alternatively, a steroid taper dose pack, such as prednisone (Sterapred DS or Sterapred DS 12 day) or methylprednisolone (Medrol Dosepack 4-mg tablets) for systemic therapy could be prescribed.**

✓ **Some suggest a sedating antipruritic agent helps with nighttime itching and scratching. The antidepressant Doxepin (Sinequan), 10 to 25 mg or the sedating antihistamine hydroxyzine (Atarax, Vistaril), 25 to 50 mg at 7 pm, may help with sleep.**

What Not To Do:

✗ Do not have the patient use hot baths or compresses. This will usually exacerbate the burning and pruritus.

✗ Do not prescribe nonsedating antihistamines. They are relatively ineffective in treating contact vulvitis and may increase discomfort by drying the vaginal mucosa.

Discussion

The major problem with managing contact vulvovaginitis is identifying the primary irritant or allergen. In many cases, more than one substance is involved, or potentially involved, and may be totally unsuspected by the patient (such as the use of scented toilet paper). For this reason, a thorough investigative history is important. Include questions about hygiene practices, clothing, and fabrics.

An allergic reaction can take 12 to 72 hours to develop, is usually very pruritic, and can often last for weeks.

Dysmenorrhea

(Menstrual Cramps)

Presentation

A young woman or female adolescent complains of crampy labor-like pains that began shortly before or at the onset of the visible bleeding of her menstrual period. The pain is focused in the lower abdomen, low back, suprapubic area, or thighs and may be associated with nausea, vomiting, increased defecation, headache, muscular cramps, or passage of clots. The pain is most severe on the first day of the menses and may last from several hours to 3 days. Often, this is a recurrent problem, dating back to the first year after menarche. Rectal, vaginal, and pelvic examinations disclose no abnormalities.

What To Do:

✓ Ask about the duration of symptoms and onset of similar episodes; onset of dysmenorrhea after adolescence or pain that is not limited to the time of the menstrual period suggests other pelvic disease. Ask about appetite, diarrhea, dysuria, dyspareunia, abnormal vaginal discharge, and other symptoms suggestive of pelvic disease.

✓ Perform a thorough abdominal and speculum and bimanual pelvic examination, looking for signs of infection, pregnancy, or uterine or adnexal disease. Perform cultures or other diagnostic tests to rule out sexually transmitted diseases (STDs) in sexually active patients. **It is appropriate to perform only an abdominal examination and forgo the pelvic examination in young adolescents with a typical history and who truly have never been sexually active.**

✓ **Confirm that the patient is not pregnant, using a urine pregnancy test (or serum beta human chorionic gonadotropin [hCG], if available).**

✓ When the history and physical examination suggest other pelvic disease, the evaluation should follow accordingly, usually with pelvic ultrasonography as the initial diagnostic test to rule out anatomic abnormalities, such as mass lesions.

✓ **For uncomplicated dysmenorrhea, nonsteroidal anti-inflammatory drugs (NSAIDs) and hormonal therapy are the mainstays of treatment. If one of these agents fails after 2 to 3 months, then consider the other.**

✓ **Try NSAIDs, such as ibuprofen (Motrin), 600 mg every 6 hours or 800 mg every 8 hours, or a fenamate, such as mefenamic acid (Ponstel) 500 mg load and 250 mg every 6 hours for 3 days (expensive), or naproxen (Naprosyn), 500 mg every 12 hours. NSAIDs may be most effective when therapy is started before the onset of menstrual pain and flow. Therapy need not be continued after the end of the flow.**

✅ **If hormonal contraception is desired, monophasic oral contraceptive pills (OCPs) and depo-medroxyprogesterone acetate (Depo-Provera) may be considered.** Extended oral contraceptive formulations (i.e., usually taking OCPs for 12 weeks followed by 1 week off) leads to less frequent menstrual periods and is associated with less menstrual pain than the monthly regimen. Both, however, are effective. A disadvantage to the longer regimen is unscheduled spotting that occurs, causing some women to discontinue use; this, however, does decrease over time.

✅ Use of the transdermal contraceptive patch in a randomized trial found dysmenorrhea more common in patch users than in oral users. Vaginal rings and intrauterine devices (IUDs) have shown variable results on dysmenorrhea symptoms. Implanted contraception has not been well studied for this issue. At this time, oral contraception appears to be the most efficacious agent for dysmenorrhea symptoms.

✅ **In women who do not desire hormonal contraception, use of topical heat appears to be as effective as oral analgesics. Systematic reviews found that exercise appears to reduce menstrual symptoms, and behavior modification with biofeedback, electromyographic training, Lamaze exercises, and relaxation training helped some women.**

✅ **Limited data demonstrate some promise in the following:**

- **Thiamine at a dosage of 100 mg daily**
- **The Japanese herbal remedy toki-shakuyaku-san (TSS)**
- **Vitamin E (500 IU per day or 200 IU twice a day) taken daily for 5 days, starting 2 days before menstruation each month (maximum effect may not be reached until 4 months of use; alternatively, start use 2 days before and continue for 3 days after onset of menses)**
- **Fish oil supplement containing 1080 mg of eicosapentaenoic acid (EPA) and 720 mg of docosahexaenoic acid (DHA) taken daily. All these supplements are relatively simple and inexpensive alternatives that can be used alone or in combination.**
- Acupuncture and acupressure have been shown to be effective in treating dysmenorrhea.

✅ If pain is not controlled with any of these approaches, pelvic ultrasonography should be performed, and gynecologic referral should be arranged for the workup of endometriosis or other secondary causes of dysmenorrhea.

What Not To Do:

❌ Do not recommend spinal manipulation for pain relief. There is reasonable evidence that it is ineffective.

❌ Do not use NSAIDs if the patient wants to get pregnant; NSAIDs have been linked to reduced ovulation. If the patient is trying to get pregnant, use of these agents should be avoided when possible.

❌ Do not continue the use of NSAIDs and oral contraceptives without further gynecologic evaluation, if the patient's symptoms persist for more than three cycles.

Discussion

Menstrual cramps affect more than half of all menstruating women, with 10% to 15% suffering enough pain to miss work, school, or home activities. It is most common during the late teens and 20s. Overproduction of prostaglandins E and F and leukotrienes in menstrual blood appears to stimulate uterine contractions and thus results in many of the symptoms of dysmenorrhea, including cramps, nausea, vomiting, bloating, and headaches. Vasopressin also may play a role by increasing uterine contractility and causing ischemic pain as a result of vasoconstriction. Risk factors for dysmenorrhea include nulliparity, heavy menstrual flow, smoking, and depression.

Most dysmenorrhea in adolescents is primary (or functional), associated with normal ovulatory cycle, with no pelvic disease, and has a clear physiologic cause.

Empirical therapy can be initiated based on a typical history of painful menses and a negative physical examination. Nonsteroidal anti-inflammatory drugs are the initial therapy of choice in patients with presumptive primary dysmenorrhea. There is no clear-cut advantage of one NSAID versus another in the treatment of dysmenorrhea. Therefore agent selection should be guided by cost, convenience, and patient preference, with ibuprofen or naproxen being good choices for most patients. Treatment with NSAIDs is most effective when initiated 1 to 2 days before the onset of menses. An adolescent who cannot predict the start of her period should be instructed to start NSAID treatment as soon as menstrual bleeding starts, or as soon as she has any menstruation-associated symptoms.

In the nonmenstruating adolescent with cyclic pain, a complete exam should be performed to evaluate for an anatomic abnormality, such as transverse vaginal septum, imperforate hymen, or noncommunicating uterine horn.

Dysmenorrhea that does not respond either to NSAIDs, administered for at least three menstrual periods, or to a combination estrogen and progestogen pill or other alternative therapies, administered for at least three ensuing menstrual cycles, should raise suspicion of secondary dysmenorrhea, and diagnostic laparoscopy should be suggested.

Primary dysmenorrhea often improves after childbirth.

Suggested Readings

French L: Dysmenorrhea, *Am Fam Physician* 71:285–291, 2005.

Harel Z: Cyclooxygenase-2 specific inhibitors in the treatment of dysmenorrhea, *J Pediatr Adolesc Gynecol* 17:75–79, 2004.

Foreign Body, Vaginal

Presentation

This can be a problem of both children and adults. Children may insert a foreign body and not tell their parents or may be the victims of child abuse. The patient is finally brought to the emergency department with a foul-smelling, bloody or brown purulent discharge, or pain. Vaginal foreign bodies in the adult may be a result of a psychiatric disorder or unusual sexual practices. Occasionally, a tampon or pessary is forgotten or lost and causes discomfort and a vaginal discharge.

What To Do:

✅ **Visualize the foreign body using a nasal speculum for the pediatric patient or a vaginal speculum for the adult. Consider using procedural sedation (see Appendix E) in a child or frightened adult.**

✅ Other noninvasive methods used to identify foreign bodies in young patients include pelvic sonography, plain abdominal radiography, and MRI, all of which are imperfect and can miss foreign bodies, such as those made of plastic.

✅ **Pediatric patients may be placed in the knee-chest position. While a rectal examination is being performed, the foreign body may be expelled from the vagina by pushing it with the examining finger in the rectum.**

✅ **Friable foreign bodies,** such as wads of toilet paper (one of the most common foreign bodies), may be flushed out using warm water or saline, an infant feeding tube, or a pediatric Foley catheter attached to a 60-mL syringe. The catheter tip is inserted into the vagina past the object, then flushed (using a moderate amount of pressure) with approximately 200 mL of fluid.

 ✅ **Lost or forgotten tampons can be removed with vaginal forceps that are first pierced through the finger of a polyvinyl glove, so that when the malodorous foreign body is extracted, the glove can immediately be pulled over it to reduce the odor before it is discarded in a sealed plastic bag. The vagina should then be swabbed with a Betadine solution.**

✅ **In difficult cases, or when large or sharp objects are involved,** young and adult patients may require general anesthesia to allow removal under direct vision. When general anesthesia is not required, conscious sedation should be considered.

✅ **With objects that are not likely to cause harm,** the patient should empty her bladder and lie in stirrups in the lithotomy position. **Insert a Foley catheter to break any suction between the foreign body and the vaginal mucosa. Most objects can then be grasped with ring forceps, a tenaculum, or the plaster and tongue blade method** (see Chapter 71).

✓ Reserve radiographs for radiopaque foreign bodies concealed in the bladder or urethra. Objects in the vagina are usually apparent on examination.

✓ When a foreign body is suspected in a child but cannot be visualized, refer the patient for examination under anesthesia and vaginoscopy, which allows the identification of foreign bodies, aids in the diagnosis of other unusual conditions, as well as allows for a complete examination and an opportunity for sexual assault forensic collection.

What Not To Do:

✗ Do not ignore a vaginal discharge in a pediatric patient or assume it is the result of benign vaginitis. Perform a bimanual or rectoabdominal examination to palpate a hard object, and then do a gentle speculum examination to look for a foreign body or signs of vaginal trauma.

✗ Do not forget to ask about possible sexual abuse, and consult with protective services if it cannot be ruled out.

Discussion

Removal of a vaginal foreign body is generally not a problem, but when large objects make removal more difficult, use the additional techniques described for rectal foreign bodies (see Chapter 71).

Vaginal discharge in children is a common gynecologic complaint. Common sources for vaginal irritation or discharge include fecal contamination from poor perineal hygiene, spread of respiratory bacteria from hand to perineal contact, and local irritants, such as bubble bath or nylon underwear. Recommended treatments have included improved hygiene measures, avoidance of irritants, oral antibiotics, and estrogen cream.

Recurrent or persistent vaginal discharge should raise concerns of an uncertain bacterial source, possible undisclosed sexual abuse, and the possibility of a foreign body. Foreign bodies are the cause for 10% of girls presenting with a complaint of bloody discharge.

If a premenarchal girl presents with vaginal discharge that does not respond to hygiene measures and medical therapy (including antibiotics)—or if the vaginal discharge is unusual, malodorous, and/or bloody or not consistent with clinical findings—a thorough investigation to rule out a foreign body must be performed.

Suggested Readings

Simon DA, Berry S, Brannian J, Hansen K: Recurrent, purulent vaginal discharge associated with longstanding presence of a foreign body and vaginal stenosis, *J Pediatr Adolesc Gynecol* 16:361–363, 2003.

Smith YR, Berman DR, Quint EH: Premenarchal vaginal discharge: findings of procedures to rule out foreign bodies, *J Pediatr Adolesc Gynecol* 15:227–230, 2002.

"Morning After" Emergency Contraception

Presentation

A woman had unprotected sexual intercourse in the past 24 to 72 hours and wants to prevent an unplanned pregnancy. Emergency contraception is not a primary form of birth control. However, this may be needed by a female who forgot to take her oral birth control pills or had the condom break during intercourse, or many other scenarios in which the usual method of birth control failed or was misused. This also may be part of the prophylactic treatment of a rape victim.

What To Do:

✅ **If there is any possibility of a preexisting pregnancy, obtain a pregnancy test. If the test is already positive, the following measures will not be effective for terminating that pregnancy.**

✅ **When a preexisting pregnancy is not an issue,** suggest or prescribe a contraceptive in large doses for a short time to prevent implantation. Note that emergency contraception is approved for sale by the U.S. Food and Drug Administration (FDA) over the counter for men and women older than the age of 17 years; a prescription is not needed unless the man or woman is age 16 or younger. In some states, the pharmacist may have special arrangements with prescribers who are seen by women younger than 16 years of age.

✅ **Emergency contraception is most effective when taken as soon as possible but will be effective up to 5 days (120 hours) after unprotected intercourse.**

✅ **Expect some nausea. Prescribe an antiemetic if needed; estrogen-containing pills do tend to have more nausea and vomiting associated with their use than progestin-only pills.**

✅ **Examples include one of the following:**

○ **Levonorgestrel tablets, 0.75 mg (Plan B or Next Choice, 2-tablet packs); take the first tablet as soon as possible within 120 hours of unprotected sex, and take the second tablet 12 hours after taking the first tablet. Plan B One-Step has been found to be just as effective as a single 1.5-mg dose; thus one could take the two 0.75-mg tablets as a single dose as well.**

○ **Patients who vomit within 1 hour of taking either dose can repeat it, but, of course, that would require buying another package.**

○ Emergency contraceptive kit (Preven Kit) contains four pills of levonorgestrel and ethinyl estradiol, along with a patient information book and urine pregnancy test.

○ When standard birth-control pills are a more available option for the patient, have her take norgestrel and ethinyl estradiol (Ovral), PO—two now and two in 12 hours, or four pills now and four in 12 hours of lower dose contraceptives (Levlen, Lo/Ovral, Nordette, Tri-Levlen, or Triphasil).

○ Ulipristal acetate (Ella, EllaOne) is not a hormone. It works on progesterone, by preventing the progesterone from having its normal effects on the uterus and ovulation. It is taken as a single 30-mg tablet. This may be more effective than the levonorgestrel tablets for those in the 72- to 120-hour postevent window.

✅ **Ask about exposure to sexually transmitted diseases, which might require separate testing and prophylaxis.**

✅ When appropriate, take this opportunity to teach about safe sex and pregnancy prevention.

✅ Arrange for follow-up if this treatment fails to prevent pregnancy.

What Not To Do:

❌ Do not prescribe emergency contraception if the patient is already pregnant; it will not work.

❌ Do not prescribe emergency contraception if the patient has unexplained vaginal bleeding. Assess for sexual assault. Consider if referral to a sexual assault nurse examiner is needed or obtain gynecologic consultation.

Discussion

Hormonal emergency contraception is a safe and effective method to prevent pregnancy after unprotected intercourse, contraceptive failure, or sexual assault. Emergency contraception involves a higher dose of combined estrogen and progestin, or progestin-only, oral contraceptive pills. The levonorgestrel-only formulation (Plan B) causes less nausea and vomiting than combination hormonal regimens. Headache, abdominal pain, and breast tenderness can also occur.

There is currently no evidence, despite numerous studies worldwide, that emergency contraception fosters unsafe sex and decreased rates of use of barrier methods of birth control, which would also protect a woman against sexually transmitted diseases, either in adolescents or in adult women.

Unprotected intercourse 3 days before ovulation results in pregnancy in approximately 15% of women, 1 or 2 days before ovulation in approximately 30%, and on the day of ovulation in approximately 12%. More than 2 days after ovulation, the probability of pregnancy approaches zero. The risk for pregnancy following sexual assault is approximately 5% in victims of reproductive age.

Emergency contraception can reduce the risk for pregnancy by at least 75%, depending on the regimen used and timing of treatment. Using the emergency contraceptive pills at any time during the cycle, research demonstrates less than a 1 in 30 chance of pregnancy (0.03%). Hormonal contraception preparations are more effective the earlier after unprotected intercourse they are taken and are recommended for use within 120 hours. The mechanism of action of hormonal contraception preparations is complex; they may interfere with ovulation, fertilization, or implantation. What is clear is that they do not interrupt an established (implanted) pregnancy, nor are they teratogenic.

Suggested Emergency Help for Clinicians and Patients

Emergency contraceptive hotline and Website: (888) NOT-2-LATE; http://www.not-2-late.com.

National Women's Health Resource Center: 877-986-9472; http://www.healthywomen.org.

Suggested Readings

Abbott J: Emergency contraception: what should our patients expect? *Ann Emerg Med* 46:111–113, 2005.

Association of Reproductive Health Professionals hotline: (800) 584–9911.

Emergency contraception OTC, *Med Lett* 46:10–11, 2004.

Emergency contraceptive kit, *Med Lett* 40:102, 1998.

Harrison T: Availability of emergency contraception: a survey of hospital emergency department staff, *Ann Emerg Med* 46:105–110, 2005.

Ovral as a morning after contraceptive, *Med Lett Drugs Ther* 31:93–94, 1989.

Trussell J, Ellertson C, Rodriguez G: The Yuzpe regimen of emergency contraception: how long after the morning after? *Obstet Gynecol* 88:150–154, 1966.

von Hertzen H, Piaggio G, Ding J, et al: Low-dose mifepristone and two regimens of levonorgestrel for emergency contraception: a WHO multicentre randomized trial, *Lancet* 360:1803–1810, 2002.

Pelvic Inflammatory Disease (PID)

Presentation

A sexually active woman (commonly 15 to 35 years of age), possibly with a new sex partner or multiple sex partners, complains of lower abdominal pain beginning with or soon after her last menstrual period. There may be associated vaginal discharge, malodor, dysuria, dyspareunia, menorrhagia, or intermenstrual bleeding. In patients with more severe infections, fever, chills, malaise, nausea, and vomiting may develop.

Women with severe pelvic pain tend to walk in a slightly bent-over position, holding their lower abdomen and shuffling their feet. Abdominal examination reveals lower quadrant tenderness, sometimes with rebound, and occasionally, there will be right upper quadrant tenderness resulting from gonococcal perihepatitis (Fitz-Hugh–Curtis syndrome). Pelvic examination demonstrates bilateral adnexal tenderness as well as uterine fundal and cervical motion tenderness.

Many women with pelvic inflammatory disease (PID) exhibit subtle or mild symptoms with absence of fever and leukocytosis as well as minimal cervical motion tenderness and adnexal tenderness.

What To Do:

✓ Always perform a pelvic examination on women with lower abdominal complaints or lower abdominal tenderness. The examination should be thorough, yet performed as gently and briefly as possible to avoid exacerbating a very painful condition. When the pain is intolerable, provide IV narcotic analgesia.

✓ Obtain urine for urinalysis and blood or urine for pregnancy testing. A catheterized urine specimen will be required when a vaginal discharge or bleeding is present.

✓ **Obtain endocervical cultures for *Neisseria gonorrhoeae* and *Chlamydia trachomatis.*** Under ideal transport conditions, gonorrheal culture is inexpensive, excellent, and, in some cases, as sensitive as nucleic acid amplification testing. **However, when the maintenance of appropriate transport conditions is not possible, nonculture nucleic acid amplified testing is superior.** Testing for *Chlamydia* has been revolutionized by the emergence of these nucleic acid amplification techniques, which has improved the sensitivity of disease detection by 25% to 30% compared with cultures. Older nonculture techniques, such as direct fluorescent antibody, enzyme immunoassay, and nonamplified nucleic acid hybridization, are even less sensitive than a culture.

✓ **When PID is strongly suspected, obtain blood for syphilis serology and hepatitis B, and recommend human immunodeficiency virus (HIV) testing, because these infections may be contracted simultaneously.**

✅ Consider obtaining a leukocyte count, sedimentation rate, and C-reactive protein level. These are indicators of clinical severity, but normal results do not rule out PID.

✅ **Determine the pH of any vaginal discharge, and make wet-mount examinations and Gram stains of endocervical secretions, looking for *Candida* organisms, *Trichomonas* organisms, leukocytes, and clue cells** (see Chapter 95). Gram stain of the cervical specimen is not adequate for diagnosing gonorrhea in women.

✅ Perform pelvic ultrasonography if there is a suspected mass, severe pain, or a positive pregnancy test. One of the most specific criteria for diagnosing PID is the finding of thickened, fluid-filled tubes, with or without free pelvic fluid, on transvaginal sonography.

✅ **Maintain a low threshold for diagnosing PID. No laboratory tests are diagnostic for PID, and the clinical diagnosis is also imprecise. In addition, the long-term sequelae of missing PID are significant and include infertility, tubo-ovarian abscess (TOA), perihepatitis, chronic pelvic pain, and ectopic pregnancy.**

✅ **Initiate empirical treatment of PID in sexually active young women and other women at risk for sexually transmitted diseases (STDs), if the following minimum criteria are present and no other causes for the illness can be identified:**

- ○ **Uterine/adnexal tenderness**
- ○ **Cervical motion tenderness**

✅ Base treatment on a patient's risk profile. More elaborate diagnostic evaluation often is needed. These **additional criteria** may be used to enhance the specificity of the minimum criteria and further support a diagnosis of PID:

- ○ Oral temperature greater than 101° F (>38.3° C)
- ○ Abnormal cervical or vaginal mucopurulent discharge
- ○ Presence of white blood cells (WBCs) on saline microscopy of vaginal secretions
- ○ Elevated erythrocyte sedimentation rate
- ○ Elevated C-reactive protein level
- ○ Laboratory documentation of cervical infection with *N. gonorrhoeae* or *C. trachomatis*

✅ **Investigate alternative causes for pain if the cervical discharge appears normal and no WBCs are found on the wet-mount preparation. Consider transvaginal sonography and spiral CT scanning to help rule out other potential gynecologic, gastrointestinal (especially appendicitis), or urologic causes.**

✅ **When in doubt, always treat.** Subtle findings may include only a history of abnormal uterine bleeding, dyspareunia, vaginal discharge, or cervical purulence.

✅ **Remove any intrauterine device (IUD).**

✅ **Treat suspected cases while awaiting diagnostic confirmation.** Prevention of long-term sequelae has been linked directly with immediate administration of appropriate antibiotics. When selecting a treatment regimen, consider availability, cost, patient compliance, and antimicrobial susceptibility.

✓ **Hospitalize** all patients with pelvic or tubo-ovarian abscess, pregnancy, high fever (38.5° C), nausea and vomiting that preclude oral antibiotics, or current use of an IUD, as well as when surgical emergencies (e.g., appendicitis) cannot be excluded. Also hospitalize when there is severe illness with septicemia or other serious disease, high risk for poor compliance, failed follow-up, or failure after 48 hours of the outpatient therapy outlined later. No data are available suggesting that adolescent women, women over 35 years of age, or HIV-infected women benefit from hospitalization for treatment of PID unless they meet the criteria as noted above.

✓ **Whether inpatient or outpatient, the Centers for Disease Control and Prevention (CDC), as of 2007, no longer recommends fluoroquinolones as therapy for *N. gonorrhoeae* as a suspected or proven pathogen in PID.** Local resistance patterns may allow use, if less than 5% of isolates are resistant; however, one must have a culture that demonstrates sensitivity, not just a positive nucleic acid amplified test (NAAT). If the NAAT is positive, one must use a cephalosporin to cover *N. gonorrhoeae*.

✓ Inpatient treatment, with or without TOA, consists of IV antibiotics. Give cefotetan, 2 g IV every 12 hours, or cefoxitin, 2 g IV every 6 hours, plus doxycycline, 100 mg orally every 12 hours. (Because of pain associated with infusion, doxycycline should be administered orally when possible, even when the patient is hospitalized.) Alternatively, clindamycin, 900 mg every 8 hours IV, plus gentamycin at a loading dose of 2 g/kg, followed by 1.5 mg/kg every 8 hours. A single daily dose of gentamycin can be substituted. Yet another alternative is ampicillin-sulbactam (3 g every 6 hours IV) with doxycycline (100 mg oral preferred). Transition to oral therapy from parenteral can start after 24 hours, with demonstrated clinical improvement.

✓ **Treat mild to moderate cases on an outpatient basis. Give ceftriaxone (Rocephin), 250 mg IM in a single dose, plus doxycycline, 100 mg PO bid for 14 days, with or without metronidazole (Flagyl), 500 mg PO bid for 14 days. (Coverage of anaerobes may require the addition of metronidazole, which will also effectively treat bacterial vaginosis and trichomoniasis, frequently associated with PID, as well as provide coverage for a patient who recently had a gynecologic instrumentation within the preceding 2 to 3 weeks).**

✓ **Arrange for follow-up examination within 72 hours.** Patients should demonstrate substantial clinical improvement (e.g., defervescence, reduction in direct or rebound abdominal tenderness, and reduction in uterine, adnexal, and cervical motion tenderness) within 3 days of initiation of therapy. Patients who do not improve within this period usually require hospitalization, additional diagnostic tests, and possible surgical intervention.

✓ **Provide analgesics as needed.**

✓ Instruct the patient to abstain from sexual intercourse for at least 2 weeks.

✓ **Unless sexual acquisition can be excluded with certainty, treat the partner for presumptive gonorrhea and chlamydia if he or she had sexual contact with the patient during the 60 days preceding the patient's onset of symptoms. Use ceftriaxone (Rocephin), 125 mg IM once, or ciprofloxacin (Cipro) 500 mg PO once (based on local resistance patterns), 500 mg PO once, PLUS either doxycycline (Vibramycin), 100 mg PO bid × 7 days, or azithromycin (Zithromax), 1000 mg PO once.**

✓ Male partners of women who have PID caused by *C. trachomatis* and/or *N. gonorrhoeae* often are asymptomatic. Sex partners should be treated empirically with regimens that are effective against both of these infections, regardless of the pathogens isolated from the infected woman. Patient-delivered treatment of sex partners was associated with a reduced risk for recurrent gonorrhea and/or chlamydia in a University of Washington (Seattle) study.

✓ **Counsel the patient about the sexually transmitted nature of PID and its risks** for infertility (8% of women after a single case, 19.5% after two episodes, and 40% in those women who had three or more episodes) and ectopic pregnancy, which is increased sixfold to tenfold. Women should also be made aware that as many as 23% of women who develop PID will be troubled with chronic pelvic pain, which is associated with a lower quality of physical and mental health. Barrier methods of contraception (condoms and diaphragms) reduce the risk. Vaginal spermicides are also bactericidal.

✓ **Rescreen the patient in 3 to 4 months,** because reinfection is common. This can be done with consideration of your population and local pattern of prevalence of disease. In one study, 15% to 23% of patients had one or more new infections, and 66% were asymptomatic.

What Not To Do:

Ⓧ Do not miss the more unilateral disorders, such as ectopic pregnancy, appendicitis, ovarian cyst or torsion, and diverticulitis. Early consultation by both a general surgeon and an obstetrician/gynecologist is sometimes necessary.

Ⓧ Do not diagnose PID in a patient with a positive pregnancy test without ruling out ectopic pregnancy, usually with a sonogram.

Ⓧ Do not ignore pelvic symptoms if the patient has gonococcal perihepatic inflammation.

Ⓧ Do not presume to treat for urinary tract infection (UTI) in a patient with lower abdominal pain and when a urine dip demonstrates leukocyte esterase. Do the pelvic exam, because the leukocytes may be from the vaginal discharge of PID.

Ⓧ Do not assume sexual activity based on age.

Ⓧ Do not talk above the educational/comprehension level of the preteen and teenage patient. Their definition of sexual activity and yours may be different.

Discussion

The clinical diagnosis of acute PID is imprecise. The positive predictive value (PPV) of a clinical diagnosis of acute PID differs, depending on epidemiologic characteristics and the clinical setting. There is a higher PPV among sexually active young women (particularly adolescents) and among patients attending STD clinics or from settings in which rates of gonorrhea or chlamydia are high. In all settings, however, no single historical, physical, or laboratory finding is both sensitive and specific for the diagnosis of acute PID (i.e., can be used both to detect all cases of PID and to exclude all women without PID).

In spite of this, prompt diagnosis and early presumptive treatment are crucial to maintaining fertility and avoiding the other complications of PID. It should be kept in mind that the diagnosis and management of other common causes of lower abdominal pain (e.g., ectopic pregnancy, acute

(continued)

Discussion continued

appendicitis, and functional pain) are unlikely to be impaired by initiating empirical antimicrobial therapy for PID.

PID is defined as salpingitis, often accompanied by endometritis or secondary pelvic peritonitis, which results from an ascending genital infection. In the United States, there is an increased risk for PID with multiple sex partners, nonbarrier contraceptive use, instrumentation of the cervix, smoking, minority race, use of an IUD, previous history of PID, and vaginal douching. The incubation period for PID varies from 1 to 2 days to weeks or months.

Gonorrheal and chlamydial infections are thought to initiate conditions that allow organisms from the lower genital tract to ascend into the upper genital tract. The resulting polymicrobial infection includes facultative and anaerobic organisms. A variety of gram-positive and gram-negative aerobic and anaerobic pathogens, such as aerobic streptococci, *Escherichia coli, Bacteroides fragilis, Proteus* spp., and *Peptostreptococcus* spp. can be recovered from the uterus, fallopian tubes, and peritoneal cavity. Gonococcal and chlamydial PID often occur within a week of the onset of menses. The absence of a positive test for *N. gonorrhoeae* or *C. trachomatis* does not rule out PID, because these microbes are only found in 25% to 40% of patients. A mixed aerobic and anaerobic infection is found in 25% to 60% of cases. PID associated with gonorrhea produces relatively rapid and more severe symptoms than chlamydia, whereas the latter is associated with more severe scarring.

Tubo-ovarian abscess (TOA) should be suspected in the setting of PID with persistent fever, despite adequate antibiotics, continued lower abdominal pain, or adnexal mass. Pelvic ultrasonography is highly sensitive (90% to 95%) in diagnosing TOA. It is usually amenable to medical therapy but requires surgical intervention in up to 25% of cases. Surgical intervention for TOA should be considered if there is an increase in the size of the abscess, persistent fever spikes, suspected abscess rupture, or lack of clinical improvement in 48 to 72 hours.

Although all of the gonorrheal isolates in the United States are susceptible to cephalosporins, resistance to quinolones has developed. Fluoroquinolones are no longer recommended for the treatment of PID. Laparoscopy is indicated in severe cases, if diagnosis is uncertain or there is inadequate response to initial antibiotic therapy.

A diagnosis of PID in children or young adolescents should prompt an evaluation for possible child abuse.

Suggested Readings

Arrendondo JL, Oyarzún E, Paz R, et al: Oral clindamycin and ciprofloxacin versus intramuscular ceftriaxone and oral doxycycline in the treatment of mild-to-moderate pelvic inflammatory disease in outpatients, *Clin Infect Dis* 24:170–178, 1997.

Braverman PK: Sexually transmitted diseases in adolescents, *Med Clin North Am* 84:869–889, 2000.

Epperly ATA, Viera AJ: Pelvic inflammatory disease, *Clin Fam Pract* 7:67–78, 2005.

Golden MR, Whittington WL, Handsfield HH, et al: Effect of expedited treatment of sex partners on recurrent or persistent gonorrhea or chlamydial infection, *N Engl J Med* 35:676–685, 2005.

Nasraty S: Infections of the female genital tract, *Prim Care* 30:193–203, vii, 2003.

Ness RB, Soper DE, Holley RL, et al: Effectiveness of inpatient and outpatient treatment strategies for women with pelvic inflammatory disease: results from the pelvic inflammatory disease evaluation and clinical health (PEACH) randomized trial, *Am J Obstet Gynecol* 186:929–937, 2002.

Simms I, Wharburton F, Weström L: Diagnosis of pelvic inflammatory disease: time for a rethink, *Sex Trans Infect* 79:491–494, 2003.

Vaginal Bleeding

Presentation

A menstruating woman complains of greater-than-usual bleeding, which is either off of her usual schedule (metrorrhagia), lasts longer than a typical period, or is heavier than usual (menorrhagia), perhaps with crampy pains and passage of clots. Prolonged bleeding is longer than 7 days duration. Profuse bleeding is generally defined as soaking a large sanitary pad or tampon every hour or two and continuing for more than 2 hours. Excessive menstrual bleeding is quantified typically as greater than 80 mL, with normal menstrual losses over a 5- to 7-day cycle on average of 30 to 45 mL.

What To Do:

✓ Establish whether or not there is hemodynamic instability, clearly identify the source of bleeding, and evaluate the volume of blood loss.

✓ **Obtain orthostatic pulse and blood pressure measurements, a complete blood count, and pregnancy test** (urine or serum beta human chorionic gonadotropin [hCG]). Measurement of beta hCG is required in all menstruating women, except when there are positive fetal heart tones, a known pregnancy, or a definite history of hysterectomy. All others should have beta hCG measured, including those with tubal ligation, Norplant, and claims of celibate lifestyle, as well as those whose doctors have told them they cannot get pregnant. (To avoid unintentionally insulting a patient, inform them that pregnancy testing is routinely required on all cases of vaginal bleeding.) Although less reliable than hemoglobin and hematocrit measurements, try to quantify the amount of bleeding by the presence of clots and the number of saturated pads used. In the United States, regular to super plus tampons hold 6 to 15 mL of blood.

✓ If the patient is deemed hemodynamically unstable, arrange for rapid transport to an acute care setting, such as an emergency department by ambulance. Start an IV line of normal saline or lactated Ringer solution and have blood ready to transfuse on short notice if there is significant bleeding—demonstrated by pallor, lightheadedness, tachycardia, orthostatic pressure changes, a pulse increase of more than 20 per minute on standing, or a hematocrit below 30%. Consider intrauterine tamponade by packing the uterus with Kerlix. Uterine curettage is first-line therapy for the unstable patient with acute or prolonged uterine bleeding. Uterine artery embolization is first-line therapy for those with uterine arteriovenous malformation. Hysterectomy is recommended when all other treatments have failed.

✅ **If the patient is hemodynamically stable, go ahead and begin to get your patient's history, including a menstrual, sexual, and reproductive history.** Are her periods usually irregular, occasionally this heavy? Does she take oral contraceptive pills, and has she missed enough to produce estrogen withdrawal bleeding? Is an intrauterine device (IUD) in place and contributing to cramps, bleeding, and infection? Was her last period missed or light, or is this period late, suggesting an anovulatory cycle, a spontaneous abortion, or an ectopic pregnancy? Ask about bruising, petechiae, or other signs suggestive of coagulopathy. Ask about use of anticoagulants, such as aspirin or warfarin (Coumadin). Ask about any history of thyroid, renal, or hepatic disease, and determine if the patient is involved in high-risk sexual activity (e.g., unprotected sexual intercourse, new and/or multiple sexual partners, trauma). Also inquire about any known structural abnormalities, such as a history of fibroid uterus.

✅ **Determine the source of bleeding by inspecting the vulva, vagina, cervical surface/os, uterus, and anus.**

✅ **Perform a speculum and bimanual vaginal examination,** looking particularly for signs of pregnancy, such as a soft, blue cervix, enlarged uterus, or passage of fetal parts with the blood. Ascertain that the blood is coming from the cervical os and not from a laceration, polyp, cervical lesion, or other vaginal or uterine disease or infection. Test for gonorrhea and chlamydia when infection may be a factor. Especially consider the young sexually active patient with intermenstrual spotting and/or prolonged menses (see Chapters 83, 93, and 95). Feel for adnexal masses as well as pelvic tenderness. Spread any questionable products of conception on gauze or suspend in saline to differentiate from organized clot. Gently press sterile ring forceps against the cervix to see whether they enter the uterus, indicating that the internal os is open (an inevitable, complete, or incomplete abortion) or closed (not pregnant or a threatened abortion, the fetus having roughly even odds of survival, which is generally treated with bed rest alone).

✅ **Obtain a transvaginal ultrasonogram and quantitative beta hCG level if the urine beta hCG is positive, or there is any uterine or adnexal abnormality on pelvic examination.** A sonogram will help assess the age and viability of the fetus in an intrauterine pregnancy. An ectopic gestational sac may be seen. A sonogram showing an empty uterus, despite a positive pregnancy test, is consistent with either a very early intrauterine pregnancy, an ectopic pregnancy, or a recent complete abortion. When the beta hCG result is positive and the patient's condition remains stable, repeat the level measurement in 48 hours.

✅ **With incomplete spontaneous abortions, deliver any products of conception that protrude from the cervical os using steady gentle traction with sponge forceps while compressing and massaging the uterus. If bleeding continues, start an IV infusion of oxytocin (Pitocin), 20 mU/min, to diminish the rate of hemorrhage. Alternatively, place 10 to 20 IU of oxytocin in 1 L of 0.9% normal saline and run it at 200 to 500 mL/hr, or give methylergonovine (Methergine), 0.2 mg IM (contraindicated in the hypertensive patient).** Obtain gynecologic consultation to consider performing a dilation and curettage (D&C) for emergent termination of the uterine bleeding. **With all bleeding while pregnant, test the mother's Rh status,** and, if negative, administer Rh immunoglobulin (RhoGAM), 50 µg IM if the uterus was less than 12 weeks' size, 300 µg IM if larger.

✅ **Send the stable patient with a threatened abortion home, as determined by an ultrasonogram positive for an intrauterine pregnancy, unless there is severe pain or hemorrhage.** Bed rest has not been shown to improve the outcome for a threatened abortion but is still usually part of the regimen.

✅ **Begin treatment for dysfunctional uterine bleeding** when the patient is hemodynamically stable and any anatomic lesions, systemic disease, infection, and pregnancy have been ruled out. **This is usually not feasible on the patient's first visit. When it is necessary to help control vaginal bleeding in the nonpregnant patient who has moderate hemorrhage, oral conjugated estrogen (Premarin), 2.5 mg PO qid can be given until the bleeding subsides. Typically, bleeding will stop within 10 to 24 hours. For mild to moderate bleeding, the dose can be bid, but is not to be continued for more than 21 to 25 days. After the estrogen, a progestin should be given, medroxyprogesterone acetate, 5 to 10 mg orally, daily for 5 to 10 days, start on day 16 or 21 of cycle.** Warn the patient that after the initial reduction of bleeding, there will be an increase in hemorrhage when the uterine lining is sloughed.

✅ **If bleeding does not subside,** consider a structural problem. Conjugated estrogen (Premarin), 25 mg, can be given IV and repeated every 4 to 6 hours (per manufacturer, every 6 to 12 hours; per ACOG [American College of Obstetricians and Gynecologists] 2000, every 4 hours for 24 hours if needed). It will take several hours to have an effect. When available, this treatment should be coordinated with a consulting gynecologist. Estrogens cause nausea and vomiting in high doses; therefore an antiemetic should also be prescribed.

✅ **Use the more convenient regimen of oral contraceptive pills with at least 35 μg ethinyl estradiol (Necon 10/11 or Ortho Novum 10/11), administered at a dose of one pill qid tapered for 3 to 5 days until the bleeding stops, and then decreased to one pill per day until the month's pack is completed.** Provide the patient with an antiemetic, and prepare her for withdrawal bleeding at the end of this new cycle. The vaginal rings and contraceptive patches have no role in treating profuse or prolonged bleeding.

✅ **Treat simple menorrhagia and mild dysfunctional uterine bleeding with standard regimens of oral contraceptives plus nonsteroidal anti-inflammatory drugs (NSAIDs)** given on the first 3 days of the menstrual period.

✅ If the cause of the uterine bleeding was missed oral contraceptive pills, advise the patient to resume the pills but use additional contraception for the first cycle to prevent pregnancy.

✅ If the cause is a new IUD, the patient may elect to have it removed and use another contraceptive technique.

✅ **In most cases, the patient should be referred for follow-up to a gynecologist for definitive diagnosis, adjustment of medications, or further treatment.** She may be evaluated by hysteroscopy, ultrasonography, and endometrial biopsy. Endometrial ablation is an option for those for whom medical therapy has been unsuccessful or is contraindicated because of thrombosis risks. This procedure is also recommended, rather than D&C, for those patients bleeding from polyps or intracavitary leiomyomas.

✅ D&C is still recommended for removing retained products of conception and for those women wishing to maintain fertility.

✅ **Medical evaluation may reveal liver disease, hypothyroidism (even when there is a minimally high thyroid-stimulating hormone [TSH] level, there may be a response to treatment), or a bleeding disorder (especially thrombocytopenia and von Willebrand disease).**

What Not To Do:

(X) Do not prescribe estrogen therapy to women at risk for intravascular thrombosis. In these women, use progestins or provide surgical intervention.

(X) Do not leap to a diagnosis of dysfunctional uterine bleeding without ruling out pregnancy.

(X) Do not rule out pregnancy or venereal infection in patients who are not at risk on the basis of a negative sexual history—confirm with physical examination and laboratory tests.

(X) Do not give aspirin for menorrhagia. It is not effective and may increase bleeding.

(X) Do not attempt to use methylergonovine in the nonpregnant patient. It has no effect.

Discussion

The patient's age should direct you to the most likely cause of her vaginal bleeding. Vaginal bleeding in a newborn may be the result of withdrawal of maternal hormones. In **prepubertal girls,** look for anatomic lesions, urethral prolapse, vulvovaginal infections, endocrinopathies, neoplasia, rectal fissures, trauma, or foreign bodies, and consider abuse. Scratching prompted by dermatoses may also cause bleeding. In **postmenarchal adolescents and women of reproductive age,** consider pregnancy-related problems first, then dysfunctional uterine bleeding (anovulatory cycles), infection with sexually transmitted diseases, anatomic lesions (fibroids, cervical polyps), and systemic illnesses (hypothyroidism, bleeding disorders). In **nonpregnant adolescents,** 50% of severe menorrhagia at the first menses is result of coagulopathy (i.e., thrombocytopenia, immune thrombocytopenic purpura, platelet dysfunction, and von Willebrand disease). In **perimenopausal and postmenopausal women,** strongly consider the possibility of malignant disease, and then evaluate for atrophic vaginitis, fibroids, polyps, anovulatory dysfunctional uterine bleeding, liver disease, anticoagulation therapy, and bleeding disorders. A third of postmenopausal bleeding is associated with common premalignant or malignant conditions of the endometrium (e.g., hyperplasia and atypia).

Dysfunctional uterine bleeding is a diagnosis of exclusion. It is usually hormonal in etiology and can be the result of abnormal endogenous hormone production or the result of problems with the administration of prescribed synthetic sex hormones, such as oral contraceptive pills. During an anovulatory cycle, there is no progesterone,

which results in a chaotic estrogen-stimulated endometrial proliferation. The uterine lining, therefore, hypertrophies and sloughs erratically, resulting in excessive or irregular uterine bleeding. This occurs most commonly around the time of menarche in girls and menopause in women. Other causes include a severely restricted diet, prolonged exercise, and significant emotional stress. Breakthrough bleeding is a form of estrogen withdrawal while taking low-dose estrogen oral contraceptives. Changing to a higher-dose pill will generally eliminate this problem. Also consider drug interactions with certain anticonvulsants and antibiotics.

The essential steps in the emergency evaluation and management of vaginal bleeding are fluid resuscitation of shock, if present; recognition of any anatomic lesion, infection, or pregnancy; and complications of pregnancy, such as spontaneous abortion or ectopic pregnancy. Treatment of the more chronic and less severe dysfunctional uterine bleeding usually consists of iron replacement and optional use of oral contraceptives to decrease menstrual irregularity (metrorrhagia) and volume (menorrhagia).

Warn the patient that after the initial reduction of bleeding, there will be an increase in hemorrhage when the uterine lining is sloughed on hormone withdrawal.

The half-life of beta hCG after the end of pregnancy is 1.5 days, and a sensitive pregnancy test may remain positive for 2 to 4 weeks after a miscarriage or abortion.

Suggested Readings

Bevan JA, Maloney KW, Hillery CA, et al: Bleeding disorders: a common cause of menorrhagia in adolescents, *J Pediatr* 138:856–861, 2001.

Falcone T, Desjardins C, Bourque J, et al: Dysfunctional uterine bleeding in adolescents, *J Reprod Med* 39:761–764, 1994.

Heller DS: Lower genital tract disease in children and adolescents—a review, *J Pediatr Adolesc Gynecol* 18:75–83, 2005.

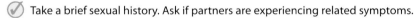

Vaginitis

Presentation

A woman complains of a vaginal discharge, possibly with itching and/or irritation of the labia and vagina. Odor, external dysuria, vague low abdominal discomfort, or dyspareunia may be present. (Suprapubic discomfort, internal dysuria, and urinary urgency and frequency suggest cystitis.)

Abdominal examination is benign, but examination of the introitus may reveal erythema of the vulva and edema of the labia, often with pustulopapular peripheral lesions (especially with *Candida* organisms). Speculum examination may disclose a diffusely red, inflamed vaginal mucosa with an adherent thick, white discharge resembling cottage cheese. These findings are also most likely the result of *Candida* organisms, especially when associated with vulvar pruritus.

A thin, homogeneous, gray-to-white milklike discharge smoothly coating the vaginal wall and having a fishy odor is characteristic of bacterial vaginosis.

Profuse yellow-green, sometimes frothy discharge with an unpleasant malodor and associated with vulvar irritation is characteristic of *Trichomonas* organisms.

Bimanual examination should show a nontender cervix and uterus, without adnexal tenderness or masses or pain on cervical motion (if present, see Chapter 93).

The appearance of the discharge is not pathognomonic and testing needs to confirm any suspicion.

What To Do:

✓ Take a brief sexual history. Ask if partners are experiencing related symptoms.

✓ Perform speculum and bimanual pelvic examination.

✓ **Collect urine for possible culture and pregnancy tests that may influence treatment.**

✓ **Swab the cervix or urethra to culture for *Neisseria gonorrhoeae* and swab the endocervix to test for *Chlamydia*** (see Chapter 83).

✓ **Touch pH indicator paper (Hydrion pH papers, ColorpHast pH Test Strips) to the vaginal mucus.** A pH greater than 4.5 suggests bacterial vaginosis or *Trichomonas* organisms, but this is only useful if there is no blood or semen to buffer vaginal secretions. A normal pH (4 to 4.5) is found with *Candida* vulvovaginitis. Normal pH for a premenarchal or postmenopausal woman is 4.7, thus a less reliable test in these patients.

✓ For wet-mount examination, dab a drop of vaginal secretions on a slide, add a drop of 0.9% NaCl and a cover slip, and examine under 400× magnification for swimming protozoa (*Trichomonas vaginalis*), epithelial cells covered by adherent bacilli ("clue cells" of bacterial vaginosis), or pseudohyphae and spores ("spaghetti and meatballs" appearance of *Candida albicans*) (Figures 95-1 and 95-2).

✓ If epithelial cells obscure the view of yeast, add a drop of 10% potassium hydroxide (KOH), smell whether this liberates the odor of stale fish (characteristic of *Gardnerella* organisms [bacterial vaginosis], *Trichomonas* organisms, and semen), and look again under the microscope for hyphae, pseudohyphae, or budding yeast.

✓ Gram stain a second specimen. This is an even more sensitive method for detecting *Candida* organisms and clue cells (see Figure 95-2, *B*), as well as a means to assess the general vaginal flora, which is normally mixed with occasional predominance of gram-positive rods.

✓ When available, culture for *T. vaginalis* using Diamond's medium, or other rapid tests available will confirm most cases of *Trichomonas* infection.

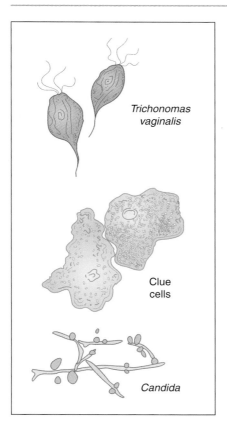

Trichonomas vaginalis

Clue cells

Candida

Figure 95-1 Test vaginal mucus on a slide with saline.

✅ If *Trichomonas vaginalis* is the cause, **prescribe metronidazole (Flagyl), 2 g, as one oral dose. A more expensive alternative that appears to be more effective and has fewer side effects is tinidazole (Tindamax), also taken as a single 2-g oral dose.** Tinidazole is considered a second-generation nitroimidazole. The patient must abstain from alcohol for 24 hours postmetronidazole and 3 days after the last dose of tinidazole because of the disulfiram-like activity of these drugs. Men infected with *T. vaginalis* may be asymptomatic or have symptoms of urethral irritation and/or discharge, or they may develop prostatitis (see Chapters 82 and 83). **Sex partners must receive the same treatment as the patient.** Advise the patient and her partner to refrain from intercourse or to use a condom until therapy has been completed and patient and partners are asymptomatic, at least 7 days. Follow-up is unnecessary for men and women who become asymptomatic after treatment or who are initially asymptomatic.

✅ Pregnant women who are symptomatic with trichomoniasis may be treated with a single 2-g dose of metronidazole, although 500 mg bid for 5 to 7 days is much better tolerated in patients already prone to nausea. Multiple studies and meta-analyses have not demonstrated a consistent association between metronidazole use during pregnancy and teratogenic or mutagenic effects in infants. The Centers for Disease Control and Prevention (CDC) no longer

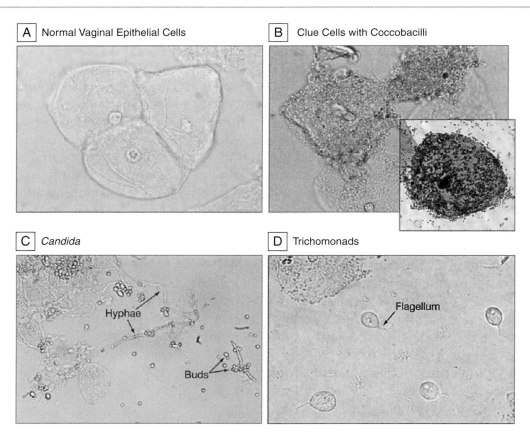

| A | Normal Vaginal Epithelial Cells | B | Clue Cells with Coccobacilli |

| C | *Candida* | D | Trichomonads |

Hyphae
Buds
Flagellum

Figure 95-2 Microscopic examination of vaginal samples. (Adapted from Anderson MR, Klink K, Cohrssen A: Evaluation of vaginal complaints. *JAMA* 291:1368–1379, 2004.)

discourages the use of metronidazole in the first trimester. However, one study did note preterm labor increased when treating with metronidazole orally, thus treatment of asymptomatic pregnant patients can be delayed until after delivery. If symptomatic, consider clotrimazole 1% intravaginally for 7 days. This will relieve symptoms but is unlikely to eradicate the organisms; thus delayed treatment postdelivery will be needed.

✓ **When the diagnosis of vulvovaginal candidiasis (VVC) is suggested clinically by a white cottage cheese–like discharge, pruritus and erythema in the vulvovaginal area, and vaginal pH less than or equal to 4.5, and when yeasts or pseudohyphae are demonstrated on either a wet preparation or a Gram stain, recommend fluconizole 150 mg PO as a single dose. It is secreted in vaginal secretions for 72 hours postingestion and is at least as effective as intravaginal treatment. In addition, it is preferred by many patients. Alternatively, if the oral route is not preferred or medication interaction precludes its use, miconazole (Monistat), 200-mg vaginal suppositories should be recommended. These are to be inserted qhs × 3 days, or alternatively, tioconazole (Monistat-1 or Vagistat-1), 6.5% cream, 5 g intravaginally can be used in a single application. (Use of cream also soothes irritated mucosa.) These treatments are available without prescription.**

✓ With severe VVC (i.e., extensive vulvar erythema, edema, excoriation, and fissure formation), have the patient use clotrimazole (Mycelex) 1% cream, 5 g intravaginally for 7 to 14 days, or prescribe 150 mg of fluconazole in two sequential doses (second dose 72 hours after the initial dose). **In patients with severe discomfort secondary to vulvitis, low-potency steroid creams used for the first 48 hours, in combination with a topical antifungal cream may be of benefit.** Women with medical conditions such as uncontrolled diabetes or those receiving corticosteroid treatment also require more prolonged (i.e., 7 to 14 days), conventional antimycotic treatment. During pregnancy, only topical azole therapies, applied for 7 days, are recommended. Sex partners need not be treated unless they have balanitis. The patient only needs to return for follow-up visits if her symptoms persist or recur within 2 months of her initial treatment.

✓ For recurrent infections, Fluconazole may be repeated and thus taken days 1, 4, and 7. Gastrointestinal side effects are fairly common, and serious side effects can occur. For recurrent *Candida,* the American Infectious Disease Society recommends 10 to 14 days of a topical or oral azole, such as miconizole or clotrimazole, followed by **6 months** of either a clotrimazole 200-mg vaginal suppository twice weekly or weekly doses of oral fluconazole 150 mg.

✓ **If the diagnosis is bacterial vaginosis, prescribe metronidazole (Flagyl), 500 mg orally bid for 7 days; or tinidazole (Tindamax) can be used orally at 1 g daily for 5 days or 2 g daily for 2 days (taken with food). Alternatively, metronidazole, 0.75% vaginal gel (MetroGel-Vaginal), one applicator intravaginally qhs for 5 days; or clindamycin, 2% vaginal cream (Cleocin), one 5-g applicator intravaginally qhs for 7 days.** Alternative therapy includes metronidazole as a single 2-g oral dose (noted to have lower efficacy than the above mentioned regimen); clindamycin, 300 mg orally bid for 7 days; or clindamycin ovules, 100 mg intravaginally qhs for 3 days. A topical single dose bioadhesive form of clindamycin is available (Clindesse); the patient uses one applicator. It is not clear as yet, but this may be less effective than other agents. Clindamycin-resistant organisms can develop in the vaginal mucosa postintravaginal treatment.

✓ Intravaginal treatment is more expensive but carries fewer gastrointestinal side effects than the oral form, and some patients prefer using intravaginal products for treating this vaginosis.

Vaginal therapy is considered more inconvenient by other patients and is associated with a high risk for vaginal candidiasis (10% to 30%). Metronidazole and timidazole cannot be used for 3 days after drinking alcohol. Sex partners need not be treated unless they have balanitis.

✓ During pregnancy, prescribe metronidazole, 500 mg orally bid or 250 mg orally tid for 7 days, or clindamycin, 300 mg orally bid for 7 days. Some prefer to use oral rather than topical therapy in pregnancy because it may also treat subclinical coinfections. Vaginal treatment is less preferred in pregnancy because of concerns about possible preterm labor.

✓ **Follow-up visits are unnecessary unless symptoms recur.**

✓ To prevent rebound *C. albicans* after antibiotics reduce the normal vaginal flora, or for treatment of mild vaginitis, consider having patients douche with 1% acetic acid (half-strength white vinegar) to maintain a normal low pH vaginal ecology.

✓ Remember that a patient may harbor more than one infection.

✓ Instruct the patient in the prevention of vaginitis. She should avoid routine douching, perfumed soaps and feminine hygiene sprays, and tight, poorly ventilated clothing.

✓ The differential

○ **Ninety percent of all cases of vaginitis are caused by bacterial vaginosis, vulvovaginal candidiasis, or trichomonal vaginitis.** However, there are noninfectious causes as well— physiologic leukorrhea, a generally nonmalodorous, mucous-like, white or yellowish discharge without other symptoms, is usually estrogen induced. Atrophic vaginitis, caused by estrogen deficiency leads to inflammation of the vagina, and topical estrogen is the treatment of choice. Desquamative inflammatory vaginitis is rare, with signs and symptoms of pain, profuse discharge, and epithelial cell exfoliation. Clindamycin, for its antibacterial as well as its anti-inflammatory effect, works well for these patients. Seminal plasma allergy is in the differential; although rare, it presents with postcoital itching, burning, edema, and erythema and can have systemic symptoms as well.

What Not To Do:

✗ Do not blindly prescribe creams or other therapies for nonspecific symptoms of vaginitis. Perform the appropriate physical examination and laboratory tests before initiating one of the treatment regimens recommended.

✗ Do not miss underlying pelvic inflammatory disease, pregnancy, or diabetes, all of which can potentiate vaginitis.

✗ Do not attempt to treat trichomoniasis with metronidazole gel. It is unlikely to achieve therapeutic levels in the urethra and perivaginal glands where infection is also located, and is considerably less efficacious than oral preparations.

✗ Do not recommend the use of commercially obtainable unstandardized *Lactobacillus* for treatment of bacterial vaginosis. Recurrence rates are high, and vaginal *Lactobacillus* replacement remains a clinical research endeavor.

✗ Do not miss candidiasis because the vaginal secretions appear essentially normal in consistency, color, volume, and odor. Nonpregnant patients may not develop thrush patches, curds, or caseous discharge.

🚫 Do not treat patients based on self-diagnosis. In one study, only 33.7% of women who self diagnosed vulvovaginal candidiasis were ultimately confirmed to have the disorder.

🚫 Do not treat sex partners of patients with bacterial vaginosis or *C. albicans* unless they show signs of infection or have had recurrent infections.

Discussion

Trichomoniasis and bacterial vaginosis are often grouped together, despite major differences in etiology, pathophysiology, and transmission implications. The reason that these two entities are frequently considered together is that they present with elevated vaginal pH, major shifts in vaginal flora, and abnormal vaginal discharge that is characteristically malodorous. Also, they frequently coexist.

Trichomonas vaginalis is a parasite that is transmitted primarily through sexual activity. In addition to the vaginal discomfort, trichomoniasis facilitates the transmission of human immunodeficiency virus (HIV). During pregnancy, infection has been associated with delivery of low-birth-weight infants and preterm deliveries. Diagnosis is typically made by identification of motile trichomonads on a saline wet preparation. It is important to note that wet-mount examination can be negative in up to 50% of culture-confirmed cases. Therefore, in suspect cases in which the wet-mount examination is negative, it is important to culture the vaginal discharge on Diamond Hollander medium or to use a DNA probe test (e.g., Affirm VPIII [Becton Dickinson and Company, Sparks, Md.]).

It is thought that bacterial vaginosis (BV) results from a disturbance in the normal vaginal flora, whereby the normal levels of *Lactobacillus* are reduced and replaced by less dominant organisms, such as *Gardnerella vaginalis, Mycoplasma, Mobiluncus, Bacteroides* spp., and *Peptostreptococcus. Lactobacillus* is necessary to maintain normal vaginal pH (<4.5) and to prevent proliferation of other organisms. Risk factors associated with BV include the number of sex partners in the previous 12 months, douching, smoking, and low socioeconomic conditions.

Patients with BV usually complain of thin, off-white, fishy-smelling discharge. However, because studies have demonstrated poor a correlation between vaginal symptoms and the final cause of vaginitis, clinicians should not treat vaginal complaints empirically based on patient history alone. BV is often diagnosed on the basis of a typical history in conjunction with clue cells on a wet preparation or an elevated vaginal pH. Although this approach to diagnosis is not unreasonable, accuracy can be improved by using complete Amsel criteria. This includes (1) milky homogeneous adherent discharge, (2) vaginal pH greater than 4.5, (3) clue cells in the vaginal fluid on light microscopy, and (4) positive whiff test. If three out of the four criteria are present, there is a 90% likelihood of BV. Cultures are not helpful in diagnosing BV. The Affirm VPIII DNA probe is a highly sensitive and specific test but is expensive, and there is a moderate delay for results. Gram staining is highly reliable and inexpensive, but it is not always available in a doctor's office.

Bacterial vaginosis has been so called because of the absence of inflammatory signs traditionally associated with *C. vaginitis.* As such, in the absence of pain, soreness, burning, and dyspareunia, BV has been considered a noninflammatory condition— hence, the term vaginosis, and not vaginitis. The lack of major inflammatory signs has correlated with the lack of polymorphonuclear leukocyte accumulation in vaginal secretions in BV.

In pregnant women, BV has been associated with an approximately twofold risk for developing preterm delivery, premature rupture of membranes, low birth weight, and postpartum endometritis. Women who have BV are more likely to have upper genital tract infections than those who do not. Similarly, women who have pelvic inflammatory disease (PID) are more likely to have BV.

C. albicans is usually implicated as the cause of yeast infection. Vulvovaginal candidiasis (VVC) may be caused by less common nonalbicans species, such as *C. glabrata* and *C. tropicalis,* which tend to be more resistant to standard treatment.

Established risk factors for VVC include uncontrolled diabetes, steroid-induced immunosuppression, recent antibiotic use, and infection with HIV. *C. albicans* is more common in the summer under tight or nonporous clothing (jeans, synthetic underwear,

(continued)

Discussion continued

and wet bathing suits). Vulvar pruritus is the most common symptom of VVC. Vaginal discharge is often minimal and sometimes absent. Although described as cottage cheese–like in character, the discharge may vary from watery to homogeneously thick.

Symptoms and signs are extremely nonspecific and can be simulated by a variety of noninfectious causes (e.g., contact and irritant dermatitis). In fact, only 20% of women presenting with pruritus have VVC. A recent assessment of the criteria for wet preparation–based diagnosis suggests that this approach is neither highly sensitive nor specific when using culture as the gold standard for diagnosis. Although costly, vaginal culture can be helpful in cases of recurrent symptoms or in women with typical symptoms and a negative KOH preparation. A reasonable approach is to reserve culture for cases of treatment failure and to

routinely use a wet mount and KOH preparation or a Gram stain of a vaginal discharge in conjunction with physical examination findings. DNA-based diagnostic tools with fairly good degrees of sensitivity and specificity are also available.

Symptoms alone do not allow clinicians to distinguish confidently between the causes of vaginitis. However, if there is no itching, candidiasis is less likely, and lack of perceived odor makes bacterial vaginosis unlikely. Similarly, physical examination signs are limited in their diagnostic power. The presence of inflammatory signs is associated with candidiasis. Presence of a "high cheese" odor on examination is predictive of bacterial vaginosis, whereas lack of odor is associated with candidiasis. Laboratory tests, particularly microscopy of vaginal discharge, are the most useful way of diagnosing the three conditions described in this chapter.

Suggested Readings

Abbott J: Clinical and microscopic diagnosis of vaginal yeast infection: a prospective analysis, *Ann Emerg Med* 25:587–591, 1995.

Anderson MR, Klink K, Cohrssen A: Evaluation of vaginal complaints, *JAMA* 291:1368–1379, 2004.

Carr PL, Rothberg MB, Friedman RH, et al: "Shotgun" versus sequential testing: cost-effectiveness of diagnostic strategies for vaginitis, *J Gen Intern Med* 20:793–799, 2005.

Clenney TL, Jorgensen SK, Owen M: Vaginitis, *Clin Fam Pract* 7:57–66, 2005.

Ferris DG, Litaker MS, Woodward L, et al: Treatment of bacterial vaginosis: a comparison of oral metronidazole, metronidazole vaginal gel, and clindamycin vaginal cream, *J Fam Pract* 41:443–449, 1995.

Klebandt MA, Carey JC, Hauth JC, et al: Failure of metronidazole to prevent preterm delivery among pregnant women with asymptomatic *Trichomonas vaginalis* infection, *N Engl J Med* 345:487–493, 2001.

Martin DH, Mroczkowski TF, Dalu ZA, et al: A controlled trial of a single dose of azithromycin for the treatment of chlamydial urethritis and cervicitis, *N Engl J Med* 327:921–925, 1992.

Schwebke JR, Hillier SL, Sobel JD, et al: Validity of the vaginal Gram stain for the diagnosis of bacterial vaginosis, *Obstet Gynecol* 88:573–576, 1996.

Sobel JD: What's new in bacterial vaginosis and trichomoniasis? *Infect Dis Clin North Am* 19:387–406, 2005.

Spence MR, Hartwell TS, Davies MC, et al: The minimum single oral metronidazole dose for treating trichomoniasis: a randomized, blinded study, *Obstet Gynecol* 85:699–703, 1997.

Swedberg J, Steiner JF, Deiss F, et al: Comparison of a single-dose vs one-week course of metronidazole for symptomatic bacterial vaginosis, *J Am Med Assoc* 254:1046–1049, 1985.

Trager JDK: What's your diagnosis? Well-demarcated vulvar erythema in two girls, *J Pediatr Adolesc Gynecol* 18:43–46, 2005.

Vazquez JA, Sobel JD: Mucosal candidiasis, *Infect Dis Clin North Am* 16:793–820, 2002.

Watson MC, Grimshaw JM, Bond CM, et al: Oral versus intravaginal imidazole and triazole antifungal agents for the treatment of uncomplicated vulvovaginal candidiasis (thrush), *Br J Obstet Gynecol* 109:85–95, 2002.

Zeger W, Holt K: Gynecologic infections, *Emerg Med Clin North Am* 21:631–648, 2003.

PART 9

Musculoskeletal Emergencies

■ Philip Buttaravoli ■ Laurel Plante ■ Wayne Misselbeck

CHAPTER

Acromioclavicular (Shoulder) Separation

96

Presentation

After a direct blow or a fall onto the tip of the shoulder with the arm adducted, the patient complains of shoulder pain increased by moderate motion of the arm. An indirect mechanism of injury commonly involves a fall onto an outstretched arm or falling back onto an elbow (Figure 96-1, *A* and *B*). Usually, patients can localize their pain to the acromioclavicular (AC) joint accurately.

Signs such as swelling, abrasions, or bruising may be evident, either on the superior shoulder, implying a direct mechanism, or on the elbow or forearm, implying an indirect mechanism. The AC joint is tender to palpation. (It is superficial and easily palpated.)

There may be no deformity, there may be a step-off between the acromion process of the scapula and the distal end of the clavicle, or the distal clavicle may be displaced superiorly and no longer connected to the acromion (Figure 96-2). These findings roughly correspond to a type I, type II (Figure 96-3), or type III (Figure 96-4) disruption of the AC joint.

Usually, the patient will come in right away because it hurts even without movement (type I or type II tear), or he may come in days later without pain, having noted that the injured shoulder hangs lower or the clavicle rides higher (type III) (see Figure 96-2). There is a 5:1 male to female injury rate.

What To Do:

✅ **Provide analgesia as needed (acetaminophen, nonsteroidal anti-inflammatory drugs [NSAIDs], and/or narcotics).**

✅ Palpate the entire shoulder girdle, including the head of the humerus. There should be tenderness only over the AC joint with varying prominence of the distal clavicle, depending on the severity of the injury. Gentle passive rotation of the humerus should not cause more pain, but there should be pain with the cross-body adduction test. This is done by elevating the

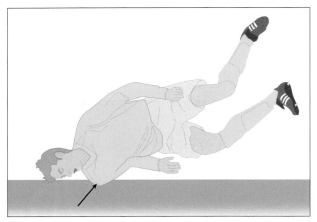

A

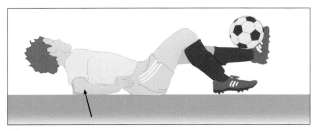

B

Figure 96-1 A, The most common mechanism of injury to the AC joint results from a direct blow onto the tip of the shoulder. **B,** An indirect force, such as a fall onto the elbow, may also disrupt the AC joint. (Adapted from Buss DD, Watts JD: Acromioclavicular injuries in the throwing athlete. *Clin Sports Med* 22:327-341, 2003.)

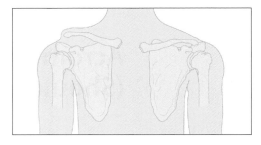

Figure 96-2 Step-off deformity of grade III injury. (Adapted from Knoop KJ, Stack LB, Storrow AB: *Atlas of emergency medicine.* New York, 1997, McGraw-Hill.) (Courtesy Frank Birinyi, MD.)

arm on the affected side to 90 degrees of forward flexion and then adducting it passively as far as possible. Pain localized over the AC joint is a positive cross-body adduction test. (It is not necessary to do this test when there is an obvious deformity.)

 Examine the patient for a possible sternoclavicular joint dislocation or clavicle fracture by palpating over the entire length of the clavicle.

 Strength may be decreased because of pain, but other bones, joints, range of motion, sensation, and circulation should be documented as being intact. Evaluation for neurologic injury is important because of the close proximity of the brachial plexus.

 Obtain a radiograph of the shoulder to be sure that there is no associated fracture of the lateral clavicle or coracoid, or fracture or dislocation of the humerus. Routine AC joint radiographs include anteroposterior (AP), 10-degree caudal tilt, and axillary views (to determine the position of the clavicle with respect to the acromion). Comparison views may be useful to allow measurements of the coracoclavicular distance and distal clavicle

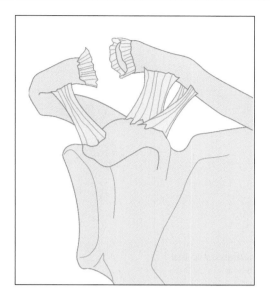

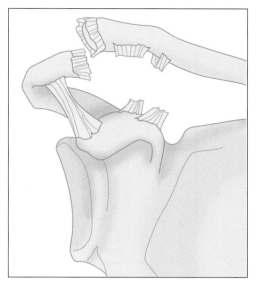

Figure 96-3 Type II injury with rupture of the AC ligament. (Adapted from Montellese P, Dancy T: The acromioclavicular joint. *Prim Care* 31:857-866, 2004.)

Figure 96-4 Type III injury with rupture of the AC and coracoclavicular ligaments. (Adapted from Montellese P, Dancy T: The acromioclavicular joint. *Prim Care* 31:857-866, 2004.)

position in the unaffected AC joint. **Weight-bearing stress views are uncomfortable and unnecessary.**

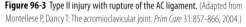 In a type I injury, the AC ligaments are sprained but intact. The coracoclavicular ligaments are intact, and the distal clavicle is stable and in normal anatomic alignment. In a type II injury, the AC ligaments are torn. The coracoclavicular ligaments are sprained but intact, and the distal clavicle is mobile in the axial plane with less than 50% subluxation.

✓ **Type I and II injuries are treated the same and differ only in the time to recovery. Provide analgesics and a sling, as needed, to provide pain relief. As quickly as tolerated, the patient should begin active range-of-motion exercises.** Once the range of motion is full and pain free, the performance of progressive strengthening and activity-specific exercises will prove that the patient is capable of returning to activity successfully and safely. This is variable and may take 2 to 12 weeks of rest and rehabilitation. With return to play, some football players may place a soft felt cut-out pad (doughnut pads or spider pads) in their shoulder pads to reduce the pain from a potential second impact.

✓ Type III injuries involve disruption of the acromioclavicular and coracoclavicular ligaments, resulting in an unstable joint. There is a 25% to 100% displacement of the AC joint. The distal clavicle is mobile in the axial and coronal planes. These are the injuries referred to in the older literature as AC dislocations.

✓ **Treatment of type III injuries remains controversial. The evidence suggests that conservative therapy is the initial treatment of choice, and that surgery should be reserved for patients who have chronic pain and weakness. Conservative treatment**

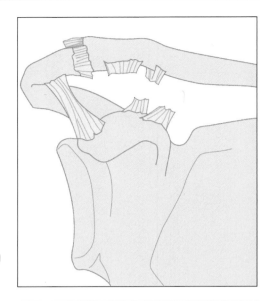

Figure 96-5 Type IV injury with posterior displacement of the distal clavicle. (Adapted from Montellese P, Dancy T: The acromioclavicular joint. *Prim Care* 31:857-866, 2004.)

is performed exactly as outlined for type I and II injuries, but the return to play or full activity will most likely be slower. Orthopedic referral should take place within 7 to 10 days or sooner if possible.

✓ Type IV injuries (Figure 96-5) include the previous findings, and, in addition, the distal clavicle tears the deltotrapezius fascia, remaining fixed posteriorly. In type V injuries, there is a 100% to 300% joint displacement and tearing of the deltotrapezius fascia. In rare type VI injuries, the clavicle is fixed beneath the acromion or coracoid and is usually accompanied by a neurologic deficit.

✓ **Type IV, V, and VI injuries require early orthopedic consultation.**

✓ Prescribe NSAIDs and narcotic analgesics as needed.

✓ **For type I, II, and III injuries, arrange for reevaluation by an orthopedic surgeon and for physical therapy to begin shoulder range-of-motion exercises within 7 to 10 days.**

What Not To Do:

✗ Do not confuse the deformity of a displaced AC ligament tear with a dislocated shoulder, which is accompanied by loss of the normal deltoid convexity and inability to rotate the shoulder internally and externally at the side.

✗ Do not bother with weight-bearing radiographs to differentiate separations based on the widening of the distance between the clavicle and scapula. These views are painful and inaccurate.

✗ Do not try to tape or strap the clavicle and scapula back into position. Patients have suffered ischemic necrosis of the skin from overzealous strapping. This includes the use of a Kenny-Howard sling.

Ⓧ Do not allow the patient to wear a sling and immobilize the shoulder for more than a week to 10 days without at least beginning pendulum exercises. The shoulder capsule may contract and restrict the range of motion.

Discussion

The AC joint is a diarthrodial synovial joint of the acromion and the distal clavicle with an intra-articular disk. This disk degenerates rapidly, resulting in narrowing of the joint space by age 40 years. The clavicle is the last bone in the body to ossify the physes; therefore Salter-Harris injuries can occur up to the age of 25 years.

The static stabilizers are the ligaments, but significant functional stability arises from the muscles attached to the shoulder girdle as well. The AC ligaments, which are incorporated into the AC joint capsule, provide most of the resistance to anteroposterior displacement and rotation of the clavicle. The two coracoclavicular ligaments, the conoid and trapezoid, prevent superior displacement of the distal clavicle. The dynamic stabilizers are the deltoid and trapezius muscles.

In patients with open physes, the physis is the weak link in the AC joint. When injured, the physis fractures and the metaphysis tears through the superior aspect of the periosteum. Because the AC joint remains in its anatomic position but the metaphysis is displaced, these injuries are called pseudodislocations. Because the inferior slip of periosteum remains in its original position, the bone it lays down is in the original orientation. Once the fracture gap is bridged, remodeling occurs, which usually brings the clavicle to its original position. Treatment for type I or III injuries is usually conservative and is the same as that described for AC joint separations.

A partial tear of the ligaments between acromion and clavicle produces pain but no widening of the joint (first-degree separation). A second-degree AC separation is visualized on radiographs as a widened joint but is otherwise the same on examination and treatment. In a third-degree or complete separation, the ligament from the coracoid process to the clavicle is probably also torn, allowing the collarbone to be pulled superior by the sternocleidomastoid muscle, but often relieving the pain of the stretched AC joint.

Nearly all patients with grade I and 90% of those with grade II injuries recover fully after 10 to 14 days of simple sling immobilization. The patient should avoid heavy lifting for 8 to 12 weeks and be referred to an orthopedic surgeon for any problems with pain or diminished range of motion.

Long-term shoulder joint stability and strength after a grade III tear remain almost normal, but patients may desire surgical repair to regain the appearance of the normal shoulder or the last few percents of function for athletics, even after being informed of the known surgical risks. Some of the literature on the treatment of AC separations listed visual prominence as a possible indication for surgery. This may be a consideration for thin patients who may have compromise of the skin or in patients who put excessive direct pressure on the AC joint, such as soldiers carrying backpacks. Caution is advised prior to surgical intervention for a cosmetic deformity, however. The surgical risks have been documented in the literature and include infection, hardware migration, failure to maintain a reduction, and scarring from the procedure.

Suggested Readings

Bradley JP, Elkousy H: Decision making: operative versus nonoperative treatment of acromioclavicular joint injuries, *Clin Sports Med* 22:277–290, 2003.

Buss DD, Watts JD: Acromioclavicular injuries in the throwing athlete, *Clin Sports Med* 22:327–341, vii, 2003.

Montellese P, Dancy T: The acromioclavicular joint, *Prim Care* 31:857–866, 2004.

Ankle Sprain

(Twisted Ankle)

Presentation

Patients usually describe stepping off a curb or into a hole. Sports-related injuries often occur after jumping and landing on another player's foot, which causes an inversion or supination of the ankle. Of all ankle sprains, 85% are inversion injuries. The sensation of a "pop" or "snap" at the time of injury with immediate loss of function suggests disruption of a ligament. Severe swelling in the first hour suggests bleeding from the torn ends. The body's response to the injury begins with inflammation, which produces swelling, warmth, pain, and stiffness that build to a maximum about 1 day after the injury.

Patients usually arrive either immediately after the injury or 1 to 2 days later, complaining of pain, swelling, and partial or complete inability to walk. Patients are usually tender around the lateral malleolus, particularly anteriorly, because the anterior talofibular ligament is the first to tear when the ankle is inverted. Although the pain during the first hours after injury is often localized to the injured area, it soon becomes diffuse during the first few days. After a few days, careful palpation will confirm which ligaments were most likely injured.

What To Do:

✓ Get a detailed description of the mechanism of injury, and ask if the patient could bear weight immediately after the injury. Ask if there have been previous injuries of the ankle. (Patients with a previous ankle injury have an increased risk for recurrence.)

✓ Document the degree and location of swelling and discoloration. Check the sensation and circulation distal to the injury. (A slight decrease relative to the uninjured foot might be attributed to the swelling.)

✓ **Palpate sites of potential injury: the fibula up to the knee, the base of the fifth metatarsal on the lateral foot, the tarsal navicular bone anteriorly, the deltoid ligament medially, and, finally, the anterior talofibular ligament in front of the lateral malleolus. Note if there is tenderness along the posterior distal 6 cm of the lateral malleolus, the posterior medial malleolus, or the tip of either malleolus.** Start palpating gently and away from the injury to overcome patients' tendency to flinch at the first touch. Save the most likely site of injury for last, because the pain may inhibit any further examination.

✓ If there is not too much pain, check joint stability with the anterior drawer test (Figure 97-1) and the talar tilt test (Figure 97-2). Perform these tests gently. For the anterior drawer test, grasp the tibia with one hand and the heel with the other hand; with the ankle in slight plantar flexion, push the leg posterior while holding the foot still or pushing anteriorly. Anterior displacement

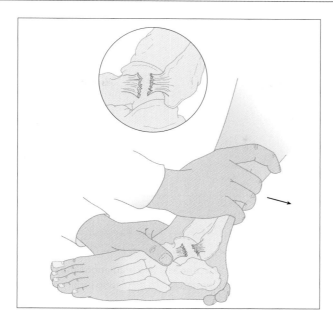

Figure 97-1 Anterior drawer test.

of the talus can be felt or seen as a dimple over the anterolateral ankle compared with the uninjured side. A positive anterior drawer indicates a significantly torn anterior talofibular ligament. The talar tilt test is also performed with the foot in the neutral position. Gently invert the ankle and compare the range of movement and the mushiness of the end point with the uninjured side. An intact calcaneofibular ligament should prevent inversion. **Often these tests cannot be accomplished because the ankle is too painful, in which case the tests may be deferred for up to 1 week.**

If there is significant medial ankle injury or severe lateral injury, perform a squeeze test to determine if there is a tear of the syndesmosis between the distal tibia and fibula. With the knee flexed at 90 degrees, place your hand over the midportion of the lower leg, with your thumb on the fibula and your fingers on the medial tibia. Squeeze the fibula and tibia together. Pain during this test signifies syndesmotic injury, predicts a prolonged recovery, and calls for an orthopedic referral. This may be associated with a fracture of the fibular head and is called a Maisonneuve fracture when there is an associated deltoid ligament tear or medial malleolus fracture.

Elevate the foot (preferably above the level of the heart), and for acute injuries apply an ice pack for 20 minutes and compress the ankle with a splint or elastic bandage.

Optional radiographs of the ankle or foot may be ordered to rule out a fracture, but radiographs are not necessary (and likely to be negative) unless there was either (1) inability to bear weight both immediately and at the initial physical examination or (2) bony tenderness to palpation of the ankle in the posterior distal 6 cm of the lateral malleolus or the posterior distal medial malleolus, or bony tenderness of the foot at the tarsal navicular or the base of the fifth metatarsal bone. The use of these decision rules must remain secondary to the judgment and common sense of the clinician. Patient satisfaction can be maintained by informing patients, "Studies show that your type of ankle sprain does not need an x-ray, and I

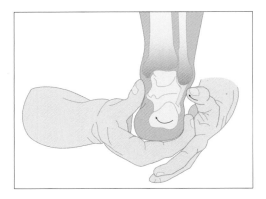

Figure 97-2 Talar tilt test.

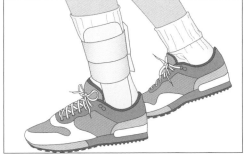

Figure 97-3 Grade I and II sprains should be fitted with a stirrup splint.

would prefer not to expose you to unnecessary irradiation." You can still give the autonomy of decision making to the patient by stating, "I'd be glad to order an x-ray if you still want it."

Be liberal in imaging patients with other distracting painful injuries, altered sensorium, intoxication, paraplegia, or bone disease. Weight bearing is defined as the ability to transfer weight twice onto each leg for a total of four steps, regardless of limping. Assess ability to bear weight after determining bony tenderness, and do not coerce the patient.

After the probability of a fracture has been ruled out, instruct the patient to elevate and rest the ankle as much as possible. When there is significant swelling, apply ice for three or four periods of 15 to 20 minutes a day for 3 days, insulating the skin from the ice with a compressive dressing to prevent frostbite and further reduce swelling. This, along with elevation, helps to minimize hemorrhage, inflammation, and pain.

Patients with mild to moderate sprains (grades I and II) should be fitted with a stirrup-type splint (Figure 97-3) **that prevents inversion and eversion of the ankle, should be given crutches and instructions how to ambulate with crutches,** and should be prescribed nonsteroidal anti-inflammatory drugs (NSAIDs), such as ibuprofen, 200 to 800 mg q6h. (Add a proton-pump inhibitor, such as omeprazole [Prilosec], or a high dose of an H_2-receptor antagonist, such as ranitidine [Zantac], to reduce NSAID-related dyspepsia.) **Acetaminophen (Tylenol) may be just as effective as NSAIDs for pain relief and completely avoids the potential for gastrointestinal (GI) side effects.** Narcotic analgesics may be required (especially at night) for the first few days. **For follow-up, instruct the patient to begin weight bearing using a stirrup splint as soon as it is tolerable, then for the next 4 to 6 weeks, and to use crutches for the shortest time possible. Once normal weight bearing and pain-free range of motion are achieved, muscle strengthening can begin.** Early phases of treatment should begin with low resistance, such as stationary cycling or swimming. Further strengthening can be accomplished using eversion exercises, which should be performed in dorsiflexion to strengthen the peroneus brevis and tertius, and in plantar flexion to strengthen the peroneus longus. These sprains can be referred to a primary care specialist for follow-up in 2 weeks.

Patients with moderate to severe sprains (grades II and III) should be placed in a soft, bulky compression dressing. If there is instability or fracture, incorporate a plaster/

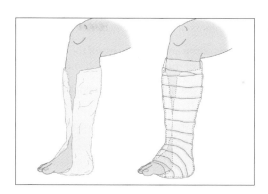

Figure 97-4 Severe sprains and fractures should be treated with a "sugar-tong" splint or Jones dressing.

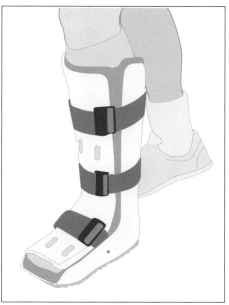

Figure 97-5 Walking boot for grade III sprains.

fiberglass sugar-tong splint (Figure 97-4) that extends almost the entire length of the tibia and fibula just below the knee. Alternatively, when available, a fracture boot or short-leg walking cast can be used with full weight bearing for the first 5 to 7 days (Figure 97-5). This allows the patient to eliminate the need for crutches and makes activities of daily living much easier. **Recovery and rehabilitation can proceed as described for grade I and II sprains.** Narcotic analgesics like hydrocodone will likely be needed for pain relief along with NSAIDs or acetaminophen.

✅ **Moderate to severe sprains, recurrent sprains, sprains with instability or syndesmotic injury, and most injuries with associated fractures should be seen by an orthopedic surgeon within 1 week.** Obtain orthopedic consultation in cases of delayed recovery, diagnostic uncertainty, neurovascular compromise, pain out of proportion to the injury (think compartment syndrome), and treatment involving competitive athletes.

✅ Tender or swollen ankle sprains in children with open growth plates are considered to be nondisplaced physeal (Salter I) fractures, even with negative radiographs, and are usually immobilized for 3 to 4 weeks. Bony structures and growth plates are often weaker than the contiguous ligaments and tendons. Care should be taken to palpate both malleoli and their respective physes, the proximal fifth metatarsal (a site of peroneus brevis avulsion), and the tarsal navicular, which may reveal an occult fracture.

✅ Patients not receiving radiographs at the initial visit should be instructed to seek follow-up if their symptoms have not improved after 1 week. Persistent ankle pain beyond 6 to 8 weeks could indicate a complication or overlooked injury. MRI, which is seldom needed at the initial presentation, may be very useful if symptoms have persisted this long.

What Not To Do:

(X) Do not have the patient apply heat during the recovery phase. It is unnecessary and increases the swelling.

(X) Do not recommend ointments or creams. They offer no benefit for ankle sprains.

(X) Do not overlook fractures of the anterior process of the calcaneus, the tarsal navicular, the talar dome or the rest of the talus, or the os trigonum, all visible on the ankle radiographs.

(X) Do not completely rule out a fracture based on a negative radiograph.

Discussion

Blunt ankle trauma is one of the most common injuries seen in emergency departments, and ankle sprains are the most common sports-related orthopedic injury, but less than 15% have associated clinically significant fractures. The old tradition of radiographic examination of all ankle injuries is no longer required, and the Ottawa decision rules described here have led to reductions in the number of negative radiographs, use of unnecessary radiation, and waiting times and costs, all without missed fractures or patient dissatisfaction.

The ankle ligaments can be divided into three groups: lateral ligaments, medial ligaments, and the ligaments of the syndesmosis. The most common injuries involve the lateral ligaments. These three groups of ligaments function as the static stabilizers of the ankle joint. The dynamic stabilizers consist of the muscles of the anterior, lateral, and posterior compartments of the leg. Mild or grade I sprains usually involve partial tearing of ligament fibers and minimal swelling, with no joint instability. Moderate or grade II sprains are characterized by some pain, edema, ecchymosis, and point tenderness over the involved structures, resulting in partial loss of joint motion. Some ligament fibers may be completely torn, but overall stability of the joint remains intact. Severe or grade III sprains exhibit gross instability with complete tearing of all ligament fibers, marked swelling, and severe pain. In general, the more extensive the ligament injury, the more difficult it is to bear weight, the more swelling noted acutely, and the more ecchymosis that develops over a few days.

Medial ligament injuries usually result from an eversion stress. Because the deltoid ligament is so strong, it is rarely injured in isolation but rather in association with lateral malleolus fracture.

Current research recommends the combination of early weight bearing and immobilization for lateral ligament injuries. Four stages characterize the biology behind functional treatment of acute lateral ankle ligament tears. Immediately after the injury, hemorrhage, swelling, inflammation, and pain are best treated with rest, ice, compression, and elevation (RICE). During the following 1 to 3 weeks, called the healing or proliferation phase, fibroblasts invade the injured area and proliferate to form collagen fibers. Protection in the form of a brace should be used during this time. Stirrup-style braces provide the best support. Three weeks after the injury, the maturation phase begins, during which the collagen fibers mature and become scar tissue. Controlled stretching of muscles and movement of the joint encourage the orientation of the collagen fibers along the stress lines, creating a stronger ligamentous repair. After 6 to 8 weeks, the new collagen fibers can withstand almost normal stress, and full return to activity is the goal. The entire maturation and remodeling of the injured ligaments lasts from 6 to 12 months. Reports indicate that up to 73% of people who sustain a lateral ankle sprain have recurrent sprains, but it is unknown how many of these participants partake in rehabilitation.

A minor sprain usually keeps an athlete out of competition for several days to 2 weeks, and a moderate sprain usually keeps an athlete out of competition for 2 to 4 weeks. Time to return to play for severe sprains will be greater than 4 weeks. Taping, lace-up braces, and air stirrup orthoses can all be helpful in the rehabilitation of ankle injuries.

When the patient reports a snapping sensation and states that it felt like something "slipped out of place," accompanied by pain in the posterolateral aspect of the ankle, consider the diagnosis of a peroneal tendon dislocation. This is seen more frequently in skiers but does occur to a lesser extent in other sport activities. Swelling and tenderness is found posteriorly and extending 6 inches proximally from

Discussion continued

the lateral malleolus. Circumduction of the ankle with palpation over the peroneal tendons may elicit a dislocation or subluxation of the peroneal tendons. These injuries require orthopedic consultation and may require acute surgical repair to prevent recurrence.

Typically, a patient with a Maisonneuve fracture will not complain of pain in the region of the proximal fibula but rather only of ankle pain in the region of the medial malleolus. Morbidity associated with proximal fibular fractures includes contusion or laceration of the common peroneal nerve (resulting in footdrop), injury to the anterior tibial artery, damage to the lateral collateral ligament of the knee, and even compartment syndrome.

The application of ice (cryotherapy) for the prevention of swelling and inflammation is generally accepted as a standard of care for the treatment of sprains. Although it is theorized that cryotherapy can be beneficial both immediately after injury and in the rehabilitation phase, the available scientific evidence does not provide much support for this belief. Therefore it is still not possible to make confident recommendations to our patients concerning the optimal type, frequency, timing, and duration of ice application. It is certainly reasonable to downplay its importance and see that a patient does not suffer further discomfort by applying such cold packs. Compression and elevation will be most effective in reducing the swelling after an ankle sprain.

A Thompson test should be performed if inspection and examination of the Achilles tendon suggests a full or partial tear there (see Figure 126-1).

Suggested Readings

Anis AH, Steill IG, Stewart, et al: Cost-effectiveness analysis of the Ottawa ankle rules, *Ann Emerg Med* 26:422–428, 1995.

Arnold BL, Docherty CL: Bracing and rehabilitation—what's new? *Clin Sports Med* 23:83–95, 2004.

Auleley GR, Kerboull L, Durieux P, et al: Validation of the Ottawa ankle rules in France: a study in the surgical emergency department of a teaching hospital, *Ann Emerg Med* 32:14–18, 1998.

Auleley GR, Ravaud P, Giraudeau B, et al: Implementation of the Ottawa ankle rules in France: a multicenter randomized controlled trial, *JAMA* 277:1935–1939, 1997.

Bachmann LM, Kolb E, Koller MT, et al: Accuracy of Ottawa ankle rules to exclude fractures of the ankle and midfoot, *BMJ* 326:417–419, 2003.

Baumhauer JF, Nawoczenski DA, DiGiovanni BF, et al: Ankle pain and peroneal tendon pathology, *Clin Sports Med* 23:21–34, 2004.

Bleakley C, McDonough S, MacAuley D: The use of ice in the treatment of acute soft tissue injury, *Am J Sports Med* 32:251–261, 2004.

Braun BL: Effects of ankle sprain in a general clinic population 6 to 18 months after medical evaluation, *Arch Fam Med* 8:143–148, 1999.

Chande VT: Decision rules for roentgenography of children with acute ankle injuries, *Arch Pediatr Adolesc Med* 149:255–258, 1995.

Cydulka RK: Accuracy of Ottawa ankle rules to exclude fractures of the ankle and midfoot, *Ann Emerg Med* 43:675–676, 2004.

Deal DN, Tipton J, Rosencrance E, et al: Ice reduces edema: a study of microvascular permeability in rat, *J Bone Joint Surg Am* 84:1573–1578, 2002.

DiGiovanni BF, Partal G, Baumhauer JF: Acute ankle injury and chronic lateral instability in the athlete, *Clin Sports Med* 23:1–19, v, 2004.

Eggli S, Sclabas GM, Eggli S, et al: The Bernese ankle rules: a fast, reliable test after low-energy, supination-type malleolar and midfoot trauma, *J Trauma* 59:1268–1271, 2005.

Eiff MP, Smith AT, Smith GE: Early mobilization versus immobilization in the treatment of lateral ankle sprains, *Am J Sports Med* 22:83–88, 1994.

Graham ID, Stiell IG, Laupacis A: Awareness and use of the Ottawa ankle and knee rules in 5 countries: can publication alone be enough to change practice, *Ann Emerg Med* 37:259–266, 2001.

Halvorson G, Iserson KV: Comparison of four ankle splint designs, *Ann Emerg Med* 16:1249–1252, 1987.

LeBlanc KE: Ankle problems masquerading as sprains, *Prim Care* 31:1055–1067, 2004.

Lucchesi GM, Jackson RE, Peacock WF, et al: Sensitivity of the Ottawa rules, *Ann Emerg Med* 26:1–5, 1995.

MacAuley D: Do textbooks agree on their advice on ice? *Clin J Sports Med* 11:67–72, 2001.

Markert RJ, Walley ME, Guttman TG, et al: A pooled analysis of the Ottawa ankle rules used on adults in the ED, *Am J Emerg Med* 16:564–567, 1998.

Pommering TL, Kluchurosky L, Hall SL: Ankle and foot injuries in pediatric and adult athletes, *Prim Care* 32:133–161, 2005.

Stiell IG, Greenberg GH, McKnight RD, et al: Decision rules for the use of radiography in acute ankle injuries: refinement and prospective validation, *JAMA* 269:1127–1132, 1993.

Stiell IG, McKnight RD, Greenberg GH, et al: Implementation of the Ottawa ankle rules, *JAMA* 271:827–832, 1994.

van Dijk CN, Lim LS, Bossuyt PM, et al: Physical examination is sufficient for the diagnosis of sprained ankles, *J Bone Joint Surg Br* 78:958–962, 1996.

Wilson DE, Noseworthy TW, Rowe BH, et al: Evaluation of patient satisfaction and outcomes after assessment for acute ankle injuries, *Am J Emerg Med* 20:18–20, 2002.

Annular Ligament Displacement, Radial Head Subluxation

(Nursemaid's Elbow)

Presentation

A toddler who is between 1 and 4 years of age has received a sudden jerk on his arm, causing enough pain that he holds it motionless against his body. Circumstances surrounding the injury may be obvious (such as a parent pulling the child up by the arm to avoid stepping into a puddle) or obscure (the babysitter who reports that the child "just fell down"). The patient and family may not be accurate about localizing the injury and think that the child has injured his shoulder or wrist. The patient is comfortable at rest, splinting his arm limply at the side with mild flexion at the elbow and pronation of the forearm. There should be no deformity, crepitation, swelling, or discoloration of the arm. There is also no palpable tenderness, except possibly over the radiohumeral joint; the child will start to cry with any movement of the elbow, especially attempted supination.

What To Do:

✓ Rule out any history of significant trauma, such as a fall from a height.

✓ Thoroughly examine the entire extremity, including the shoulder girdle, hand, and wrist. To avoid obtaining a false-positive examination, special effort should be made to keep the elbow joint perfectly immobile while evaluating for tenderness.

✓ If there is significant trauma, point tenderness, swelling, ecchymosis, or any suspicion of a fracture, get a radiograph.

✓ **When nursemaid's elbow is suspected,** place the patient in the parent's lap and inform the mother or father that it appears that a ligament in their child's elbow is slightly out of place and that you are going to put it back in place. Warn them that this is going to hurt for a few moments.

✓ **Put your thumb over the head of the radius with your fingers supporting the elbow and press down with your thumb while you smoothly and fully supinate the forearm and extend the elbow. Complete the procedure by fully flexing the elbow while your thumb remains pressing against the radial head and the forearm remains supinated** (Figure 98-1). At some point, you should feel a click beneath your thumb. The patient will usually scream for a while at this point. **Leave for about 10 minutes, then return and reexamine the elbow to see that the child has fully recovered.** This recovery may take as much as 30 minutes. Postreduction immobilization is unnecessary.

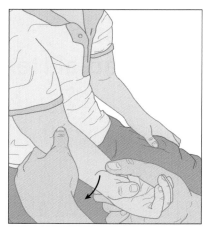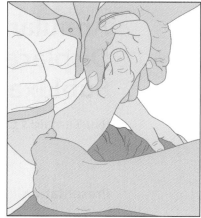

Figure 98-1 Supination technique for annular ligament displacement (ALD) reduction.

Figure 98-2 "Handshake" or hyperpronation maneuver. Simultaneous pronation of the wrist and extension of the elbow (**A**), followed by flexion of the elbow with the forearm maintained in pronation (**B**). (Adapted from Kaplan RE, Lillis KA: Recurrent nursemaid's elbow [annular ligament displacement] treatment via telephone. *Pediatrics* 110:171-174, 2002.)

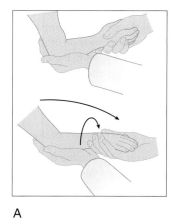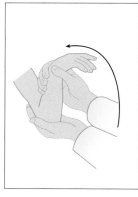

A   B

✓ **An alternative maneuver that some believe is more effective is the "handshake" or hyperpronation maneuver. Grasp the hand of the patient's affected arm as if to shake it, place your other hand under the affected elbow with your thumb over the radial head, and slowly pronate the wrist. This can be done alone or while simultaneously extending the elbow, followed by fully flexing the elbow while still maintaining pronation of the forearm** (Figure 98-2).

✓ Initial attempts at reduction using either technique are usually successful.

✓ Failure is more likely to occur if reduction is attempted 12 or more hours after the injury has occurred.

✅ **If there is not full recovery, a repeated attempt using the alternative maneuver may be warranted. If this is also unsuccessful, radiography should be obtained.** Examine again for possible injury to the clavicle or humerus (particularly the lateral condyle), and consider other bone and joint disorders. Differential diagnosis includes fracture, soft tissue injury, infection, arthritis, tumor, neurologic injury, and vasoocclusive crisis in sickle cell.

✅ Place these children in a sling, with or without posterior splinting. (The elbow should be kept at 90-degree flexion with as much supination of the forearm as comfort will allow.) Provide pediatric or orthopedic follow-up within 24 to 48 hours. Self-reduction almost always occurs during the period of immobilization.

✅ **When full recovery has been obtained, reassure the parents, explain the mechanism involved in the injury, and teach them how to prevent and treat recurrences.**

What Not To Do:

❌ Do not attempt to reduce an elbow where the possibility exists of fracture or dislocation.

❌ Do not get unnecessary radiographs when all the findings are consistent with nursemaid's elbow. The radiographs will appear normal.

❌ Do not confuse nursemaid's elbow with the more serious brachial plexus injury, which occurs after much greater stress and results in a flaccid paralysis of the arm.

Discussion

Nursemaid's elbow or annular ligament displacement (ALD), formerly called radial head subluxation (RHS), is a common pediatric orthopedic problem. It is most often seen in children who are between 1 and 4 years of age and is extremely rare in children who are older than 5 years of age. This displacement usually occurs as the result of a sudden forceful longitudinal traction on the hand while the forearm is pronated and the elbow is extended, as when one pulls the forearm of a resisting child.

This condition is actually a displacement of the annular ligament between the capitulum of the distal humerus and the radial head. The annular ligament is displaced from its normal position, covering the radial head, into the radiohumeral joint (Figure 98-3). Radiographs of an untreated nursemaid's elbow are normal without any evidence of abnormal positioning of the radial head. Although there is a transient subluxation of the radial head, prolonged subluxation does not occur. ALD is more common in girls and in the left arm. About one third have had a previous episode.

The assessment of the young child is especially challenging, because the child cannot relate a coherent history, has difficulty localizing pain, and often is frightened and uncooperative, hindering physical examination. The classic history of a child being pulled up by the arm while falling or lifted by the arm is obtained in only 50% of patients. The diagnosis is nonetheless made by history and physical examination and confirmed by prompt reuse of the affected arm following reduction. Supination or pronation of the forearm usually causes reduction of the annular ligament back into its normal position. The reported recurrence rate involving either the same or contralateral arm is extremely variable, ranging from 5% to 39%.

ALD should be considered in any toddler presenting with arm injury without obvious evidence of trauma. The key to diagnosis is the observation that the child is not in pain; has no swelling, ecchymosis, or deformity; holds the elbow in a slightly flexed position with wrist pronated; refuses to use the arm; and resists supination. When history and physical examination suggest ALD, it is appropriate to attempt reduction without obtaining radiographs. Successful reduction is more likely when a click is felt. On occasion, if the

(continued)

Discussion continued

injury has been present for several hours, edema, pain, and natural splinting will continue even after reduction or may prevent reduction.

Although not fully proven safe, parents or caretakers can be instructed by telephone to treat ALD, especially in those cases in which there is a previous history and in which the history is typical of recurrent ALD. Instruct the caregiver to restrain the

child by placing her in a second adult's lap and then have him grasp the child's hand. With the treating adult's other hand under the child's affected elbow, straighten out the arm with the palm of the child's hand facing upward. Then, have the child bend the elbow up, touching the palm of her hand to the same shoulder. After 20 minutes, the child should be moving the arm normally.

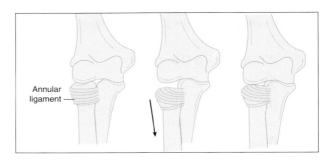

Figure 98-3 Annular ligament displacement (nursemaid's elbow). (Adapted from Kaplan RE, Lillis KA: Recurrent nursemaid's elbow [annular ligament displacement] treatment via telephone. *Pediatrics* 110:171-174, 2002.)

Suggested Readings

Frumkin K: Nursemaid's elbow: a radiographic demonstration, *Ann Emerg Med* 14:690–693, 1985.

Meiner EM, Sama AE, Lee DC: Bilateral nursemaid's elbow, *Am J Emerg Med* 22:502–503, 2004.

Quan L, Marcuse EK: The epidemiology and treatment of radial head subluxation, *Am J Dis Child* 139:1194–1197, 1985.

Schunk JE: Radial head subluxation: epidemiology and treatment of 87 episodes, *Ann Emerg Med* 19:1019–1023, 1990.

Schutzman SA, Teach S: Upper-extremity impairment in young children, *Ann Emerg Med* 26:474–479, 1995.

Boutonnière Finger

Presentation

After jamming the tip of a partially or fully extended finger (resulting in hyperflexion of the proximal interphalangeal [PIP] joint) or with direct trauma over the joint, the patient develops a painful, swollen PIP joint. These injuries are seen in basketball players and martial artists, who use open-hand blocking techniques, as well as when an athlete's hand is stepped on. Tenderness is greatest over the dorsum of the base of the middle phalanx, and there is diminished extensor tendon strength with pain when the middle phalanx is extended against resistance. The classic boutonnière deformity is rarely present immediately after injury. Radiographs are usually normal.

What To Do:

✓ Obtain a detailed history of the mechanism of injury.

✓ Perform a complete examination, palpating for point tenderness of the dorsum of the joint, the collateral ligaments, and the volar plate. Test for joint stability in all directions, test sensation, and check for injuries proximal and distal to the PIP joint.

✓ **Check for a possible tear of the central slip of the extensor digitorum communis tendon. With the patient's PIP joint flexed at 90 degrees over a straight edge (such as a countertop), apply resistance to active extension over the middle phalanx. If the central slip is disrupted, the patient will not be able to apply pressure against resistance** (Figure 99-1, *A* to *C*). It is possible for the patient to extend the injured finger without resistance using the lateral bands of the extensor tendon, causing the distal phalanx to hyperextend. Full passive extension is easily obtained. The distal interphalangeal (DIP) joint is in slight hyperextension at rest.

✓ When available, diagnostic high-frequency ultrasonography is a very accurate noninvasive study that can identify central slip injuries in the extensor mechanism of the finger. This can confirm the diagnosis and either allow early initiation of splinting or eliminate the need for prolonged splinting.

✓ Test for collateral ligament stability with varus and valgus stress (Figure 99-1, *D*).

✓ **If avulsion of the central slip of the extensor tendon is suspected, splint the PIP joint in extension. The splint should leave the DIP and metacarpophalangeal (MCP) joints completely mobile, or the collateral ligaments will contract.** Active DIP flexion should be encouraged. This action pulls the PIP extensor hood mechanism distally, thereby further approximating the two ends of the ruptured central slip. The PIP joint should remain constantly splinted for 6 to 8 weeks—3 to 4 weeks of static extension splinting (Figure 99-2), followed by 2 to 3 weeks of dynamic extension splinting. Occasionally, it should be splinted for another 8 to 10 weeks, whenever the patient engages in any activity that is likely to cause reinjury.

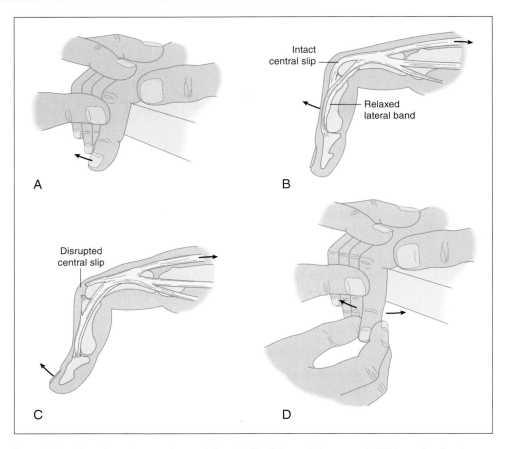

Figure 99-1 Extension against resistance tests for a central slip avulsion (**A** to **C**). Varus and valgus stress at the PIP joint tests for collateral ligament instability (**D**).

✓ Prompt referral should be made to a hand surgeon to evaluate for potential acute operative repair.

✓ Provide standard acetaminophen or nonsteroidal anti-inflammatory drugs (NSAIDs) along with initial cold compresses and elevation.

What Not To Do:

✗ Do not assume that posttraumatic swelling of a PIP joint represents a simple sprain until testing for extension against resistance.

✗ Do not overlook associated injuries that may cause joint instability. Such injuries may require immediate orthopedic consultation.

✗ Do not be fooled by the patient's ability to actively extend the PIP joint. In the acute setting, the patient may be able to fully extend through the action of the lateral bands, despite a complete rupture of the central slip.

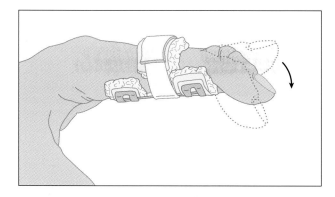

Figure 99-2 Suspected avulsion of the central slip of the extensor tendon necessitates splinting of the PIP joint in extension, while allowing the DIP joint to go through a full range of motion. (Adapted from Ruiz E, Cicero JJ: *Emergency management of skeletal injuries.* St Louis, 1995, Mosby.)

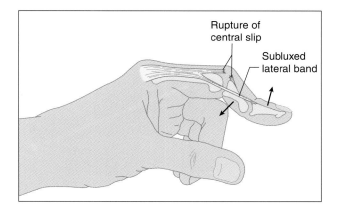

Rupture of
central slip

Subluxed
lateral band

Figure 99-3 Boutonnière deformity.

Discussion

The boutonnière (buttonhole) injury or deformity refers to a rupture of the central slip of the extensor tendon at the PIP joint. Similar to the mechanism of injury in mallet finger, there is forced PIP flexion at the same time the PIP joint is held rigidly in extension.

Although the acute manifestations of a disrupted central slip may be limited to swelling and tenderness over the PIP joint, with time the central slip retracts. The lateral bands will slip and displace volarly, becoming flexors of the PIP joint and allowing the joint to herniate dorsally through the defect in the tendon (like a button through a buttonhole), thereby creating a flexed PIP joint. Eventually, a position of flexion at the PIP joint

and hyperextension at the DIP joint become fixed, producing the classic buttonhole or boutonnière deformity (Figure 99-3).

Early diagnosis is clearly the key to prevention. Because the acute injury may suggest nothing more than a contusion or sprain, any injury around the PIP joint should be viewed with suspicion.

A boutonnière finger, like a mallet finger, requires complete and prolonged immobilization. Unfortunately, many people do not seek help for a central slip avulsion until a deformity has developed; at that point, surgery may be required to correct the retinacular structures and the subluxed lateral

(continued)

Discussion continued

bands. Once a deformity becomes chronic or fixed, it presents a difficult surgical challenge with potentially permanent functional deficits.

A hyperextension injury at the PIP joint that disrupts the volar plate and tears the accessory collateral ligaments may lead to chronic pseudoboutonnière

deformity if there is a delay in diagnosis. This pseudoboutonnière is generally less severe than a true boutonnière deformity. Treatment of a pseudoboutonnière deformity consists of progressive stretching of the contracture with dynamic splinting before considering surgical release.

Suggested Readings

Hong E: Hand injuries in sports medicine, *Prim Care* 32:91–103, 2005.

Patel D, Dean C, Baker RJ: The hand in sports: an update on the clinical anatomy and physical examination, *Prim Care* 32:71–89, 2005.

Perron AD, Brady WJ: Evaluation and management of the high-risk orthopedic emergency, *Emerg Med Clin North Am* 21:159–204, 2003.

Westerheide E, Failla JM, van Holsbeeck M, et al: Ultrasound visualization of central slip injuries of the finger extensor mechanism, *J Hand Surg* 28:1009–1013, 2003.

Boxer's Fifth Metacarpal Fracture

CHAPTER 100

Presentation

The patient seeks help for painful swelling of the hand over the distal fifth metacarpal (MC) after punching an object or another person with a closed fist. It occurs commonly during fistfights or from punching a hard object, such as a wall or a filing cabinet, and may be an act of deliberate self-harm.

What To Do:

✓ Obtain a clear history regarding the mechanism of injury and the circumstances that led up to the punching incident.

✓ Examine the patient's hand, with attention to inspection and palpation of the fifth MC. The normal prominence of the fifth knuckle may be lost, and most often there will be tenderness at the neck of the fifth MC, where the shaft meets the head.

✓ **Obtain routine radiographs of the injured hand to determine the exact nature and degree of angulation of any fracture.**

✓ **Also, assess for malrotation by examining the direction of the fingers in flexion. All of the fingertips should be aligned parallel to one another** (Figure 100-1).

✓ No malrotation is acceptable. If any malalignment is present (Figure 100-2), inject the fracture hematoma with a long-acting local anesthetic (e.g., bupivacaine [Marcaine] 0.5%), and, with traction and counterrotation, reduce any malrotation. Buddy-tape the fifth finger to the fourth finger to maintain normal alignment.

✓ Most fractures occur just below the metacarpal head without rotation but are usually displaced in a volar direction. **Up to 70 degrees of volar angulation is acceptable in the nonoperative management of a boxer's fracture.**

✓ Patients with a rotational deformity (with or without reduction) should be placed in an ulnar gutter splint with the fourth and fifth metacarpophalangeal (MCP) joints in a 90-degree flexed position and given orthopedic follow-up within 1 week.

✓ **Patients with up to 70 degrees of volar angulation without rotation can be treated with a simple pressure bandage (e.g., bulky cotton padding wrap covered with an elastic bandage) along with adequate analgesics, such as acetaminophen alone or nonsteroidal anti-inflammatory drugs (NSAIDs) and/or hydrocodone/acetaminophen (Lorcet, Lortab, Vicodin).**

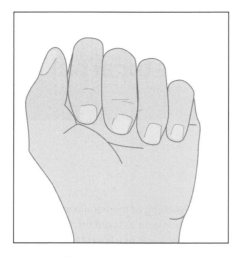

Figure 100-1 Normal alignment.

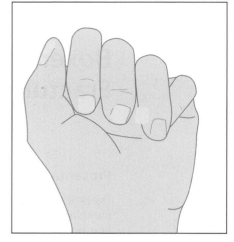

Figure 100-2 Rotational deformity.

✓ After 1 week, these patients are allowed immediate mobilization within the limits imposed by pain.

✓ Self-harmers and patients who are having problems controlling their anger should be considered for psychiatric assessment and referral.

What Not To Do:

✗ Do not overlook a so-called "fight bite" injury. All open wounds over the MCP joints should be considered "fist-to-mouth" human bite wounds, which have the highest incidence of infectious complications of any closed-fist injury and of any type of bite wound (see Chapter 144).

Discussion

An isolated fracture of the distal fifth metacarpal bone, known as a boxer's fracture, is the most common type of metacarpal fracture. Boxer's fractures received their name from one of their most common causes—punching an object with a closed fist. This is somewhat of a misnomer, because boxers learn not to punch this way, and the injury is seen more commonly in a lay person striking a hard object with a closed fist.

Reduction of angulated fractures of less than 70 degrees appears to be of no value with respect to range of motion (ROM) of the fifth MCP joint. Patients with less than 70 degrees of volar angulation and no rotational deformity who

were treated with a pressure bandage for 1 week, followed by immediate mobilization, showed no statistical differences with respect to ROM, satisfaction, pain perception, return to work/hobby, and need for physiotherapy when compared with patients treated for 3 weeks with a plaster ulnar gutter splint.

This injury has been described as "a tolerable fracture in an intolerable patient." Anxiety symptoms and maladaptive personality traits are very common in patients with boxer's fractures. Psychiatric assessment and counseling should be strongly considered in these patients, who actually have a high risk for recurrence of self-harm or aggressive acts.

Suggested Readings

Hong E: Hand injuries in sports medicine, *Prim Care* 32:91–103, 2005.

Mercan S, Uzun M, Ertugrul A, et al: Psychopathology and personality features in orthopedic patients with boxer's fractures, *Gen Hosp Psych* 27:13–17, 2005.

Muller MG: Immediate mobilization gives good results in boxer's fractures with volar angulation up to 70 degrees: a prospective randomized trial comparing immediate mobilization with cast immobilization, *Arch Orthop Trauma Surg* 123:537, 2003.

Patel D, Dean C, Baker RJ: The hand in sports: an update on the clinical anatomy and physical examination, *Prim Care* 32:71–89, 2005.

Perron AD, Brady WJ: Evaluation and management of the high-risk orthopedic emergency, *Emerg Med Clin North Am* 21:159–204, 2003.

Bursitis

Presentation

Following minimal trauma or repetitive motion, a nonarticular synovial sac or bursa protecting a tendon or prominent bone becomes swollen, possibly fluctuant, and possibly painful and inflamed. It may be nontender or tender. The elbow, hip, knee, and shoulder are most commonly involved unilaterally.

Olecranon bursitis can be caused by trauma from a direct blow (often only causing acute hemorrhage into the bursa), chronic crushing friction from prolonged leaning on the elbows, crystal deposition (gout), systemic diseases (rheumatoid arthritis, diabetes, systemic lupus erythematosus [SLE], alcoholism, uremia), or infection (usually from an overlying skin lesion or wound).

Trochanteric bursitis causes pain and tenderness that is greatest over the area of the greater trochanter of the hip. Active resistance to abduction of the hip may increase the pain.

Ischial bursitis can result from trauma or prolonged sitting on a hard surface. This causes buttock pain that may radiate down the back of the thigh. Palpation will reveal point tenderness over the ischial tuberosity.

Prepatellar bursitis, also known as "housemaid's knee," is caused by frequent or prolonged kneeling on hard surfaces. There may be marked swelling and tenderness over the anterior surface of the patella.

Pes anserine bursitis is located on the medial inferior aspect of the knee at the inferior margin of the medial collateral ligament about 4 to 5 cm below the joint margin and just superior to the pes anserinus tendon. Inflammation of this bursa is common in overweight patients and those beginning an exercise program. The knee pain is worsened when climbing stairs, and there is tenderness to direct palpation over the area of the bursa.

Subdeltoid (or subacromial) bursitis can be the result of traumatic injury or chronic overuse, and it frequently accompanies other shoulder problems. A history of pain in the lateral shoulder, which can be severe with acute onset, and tenderness to palpation along the acromial border help make the diagnosis.

Because there is no joint involved, there is usually little decreased range of motion, except in the shoulder, where bursitis can produce dramatic limitation. If the tendon sheath is involved, there may be some stiffness and pain with motion. Swelling is less evident when the bursa is deep, such as in the case of ischial bursitis.

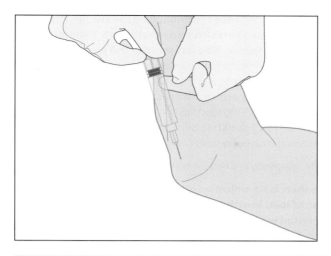

Figure 101-1 Technique for draining olecranon bursitis.

What To Do:

✓ Obtain a detailed history of the injury or precipitating activity, document a thorough physical examination, and rule out a joint effusion (see Chapter 120).

✓ Obtain a radiograph or ultrasound study if the possibility of a foreign body exists.

✓ **Primarily pertaining to olecranon and prepatellar bursitis, swelling and fluctuance suggest an effusion in the bursa, and cellulitis-like erythema, fever, warmth, and tenderness with an overlying skin lesion suggest infection. Prepare the skin with alcohol and povidone-iodine antiseptic solution, and either anesthetize the skin with 1% lidocaine using a 30-gauge needle or spray with ethyl chloride. Puncture the swollen bursa with an 18- or 20-gauge needle using aseptic technique, withdraw some fluid to drain the effusion, and have the fluid analyzed to rule out a bacterial infection.** A tangential approach to the olecranon bursa can be performed by keeping the barrel of your 10-mL syringe parallel to the ulna over the forearm while puncturing the bursa (Figure 101-1). The elbow can be held in extension or up to 90 degrees of flexion.

✓ A tangential approach to the prepatellar bursa can be obtained by keeping the barrel of your syringe parallel to the long axis of the tibia.

✓ **Relatively clear yellow or serosanguineous fluid** drained from a minimally inflamed bursa **needs to be sent only for culture,** because clear fluid indicates nonseptic bursitis. Using a hemostat to grasp the needle hub to twist off and remove the syringe, the needle can be left within the bursa for later instillation of a corticosteroid. **When the fluid appears purulent or cloudy,** or if the clinical picture is unclear, the needle can be removed. **This fluid should be sent for leukocyte count, Gram stain, culture, and sensitivity; it should also be analyzed for crystals when there is suspicion of gout.**

✓ Examine a Gram stain of the effusion. This may be negative in about 30% of patients with septic bursitis. Leukocyte counts greater than 2000/mm³ have a high sensitivity and specificity for bursal infections. The white blood cell (WBC) count for the nonseptic bursitis will usually be only a few hundred/mm^3. **With or without fluid to examine, it is often difficult to clinically distinguish an inflamed bursa from an infected one. Therefore, if there is any suggestion or sign of a bacterial infection, hold any steroids and prescribe appropriate oral antibiotics.** Bacterial infections tend to be gram-positive cocci, specifically *Staphylococcus aureus,* and respond well to dicloxacillin (Dynapen), 500 mg qid for 2 to 3 weeks. Alternatively, prescribe drugs that are active against community-acquired, methicillin-resistant *S. aureus* (CAMRSA), such as trimethoprim-sulfamethoxazole (TMP/SMX) (Bactrim DS), sulfamethoxazole 800 mg, trimethoprim 160 mg bid × 14 days; doxycycline 100 mg bid × 14 days; clindamycin (Cleocin), 300 mg qid × 14 days; or, in the most worrisome cases, linezolid (Zyvox), 600 mg bid for 2 to 3 weeks (extremely expensive).

✓ Initially, reaspirate any recurrent infected effusion on a daily basis.

✓ **When there is no indication of a bacterial infection, inflammatory bursitis may respond to injection of local anesthetics such as lidocaine (Xylocaine) 1% or bupivacaine (Marcaine), 5 to 9 mL, mixed with corticosteroids, such as methylprednisolone (Depo-Medrol) 0.25%, 40 mg, or betamethasone (Celestone Soluspan), 1 mL. Use the 18- or 20-gauge aspiration needle that you left in place. Alternatively, use a 25-gauge, 1¼-inch needle** and review the anatomy so that the needle can be carefully pushed through the lowest density tissue and the shortest pathway, causing the least amount of pain while probing for the bursa sac. For olecranon bursitis, perform the injection with the arm in extension, and penetrate the sac parallel to the ulna on the lateral side, away from the ulnar nerve. Approach the greater trochanteric bursae from the lateral and posterior side. For the subacromial bursa, insert the needle just inferior to the posterolateral edge of the acromion and then direct the needle toward the opposite nipple. **The anesthetic and steroid should flow freely into the space without any resistance or significant discomfort to the patient.** After injection, it may take several minutes or longer for patients to perceive pain relief and regain lost range of motion. The literature suggests that the instillation of a long-acting cortisone solution is associated with a significantly better cure rate than aspiration or nonsteroidal anti-inflammatory drugs (NSAIDs) alone or in combination.

✓ **For knee and elbow, apply a bulky compressive dressing for protection and comfort. Construct a splint, and instruct the patient in rest, elevation, and ice packing. A sling should suffice for the shoulder.**

✓ Prescribe NSAIDs if tolerated, and arrange for follow-up. When a long-acting cortisone solution has been used, NSAIDs can be avoided.

✓ Fluid may reaccumulate and require additional aspiration.

✓ When symptoms have subsided, prior to returning to any previous activity, have the patient add appropriate padding to prevent further bursal irritation.

✓ Septic bursitis resolves slowly and may take weeks to get better. Two to 3 weeks of antibiotics are required, and close follow-up is mandatory.

What Not To Do:

✗ Do not inject corticosteroids into an infected bursa. The infection is likely to worsen and spread.

✗ Do not puncture an area of olecranon bursitis by needling perpendicular to the ulna. Flexion and trauma may produce a chronic sinus.

(X) Do not routinely obtain radiographs when there is minimal trauma involved. They are generally not helpful or necessary in acute bursitis.

Discussion

Common sites for bursitis include the subacromial bursa of the shoulder, the prepatellar bursa of the knee, the olecranon bursa of the elbow, and the trochanteric bursa of the hip. In shoulder bursitis, radiographs may reveal calcific bursitis. There may be bony spurs in olecranon bursitis, but these images are not needed for routine emergency therapy.

Burning pain and sometimes numbness in the anterolateral thigh, which may be worsened by prolonged standing or walking, may be caused by compression of the lateral femoral cutaneous nerve in the area of the anterior superior iliac spine **(meralgia paresthetica).** Obese, pregnant, or diabetic patients or workers who carry a heavy tool belt are commonly affected. Tightly fitting garments may also precipitate the syndrome. There is no tenderness over the greater trochanter of the hip, and this should not be confused with bursitis. Meralgia paresthetica usually resolves after conservative treatment, such as weight loss and the wearing of loose-fitting clothes.

Patients with septic bursitis, unlike those with septic arthritis, can often be safely discharged on oral antibiotics, because the risk for permanent damage is much less when there is no joint involvement. Severe cases with extensive cellulitis or lymphangitis, however, may require hospitalization and IV antibiotics. Immunocompromised patients may require longer courses of antibiotics. Grossly purulent fluid that reaccumulates must be repeatedly reaspirated on a daily basis.

Some long-acting corticosteroid preparations can produce rebound bursitis several hours after injection, after the local anesthetic wears off but before the corticosteroid crystals dissolve. Patients should be so informed. Patients should prevent recurrence by wearing knee or elbow pads at work, avoiding pressure and trauma to vulnerable areas, and caring for skin wounds near bursae.

Suggested Readings

Deu RS, Carek PJ: Common sports injuries: upper extremity injuries, *Clin Fam Pract* 7:249–265, 2005.

McFarland EG, Gill HS, Laporte DM, et al: Miscellaneous conditions about the elbow in athletes, *Clin Sports Med* 23:743–763, xi-xii, 2004.

Pien FD, Ching D, Kim E: Septic bursitis: experience in a community practice, *Orthopedics* 14:981–984, 1991.

Smith DL, McAfee JH, Lucas LM, et al: Treatment of nonseptic olecranon bursitis, *Arch Intern Med* 149:2527–2530, 1989.

Tallia AF, Cardone DA: Diagnostic and therapeutic injection of the shoulder region, *Am Fam Physician* 67:2147–2152, 2003.

Carpal Tunnel Syndrome

Presentation

The patient complains of pain, tingling, or a "pins and needles" sensation in the hand or fingers. Onset may have been abrupt or gradual, but the problem is most noticeable after extended use of the hand or when driving or holding up a newspaper. Symptoms are usually worse at night and commonly awaken the patient. Sports such as racquetball and handball or activities such as assembly-line work and use of vibratory tools (e.g., jackhammers) are frequently associated with carpal tunnel syndrome (CTS). CTS has also been associated with a number of systemic conditions, including rheumatoid arthritis, diabetes, hypothyroidism, acromegaly, gout, renal failure, obesity, pregnancy, and menopause. The sensation may be bilateral, may include pain in the wrist or forearm, and is usually ascribed to the entire hand until specific physical examination localizes it to the median nerve distribution. Strenuous use of the hand almost always aggravates the symptoms. To relieve the symptoms, patients often "flick" their wrist as if shaking down a thermometer (flick sign). More established cases may include weakness of the thumb and atrophy of the thenar eminence. Although one hand typically has more severe symptoms, both hands often are affected.

Physical examination localizes paresthesia and decreased sensation to the median nerve distribution (which may vary) (Figure 102-1). Motor weakness, if present, is localized to intrinsic muscles with median innervation. Innervation varies widely, but the muscles most reliably innervated by the median nerve are the abductors and opponens of the thumb (Figure 102-2). CTS typically occurs after 30 years of age and is 3 times more common in women than in men.

What To Do:

✓ Perform and document a complete examination, sketching the area of decreased sensation and grading (on a scale of 1 to 5) the strength of the hand. **One clinical finding that best identifies patients with electrodiagnostic studies that are positive for CTS is hypalgesia (diminished perception of painful stimuli) along the palmar aspect of the index finger, compared with the ipsilateral little finger. Another typical finding is weakness of resistance to downward pressure applied to the distal phalanx of the thumb, while the patient rests the dorsal surface of her hand on a hard surface with the thumb raised perpendicular to her palm** (see Figure 102-2).

✓ Although the Tinel sign and a positive Phalen maneuver are classic clinical signs of CTS, their actual utility in the diagnosis has been less clear.

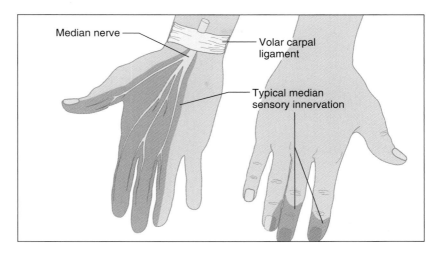

Figure 102-1 Sensory abnormalities are found along the median nerve distribution.

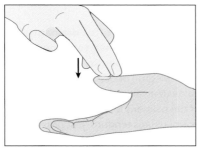

Figure 102-2 Testing thumb abduction.

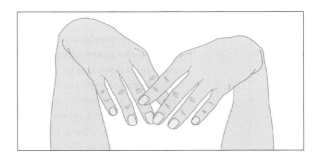

Figure 102-3 The Phalen test.

Have the patient passively drop both wrists to 90 degrees of flexion for 60 seconds to see if this reproduces symptoms. This is known as the Phalen test (Figure 102-3); it is more sensitive than the reverse (hyperextending the wrist), and more specific than tapping over the volar carpal ligament to elicit paresthesia in the distribution of the median nerve (Tinel sign).

The hand elevation test is comparable in accuracy to the Phalen test and only requires the patient to hold her arm over her head as high as comfortably possible. Reproduction of CTS symptoms within 1 minute is considered a positive test.

Patients should be told to avoid repetitive wrist and hand motions that may exacerbate symptoms or make symptom relief difficult to achieve. If possible, they should not use vibratory tools (e.g., jackhammers, floor sanders).

Wrist splints that maintain the wrist in a neutral position may be helpful for patients who engage in repetitive wrist motion often.

A 4-week course of oral prednisone (e.g., 20 mg daily for 2 weeks, then 10 mg qd for another 2 weeks) may offer short-term relief in mild to moderate cases.

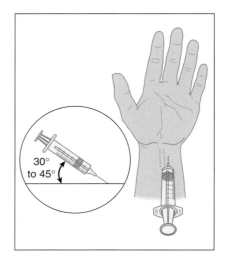

Figure 102-4 Location for needle insertion.

✅ **Alternatively, injections of corticosteroids can often dramatically alleviate symptoms and may improve symptoms for a longer period. When combined with a local anesthetic, such injections can be diagnostic as well as therapeutic.** Using a 1-inch, 25-gauge needle with 20 mg of methylprednisolone (Depo-Medrol) or 0.5 mL of betamethasone (Celestone Soluspan) along with 5 mL of bupivacaine (Marcaine), 0.25%, with the hand positioned on a rolled towel, inject on the ulnar side of the palmaris longus tendon, which is midway between the flexor carpi radialis and the flexor carpi ulnaris tendons, just proximal (1 cm) to the flexor crease of the wrist, distally into the central portion of the flexor tendon mass (Figure 102-4). The palmaris longus tendon can be identified by having the patient pinch the thumb and fifth fingers together while slightly flexing the wrist. Avoid injecting either the median or ulnar nerve or radial or ulnar artery. If injection produces paresthesia in the distribution of the median or ulnar nerve, withdraw the needle and redirect it to avoid intraneural injection. If the patient gets immediate relief of her symptoms, the diagnosis of CTS is very likely. When the local anesthetic wears off and after 1 day of wrist splinting, the patient can expect symptomatic relief, but the maximum effect may not come until a few days later. Warn the patient that her hand will feel somewhat numb for a few hours, and that a rebound phenomenon or flare may develop within 12 hours after the injection. Nonsteroidal anti-inflammatory drugs (NSAIDs), elevation, and ice packs will help if this rebound pain occurs.

✅ **If the first injection is successful, a repeat injection can be considered after a few months.** Surgery should be considered if a patient needs more than two injections.

✅ Explain the nerve-compression causative factor to the patient and arrange for additional evaluation and follow-up.

✅ Borderline diagnoses may be established with electrodiagnostic studies (nerve conduction and electromyography [EMG]), but they have significant false-positive and false-negative results. If symptoms are refractory to the above conservative measures or if nerve conduction studies show severe entrapment, surgical referral for open or endoscopic carpal tunnel release may be necessary.

✓ **Carpal tunnel syndrome should be treated conservatively in pregnant women, because spontaneous postpartum resolution is common.**

What Not To Do:

✗ Do not rule out thumb weakness just because the thumb can touch the little finger. Thumb flexors may be innervated by the ulnar nerve.

✗ Do not diagnose carpal tunnel syndrome solely on the basis of a positive Tinel sign. Paresthesia can be produced in the distribution of any nerve if one taps hard enough.

✗ Do not perform the Phalen test for more than 60 seconds; maintaining a flexed wrist for longer may produce paresthesia in a normal hand.

✗ Do not prescribe or recommend NSAIDs, pyridoxine (vitamin B_6), diuretics, or chiropractic therapy. They have been shown to be no more effective than a placebo in relieving the symptoms of CTS.

Discussion

Carpal tunnel syndrome is one of the most common causes of hand pain, particularly in middle-aged women. There is little space to spare where the median nerve and digit flexors pass beneath the volar carpal ligament, and very little swelling may produce this specific neuropathy. There is no single reference standard for the diagnosis of CTS. Whether carpal tunnel syndrome is a clinical or electrophysiologic diagnosis remains somewhat controversial. Professional consensus committees have recognized nerve conduction studies as the diagnostic standard for CTS. It must still be appreciated that although electrodiagnostic studies may assist in confirming the diagnosis, they unfortunately have significant false-positive and false-negative results.

Although most cases are idiopathic or the result of nonspecific flexor tenosynovitis, CTS is also associated with trauma and a number of systemic conditions previously mentioned. There is also strong evidence of a positive association of CTS with exposure to forceful work and repetition—for example, in meat packers, poultry processors, and automobile assembly workers.

Although the incidence of diagnosed CTS has increased during the past 20 years, and public attention has focused on excessive keyboard use, frequent computer use has not yet been established as a cause of CTS. Although 30% of frequent computer users complain of hand paresthesias, only 10% meet clinical criteria for carpal tunnel syndrome, and nerve conduction studies are abnormal in only 3.5% of these persons.

Usually, the initial diagnosis of CTS is made on clinical grounds. Because about 50% will resolve spontaneously, not all need to be referred for nerve conduction studies or surgical assessment.

Patients with mild symptoms should be offered conservative treatment. In those cases clearly related to occupational job tasks, such as highly repetitive forceful work or work involving hand and wrist vibration, the patient should be advised to modify the activities or movements that caused the CTS.

Splinting is a low-cost option that may provide benefit and certainly warrants an initial trial. Compared with nighttime-only splint use, full-time use has been shown to provide greater improvement of symptoms and electrophysiologic measures; however, compliance with full-time use is more difficult.

Steroid injection and, to a lesser extent, oral corticosteroids provide the most effective nonsurgical treatment.

Surgical referral should be considered in patients with symptoms that are causing persistent sleep disturbance, interfering with their ability to work, or otherwise adversely affecting their lifestyle.

In general, the management is surgery for persistent symptoms (not resolving after 1 year)

(continued)

Discussion continued

or deteriorating symptoms (worsening clinical plus or minus deterioration on nerve conduction studies). Indications for surgery also include severe symptoms, persistent dysesthesia, thenar weakness or atrophy, and acute median neurapraxia caused by the closed compartment compression. One study showed that patients who had surgery within 3 years of the initial diagnosis were twice as likely to have symptom relief than were those whose surgery was delayed more than 3 years. Endoscopic carpal tunnel release is a newer procedure that allows division of the transverse carpal ligament, with the overlying structures left intact. Use of this procedure purportedly lessens scar formation and allows an earlier return to work and activities of daily living. Neither open nor endoscopic technique has been conclusively proven superior. The wrist is generally splinted for 3 to 4 weeks after surgery.

Less often, the median nerve can be entrapped more proximally, where it enters the medial antecubital fossa through the pronator teres. Symptoms of this type of entrapment syndrome may be reproduced with elbow extension and forearm pronation.

Suggested Readings

Atroshi I, Gummesson C, Johnsson R, et al: Prevalence of carpal tunnel syndrome in a general population, *JAMA* 282:153–158, 1999.

Burke DT, Burke MM, Stewart GW, et al: Splinting for carpal tunnel syndrome: in search of the optimal angle, *Arch Phys Med Rehab* 75:1241–1244, 1994.

Chang MH, Chiang HT, Lee SS, et al: Oral drug of choice in carpal tunnel syndrome, *Neurology* 51:390–393, 1998.

D'Arcy C, McGee S: Does this patient have carpal tunnel syndrome? *JAMA* 283:3110–3117, 2000.

De Smet L: Value of some clinical provocative tests in carpal tunnel syndrome: do we need electrophysiology and can we predict the outcome? *Hand Clin* 19:387–391, 2003.

Deu RS, Carek PJ: Common sports injuries: upper extremity injuries, *Clin Fam Pract* 7:249–265, 2005.

Dias JJ, Burke FD, Wildin CJ, et al: Carpal tunnel syndrome, *J Hand Surg Br* 29:329–333, 2004.

Goodyear-Smith F, Arroll B: What can family physicians offer patients with carpal tunnel syndrome other than surgery? A systematic review of nonsurgical management, *Ann Fam Med* 2:267–273, 2004.

Hui ACF, Wong S, Leung CH, et al: A randomized controlled trial of surgery vs steroid injection for carpal tunnel syndrome, *Neurology* 64:2074–2078, 2005.

Kamath V, Stothard J: A clinical questionnaire for the diagnosis of carpal tunnel syndrome, *J Hand Surg Br* 28:455–459, 2003.

Kele H, Verheggen R, Bitterman H, et al: The potential value of ultrasonography in the evaluation of carpal tunnel syndrome, *Neurology* 61:389–391, 2003.

Kuhlman KA, Hennessey WJ: Sensitivity and specificity of carpal tunnel syndrome signs, *Am J Phys Med Rehab* 76:451–457, 1997.

Tallia AF, Cardone DA: Diagnostic and therapeutic injection of the wrist and hand region, *Am Fam Physician* 67:1356–1362, 2003.

Viera AJ: Management of carpal tunnel syndrome, *Am Fam Physician* 68:265–272, 2003.

Cervical Strain

(Whiplash)

Presentation

The patient may arrive directly from a motor vehicle collision complaining of acute neck pain, arrive the following day (complaining of increased neck stiffness and pain), or arrive anytime afterward (to have the injuries "documented"). The injury was incurred when the neck was subjected to sudden extension and flexion when the car was struck from the rear, possibly injuring intervertebral joints, disks, and ligaments; cervical muscles; or even nerve roots.

Sports injuries are another source of neck injury and pain. As is common with other strains and sprains, the stiffness and pain tend to peak on the day after the injury.

What To Do:

✓ Obtain a detailed history to determine the mechanism and severity of the injury. Was the patient wearing a seat belt? Was the headrest up? Were eyeglasses thrown into the rear seat? Was the seat broken? Was the car damaged? Was the car drivable afterward? Was the windshield shattered? Was there intrusion into the passenger compartment?

✓ Did a sports injury include a worrisome mechanism of injury, such as axial loading with the neck flexed or hyperextended, or did it involve spear tackling (using the helmet as the point of impact when tackling)?

✓ **Historical red flags that suggest a serious spinal injury include any dangerous mechanism of injury (e.g., a fall from a height of more than 1 meter; an axial loading injury, as described above or a diving injury; high-speed [>60 m/hr or 100 km/hr] motor vehicle collision rollover or ejection; motorized recreational vehicle or bicycle collision) or the presence of paresthesias in the extremities, severe neck pain, or persistent patient apprehension.**

✓ To evaluate the possibility of head trauma, ask about loss of consciousness or amnesia, headache, and nausea or vomiting (see Chapter 10).

✓ Examine the patient for involuntary splinting, point tenderness over the spinous processes of the cervical vertebrae, cervical muscle spasm or tenderness, and strength, sensation, and reflexes in the arms (to evaluate the cervical nerve roots).

✓ **Physical red flags that suggest a serious spinal injury include age of 65 years or older, inability of the patient to actively rotate his neck 45 degrees to the left and to the right, any focal neurologic findings, or midline cervical tenderness.**

✅ If there is any question at all of an unstable neck injury because of historical or physical red flags mentioned previously or if there is altered mentation, intoxication, or painful distracting injuries, start the evaluation with a cross-table lateral radiograph of the cervical spine while maintaining cervical immobilization with a rigid collar. If necessary, the anteroposterior (AP) view and open-mouth view of the odontoid can also be obtained before the patient is moved.

✅ Use of plain films is adequate for low-risk patients, but there are no identifiable factors that predict false-negative cervical spine radiographs. Therefore a CT scan of the cervical spine should be obtained when plain films are inadequate or because of difficult clinical circumstances, such as obesity. A CT scan of the cervical spine should also be obtained when you are dealing with a high- or moderate-risk patient who is having CT scanning of other body parts.

✅ **Most minor neck injuries can be safely cleared without obtaining any radiologic studies.** Using the **"Canadian C-spine rule,"** if there are no historical or physical high-risk factors (red flags noted previously), and the patient has low risk factors that allow a safe assessment of neck range of motion (e.g., simple rear-end motor vehicle collision, ability to sit at the time of the examination, ability to ambulate at any time after the injury, or delayed onset of neck pain) and is able to actively rotate his neck 45 degrees to the left and to the right, then he does not need radiographs or CT scanning.

✅ Alternatively, the **National Emergency X-ray Use Study (NEXUS)** can be applied to safely clear the cervical spine without any imaging studies in patients who have normal alertness, are not intoxicated, have no painful distracting injuries, and, on examination, have no midline cervical tenderness or focal neurologic deficits.

✅ **If (1) the C-spine has been cleared clinically or if radiographs or CT scans show no fracture or dislocation, and (2) history and physical examination are consistent with mild to moderate stable joint, ligament, and/or muscle injury, explain to the patient that the stiffness and pain are often worse after 24 hours but usually begin to resolve over the next 3 to 5 days.** Most patients are back to normal in 1 week, although some have persistent pain for 6 weeks.

✅ **When there is significant discomfort, provide 1 or 2 days of intermittent immobilization by fitting a soft cervical collar to wear when out of bed.** Place the wide side of the cervical collar either anterior or posterior, based on the position of maximum comfort. When worn in reverse, the collar allows neck flexion and may be valuable, particularly when carrying out certain activities of daily living, such as driving. If neither position improves comfort, omit the collar. **Under any circumstances, a collar should be used for as brief a time as possible, because early mobilization has been shown to speed recovery.**

✅ Instruct the patient to apply heat or cold if either is found to be beneficial, and take over-the-counter (OTC) acetaminophen or anti-inflammatory analgesics, such as ibuprofen or naproxen.

✅ **Have the patient begin gentle range-of-motion exercises as soon as possible.** One exercise and mobilization protocol consists of small-range and amplitude rotational movements of the neck, first in one direction, then the other, to be repeated 10 times in each direction every waking hour. The movements should be performed up to a maximum comfortable range. These home exercises can be done in the sitting position, if symptoms are not too severe or in the unloaded supine position when the sitting position is too painful.

✓ The athlete must demonstrate a full pain-free range of motion and at least 90% strength before return to play can be advised.

✓ Arrange for follow-up for all patients, as necessary.

What Not To Do:

✗ Do not forget to tell the patient her symptoms may well be worse the day after the injury.

✗ Do not refer the patient for chiropractic manipulation of the cervical spine. There is risk for cervical myelopathy, cervical radiculopathy, and vertebral basilar artery strokes, with little chance of any improvement.

✗ Do not be slack in recording the history and physical examination. This sort of injury may end up in litigation, and a detailed record can obviate the physician being subpoenaed to testify in person.

✗ Do not check neck movement by using passive range-of-motion testing. This has the potential for causing serious neurologic injury.

✗ Do not obtain a radiograph of every neck. A thousand negative cervical spine radiographs are cost effective if they prevent one paraplegic from an occult unstable fracture, but with the Canadian C-spine rules and NEXUS establishing a standard of care for the evaluation of neck injuries, not all patients need radiography just because they were in a motor vehicle collision, fell, or hit their head.

✗ Do not remove shoulder pads and helmets in football and hockey players until the cervical spine has been cleared, unless there is airway compromise or the helmet prevents cervical immobilization. To safely remove this equipment, the patient's torso, head, and neck are elevated about 30 to 40 degrees by a four-person team. With manual stabilization of the neck, the helmet and shoulder pads are removed simultaneously, and the patient is lowered to the supine position.

Discussion

Most injuries to the cervical spine are minor. The most commonly encountered injuries are soft tissue trauma and include ligament sprains, muscle strains, and soft tissue contusions. Fortunately, these injuries generally heal without producing long-term problems.

The cervical spine is made up of seven specialized vertebrae, which together provide a wide range of motion to the head. As with other joints, the large range of motion afforded by the cervical spine comes at the cost of stability, because the cervical region has relatively little intrinsic bony stability and relies on ligament restraints to avoid excessive or pathologic mobility.

The primary static stabilizers of the neck include the anterior longitudinal ligament, intervertebral disk,

posterior longitudinal ligament, ligamentum flavum, facet capsules, and interspinous and supraspinous ligaments. Important dynamic stabilizers consist of the sternocleidomastoid, trapezius, strap, and paraspinal muscles. This muscular envelope functions as a dynamic splint and protects the cervical spine during the full range of motion, whereas the ligamentous structures act as a check rein, limiting motion at the end points.

Strains are defined as stretch injuries occurring at the musculotendinous junction or within the muscle substance. Sprains involve a stretch injury to a ligamentous structure. Cervical contusions involve a blunt-force injury to the soft tissues. Sprains occur with

(continued)

Discussion continued

a spectrum of ligamentous disruptions, ranging from mild pain without instability to gross ligamentous disruption. Injuries to the facet joints and capsular ligaments have been blamed for chronic neck pain following forced flexion injuries, such as whiplash.

Typically, patients who have sustained a cervical sprain, strain, or contusion present with painful, limited cervical motion and tenderness over the involved structure. The management of cervical sprains, strains, and contusions is similar, although ligament injuries usually take more time to heal.

Whiplash, in contrast with most other injuries, has a female preponderance of 2:1. Some have speculated that this gender difference reflects a woman's smaller, less muscular neck. Most patients presenting for evaluation at some point after the injury have less specific symptoms, however, and few "hard" signs on examination. Localized neck pain, neck stiffness, occipital headache, dizziness in all of its forms, malaise, and fatigue are common whiplash symptoms. Localized paracervical tenderness to palpation, reduced range of neck motion, and weakness of the upper extremities secondary to guarding are common findings.

Although most patients with myofascial symptoms recover in several months, 20% to 40% complain of debilitating symptoms for extended periods, sometimes years.

When litigation is involved, some patients exaggerate or lie about persisting symptoms to help make their legal cases. Most plaintiffs who have persistent symptoms at the time of settlement of their litigation, however, are not cured by a verdict. The clinician should evaluate the merits of each case individually. The available evidence does not support bias against patients just because they have pending litigation.

The term *whiplash* is probably best reserved for describing the mechanism of injury and is of little value as a diagnosis. Because of the many undesirable legal connotations that surround this term, it may be advisable to substitute "flexion/extension injury."

Brachial plexus injuries, which are commonly referred to as "stingers" or "burners," are a common occurrence in athletics, especially in football. Either traction on the brachial plexus or compression of the dorsal nerve roots can cause these injuries.

When the neck is flexed laterally and the contralateral shoulder is depressed, a traction force is created on the brachial plexus. Conversely, extreme lateral flexion of the neck can cause cervical nerve root compression by narrowing the neural foramen. Both types of stingers usually result in transient neuropraxia, manifested in the injured athlete as a burning sensation down the affected arm and weakness of C5-6–innervated muscles (deltoid, biceps, supraspinatus, infraspinatus). The athlete is usually seen coming off the field or mat shaking his arm, which may be hanging limply at the side, and leaning toward the side of injury.

Usually, a stinger is a self-limited injury that does not require anything more than keeping the athlete out of the game until the neurologic symptoms have resolved. (Pain usually resolves in less than 15 minutes; strength returns in 24 to 48 hours.)

The athlete should not return to play if there is any cervical pain, limited cervical range of motion, bilateral limb involvement, or persistent neurologic deficits.

Suggested Readings

Bandiera G, Stiell IG, Wells GA, et al: The Canadian C-spine rule performs better than unstructured physician judgment, *Ann Emerg Med* 42:395–402, 2003.

Borchgrevink GE, Kaasa A, McDonagh D, et al: Acute treatment of whiplash neck sprain injuries: a randomized trial of treatment during the first 14 days after a car accident, *Spine* 23:25–31, 1998.

Daffner RH: Identifying patients at low risk for cervical spine injury: the Canadian C-spine rule for radiography, *JAMA* 286:1893–1894, 2001.

Demetriades D, Charalambides K, Chahwan S, et al: Nonskeletal cervical spine injuries: epidemiology and diagnostic pitfalls, *J Trauma* 48:724–727, 2000.

Devereaux MW: Neck pain, *Prim Care* 31:19–31, 2004.

Dickinson G, Stiell IG, Schull M, et al: Retrospective application of the NEXUS low-risk criteria for cervical spine radiography in Canadian emergency departments, *Ann Emerg Med* 43:507–514, 2004.

Dorshimer GW, Kelly M: Cervical pain in the athlete: common conditions and treatment, *Prim Care* 32:231–243, 2005.

Evans RW: The postconcussion syndrome and whiplash injuries; a question-and-answer review for primary care physicians, *Prim Care* 31:1–17, 2004.

Gennis P, Miller L, Gallagher J, et al: The effect of soft cervical collars on persistent neck pain in patients with whiplash injury, *Acad Emerg Med* 3:568–573, 1996.

Griffen MM, Fryberg ER, Kerwin AJ, et al: Radiographic clearance of blunt cervical spine injury: plain radiograph or computed tomography scan? *J Trauma* 55:222–227, 2003.

Hoffman JR, Mower WR, Wolfson AB, et al: Validity of a set of clinical criteria to rule out injury to the cervical spine in patients with blunt trauma, *N Engl J Med* 343:94–99, 2000.

Kerr D, Bradshaw L, Kelly A: Implementation of the Canadian C-spine rule reduces cervical spine x-ray rate for alert patients with potential neck injury, *J Emerg Med* 28:127–131, 2005.

Mower WR, Hoffman JR, Pollack CV, et al: Use of plain radiography to screen for cervical spine injuries, *Ann Emerg Med* 38:1–7, 2001.

Richell-Herren K: Mobilization of neck sprains, *J Accid Emerg Med* 16:363, 1999.

Rosenfeld M, Gunnarsson R, Borenstein P: Early intervention in whiplash-associated disorders, *Spine* 25:1782–1787, 2000.

Stiell IG, Wells GA, Vandemheen KL, et al: The Canadian C-spine rule for radiography in alert and stable trauma patients, *JAMA* 286:1841–1848, 2001.

Stiell IG, Clement CM, McKnight RD, et al: The Canadian C-spine rule versus the NEXUS low-risk criteria in patients with trauma, *N Engl J Med* 349:2510–2518, 2003.

Viccellio P, Simon H, Pressman BD: A prospective multicenter study of cervical spine injury in children, *Pediatrics* 108:E20, 2001.

Zmurko MG, Tannoury TY, Tannoury CA, Anderson DG: Cervical sprains, disc herniations, minor fractures, and other cervical injuries in the athlete, *Clin Sports Med* 22:513–521, 2003.

Cheiralgia Paresthetica

(Handcuff Neuropathy)

Presentation

The patient may complain of pain around the thumb caused by tight handcuffs. The pain decreases with handcuff removal, but there is residual paresthesia or decreased sensation over the radial side of the thumb metacarpal (or a more extensive distribution). Pulling on a ligature around the wrist or wearing a tight watchband may also produce the same injury.

What To Do:

✅ Carefully examine and document the motor and sensory function of the hand. Draw the area of paresthesia or decreased sensation as demonstrated by light touch or two-point discrimination. Document that there is no weakness or area of complete anesthesia.

✅ **Explain to the patient that the nerve has been bruised and that its function should return as it regenerates, but that the process is slow, requiring about 2 months.**

✅ Arrange for follow-up if needed. Bandages, splints, or physical therapy are usually not necessary.

What Not To Do:

❌ Do not overlook more extensive injuries, such as a complete transection of the nerve (with complete anesthesia) or more proximal radial nerve palsy (see Chapter 129). Do not forget alternative causes, such as peripheral neuropathy, de Quervain tenosynovitis (see Chapter 108), carpal tunnel syndrome (see Chapter 103), scaphoid fracture (see Chapter 130), or a gamekeeper's thumb (see Chapter 135).

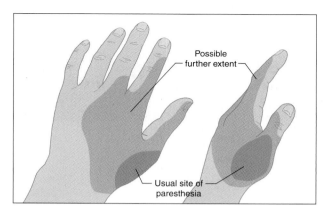

Figure 104-1 *Darkest shading* shows the usual site of paresthesia. *Lighter shading* shows possible further extent.

Discussion

A superficial, sensory, cutaneous twig of the radial nerve is the branch most easily injured by constriction of the wrist. Its area of innervation can vary widely (Figure 104-1). Axonal regeneration of contused nerves proceeds at about 1 mm per day (or about an inch per month). Recovery may require 2 months (measuring from site of injury in wrist to end of area of paresthesia). Patients may want this injury documented as evidence of "police brutality," but it can be a product of their own struggling as much as too-tight handcuffs.

Suggested Reading

Younger DS: Entrapment neuropathies, *Prim Care* 31:53–65, 2004.

Clavicle (Collarbone) Fracture

Presentation

The patient has fallen onto his shoulder or, less commonly, an outstretched arm, or has received a direct blow to the clavicle and now presents with anterior shoulder pain. With distal clavicle fractures, patients may complain of pain on the top of the shoulder. There may be deformity of the bone with swelling, abrasion, and/or ecchymosis. This is usually seen in the midclavicle and is exquisitely tender if palpated. The deformity may appear similar to an acromioclavicular (AC) joint separation with distal clavicle fractures, but the tenderness is usually more medial along the clavicle than with AC injuries (see Chapter 96). The affected shoulder may appear slumped inward and downward compared with the contralateral shoulder, and the patient is usually supporting the injured side by holding his arm close to his body. Paresthesias in the distribution of the supraclavicular nerves can occur.

An infant or small child might present not moving the arm after a fall, but examination of the arm will be normal, and only further examination of the clavicle will reveal the actual site of the injury.

What To Do:

✓ Perform a detailed history and physical examination. A high-energy mechanism of injury should raise the suspicion of associated injuries. A motorcycle collision or fall from a great height should lead to suspicion of ipsilateral rib fractures and/or pulmonary injury. All patients with suspected clavicle fractures should be questioned with respect to any neck pain, numbness or paresthesias, chest pain, or shortness of breath. Palpation of the ribs and assessment of chest excursion are essential. Cervical motion should be full and pain free.

✓ After completing a musculoskeletal examination, including gentle palpation along the entire length of the clavicle and proximal humerus, evaluate the neurovascular status of the arm.

✓ **Obtain radiographs to rule out or accurately define a suspected clavicle fracture. A simple anteroposterior (AP) view of the clavicle will demonstrate most midclavicle fractures. An acromioclavicular (Zanca) view, which is a 20-degree cephalad view, is normally included.** If there is suspicion of glenohumeral joint injury, shoulder radiographs should be added. If there is any shortness of breath, a chest radiograph should be performed. Occasionally, a **CT scan can be useful for evaluation of comminution, position of fracture fragments, and, most important, evaluation of a suspected sternoclavicular (SC) joint injury.** Fractures or dislocations at the sternal end of the clavicle are often difficult to see on plain radiographs but are well visualized on CT scans.

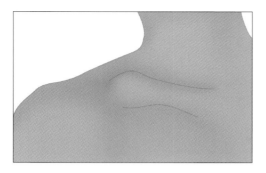

Figure 105-1 Clinical appearance of a type II distal clavicle fracture.

Obtain orthopedic consultation if there is any evidence of neurovascular compromise. Consultation should also be obtained with open fractures or if there is significant displacement (> 2 cm) between fracture fragments or if the overlying skin is tented and appears to be under tension. Fractures of the distal third of the clavicle medial to the acromioclavicular joint, where the proximal fragment is detached from the coracoclavicular ligaments and is unstable (type II; Figure 105-1), also require orthopedic consultation to consider surgical reduction. Additionally, fractures with complete displacement (displacement greater than one bone width) also need orthopedic consultation.

All uncomplicated fractures can simply be treated with a sling to provide comfort and appropriate immobilization. Rotation at the glenohumeral joint should be encouraged. The sling can be discontinued when the pain is resolved. Passive and active range-of-motion exercises can begin as soon as the patient's comfort allows.

Prescribe analgesics, usually acetaminophen or anti-inflammatories such as ibuprofen or naproxen, but generously add narcotics when significant pain is present or anticipated.

Inform the patient that he may be more comfortable sleeping in a semiupright position, with a sling.

Arrange for orthopedic follow-up in 1 week to evaluate healing and begin pendulum exercises of the shoulder. Resistive strengthening can commence when the fracture site is nontender and full pain-free motion exists.

Contact sports are to be avoided until the fracture appears clinically and radiographically to be healed.

Inform the patient that the bone will likely heal with a noticeable callus (visible lump).

What Not To Do:

Do not apply a figure-of-eight dressing or a Kenny-Howard–type splint. They are not necessary and often cause greater patient discomfort.

Do not leave an arm fully immobilized in a sling for more than 7 to 10 days. This can result in loss of range of motion or "frozen shoulder."

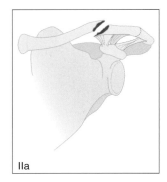
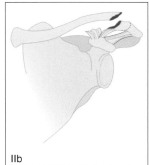

IIa

IIb

Figure 105-2 Type IIa and IIb clavicle fractures.

Discussion

The clavicle connects the shoulder girdle to the axial skeleton and articulates with the acromion laterally and the sternum medially. Clavicle fractures are classified by the location of the fracture, with the clavicle divided into thirds. Most fractures involve the middle segment of the clavicle (approximately 69%). The distal third of the clavicle is fractured roughly 28% of the time, and the proximal third is the least common site of fracture (about 5%, but in some studies, up to 22%).

Distal clavicle fractures are classified into five categories. A type I distal clavicle fracture is minimally displaced and occurs lateral to the coracoclavicular (CC) ligaments. Type II fractures may be medial to the CC ligaments (IIa) or lateral to the CC ligaments with CC ligament disruption from the proximal fragment (IIb) (Figure 105-2), which in both cases results in the proximal segment being detached from the CC ligaments and, therefore, more prone to distraction of the fracture fragments. Type III distal clavicle fractures extend into the AC joint, type IV involves periosteal sleeve disruption (seen in younger patients), and type V involves an avulsion fracture that leaves only an inferior cortical fragment attached to the CC ligaments and is functionally similar to type II. **Only the type II and type V distal clavicle fractures are considered unstable and warrant early orthopedic consultation.**

The management of type II distal clavicle fractures is controversial. Although many authors advocate a surgical approach, because of the relatively high risk of nonunion (approximately 30%), only a small minority of those nonunions have significant functional limitation.

One approach to surgical intervention in both midclavicular and distal clavicular fractures is to treat marked displacement, high-energy injuries, and potential skin compromise with acute surgical fixation. Otherwise, nonsurgical treatment is selected. With distal clavicle fracture, the patient is counseled about the anticipated 20% to 30% nonunion rate but is also informed of the expectation that the chance for persistent pain or functional loss is low.

Proximal clavicle fractures are the least common but are associated with subluxation or dislocation of the corresponding sternoclavicular (SC) joint. CT scans are far superior to plain radiographs in determining the extent of these injuries. **In general, most isolated, minimally displaced, proximal fractures are treated in the same manner as midclavicular fractures. Significant displacement and SC dislocation require rapid orthopedic consultation. Fractures of the proximal clavicle should always prompt a thorough examination to look for other injuries, because approximately 90% have an associated injury.**

In children, fracture of the clavicle requires very little force and usually heals rapidly and without complication. In adults, however, this fracture usually results from a greater force and is associated with other injuries and complications. Clavicle fractures are sometimes associated with a hematoma from the subclavian vein. However, other nearby structures, including the carotid artery, brachial plexus, and lung, are usually protected by the underlying anterior scalene muscle as well as the tendency of the sternocleidomastoid muscle to pull up the medial fragment of bone.

Discussion continued

A great deal of angulation deformity and distraction on radiographs of midshaft fractures are usually acceptable, because the clavicle mends and re-forms itself so well and does not have to support the body in the meantime. As with rib fractures, respiration prevents full immobilization, and therefore the relief that comes with callus formation may be delayed.

Suggested Readings

Anderson K, Jensen PO, Lauritzen J: Treatment of clavicular fractures: figure-of-eight bandage versus a simple sling, *Acta Orthop Scand* 58:71–74, 1987.

Eskola A, Vainionpaa S, Myllynen P, et al: Outcome of clavicular fracture in 89 patients, *Arch Orthop Trauma Surg* 105:337–338, 1986.

Shuster M, Abu-Laban RB, Boyd J, et al: Prospective evaluation of clinical assessment in the diagnosis and treatment of clavicle fracture: are radiographs really necessary? *Can J Emerg Med* 5:309–313, 2003.

Stanley D, Norris SH: Recovery following fractures of the clavicle treated conservatively, *Injury* 19:162–164, 1988.

Coccyx Fracture

(Tailbone Fracture)

Presentation

The patient slipped and fell on his buttocks or tailbone, was kicked or injured during an athletic activity, directly impacting the sacrococcygeal synchondrosis, and now complains of pain at the tip of his spine that is worse with sitting and perhaps with defecation. There should be little or no pain with standing, but walking may be uncomfortable. On physical examination, there is point tenderness and perhaps deformity of the coccyx that may be best palpated by examining through the rectum with a gloved finger (Figure 106-1).

What To Do:

⊘ Verify the history (was this actually a straddle injury?) and examine thoroughly, including the lumbar spine, pelvis, and legs. **Palpate the coccyx** from inside and out, feeling primarily for point tenderness and/or pain on motion. Often, with gentle examination with a gloved hand, the entire coccyx can be examined and tested for stability without the discomfort of a rectal examination.

⊘ **Radiographs are optional and probably should be avoided.** Any noticed variation can be an old fracture or an anatomic variant, and a fractured coccyx can appear within normal limits.

⊘ **The diagnosis can usually be made clinically. If there is a tender deformity, especially if accompanied by movement or crepitus of the distal segment, a fracture of the coccyx is most probable.** Exquisite tenderness alone is an indication of contusion or a stable nondisplaced fracture. **The therapy is the same for both contusion and fracture.**

⊘ **Reassurance and an explanation of your findings and presumed diagnosis will be satisfying to most patients without having to get radiographs,** especially when the patients are informed about the frequent inaccuracy of radiographs and the fact that you do not want to expose their genital area to any unnecessary irradiation.

⊘ **Instruct the patient in how to sit forward, resting his weight on ischial tuberosities and thighs, instead of on the coccyx. A foam-rubber doughnut cushion or gel cushion may help. If necessary, prescribe or recommend acetaminophen or anti-inflammatory pain medications and stool softeners. Cold packs or hot sitz-type baths may provide further comfort. Avoid narcotics when possible, because constipation may aggravate the coccygeal pain.**

⊘ Inform the patient that the pain will gradually improve over 1 to 4 weeks as bony callus forms and motion decreases, and arrange for follow-up as needed.

⊘ If pain persists for a minimum of 2 months, consider injection of corticosteroid (i.e., methylprednisolone [Depo-Medrol] 20 mg) or therapeutic ultrasound. Chronic pain is rare, but treatable, by surgically removing the coccyx.

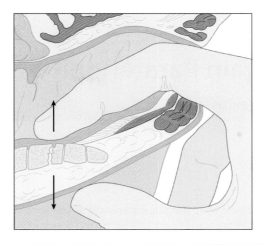

Figure 106-1 Finger palpating the coccyx by rectal examination.

Discussion

The term *coccyx* actually comes from the Greek term *kokkoux* (for cuckoo) because it resembles the shape of a cuckoo's beak.

A fracture, contusion, or partial dislocation of the sacrococcygeal junction can cause painful, abnormal movement of the coccyx, especially when sitting pressure is applied to this region. Resulting pain can involve use of the levator ani muscle and the anococcygeal, sacrotuberal, and sacrospinal ligaments, as well as the gluteus maximus muscles.

De Quervain Paratenonitis

(Thumb Tenosynovitis)

Presentation

The patient, usually a middle-aged woman, experiences an insidious onset of difficulty with tasks such as opening jars because of pain localized to the dorsoradial aspect of the wrist that is exacerbated with thumb and wrist motion, and which may also be present on awakening. Mothers of infants aged 6 to 12 months and daycare workers are frequently affected because of repetitive lifting of infants. De Quervain disease is also common in racquet sports, fishing, and golf.

On examination, the first dorsal compartment over the radial styloid is thickened and tender to palpation. Crepitus of the tendon may be felt on active and passive thumb motion. Tenderness will be elicited on palpating or stretching the extensor pollicis brevis and abductor pollicis longus tendons bordering the palmar side or, less commonly, the extensor pollicis longus tendon bordering the dorsal side of the anatomic snuff box (Figure 107-1).

What To Do:

✅ Obtain a careful history to reveal the underlying causative activity as well as to inquire into the patient's general health. An alternate source of this paratendinopathy may be uncovered, such as gonococcal tenosynovitis or fluoroquinolone-induced tendinopathy.

✅ Perform a physical examination to determine the exact source of pain and tenderness.

✅ Document normal circulation and sensation. Compress the thumb metacarpal onto the scaphoid (axial loading of the carpometacarpal joint) to rule out arthritis at the joint with a painless maneuver.

✅ **Have the patient fold the thumb into the palm, close the fingers over it into a fist, then passively ulnar deviate the wrist. This is known as the Finkelstein test** (Figure 107-2) **and reproduces the pain of de Quervain tenosynovitis of the extensor pollicis brevis and abductor pollicis longus tendons.** A positive test causes sharp pain over the first dorsal compartment.

✅ **Acute de Quervain paratenonitis responds best to corticosteroid injection into the tendon sheath** (Figure 107-3). Results of a recent meta-analysis of treatments for de Quervain tenosynovitis showed that there was an 83% cure rate with injection alone. This rate was much higher than any other therapeutic modality (61% for injection and splint, 14% for splint alone, and 0% for rest or nonsteroidal anti-inflammatory drugs [NSAIDs]). **Tendon-sheath injection is a technique that can be used by the more experienced clinician.** Using a

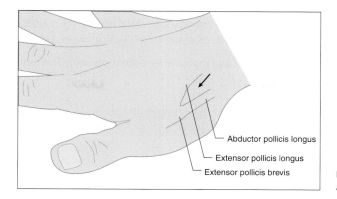

Figure 107-1 First dorsal wrist compartment and the extensors of the thumb.

Abductor pollicis longus

Extensor pollicis longus

Extensor pollicis brevis

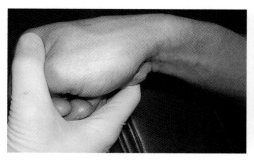

Figure 107-2 Demonstration of the Finkelstein test. (Adapted from Parmelee-Peters K, Eathorne SW: The wrist: common injuries and management. *Prim Care* 32:35-70, 2005.)

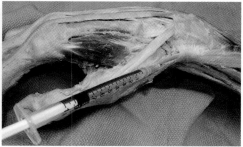

Figure 107-3 Inject site for de Quervain tenosynovitis. (Adapted from Parmelee-Peters K, Eathorne SW: The wrist: common injuries and management. *Prim Care* 32:35-70, 2005.)

27-gauge, ½- to 1-inch needle, slowly penetrate the skin and soft tissue, aiming for the middle of the tendon. When the tendon is hit, it may produce a muscle reflex, increased resistance to advancement of the needle, and pain, which are signals to withdraw the needle slightly. Move the muscle-tendon unit so it slides back and forth, and readvance the needle until the tendon is felt slightly scraping the point. Back off 1 mm, steady the syringe and needle, and inject 1 mL of betamethasone (Celestone) or 20 mg of triamcinolone (Aristocort) along with 2 mL of bupivacaine (Marcaine) 0.5%. While injecting, palpate the tendon, feeling for a "sausaging" effect as the mixture inflates the sheath. Warn the patient that there may be a transient flare in pain when the anesthetic wears off, which may last 24 to 48 hours. The corticosteroid should begin to have a noticeable therapeutic effect within a few days.

What Not To Do:

Ⓧ Do not allow NSAIDs to be used. They have been shown to be of no value in this condition and have potentially hazardous side effects.

Ⓧ Do not inject directly into the tendon. This may weaken the tendon and lead to future rupture.

(X) Do not inject steroids into the very superficial layer of the subcutaneous tissue. This may cause skin depigmentation, which is particularly noticeable in dark-skinned individuals.

(X) Do not splint the wrist and thumb after steroid injection. This reduces the cure rate over injection alone.

Discussion

Symptoms of de Quervain syndrome are related to overuse. The involved tendons course under the extensor retinaculum in a groove along the radial styloid process. Repetitive wrist motion causes shear stress on the tendons in their small compartment, which results in inflammation of the tenosynovium. This is more accurately called paratenonitis. The term includes what was previously called peritendinitis, tenosynovitis (single layer of areolar tissue covering the tendon), and tenovaginitis (double-layer tendon sheath). Clinically, paratenonitis presents with acute edema and hyperemia of the paratenon with infiltration of inflammatory cells. After a few hours to a few days, a fibrinous exudate fills the tendon sheath and causes the crepitus that can be felt on clinical examination.

This condition is often seen in supermarket cashiers and piecework factory workers and after intensive computer keyboarding. De Quervain disease is approximately 6 times more common in women than in men. It is important to have the patient avoid the activity that brought on the condition.

Tendon sheath injections are well tolerated and can be repeated safely at least three times, spaced several months apart. Most often, one injection is effective. One small study suggested that postpartum women with de Quervain disease respond well to conservative management without steroid injection.

Suggested Readings

Carek PJ, Hunter MH: Joint and soft tissue injections in primary care, *Rheumatology* 7:359–378, 2005.

Maffulli N, Wong J, Almekinders LC: Types and epidemiology of tendinopathy, *Clin Sports Med* 22:675–692, 2003.

Rajwinder SD, Carek PJ: Common sports injuries: upper extremity injuries, *Clin Fam Pract* 7 (2), 2005.

Richie CA: Corticosteroid injection for treatment of de Quervain's tenosynovitis: a pooled quantitative literature evaluation, *J Am Board Fam Pract* 16:102–106, 2003.

Weiss APC, Akelman E, Tabatabai M, et al: Treatment of de Quervain's disease, *J Hand Surg* 19:595–598, 1994.

Extensor Tendon Avulsion—Distal Phalanx

(Baseball or Mallet Finger)

Presentation

There is a history of a sudden resisted flexion of the distal interphalangeal (DIP) joint, such as when the finger tip is struck by a ball or jammed against a stationary object, resulting in pain and tenderness over the dorsum of the base of the distal phalanx. This injury can occur with relatively minor trauma (such as jamming a finger while reaching for a light switch in the dark) or even as a result of a direct blow to the dorsum of the finger. It may or may not be accompanied by swelling and ecchymosis over the DIP joint. When the finger is at rest or held in extension, the injured DIP joint remains in slight or moderate flexion (Figure 108-1).

What To Do:

✓ **Obtain a radiograph** with anteroposterior and lateral views, which may or may not demonstrate an avulsion fracture. The lateral view will allow visualization of a bony avulsion at the dorsal base of the distal phalanx (Figure 108-2).

✓ Test for stability of the collateral ligaments of the DIP joint with varus and valgus stress.

✓ While stabilizing the metacarpophalangeal (MCP) and the proximal interphalangeal joint (PIP) in extension, **ask the patient to extend the DIP joint. There should be a loss of full active extension while active flexion and passive range of motion remain intact.**

✓ **If the avulsion fragment is small or there is no bone involvement, nonoperative treatment is preferred. Apply a finger splint that will hold the DIP joint in neutral position or slight hyperextension and gently secure it in place with tape.** Either a dorsal or a volar splint of aluminum and foam may be used. Plastic fingertip splints are manufactured in various sizes (e.g., Stax extension splints) (Figures 108-3 to 108-5).

✓ **Instruct the patient to keep the DIP joint in full extension continuously and seek hand specialist or orthopedic follow-up care within 1 week.**

✓ **Closed mallet fingers should be immobilized in extension full time for 8 weeks. Patients must understand that if they take the finger out to wash or air it out, they cannot let the DIP joint fall into flexion. Each time the DIP joint flexes, the treatment clock starts over again at time zero.**

✓ Skin breakdown can be a significant problem, and patients should be instructed to remove the splint daily while holding the joint in extension, resting the joint on a flat surface to allow the skin to dry and reduce the chance of maceration. **One splint that is well tolerated and can**

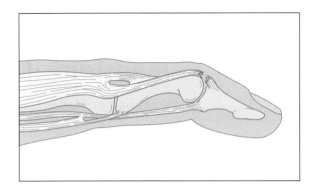

Figure 108-1 Injured distal interphalangeal joint in slight flexion.

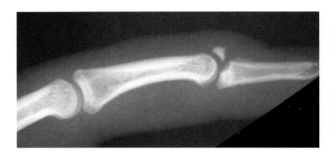

Figure 108-2 Radiograph showing avulsion fracture. (Adapted from Raby N, Berman L, de Lacey G: *Accident and emergency radiology.* Philadelphia, 2005, WB Saunders.)

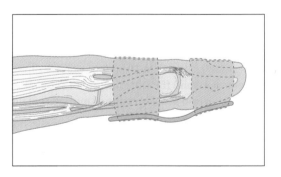

Figure 108-3 Commercial concave aluminum splint.

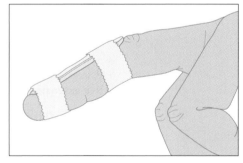

Figure 108-4 Dorsal aluminum splint.

be left on continuously (but is moderately expensive and somewhat difficult to learn how to mold) is the MEALS splint (George Tiemann & Co., Hauppauge, N.Y.).

An additional 6 weeks of splinting can follow if there is not a full ability to extend against resistance. After full active DIP extension is achieved, a gradual withdrawal of the splint can be instituted, with wearing of the splint only at night and with sports for another 6 weeks. Participation in sports is acceptable so long as the DIP joint is firmly immobilized in extension and is protected against further injury.

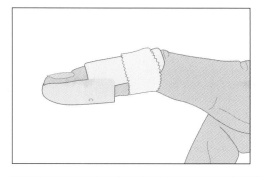

Figure 108-5 Commercial Stax extension splint.

✓ Prescribe an analgesic as needed.

✓ **Surgery is recommended for displaced avulsion fractures with a large articular component** (more than 50% of the articular surface), volar subluxation of the distal phalanx, or failure of splinting.

What Not To Do:

✗ Do not assume that there is no significant injury if the radiograph is negative. The clue to this injury is persistent drooping of the distal phalanx and tenderness over the bony insertion of the extensor tendon. With or without a fracture, the tendon avulsion requires splinting.

✗ Do not forcefully hyperextend the joint beyond the point of skin blanch or pain. This can result in ischemia and dorsal skin necrosis over the joint.

✗ Do not unnecessarily impair the movement of the PIP joint.

Discussion

Mallet finger, also known as "baseball finger" or "drop finger," involves disruption of the extensor tendon or an avulsion fracture of the distal phalanx. The classic mechanism involves a direct blow to the tip of the finger while the DIP joint is held in extension. Although this injury is commonly caused during participation in athletic activities (e.g., by contact with a baseball, volleyball, or basketball), mallet finger may occur with household activities, such as pushing off a sock or tucking in bed sheets. Given the mechanism, it makes sense that the middle finger, the longest one, is most commonly involved, although a mallet finger may involve any of the digits, including the thumb.

Swelling and tenderness may be found on the dorsum of the DIP joint, but commonly the injury is painless, and the loss of extension may not appear for several days to weeks.

Patients may wait weeks to months before being seen and may present with a subsequent swan neck deformity. This is caused by the unopposed extensor mechanism on the middle phalanx leading to hyperextension of the PIP joint.

With a chronic mallet finger presentation without significant bone involvement, splinting in extension should still be attempted but must be done for anywhere from 2 to 3 months.

Many splints are commercially available for splinting this injury (e.g., Stax hyperextension splints, padded aluminum, and frog splints), but, in a pinch, a paper clip will do (Figure 108-6). A dorsal splint allows more use of the finger but requires more padding and may contribute to ischemia of the skin

(continued)

overlying the DIP joint. Figure-of-eight taping can also provide some limitation of flexion. A Cochrane review looking at interventions for treating mallet finger injuries found insufficient evidence to establish the effectiveness of different finger splints in determining when surgery is indicated. The MEAL splint noted earlier must be heated in hot water in a nonstick container before it can be molded and stretched to fit the finger. It is very comfortable for the patient, has no absorbent surfaces, and can

be worn after washing without having to remove it to prevent skin maceration. (Patients have to be warned that the MEAL splint may slide off when they are showering.)

Mallet thumb can be treated similarly to mallet finger, with a trial of splinting in extension; however, because larger forces are required to cause mallet thumb, consider earlier surgical intervention than with the same injury in a triphalangeal digit.

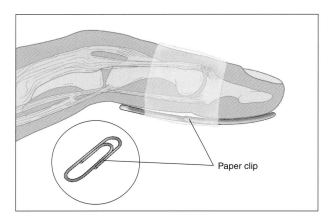

Paper clip

Figure 108-6 Paper-clip splint.

Suggested Reading

Hong E: Hand injuries in sports medicine, *Prim Care* 32:91–103, 2005.

Finger Dislocation

(PIP Joint)

Presentation

The patient will have jammed his finger, causing a hyperextension injury that forces the middle phalanx dorsally and proximally out of articulation with the distal end of the proximal phalanx. An obvious swollen, painful deformity of the proximal interphalangeal (PIP) joint will be present, unless the patient or a bystander has reduced the dislocation on his own.

There should be no sensory or vascular compromise.

What To Do:

✓ When a deformity is present, unless there is crepitus or bony instability and a shaft fracture is suspected, **radiographs may be deferred,** and joint reduction can be carried out first. **If the nature of the injury is at all unclear, obtain radiographs before attempting a reduction.**

✓ **If there has been significant delay in seeking help or if the patient is suffering considerable discomfort,** a digital block over the proximal phalanx or, most effectively, **1% lidocaine injected directly into the joint will allow a more comfortable reduction. The patient may be allowed the choice of whether to use this anesthesia or not.**

✓ **To reduce a dorsal dislocation, do not just pull on the fingertip; instead, with the joint slightly extended, push the base of the middle phalanx distally using your thumb while holding the patient's distal phalanx with your other thumb and index finger. Then, apply traction and gently flex the middle phalanx until it slides smoothly into its natural anatomic position** (Figure 109-1).

✓ Lateral PIP dislocations are dramatic in appearance (pointing laterally at a very unnatural angle), and often they have been self-reduced. When this type of dislocation requires reduction, grasp the end of the affected finger between your thumb and index finger and apply steady traction along the long axis. Bring the middle phalanx into line with the proximal phalanx and squeeze the sides of the PIP joint to correct any residual lateral displacement. A collateral ligament rupture with resultant ulnar or radial joint instability generally accompanies these dislocations.

✓ Volar PIP dislocations are uncommon but are almost always accompanied by an injury to the central slip of the extensor tendon, which can lead to a disabling boutonnière deformity if not properly treated (see Chapter 99). These dislocations can be reduced by applying the same principles used for the dorsal dislocation but in reverse. With mild flexion, push the proximal end of the middle phalanx distally with one thumb, while applying traction on the distal phalanx held between your other thumb and index finger until finally pushing and pulling the middle phalanx dorsally into its normal position.

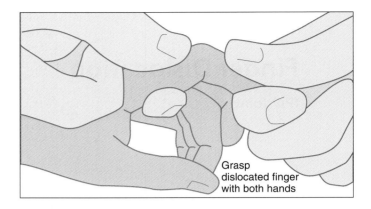

Grasp
dislocated finger
with both hands

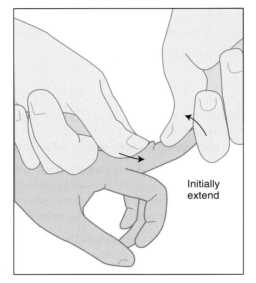

Initially
extend

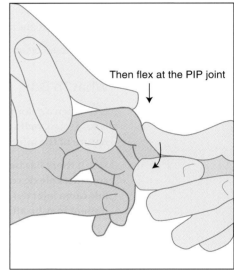

Then flex at the PIP joint

Figure 109-1 Proximal interphalangeal joint reduction for dorsal dislocation.

Irreducible dislocations may be caused by avulsion and entrapment of the volar plate in the joint, entrapment of the long flexor tendon in the joint, or entrapment of an osteochondral fragment. These and all open dislocations necessitate immediate consultation with an orthopedist or hand surgeon. Surgical repair will also be required if there is an avulsion fracture of more than 33% of the articular surface area.

When the joint is reduced, test the PIP joint for collateral ligament instability by applying varus and valgus stress in full extension and 20 degrees of flexion. A partial ligament tear allows no laxity, but there is little or no resistance to stress if the collateral ligament tear is complete. **Test for avulsion of the central extensor tendon slip by having the patient attempt to extend the middle phalanx against resistance** (see Chapter 99). If the patient cannot extend his finger at the PIP joint, a central slip extensor injury should be suspected.

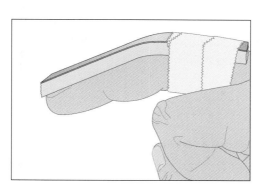

Figure 109-2 Dorsal extension block splint for proximal interphalangeal dislocation.

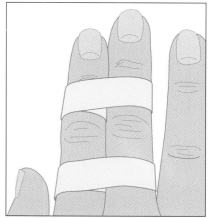

Figure 109-3 Buddy taping.

Testing for avulsion of the volar carpal plate, you will be able to hyperextend the PIP joint more than that of the same finger on the uninjured hand if a disruption is present. Delayed diagnosis of volar plate disruption may lead to chronic pseudoboutonnière deformity (see Chapter 99). **If any of these associated injuries exist, orthopedic consultation should be sought, and prolonged splinting and rehabilitation may be required.**

✓ **Postreduction radiographs should be taken.** "Chip fractures" may represent tendon or ligament avulsions. Radiographs will also allow you to detect an incomplete reduction. The true lateral view is most helpful in detecting subtle subluxation and small avulsion fractures on the volar surface. In an unsatisfactory reduction, the joint's surfaces will be misaligned.

✓ **If the joint feels unstable with a tendency to dislocate when extended, or there are minor fractures present, then splint the finger 20 to 30 degrees short of full extension with a padded dorsal splint for 3 to 4 weeks** (Figure 109-2). Follow up the splinting with buddy taping (Figure 109-3) to the adjacent finger for another 2 to 4 weeks, and provide follow-up for active range-of-motion exercises to restore normal joint mobility. When collateral ligament instability is present, buddy tape the affected finger to the finger adjacent to the ruptured ligament.

✓ When a central extensor tendon slip injury is suspected, splint the PIP joint in full extension without immobilizing the distal interphalangeal or metacarpophalangeal joints (see Chapter 99).

✓ **If the joint feels stable, "buddy taping" to adjacent digits for 7 to 10 days is an acceptable immobilization technique** (see Figure 109-3). **The tape should be removed at night or if the skin becomes wet (to prevent skin maceration). Have the patient dry the skin thoroughly prior to re-taping.** Cotton padding placed between fingers can also be used to prevent skin breakdown.

✓ Inform the patient that joint swelling and stiffness with loss of motion may persist for several months after the initial injury. Prophylactic nighttime PIP extension splinting can be used to prevent the mild PIP joint flexion contractures that are common consequences of these injuries. Active range-of-motion exercises performed by squeezing a soft foam ball can be helpful.

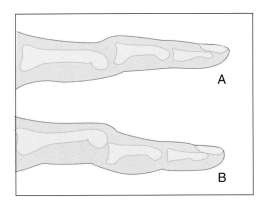

Figure 109-4 A, Dorsal dislocation. **B,** Volar dislocation.

☑ Remind the patient to keep the injured finger elevated. If it provides comfort, you can recommend ice application for 20 minutes three to four times over the next 24 hours and acetaminophen or nonsteroidal anti-inflammatory drugs (NSAIDs) for pain.

What Not To Do:

✗ Do not immobilize the PIP joints by taping over them when buddy taping. Early mobilization of this joint is an important benefit.

Discussion

Proximal interphalangeal dislocations are often simple and easily reduced. However, they may also lead to severely restricted hand function. Most are dorsal dislocations, with the middle phalanx dislocating dorsally, and involve disruption of the volar plate. Often, an athlete reduces the finger himself, or a coach does it (hence the term "coach's finger").

Early recognition of instability—either dorsal, volar, or lateral—offers the best possibility of closed treatment leading to satisfactory functional healing. The main goals are to enable volar plate, collateral ligament, or central slip healing, and to restore normal joint function.

Fracture dislocation is the most disabling PIP joint injury and can result in both dorsal and volar instability (Figure 109-4).

Suggested Readings

Hong E: Hand injuries in sports medicine, *Prim Care* 32:91–103, 2005.

Patel D, Dean C, Baker RJ: The hand in sports: an update on the clinical anatomy and physical examination, *Prim Care* 32:71–89, 2005.

Singer AJ: Comparison of patient and practitioner assessments of pain from commonly performed emergency department procedures, *Ann Emerg Med* 33:652–658, 1999.

Finger Sprain

(PIP Joint)

Presentation

During a sports activity or a fall, the patient's finger is jammed or hyperextended, resulting in a painful, swollen, possibly ecchymotic proximal interphalangeal (PIP) joint. There may have been an initial dislocation, which was reduced by the patient or a bystander (see Chapter 109).

What To Do:

✓ Get a detailed history of the exact mechanism of injury.

✓ Palpate to locate precise areas of tenderness. Pay particular attention to the collateral ligaments, the volar plate, and the dorsal insertion of the central slip of the extensor tendon at the base of the middle phalanx. Note any associated injuries above and below the PIP joint.

✓ **Obtain anteroposterior and lateral radiograph views of the finger.** "Chip fractures" may represent tendon or ligament avulsions. Surgical repair and orthopedic consultation are required if there is an avulsion fracture of more than 33% of the articular surface.

✓ If pain precludes active motion testing or passive stressing of the joint ligaments, consider using a 1% lidocaine digital block or, more effectively, direct joint injection. The patient may decide if this anesthesia is used or not. (He may prefer feeling the pain of the examination than the pain of injection.)

✓ **Assess collateral ligament stability by stress testing the injured joint both radially and ulnarly—performed with the joint at about 20 degrees of flexion. A partial ligament tear allows no laxity, but there is little or no resistance to stress if the collateral ligament tear is complete.**

✓ **Test for** avulsion of the central anterior tendon slip **by having the patient attempt to extend the middle phalanx against resistance** (see Chapter 99). **If the patient is unable to extend his finger at the PIP joint, a central-slip extensor injury should be suspected.**

✓ **Test for an** avulsion of the volar carpal plate **by passively attempting to hyperextend the PIP joint.** If hyperextension is greater than that of the same finger on the uninjured hand, a disruption of the volar plate must be considered, because delay in making this diagnosis may lead to chronic pseudoboutonnière deformity (see Chapter 99).

✓ If any of these associated injuries exist, orthopedic consultation should be sought, and prolonged splinting and rehabilitation may be required.

✅ **When there is no loss of function and no significant joint instability or fracture, immobilize the joint by buddy taping adjacent digits.** Have the patient remove the tape while sleeping or if the hand becomes wet (to prevent maceration of the skin), and have him dry the skin thoroughly prior to re-taping. **Prophylactic nighttime PIP extension splinting can be used with the more serious sprains to prevent the mild PIP joint flexion contractures that are common consequences of these injuries.** Very minor sprains may not require any special splinting.

✅ When a central extensor tendon slip injury is suspected, splint the PIP joint in full extension without immobilizing the distal interphalangeal or metacarpophalangeal joints (see Chapter 99).

✅ **Disruption of the volar plate with abnormal hyperextension at the PIP joint and injuries with minor fractures require splinting with a padded dorsal splint 20 to 30 degrees short of full extension for 3 to 4 weeks with buddy taping to the adjacent finger for another 2 to 4 weeks.** Provide follow-up for active range-of-motion exercises to restore normal joint mobility.

✅ **When collateral ligament instability is present, splint the affected finger to the finger adjacent to the ruptured ligament.**

✅ Instruct the patient to use elevation and acetaminophen or nonsteroidal anti-inflammatory drugs (NSAIDs) for pain. Ice may be used if it provides comfort.

✅ Inform the patient that swelling, stiffness, and discomfort may persist for several months, and provide follow-up for continued care or physical therapy. Active range-of-motion exercises performed by squeezing a soft foam ball can be helpful.

What Not To Do:

❌ Do not miss joint instability or tendon avulsion—these injuries require special splinting and orthopedic referral.

❌ Do not immobilize the PIP joints when buddy taping by taping over the PIP joints. Early mobilization is an important benefit.

Discussion

Most PIP joint sprains are stable and heal well with minimal splinting and early mobilization.

The major complications of the more severe PIP joint injuries are stiffness, joint enlargement, ligamentous laxity, and boutonnière deformity. Temporary stiffness and joint enlargement are to be expected for most PIP joint sprains. Boutonnière deformity (see Chapter 99) can be prevented by adequate examination and diagnosis of volar-plate disruption and central-slip injuries. Ligamentous laxity is not common, but if there is significant laxity, which usually affects the index or small finger, the ligament may need to be surgically reattached or reconstructed.

Early recognition of instability—either dorsal, volar, or lateral—as well as discovering weakness to extension against resistance, offers the best possibility of closed treatment leading to satisfactory functional healing. The main goals are to enable volar-plate, collateral-ligament, or central-slip healing, and to restore normal joint function.

Fingertip (Tuft) Fractures

Presentation

The patient seeks help after a crushing injury to the fingertip, such as catching it in a closing car door. The finger tip will be swollen and painful, with ecchymosis. There may or may not be a subungual hematoma, open nail bed injury, or fingerpad laceration.

What To Do:

✓ Assess for associated injuries and distal interphalangeal (DIP) joint instability.

✓ **Obtain finger radiographs with anteroposterior and lateral views.**

✓ **If there are open wounds, perform a digital block** (see Appendix B), **thoroughly cleanse and débride any open wounds, and repair any nail bed lacerations** (see Chapter 146).

✓ **For open-tuft fractures with clean wounds, prophylactic antibiotic coverage is not indicated. Early aggressive local wound care has been found to be the best prevention against infection in open fingertip fractures.** When there is gross contamination with marginally viable tissue, prophylactic antibiotics such as cefazolin (Ancef), 1000 mg IV, followed by cephalexin (Keflex), 500 mg qid PO × 5 days, may be appropriate.

✓ Provide tetanus prophylaxis for open fractures (see Appendix H).

✓ Treat painful subungual hematomas (see Chapter 156).

✓ **Apply a sterile, nonadhesive protective dressing to open wounds** (see Appendix C), **and with or without an open wound, provide an aluminum fingertip splint** (Figure 111-1) **to prevent further injury and pain.**

✓ **If necessary, provide oral analgesics and advise the patient to elevate the injury above the heart to minimize swelling.**

✓ Ensure follow-up to monitor the patient's recovery, and in the case of open fracture, to intervene in the event of infection.

What Not To Do:

✗ Do not splint the proximal interphalangeal joint.

✗ Do not prescribe prophylactic antibiotics for clean and uncomplicated open fractures of the distal tuft. Prophylactic antibiotics have been shown to be of no benefit when aggressive irrigation and débridement have been provided.

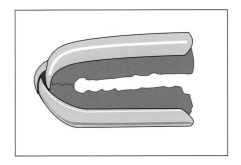

Figure 111-1 Aluminum fingertip splint.

(X) Do not obtain cultures from acute open-tuft fractures. They have not been shown to be helpful in making therapeutic decisions.

Discussion

Distal phalanx fractures are the most frequently seen fractures of the hand, with the tuft being the most common site. Fractures at the base of the distal phalanx may lead to chronic pain and degenerative changes in the distal interphalangeal joint if there is significant intra-articular involvement, and require referral to an orthopedic or hand surgeon

Suggested Readings

Sloan JP, Dove AF, Maheson M, et al: Antibiotics in open fracture of the distal phalanx? *J Hand Surg Br* 12:123–124, 1987.

Stevenson J, McNaughton G, Riley J: The use of prophylactic flucloxacillin in treatment of open fractures of the distal phalanx within an accident and emergency department: a double-blind randomized placebo-controlled trial, *J Hand Surg Br* 28:388–394, 2003.

Suprock MD, Hood JM, Lubahn JD: Role of antibiotics in open fractures of the finger, *J Hand Surg Am* 15:761–764, 1990.

Flexor Digitorum Profundus Tendon Avulsion—Distal Phalanx

(Splay Finger)

Presentation

The patient has injured his finger tip by falling backward and striking it on the floor or hitting it in some other way, causing sudden and forceful hyperextension at the distal interphalangeal (DIP) joint against resistance. Alternatively, this injury can befall a football player trying to tackle the ball carrier but only catching the jersey or belt with the distal phalanx of one finger (Figure 112-1). Both mechanisms can avulse the insertion of the flexor tendon on the distal phalanx. The patient may feel a pop, followed by immediate pain and swelling. The distal fingerpad becomes markedly swollen, often with ecchymosis. The patient is often unaware that he cannot flex the DIP joint.

What To Do:

✓ Have the patient try to close the fingers against the palm in a loose fist. All the fingers will readily flex into the palm, but the DIP joint of the injured digit is unable to bend, and the patient cannot bring the finger tip into the palm. The patient will have full range of motion of the proximal interphalangeal joint.

✓ Neurovascular examination reveals intact function.

✓ **Obtain radiographs of the finger with anteroposterior and lateral views.** The radiograph is usually normal, although occasionally a small avulsion fracture may be visible on the proximal volar aspect of the distal phalanx.

✓ **Request consultation from a hand surgeon for early surgical repair.** If this injury is not treated within 3 weeks, the tendon will shorten and retract into the palm.

✓ **A protective dorsal splint (positioned for greatest comfort) incorporating the adjacent finger and extending to the mid-forearm can be applied to reduce pain and help prevent further injury.**

✓ Provide necessary analgesia with nonsteroidal anti-inflammatory drugs (NSAIDs) or acetaminophen.

What Not To Do:

✗ Do not assume a simple sprain exists because of negative radiographs. When there is marked swelling of the distal finger pad following a grabbing injury, be mindful of the possibility of a flexor digitorum profundus avulsion.

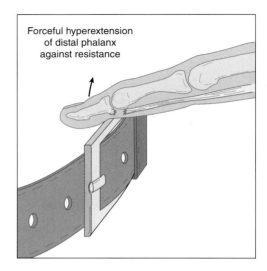

Forceful hyperextension
of distal phalanx
against resistance

Figure 112-1 Avulsion of the flexor digitorum profundus tendon.

Discussion

Avulsion of the insertion of the flexor digitorum profundus tendon results from the sudden forced extension of a finger during resisted flexion of the digit with the metacarpophalangeal joint in extension. Unless the clinician specifically examines for active flexion of the DIP joint, the opportunity to repair the tendinous insertion may be lost.

Suggested Reading

Grant I, Berger AC, Ireland DC: Rupture of the flexor digitorum profundus tendon to the small finger within carpal tunnel, *Hand Surg* 10:109–114, 2005.

Ganglion Cysts

Presentation

The patient is concerned about a rubbery, rounded swelling most commonly emerging from the dorsal or volar aspect of the wrist or the flexor tendon sheath of the hand. It may have appeared abruptly, been present for years, or fluctuated, suddenly resolving and gradually returning in pretty much the same place. The patient often first notices it when a minor injury brings it to their attention and frightens them. There is usually little tenderness, inflammation, or interference with function, but ganglion cysts may be bothersome with symptoms that include pain, paresthesias, limitation of motion, or weakness. Often, the patient is only disturbed by its unsightly appearance.

What To Do:

✓ Take a thorough history and physical examination of the hand to ascertain that everything else is normal. These cysts are usually self-evident and generally no larger than 2 cm in diameter. They are soft and ballotable and appear on the dorsal or volar aspect of the wrist.

✓ **It is unnecessary to obtain a radiograph of a classic, asymptomatic ganglion cyst.** Standard radiographs will not demonstrate the cyst and need only be obtained when the cyst is symptomatic and there is a question of underlying bony disease or injury.

✓ **Although most ganglions can be diagnosed easily on physical examination, ultrasonography may be helpful in diagnosing a small or questionable lesion. Transillumination with an otoscope light will demonstrate its clear cystic nature.**

✓ **Explain to the patient that this is a fluid-filled cyst, spontaneously arising from bursa, ligament, or tendon sheath and poses no particular danger. Treatment options include the following: (1) doing nothing; (2) draining the contents of the cyst with an 18- or 22-gauge needle to reduce its size, with or without injecting it afterward with a corticosteroid; or (3) arranging for a surgical excision, which will provide a definitive pathologic diagnosis.**

✓ **Most ganglia resolve spontaneously and do not require treatment.**

✓ If the patient has symptoms, including pain or paresthesias, or is disturbed by the appearance, aspiration with or without injection of a corticosteroid is effective, without recurrence, in 27% to 67% of patients. Surgical treatment involves total ganglionectomy, with removal of a modest portion of the attached capsule. Recurrence after surgical treatment is between 5% and 15%.

✓ Follow the wishes of the patient regarding treatment, and arrange for follow-up.

If the patient requests immediate decompression, prepare the skin and anesthetize the skin and cyst wall using a 30-gauge needle with 1% lidocaine. With an 18- or 22-gauge needle on a 10-mL syringe, aspirate the mucinous contents. Optionally, instill a long-acting corticosteroid, such as 1 mL betamethasone (Celestone Soluspan) or 10 to 20 mg of triamcinolone (Kenalog-10), along with 2 mL of 0.25% or 0.5% bupivacaine (Marcaine). When injecting a corticosteroid after aspiration, a hemostat is used to stabilize the needle while the syringe is changed.

Provide appropriate follow-up care.

What Not To Do:

Do not ignore a cyst that drains spontaneously. With external drainage, there is the risk for developing a serious joint or soft tissue infection.

Discussion

Ganglion cysts are outpouchings of bursae, ligament, or tendon sheaths, with no clear cause and no relation to nerve ganglia. Perhaps ganglion cysts got their name because their contents are like "glue."

Ganglion cysts may be caused by trauma or tissue irritation when modified synovial cells lining the synovial-capsular interface are stimulated to produce mucin. This mucin dissects along the attached joint ligament and capsule to form capsular ducts and dilatations (lakes) of mucin. The ducts and lakes of mucin coalesce to form a solitary ganglion cyst. Their viscous mucin consists of hyaluronic acid, albumin, globulin, and glucosamine.

Dorsal wrist ganglia represent 60% to 70% of all ganglia. Twenty percent of all ganglia occur in the volar wrist. The flexor tendon sheath of the fingers is involved in 10% to 12% of ganglia.

A dorsally located ganglion of the distal interphalangeal joint is also known as a mucous cyst. Reassurance about their insignificance is often the best we can offer patients.

Suggested Readings

Tallia AF: Diagnostic and therapeutic injection of the wrist and hand region, *Am Fam Physician* 67:745–750, 2003.

Zubowicz VN, Ishii CH: Management of ganglion cysts of the hand by simple aspiration, *J Hand Surg Am* 12:618–620, 1987.

Gouty Arthritis, Acute

Presentation

Usually, a middle-aged male patient with an established diagnosis of gout or hyperuricemia rapidly develops an intensely painful monarticular arthritis, often in the middle of the night, but sometimes a few hours following a minor trauma. Any joint may be affected, usually of the lower limb, including the ankle, knee, and tarsal joints, but most common is the metatarsophalangeal joint of the great toe (podagra). The joint is red, hot, swollen, and intensely tender to touch or movement. There is usually no fever, rash, or other sign of systemic illness, although low-grade fever, leukocytosis, and an elevation of the erythrocyte sedimentation rate may occur. The patient may have predisposing factors that increase his risk for developing gout, such as obesity, moderate to heavy alcohol intake, high blood pressure, diabetes, and abnormal kidney function, or he may be taking certain drugs, including thiazide diuretics, low-dose aspirin, and tuberculosis medications (pyrazinamide and ethambutol).

What To Do:

✅ **If the patient has not been previously diagnosed by arthrocentesis that showed crystals, tap the involved joint as described for acute monarticular arthritis** (see Chapter 120). In addition to ruling out infection, look under the microscope for crystals in the joint fluid. Urate crystals look like needles and may be in white cells. The calcium pyrophosphate dihydrate crystals of pseudogout are rhomboids. Polarizing filters above and below the sample help distinguish the strongly negative birefringent crystals of sodium urate from the weakly positive birefringent calcium pyrophosphate dehydrate (Figure 114-1). The synovial fluid is typically inflammatory with a white blood cell (WBC) count ranging from 5000 to 50,000/mL, predominantly neutrophils. Higher counts should always raise the question of an infection.

✅ Radiographs may be obtained but are only likely to be helpful in the late stages of the disease (Figure 114-2) or if other underlying disease is in question (e.g., pseudogout, tumor).

✅ **In most middle-aged patients with acute gout who are otherwise healthy, nonsteroidal anti-inflammatory drugs (NSAIDs) are the treatment of choice.**

✅ Provide rapid pain relief with loading doses of NSAIDs, such as ketorolac (Toradol), 60 mg IM; indomethacin (Indocin), 50 mg PO tid; ibuprofen (Motrin), 800 mg PO qid; or naproxen sodium (Anaprox), 550 mg PO bid, then tapering after 24 to 48 hours, once pain has subsided, to maintenance doses for the next 5 to 7 days (e.g., indomethacin, 25 mg tid; ibuprofen, 600 mg qid; naproxen, 275 mg bid). Excruciating pain may require one dose of narcotics while the anti-inflammatory drugs take effect. **All NSAIDs have been shown to be equally effective.**

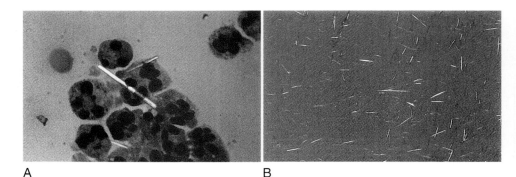

A B

Figure 114-1 A and **B,** Microscopic example of monosodium urate monohydrate microcrystals under polarized light and under light microscopy. (Adapted from Knoop KJ, Stack LB, Storrow AB: *Atlas of emergency medicine,* ed 2. New York, 2002, McGraw-Hill.)

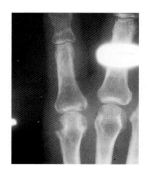

Figure 114-2 The fifth metacarpophalangeal joint in this radiograph is fairly characteristic of the late stages of gout. Marginal erosions of the metacarpal head result in prominent "overhanging" edges. (Adapted from Yu J: *Musculoskeletal imaging.* St Louis, 2001, Mosby.)

The choice of NSAID is not as important as initiating therapy early in an attack. They should be used with caution or not at all in patients with any of the following: significant renal impairment (creatinine > 2), poorly controlled congestive heart failure, history of or active peptic ulcer disease, anticoagulation therapy, or hepatic dysfunction.

✅ **Corticosteroids are effective in the treatment of gout. When used appropriately for a short duration, they are a safe alternative for patients in whom NSAIDs are contraindicated.** Care must be used in patients with diabetes, but in recent years, corticosteroids have been used more often in older patients with multiple comorbid conditions because of their low-toxicity profile.

✅ **For a monoarticular flare-up, an intra-articular injection of a long-acting corticosteroid is often the safest treatment.** Delay injecting corticosteroids into the joint until the possibility of infection is eliminated (see Chapter 120). After draining as much fluid as possible from the joint, using aseptic techniques, inject betamethasone (Celestone Soluspan), 1 mg (small joints) to 4 mg (large joints), or methylprednisolone (Depo-Medrol), about 20 to 40 mg mixed in an appropriate volume (depending on joint size) of bupivacaine (Marcaine) 0.5% to provide immediate pain relief.

✅ **Oral corticosteroids may also be used.** Start with 20 to 40 mg of prednisone (Deltasone) and then taper throughout 8 days. If tapered too rapidly, a rebound flare-up of gout may occur.

✓ An alternative to oral steroids is a single intramuscular injection of methylprednisolone (Depo-Medrol), 40 mg. This has no therapeutic advantage over oral dosing but is useful if the patient cannot take oral medications.

✓ **Adrenocorticotropic hormone (ACTH), 80 units IM, is also effective and can be used in patients with multiple medical problems, including congestive heart failure, chronic renal insufficiency, and peptic ulcer disease.** Its use is limited by patient comfort (IM administration), cost, and availability.

✓ An alternative treatment for acute gouty arthritis within the first 12 to 24 hours of an attack is colchicine, 0.6 mg PO qh, until pain is relieved, the patient develops nausea, vomiting, or diarrhea, or a maximum dose of 6 mg is reached. Often patients experience adverse gastrointestinal (GI) effects before relief of gout symptoms. Colchicine can also be given IV, 2 mg q6h to a maximum of 4 mg. After these maximum doses, no more colchicine should be prescribed for 1 week to avoid toxicity. IV administration can cause anaphylaxis, and extravasation can cause tissue necrosis. At high doses, colchicine is bone marrow–suppressive and with renal insufficiency or patients taking cyclosporine or statins, colchicine can cause neuromyopathy. **Because of its small benefit-to-toxicity ratio, colchicine should only be considered if there is no alternative therapy.**

✓ Colchicine is usually used at low doses, 0.6 mg once or twice daily, to prevent attacks or rebound flare-ups in patients in whom steroids are being tapered or urate-lowering therapy is being started. It should still be used with caution in older patients with reduced renal function.

✓ **It should be remembered that gout is a self-limited disease. At times, the risks of certain treatments may outweigh the benefits, especially in elderly patients.**

✓ Instruct the patient to elevate and rest the painful extremity, apply ice packs, and arrange for follow-up. In gouty arthritis, cold applications, in addition to being a useful adjuvant treatment, are helpful for discriminating gout from other forms of inflammatory arthritis. **Topical ice has been shown to help relieve joint pain in patients with gouty arthritis but not in patients with other inflammatory arthritides.**

✓ Patients should be informed about the factors contributing to their hyperuricemia, such as obesity, a high-purine diet, regular alcohol consumption, and diuretic therapy, which may all be correctable.

✓ Urate-lowering therapy with probenecid or allopurinol is considered cost effective for patients who have two or more attacks of gout per year. Some physicians advocate using this treatment in patients who experience more than four attacks per year.

✓ Most patients will note improvement within the first 12 to 24 hours, with resolution of symptoms in the next 7 to 10 days.

What Not To Do:

✗ Do not depend on serum uric acid to diagnose acute gouty arthritis—it may or may not be elevated (>8 mg/dL) at the time of an acute attack. Hyperuricemia will be found in 70% of patients with their first attack of gout.

Ⓧ Do not use NSAIDs when a patient has a history of active peptic ulcer disease with bleeding. Relative contraindications include renal insufficiency, volume depletion, gastritis, inflammatory bowel disease, asthma, and congestive heart disease.

Ⓧ Do not insist on reconfirming an established diagnosis of gout by ordering serum uric acid levels (which are often normal during the acute attack) or tapping an exquisitely painful joint at every attack in a patient with known gout and a typical presentation.

Ⓧ Do not, on the other hand, miss a septic arthritis in a patient with gout who is toxic and has a high fever, an elevated WBC count, an identified source of infection, or comorbidities, such as diabetes, alcohol abuse, and advanced age. Septic arthritis carries the potential for a high morbidity and mortality.

Ⓧ Do not attempt to reduce the serum uric acid level with probenecid or allopurinol during an acute attack of gouty arthritis. This will not help the arthritis and may even be counterproductive. Leave it for follow-up. Because of the high frequency of comorbid conditions and decreased life expectancy in elderly patients, it may be less important to institute urate-lowering therapy in these patients than in younger patients with many years of cumulative attacks and joint damage in their future.

Ⓧ Do not stop urate-lowering maintenance therapy during an acute attack. In these cases, therapy should be continued, and the acute gouty flare treated in the usual manner.

Discussion

Among mammals, only humans and other primate species excrete uric acid as the end product of purine metabolism. This is because humans and primates lack the enzyme uricase, which converts uric acid to allantoin, a more soluble excretory product.

When overproduction or underexcretion of uric acid occurs, the serum urate concentration may exceed the solubility of urate (a concentration of approximately >6.8 mg/dL), and supersaturation of urate in the serum and other extracellular spaces results. This state (called hyperuricemia), increases the risk for crystal deposition of urate, from the supersaturated fluids, in tissues. Hyperuricemia is defined as a serum uric acid level of more than 7.0 mg/dL in men or more than 6.0 mg/dL in women.

Hyperuricemia is clearly associated with an increased risk for the development of gout, although most patients with hyperuricemia are asymptomatic and never develop gout. In the general population, 80% to 90% of gout patients are underexcreters, although renal function is otherwise normal. The risk for the development of gout increases with increasing serum uric acid level.

In younger patients, hyperuricemia and gout are overwhelmingly observed in men. The initial attack

of gout is monarticular in 85% to 90% of patients. Lower-extremity joints are usually affected, with approximately 60% of first attacks involving the first metatarsophalangeal joints. Attacks may last from a few days to 2 to 3 weeks without treatment, with a gradual resolution of all inflammatory signs and a return to apparent normalcy. An "intercritical" period, lasting weeks to months, may elapse before a new attack occurs in the same or another joint. Without specific therapy, a second attack will occur in 78% of patients within 2 years, and in 93% within 10 years. Over subsequent years, attacks occur more frequently and may be polyarticular and associated with fever and constitutional symptoms. Tophaceous deposits become apparent over the elbows, fingers, or other areas over the years (tophaceous gout), and chronic polyarticular arthritis may develop, which is often less severe, sometimes resembling rheumatoid arthritis or degenerative joint disease. Distal interphalangeal (DIP) joint involvement is a little more common than proximal interphalangeal (PIP) involvement, and tophaceous deposits on Heberden nodes can often be confused with osteoarthritis.

In patients older than 60 years with newly diagnosed gout, approximately 50% are women. Elderly women may have more finger involvement

Discussion continued

than men; 25% of women present with hand involvement and polyarticular disease.

Obesity, genetic predisposition, high intake of meat and seafood, hyperlipidemia, hypertension, and heavy alcohol use are associated with younger gout patients, whereas renal insufficiency, low-dose salicylates, and thiazide diuretic use are more often associated with elderly onset gout.

Transplant patients and patients on cyclosporine therapy are also at increased risk for developing gout, as are patients with myeloproliferative disorders, polycythemia vera, myeloid metaplasia, and chronic myelogenous leukemia.

Trauma, surgery, infection, and starvation as well as alcoholic or dietary indiscretions may provoke acute attacks. Acute attacks have been known to follow a game of golf, a long walk, or a hunting trip, leading to the name "pheasant hunter's toe." The solubility of uric acid decreases with a lower body temperature and in a lowering pH. These properties may provide an explanation for the increase in gouty attacks in the peripheral joints in cold weather.

Radiographs in gout characteristically demonstrate normal bone mineral density until the late stages of the disease. Well-marginated para-articular erosion with overhanging edges or margins is the characteristic lesion of chronic gouty arthritis.

The gold standard for establishing a definite diagnosis of gout is the presence of monosodium urate crystals in aspirated joint fluid or tophus.

Physicians often opt to reach a diagnosis based on clinical features and demonstration of hyperuricemia. No studies have been published on the usefulness or validity of any diagnostic clinical criteria. Serum uric acid levels are commonly elevated in patients without gout and can be normal or even low in patients with gout.

When it is impractical or not possible to obtain joint fluid, supportive data that can be used to make a diagnosis of gout include a history of gout; a typical clinical history of sudden onset of an exquisitely painful joint, classically the first metatarsophalangeal joint; a history of underlying renal disease or use of medications that cause hyperuricemia; an elevated serum urate level; radiologic evidence suggestive of gouty arthritis; and a favorable response to topical cold applications.

Suggested Readings

Monu JU, Pope TL: Gout: a clinical and radiologic review, *Radiol Clin North Am* 42:169–184, 2004.

Rott KT, Agudelo CA: Gout, *JAMA* 289:2857–2860, 2003.

Wise CM: Crystal-associated arthritis in the elderly, *Clin Geriatr Med* 21:491–511, 2005. v–vi.

Knee Sprain

Presentation

After twisting the knee from a slip and fall or sports injury, the patient complains of knee pain and variable ability to bear weight. There may be an effusion or spasm of the quadriceps, forcing the patient to hold the knee at 10 to 20 degrees of flexion. See Figure 115-1 for normal anatomy.

With an anterior cruciate ligament (ACL) tear, there will most likely be a noncontact injury involving a sudden deceleration (landing from a jump, cutting, or sidestepping), hyperextension, or twisting, as is common in basketball, football, and soccer. This may be accompanied by the sensation of a "pop," followed by significant nonlocalizing pain and subsequent swelling and effusion. Significant injuries will have a positive Lachman examination.

The other common knee injury involves the medial collateral ligament (MCL). This may be torn with a direct blow to the lateral aspect of a partially flexed knee, such as being tackled from the side in football, or by an external rotational force on the tibia, which can occur in snow skiing when the tip of the skin is forced out laterally. There may also be an awareness of a "pop" during the injury, but unlike the ACL tear, it is localized to the medial knee, along with more focal pain and swelling. Significant injuries cause laxity of the MCL with valgus stress testing at 30 degrees of flexion.

The meniscus can be torn acutely with a sudden twisting injury of the knee while the knee is partially flexed, such as may occur when a runner suddenly changes direction or when the foot is firmly planted, the tibia is rotated, and the knee is forcefully extended. Pain along the joint line is felt immediately, and there is often a mild effusion with tenderness to palpation along either that medial or lateral joint line. There may be a positive McMurray test.

Posterior cruciate ligament (PCL) injuries occur with forced hyperflexion, as can occur in high-contact sports, such as football and rugby. Tears of the PCL can also occur with a posterior blow to the proximal tibia of a flexed knee, as occurs with dashboard injuries to the knee during motor vehicle collisions. Hyperextension, most often with an associated varus or valgus force, can also cause PCL injury. There is no report of a tear or pop, only vague symptoms, such as unsteadiness or discomfort. There is commonly a mild to moderate knee effusion, and a significant injury will have a positive posterior drawer test, and a posterior sag sign will be present.

Injury of the lateral collateral ligament (LCL) is much less common than injury of the MCL. This usually results from varus stress to the knee, as occurs when a runner plants his foot and then turns toward the ipsilateral knee or when there is a direct blow to the anteromedial knee. The patient reports acute onset of lateral knee pain that requires prompt cessation of activity.

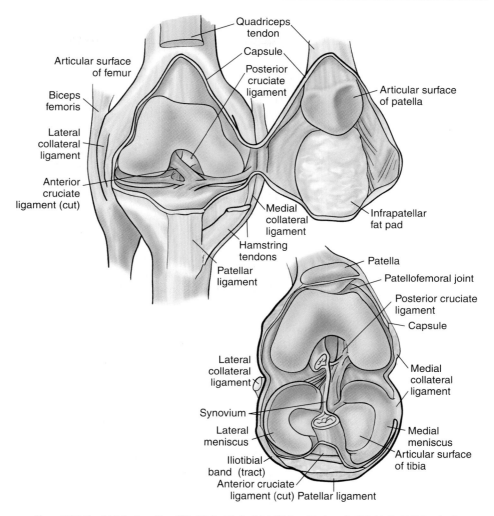

Figure 115-1 Knee joint structures. (From Miller MD, Hart JA, MacKnight JM: *Essential orthopaedics.* Philadelphia, 2010, Saunders.)

What To Do:

☑ If there is going to be any delay in examining the knee, provide ice, a compression dressing, and elevation above the level of the heart.

☑ **For severe pain, provide immediate analgesia with nonsteroidal anti-inflammatory drugs (NSAIDs), such as ibuprofen (Motrin), 800 mg PO, along with a narcotic such as oxycodone (Percocet, Tylox).** Parenteral narcotics may be required.

☑ **Ask about the mechanism of injury, which is often the key to the diagnosis.** The position of the joint and direction of traumatic force dictates which anatomic structures are at greatest risk for injury. The patient can usually re-create exactly what happened by using the uninjured knee to demonstrate.

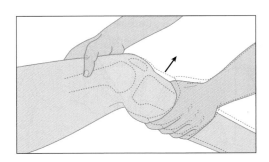

Figure 115-2 The Lachman test.

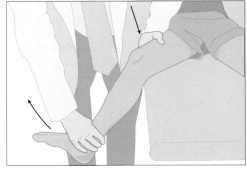

Figure 115-3 Valgus stress test.

✓ Obtain information about associated symptoms. Knee buckling/instability with pivoting or walking is associated with ACL tear. A knee-joint effusion within 4 to 6 hours of injury suggests an intra-articular injury, such as ACL, meniscus, or osteochondral fracture. Sensations of locking or catching inside the knee may be associated with meniscal tears.

✓ **During inspection and examination of the injured knee, comparison with the normal knee is important.** Initiate the examination by focusing first on the leg that is healthy. This helps to create trust and allows the patient to relax for a more accurate examination. Inspect the knee for swelling, ecchymosis, malalignment, or disruption of skin. Palpate the bony and ligamentous structure on the medial and lateral aspect of the knee, and palpate along both joints to elicit any point tenderness. With the patient supine, feel for an effusion and discomfort with patellar motion. Determine if there is any crepitus or limitation in range of motion by gently attempting to fully flex and extend the knee. Look for injuries of the back and pelvis. Check hip flexion, extension, and rotation. Thump the sole of the foot as an axial loading clue to a tibia or fibula fracture.

✓ Document any effusion, discoloration, heat, deformity, or loss of function, circulation, sensation, or movement.

✓ **Stress the four major knee ligaments, comparing the injured with the uninjured knee to determine if there is any instability.** A complete knee examination will help to detect isolated ligamentous injuries but will also help the examiner find coexisting injuries.

✓ **Perform a Lachman test to diagnose injury of the ACL** (Figure 115-2). With the knee flexed 20 to 30 degrees, place one hand on the proximal tibia and the other on the distal femur, with the patient's heel on the examination table. Stabilize the femur, grasp the tibia, and pull it anteriorly with a brisk tug. ACL tears will have increased anterior translation, at least 3 mm greater than the noninjured side, and a soft or nonexistent end point.

✓ **Test MCL stability with the valgus stress test** (Figure 115-3). With the knee still flexed 20 to 30 degrees, grasp the tibia distally to stabilize the lower leg, then apply direct, firm pressure in a medial direction from the lateral femoral condyle. Pain in the location of the MCL during valgus stressing, but no laxity, is called a grade I sprain. Grade II sprains have some laxity during valgus load; however, there is still a solid end point. When there is a soft or nonexistent end point, this is called a grade III MCL sprain, which represents a complete tear of the ligament.

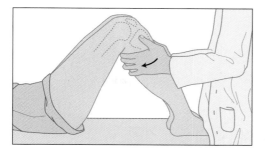

Figure 115-4 Posterior drawer test.

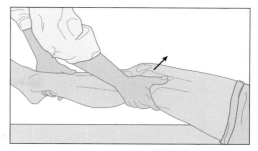

Figure 115-5 Varus stress test. (The valgus stress test is the opposite of this test.)

Repeat valgus stress testing in full extension. If there is joint laxity when the knee is locked in full extension, there is a strong possibility of an accompanying ACL, posterior oblique ligament, or posteromedial capsular tear.

✓ **Test the integrity of the PCL and posterior capsule with the posterior drawer test** (Figure 115-4). The test is performed with the patient supine and the hip flexed to 45 degrees. Flex the knee to 90 degrees and apply firm, direct pressure in a posterior direction to the anteroproximal tibia with your thumbs located on the medial and lateral joint lines. If the force displaces the anterior superior tibial border beyond the medial femoral condyle, this suggests a complete PCL injury; posterior displacement of the tibia more than 5 mm posterior to the femur suggests a combined PCL and posterolateral-corner injury. Look for increased posterior displacement of the tibia and a soft or mushy end point. When the knee is in 90 degrees of flexion, the proximal tibia normally sits about 10 mm anterior to the femoral condyles. If no step-off is present, a posterior sag sign exists and is also associated with PCL injury. These tests may be difficult to perform if there is a large effusion. Fifteen percent of patients with posterolateral knee injuries have a common peroneal nerve injury. It is important to ask patients about sensory changes or muscle weakness and to examine ankle dorsiflexion and great-toe extension.

✓ **Test LCL stability with the varus stress test** (Figure 115-5), pressing laterally on the medial femoral condyle with the knee flexed to 20 to 30 degrees and in full extension. Grading is the same as for MCL sprains. Lateral joint line opening in full extension typically indicates a multiligament injury. Grade III tears are indicative of complete LCL tear and have a high association with posterolateral corner injury or cruciate tears. If there is varus laxity, also check the function of the peroneal nerve by asking the patient to dorsiflex the big toe.

✓ **Examine for an injury to the medial or lateral meniscal cartilage with the McMurray test** (Figure 115-6). With the patient supine, hold the knee anteriorly at the femoral condyle with one hand, fingers positioned along the joint line, and while applying a valgus force to the knee, hold the foot with the other hand. Then, while externally rotating the lower leg, fully flex the knee and hip, slowly extend, and then repeat with the lower leg internally rotated. Pain associated with audible sounds or palpable crepitus suggests a tear of the meniscus. This test may be difficult to complete if there is acute pain and muscle spasm.

✓ **A negative test does not rule out a meniscal tear.** Tenderness from meniscal tears is localized along the joint line, most prominently at or posterior to the collateral ligament. The medial meniscus is more susceptible to injury.

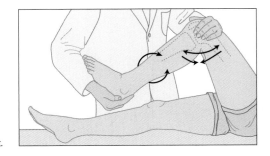

Figure 115-6 The McMurray test.

✅ **Palpate the patella and head of the fibula, looking for tenderness associated with fracture.**

✅ **Assess for effusion** by placing a finger lightly on the patella with the knee relaxed and fully extended and, with the other hand, gently pinching the soft tissue on both sides of the patella, feeling for a fluid wave. In the presence of an intra-articular effusion, the patella can also be bounced or balloted against the underlying femoral condyle.

✅ **Radiographs to rule out fracture may be deferred or avoided if the patient does not meet one of the following Ottawa knee rules:**

- ⚪ Fifty-five years of age or older
- ⚪ Tenderness at the head of the fibula
- ⚪ Isolated tenderness of the patella
- ⚪ Inability to flex the knee to 90 degrees
- ⚪ Inability to bear weight (four steps) both immediately after injury and at initial physical assessment

✅ **These criteria do not apply to patients younger than 5 years of age or patients with an altered level of consciousness, multiple painful injuries, paraplegia, or diminished limb sensation.**

✅ **Minor (grade I) sprains that do not exhibit any joint instability or intra-articular effusion can be treated with rest, elevation, and, if comfort is improved, ice (20-minute periods three or four times a day for 3 days), and acetaminophen or nonsteroidal anti-inflammatory (NSAIDs) (ibuprofen, naproxen).** The patient can usually return to his previous activities as rapidly as pain allows. Provide follow-up if symptoms do not improve in 5 to 7 days.

✅ **Moderate (grade II) and severe (grade III) sprains with partial or complete ligament tears, meniscal tears, joint effusion, or instability should be treated with rest and ice, as above, but also immobilized with a bulky compression splint or knee immobilizer and made non–weight-bearing with crutches.** Patients should keep the leg elevated above the heart as much as possible to minimize swelling. Narcotic analgesics may be added to acetaminophen and/or NSAIDs, and **patients should be referred for orthopedic assessment within 5 to 7 days.**

✅ Instruct the patient that additional injuries may become apparent as the spasm and effusion abate.

What Not To Do:

(X) Do not assume that a negative radiograph means a major injury does not exist.

(X) Do not rely on MRI to assess all injured knees. MRI is not cost-effective or superior to clinical assessment in accuracy. MRI is a useful tool for assessing a knee before operative intervention, especially with posterolateral corner injuries, which may require the reconstruction of multiple ligaments and the lateral meniscus.

(X) Do not inject or prescribe corticosteroids for acute knee injuries. These drugs may retard soft tissue healing.

(X) **Do not miss vascular injuries with bicruciate ligament injuries. These injuries are equivalent to knee dislocations with regard to mechanism of injury, severity of ligamentous injury, and frequency of major arterial injuries.**

Discussion

The ACL, PCL, MCL, and LCL, make up the main static stabilizers of the knee. Together, the four ligaments enable the knee to function as a complex hinge joint, with rotational capabilities that allow the tibia to rotate internally and glide posteriorly on the femoral condyles during flexion and to rotate externally 15 to 30 degrees during extension.

The menisci are crescent-shaped cartilaginous structures that provide a cushioning congruous surface for the transmission of 50% of the axial forces across the knee joint. The menisci increase joint stability, facilitate nutrition, and provide lubrication and shock absorption for the articular cartilage.

Most patients with a knee injury suffer soft tissue damage, including ligament, tendon, meniscal cartilage, and muscle tears. In most cases, plain radiographs do little to aid diagnosis of soft tissue injury. Plain radiographs can show findings suggestive of ACL injury, such as an avulsion of the lateral capsule, known as a Segond fracture or a tibial spine avulsion. They can also show subtle fractures of the posterior tibial plateau or associated fibular head avulsion fractures. However, clinicians must rely on physical examination to identify patients with serious knee injuries that require splinting and/or orthopedic referral.

Joint aspiration of hemarthrosis to reduce severe pain should be reserved for patients with very large or tense effusions and should be performed with sterile technique. Fat globules in bloody joint fluid suggest occult fracture.

Conservative treatment versus surgical reconstruction is the main treatment decision when managing an ACL tear. ACL reconstruction is the preferred treatment for adolescents and most young adults who are unwilling to modify their physical activity levels. In older patients, there is support for both conservative and operative treatment. Patients with a sedentary or low-impact lifestyle are ideal candidates for conservative or nonoperative management. Patients who compete in jumping or cutting sports are likely to benefit from ACL reconstruction.

A medial stabilizing brace can be prescribed for grade II and grade III MCL injuries. Select the longest brace that fits the patient to provide maximum MCL protection. Currently, surgical repair of a grade III MCL tear is reserved for the patient who has associated damage to the ACL or meniscus.

A long-leg knee brace can be prescribed for grade II LCL sprains. One such brace is the extension locking splint, which allows a full range of motion in flexion and extension, but will give support to varus and valgus stresses. This brace can also be locked in extension for ambulation during the first 1 to 2 weeks of rehabilitation.

The standard now for grade III LCL and posterolateral corner injuries with or without PCL involvement is surgical repair, and more often reconstruction, which should be completed within the first 1 to 2 weeks following the injury.

In general, a patient who has had a knee injury can be given the go-ahead to resume sports activities when examination demonstrates that the cruciate and collateral ligaments are intact, the knee is capable of moving from full extension to flexion of 120 degrees, and there is no effusion. The patient's pain should be markedly diminished, and there should be no locking, instability, or limp.

Suggested Readings

Bauer SJ, Hollander JE, Fuchs SH, et al: A clinical decision rule in the evaluation of acute knee injuries, *J Emerg Med* 13:611–615, 1995.

Brown JR, Trojian TH: Anterior and posterior cruciate ligament injuries, *Prim Care* 31:925–956, 2004.

Bulloch B, Neto G, Plint A, et al: Validation of the Ottawa knee rule in children: a multicenter study, *Ann Emerg Med* 42:48–55, 2003.

Emparanza JI, Aginaga JR: Validation of the Ottawa knee rules, *Ann Emerg Med* 38:364–368, 2001.

Gelb HJ, Glasgow SG, Sapega AA, et al: Magnetic resonance imaging of knee disorders: clinical value and cost-effectiveness in a sports medicine practice, *Am J Sports Med* 24:99–103, 1996.

Johnson LL, Johnson AL, Colquitt JA, et al: Is it possible to make an accurate diagnosis based only on a medical history? A pilot study on women's knee joints, *Arthroscopy* 12:709–714, 1996.

Muellner T, Weinstabl R, Schabus R, et al: The diagnosis of meniscal tears in athletes: a comparison of clinical and magnetic resonance imaging investigations, *Am J Sports Med* 25:7–12, 1997.

Nichol G, Stiell IG, Wells GA, et al: An economic analysis of the Ottawa knee rule, *Ann Emerg Med* 34:438–447, 1999.

O'Shea KJ, Murphy KP, Heekin RD, Herzwurm PJ: The diagnostic accuracy of history, physical examination and radiographs in the evaluation of traumatic knee disorders, *Am J Sports Med* 24:164–167, 1996.

Quarles JD, Hosey RG: Medial and lateral collateral injuries: prognosis and treatment, *Prim Care* 31:957–975, ix, 2004.

Scholten RJ, Devillé, Opstelten W, et al: The accuracy of physical diagnostic tests for assessing meniscal lesions of the knee: a meta-analysis, *J Fam Pract* 50:938–944, 2001.

Seaberg DC, Yealy DM, Lukens T, et al: Multicenter comparison of two clinical decision rules for the use of radiography in acute, high-risk knee injuries, *Ann Emerg Med* 32:8–13, 1998.

Solomon DH, Simel DL, Bates DW, et al: Does this patient have a torn meniscus or ligament of the knee? *JAMA* 286:1610–1620, 2001.

Stiell IG, Greeberg GH, Wells GA, et al: Derivation of a decision rule for the use of radiography in acute knee injuries, *Ann Emerg Med* 26:405–414, 1995.

Stiell IG, Greeberg GH, Wells GA, et al: Prospective validation of a decision rule for the use of radiography in acute knee injuries, *JAMA* 275:611–615, 1996.

Stiell IG, Wells GA, Hoag RH, et al: Implementation of the Ottawa knee rule for the use of radiography in acute knee injuries, *JAMA* 278:2071–2079, 1997.

Strayer RJ, Lang ES: Does this patient have a torn meniscus or ligament of the knee? *Ann Emerg Med* 47:499–501, 2006.

Wascher DC, Dvirnak PC, DeCoster TA: Knee dislocation: initial assessment and implications for treatment, *J Ortho Trauma* 11:525–529, 1997.

Weber JE, Jackson RE, Peacock WF, et al: Clinical decision rules discriminate between fractures and nonfractures in acute isolated knee trauma, *Ann Emerg Med* 26:429–433, 1995.

Lateral Epicondylitis and Medial Epicondylitis

(Tennis Elbow, Golfer's Elbow)

Presentation

In lateral epicondylitis, the patient complains of pain in the lateral elbow that frequently radiates down the lateral aspect of the forearm. Because the lateral epicondyle is the bony origin of wrist extensors, patients are usually involved in an activity that requires repetitive wrist extension, such as tennis or mechanical work. Occasionally, the patient can recall a specific injury to the area, but more often the pain is of gradual, insidious onset. Most patients relate symptoms to activities that stress the wrist extensor and supinator muscles, and especially to activities that involve forceful gripping or lifting of heavy objects. Even holding lightweight objects such as a cup may be difficult. There is tenderness to palpation over the origin of the extensor carpi radialis brevis tendon immediately anterior, medial, and distal to the lateral epicondyle. This tenderness is more pronounced with resisted wrist extension while the elbow is in extension or when the forearm is pronated.

Patients with medial epicondylitis complain of pain over the medial epicondyle and the proximal forearm. The pain may radiate down the medial aspect of the forearm. Medial epicondylitis has been associated with activities involving repetitive forearm pronation and wrist flexion, again related to this being the insertion point for wrist flexors. It occurs frequently in baseball pitchers and is also related to golf, tennis, bowling, racquetball, archery, weightlifting, and javelin throwing. It is also associated with occupations such as carpentry, plumbing, and meat cutting. Onset is usually insidious, but there may be an inciting event. The patient may also complain of a weak grasp and pain with repetitive wrist flexion and pronation. There will be tenderness to palpation just anterior to the medial epicondyle at the origin of the pronator teres and flexor carpi radialis muscles. Resisted wrist flexion and forearm pronation while the patient's elbow is in extension will reproduce symptoms.

What To Do:

✓ Obtain a careful history that includes inquiry into activities that may be causing overuse injury to the elbow. Also ascertain information about the patient's general health that may reveal an alternate source of tendinopathy, such as psoriasis, a sexually transmitted disease, gout, or the use of a fluoroquinolone within the past 3 months.

✓ Physical examination should concentrate on localizing the precise site of musculotendinous tenderness but should also include neck examination to help rule out cervical disease.

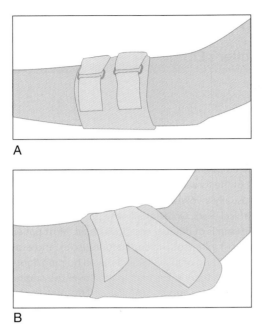

Figure 116-1 A, Lateral elbow brace. **B,** Medial elbow brace.

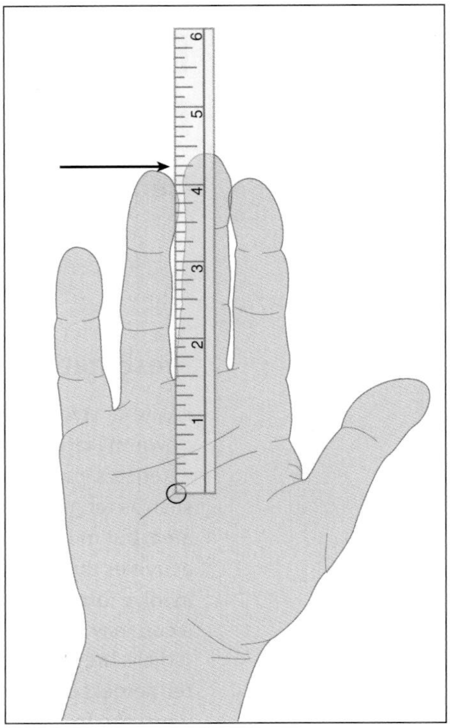

Figure 116-2 Hand-size measurement to determine proper grip handle size—Nirschl technique. (Adapted from Nirschl RP: Elbow tendinosis/tennis elbow. *Clin Sports Med* 11:851-870, 1992.)

✓ **Initial treatment begins with the immediate, temporary cessation of offending activities. Complete immobilization or inactivity is not recommended. The affected elbow is iced or ice massaged for 5 to 15 minutes, two to four times per day, for its local vasoconstrictive and analgesic effects.**

✓ **Prescribe a nonsteroidal anti-inflammatory drug (NSAID) if it is not contraindicated by allergy, bleeding, gastritis, or renal insufficiency. One recent trial suggests that a 7-day treatment course with a once-daily, 100-mg ketoprofen topical patch can provide pain relief without the adverse events associated with systemic delivery of an NSAID (at a much higher cost to the patient). Always advise patients to take NSAIDS with food and plenty of clear fluids to help alleviate stomach discomfort and to protect kidney function. Prescribing a histamine blocker or proton pump inhibitor can also be helpful.**

✓ When comfort allows, deep friction massage, muscle stretching, and grip strengthening may help with early rehabilitation.

✓ If the patient does not respond to these measures, consider injecting the area with bupivacaine and a steroid. Conflicting data have been published regarding the efficacy of such corticosteroid injections, and although there is likely to be significant pain reduction at 6 weeks after the injection, there appears to be no difference from preinjection pain and pain at

3 months and 1 year. When this modality is elected, you can inject bupivacaine 0.5% (Marcaine), 3 mL, and methylprednisolone (Depo-Medrol), 10 to 20 mg, using a 1¼-inch, 25-gauge needle. Forewarn patients of a possible flare-up of pain when the local anesthetic wears off, which may last for 24 to 48 hours.

✓ **The counterforce brace has been found to be helpful and is thought to reduce the load at the lateral or medial epicondyle by preventing the forearm muscles from fully expanding. Braces placed just distal to the epicondyles reduce loads greater than pads placed over the epicondyles** (Figure 116-1, *A* and *B*).

✓ Patients should be informed that recovery often takes several months but that most patients treated with conservative therapy respond successfully without recurrent symptoms. Physical therapy may be considered, but keep in mind that there are no published data proving its efficacy.

What Not To Do:

✗ Do not order radiographs for a classic presentation. Reserve them for questions of bony disease.

✗ Do not inject corticosteroids repeatedly into the tendon. They cause it to weaken or possibly rupture.

Discussion

The characteristics most likely to result in elbow tendon overuse are age older than 35 years, high activity level (sports or occupational), and demanding activity technique. Medial epicondylitis, commonly referred to as "golfer's elbow," occurs much less frequently than lateral epicondylitis, which is diagnosed 7 to 10 times more often.

Although the precise universal pathophysiology of epicondylitis has yet to be established, it is now generally accepted that the injury results from microtearing of the tendon origin at the epicondyle. This progresses to a failed reparative response and subsequent tendon degeneration that ultimately alters the typical musculotendinous biomechanics of the elbow. Because of its relationship to other overuse tendinopathies (see Chapter 132), the more appropriate descriptive terms for lateral and medial epicondylitis are lateral elbow tendinosis and medial elbow tendinosis.

Both tennis elbow and golfer's elbow usually affect patients who are between 30 and 60 years of age, with a peak incidence in the 40s. An acute onset of symptoms occurs more often in young athletes, and chronic, recalcitrant symptoms typically occur in older patients.

Poor form for the backhand stroke, extending the wrist when striking the ball instead of holding the wrist and elbow immobile, and swinging from the shoulder increase one's risk for lateral elbow tendinosis. There is some evidence to support that a two-handed backstroke may decrease risk because of improved stroke mechanics. Patients with medial elbow tendinosis who regularly play tennis often exhibit an improper serve and forehand stroke.

Equipment that is properly sized to the athlete is essential, especially in racquet sports, to prevent subsequent bouts of epicondylitis. Correct grip size is calculated by measuring from the proximal palm crease to the tip of the ring finger along its radial border (Figure 116-2). Lighter graphite frames, racquets less tightly strung (manufacturer's low-range recommendations), racquets with higher string counts per unit area, and a larger racquet head (90 to 100 square inches of hitting zone) will help to minimize injurious vibration and help prevent stressful off-center contact. In golf, clubs of proper weight, length, and grip are similarly important and can significantly reduce the injurious forces generated within the elbow.

Continued conditioning of the entire body along with the affected extremity is vital to a patient's successful recovery. Conditioning, including flexibility, strength, and endurance, is best performed with a slow, structured interval program.

Suggested Readings

Ciccotti MC, Schwartz MA, Ciccotti MG: Diagnosis and treatment of medical epicondylitis of the elbow, *Clin Sports Med* 23:693–705, xi, 2004.

Giangarra CE, Conroy B, Jobe FW, et al: Electromyographic and cinematographic analysis of elbow function in tennis players using single- and double- backhand strokes, *Am J Sports Med* 21:394–399, 1993.

Hay EM, Paterson SM, Lewis M, et al: Pragmatic randomised controlled trial of local corticosteroid injection and naproxen for treatment of lateral epicondylitis elbow in primary care, *BMJ* 319:964–968, 1999.

Mazières B, Rouanet S, Guillon Y, et al: Topical ketoprofen patch in the treatment of tendinitis: a randomized, double blind, placebo controlled study. *J Rheumatol* 32:1563–1570, 2005.

Mellor S: Treatment of tennis elbow: the evidence, *BMJ* 327:330, 2003.

Nirschl RP, Ashman ES: Elbow tendinopathy: tennis elbow, *Clin Sports Med* 22:587–598, 2003.

Sellards R, Kuebrich C: The elbow: diagnosis and treatment of common injuries, *Prim Care* 32:1–16, 2005.

Smidt N, van der Windt DA, Assendelft WJ, et al: Corticosteroid injections, physiotherapy, or a wait-and-see policy for lateral epicondylitis, *Lancet* 359:657–662, 2002.

Whaley AL, Baker CL: Lateral epicondylitis, *Clin Sports Med* 23:677–691, x, 2004.

Ligament Sprains

(Including Joint Capsule Injuries)

Presentation

Ligament strains occur when a joint is distorted beyond its normal anatomic limits (as when an ankle is inverted or a shoulder is dislocated and reduced). The patient may complain of a snapping or popping noise at the time of injury, immediate swelling, and loss of function (suggestive of grade II or III sprains or a fracture). Alternatively, the patient may come to your office hours to days after the injury with a report of gradually increasing swelling resulting in pain and stiffness (suggestive of a grade I or II sprain and development of a traumatic effusion).

What To Do:

✓ Obtain a detailed history of the mechanism of injury, and examine the joint for structural integrity, function, and point tenderness. Inability to fully extend an elbow is a strong indicator of significant injury. Use the uninjured limb as a control. **Ligamentous injuries are classified as grade I sprains (minimal stretching causing pain without swelling or laxity); grade II sprains (a partial tear with pain, functional loss and bleeding with swelling and slight laxity), which can be managed conservatively; and grade III sprains (complete tear with significant pain, marked swelling, and gross instability), often requiring a rigid splint and possible surgical intervention.** A tense joint effusion will limit the physical examination (and is one reason to require reevaluation after the swelling has decreased) but also suggests less than a third-degree ligamentous injury, which is normally accompanied by a tear of the joint capsule, and release of any tense effusion.

✓ **Obtain radiographs (these can be deferred if findings are minimal with full range of motion without bony tenderness or if specific criteria are not met, as for ankle and knee sprains)** (e.g., Ottawa Ankle and Knee Rules—see Chapters 97 and 115).

✓ **For first- and second-degree sprains, gently immobilize the joint using an elastic bandage alone or in combination with a cotton roll or plaster splint, as discomfort demands. Dynamic bracing (such as ankle stirrup splints and hinge knee braces) should be used with stable injuries when available. Most upper-extremity injuries can be immobilized by a sling alone or in combination with a soft or rigid splint.**

✓ Consider prescribing acetaminophen or anti-inflammatory pain medication when the patient complains of pain at rest, and provide crutches when discomfort will not allow weight bearing.

✅ **If there is a fracture or ligament tear with instability (third-degree sprain), the limb is usually best immobilized in a splint or cast—splint ankles at 90 degrees, wrists in extension, and fingers at slight flexion.**

✅ **Provide narcotic analgesics when indicated.**

✅ Instruct the patient in rest, elevation above the level of the heart, and, when it provides comfort, application of ice 10 to 20 minutes each hour for the first few hours then three or four times a day for 3 days. Minor injuries may need only 1 day of treatment.

✅ Explain to the patient that swelling in acute musculoskeletal injuries usually increases for the first 24 hours, and then decreases over the next 2 to 4 days (longer if the treatment above is not employed). Also inform the patient that some swelling and discomfort may persist for several weeks and at times for several months.

✅ **Advocate early mobilization and early return to normal functions for first- and second-degree sprains.**

✅ Explain the possibility of occult injuries, the necessity for follow-up, and the slow healing of injured ligaments (usually 6 months until full strength is regained).

What Not To Do:

❌ Do not obtain radiographs before the history or physical examination. Films of the wrong spot can be very misleading. For example, physicians have been steered away from the diagnosis of an avulsion fracture of the base of the fifth metatarsal by the presence of normal ankle films.

❌ Do not base the diagnosis on radiographs. They should be used as confirmatory evidence.

❌ Do not obtain routine comparison views on pediatric patients. They usually do not improve diagnostic accuracy.

Discussion

A tense joint effusion will limit the physical examination (and is one reason to require reevaluation after the swelling has decreased) but also suggests less than a third-degree ligamentous injury, which is normally accompanied by a tear of the joint capsule, and release of any tense effusion.

The benefit of cryotherapy for acute ligamentous injuries is controversial. For this reason, the use of ice should not be mandatory but should be used only when it is comforting to the patient.

Suggested Readings

Bleakley C, McDonough S, MacAuley D, et al: The use of ice in the treatment of acute soft tissue injury, *Am J Sports Med* 32:251–261, 2004.

Carr KE: Musculoskeletal injuries in young athletes, *Clin Fam Pract* 5:385–415, 2003.

Hocutt JE Jr, Jaffe R, Rylander CR, Beebe JK: Cryotherapy in ankle sprains, *Am J Sports Med* 10:316–319, 1982.

MacAuley D: Do textbooks agree on their advice on ice? *Clin J Sport Med* 11:67–72, 2001.

Locked Knee

Presentation

The patient, usually with a history of a previous knee injury, and often with previous knee locking, suddenly develops a mechanical inability to extend her knee fully. The knee may flex but not extend and may be causing mild to moderate pain.

What To Do:

✓ Perform a complete knee examination, checking for point tenderness, effusion, meniscal tear, and joint stability. **If comfort allows, gently and repeatedly perform the maneuvers of the McMurray test** (see Chapter 115). This alone may release the locked knee. If not, continue as described below.

✓ **Obtain knee radiographs, looking for an osteocartilaginous loose body or other disease.**

✓ **With pain and persistent locking,** prepare the knee with povidone-iodine solution and, at a point just superior and lateral or medial to the patella, using a 25-gauge, 1-inch needle, inject 10 mL of 0.5% bupivacaine (Marcaine) into the joint space (see Figure 120-1, A, p. 460.)

✓ **With the knee thus anesthetized, place a roll of towels under the heel and ankle to serve as a fulcrum. Leave the patient supine so that gravity will aid in extension and have the patient gently rock and rotate the knee for approximately 20 minutes or until the locked knee has released. Repeated McMurray maneuvers may again be gently performed if joint reduction has not occurred. Alternatively, longitudinal traction can be applied with gentle rotation of the knee internally and externally.**

✓ When the mechanical block is dislodged and the knee extended, place the patient in a knee immobilizer, keep the patient non–weight-bearing with crutches, and refer the patient to an orthopedic surgeon for early arthroscopic examination and definitive treatment.

What Not To Do:

✗ Do not forcefully manipulate the knee. This may produce further intra-articular injury.

Discussion

Knee locking is usually caused by previous injuries that include meniscal tears, partial or complete anterior cruciate ligament tears, osteocartilaginous loose bodies, pathologic medial plicae, and foreign bodies. Less commonly, locking can occur without a history of trauma. In such cases, the cause may be torsion of the infrapatellar fat pad or an intra-articular tumor, such as a ganglion. Locking of the knee occurs when one of these structures has become entrapped between the tibial plateau and the femoral condyles, mechanically blocking extension of the joint. This may happen suddenly, and may resolve suddenly.

If full extension cannot be obtained, the patient can be placed in a soft, bulky, partially immobilizing dressing (thick cotton roll covered with an elastic wrap) and placed on crutches until orthopedic follow-up can be obtained.

Lumbar Strain, Acute

("Mechanical" Low Back Pain, Sacroiliac Dysfunction)

Presentation

Suddenly or gradually, after lifting, sneezing, bending, or other movement, the patient develops a steady pain in one or both sides of the lower back. At times, this pain can be severe and incapacitating. It is usually better when lying down, worse with movement, and will perhaps radiate around the abdomen or down the thigh but no farther. There is insufficient trauma to suspect bony injury (e.g., a fall or direct blow) and no evidence of systemic disease that would make bony disease likely (e.g., osteoporosis, metastatic carcinoma, multiple myeloma). On physical examination, there may be spasm in the paraspinous muscles (i.e., contraction that does not relax, even when the patient is supine or when the opposing muscle groups contract, as with walking in place), but there is no point tenderness over the spinous processes of lumbar vertebrae and no nerve root signs, such as pain or paresthesia in dermatomes below the knee (especially with straight-leg raising), no foot weakness, and no loss of the ankle jerk. There may be point tenderness to firm palpation or percussion over the sacroiliac joint (SIJ), especially if the patient complains of pain toward that side of his lower back.

What To Do:

✓ Perform a complete history and physical examination of the abdomen, back, and legs, looking for alternative causes for the back pain. Pay special attention to red flags, such as a history of significant trauma, cancer, weight loss, fever, night sweats, injection drug use, compromised immunity, recumbent night pain, severe and unremitting pain, urinary retention or incontinence, saddle anesthesia, and severe or rapidly progressing neurologic deficit. Red flags on physical examination include elderly patients, fever, spinous point tenderness to percussion, abdominal tenderness or mass, and lower extremity motor weakness.

✓ **Radiographs are generally not required,** but consider obtaining plain radiographs of the lumbosacral spine on patients who have suffered injury that is sufficient to cause bony injury. Mild trauma in patients who are older than 50 years, patients younger than 20 years of age with nontraumatic pain, or patients older than 50 years of age who have had pain for more than a month warrant radiographs. Radiographs should also be ordered for patients who are on long-term corticosteroid medication, patients with a history of osteoporosis or cancer, and patients who are older than 70 years of age. A negative radiograph does not rule out disease.

✓ **Laboratory investigation is generally not indicated,** but order a complete blood count (CBC) and an erythrocyte sedimentation rate (ESR) on patients with a history of immune deficiency, cancer or IV drug abuse, or signs or symptoms of underlying systemic disease (e.g., unexplained weight loss, fatigue, night sweats, fever, lymphadenopathy, and back pain at night or that is unrelieved by bed rest) or children who are limping, refuse to walk, or bend forward. Bone scans, CT scans, or MRI may be better than plain radiographs in these patients. Consider diagnoses such as multiple myeloma, vertebral osteomyelitis, spinal tumor, diskitis, or spinal subdural abscess. Bedside ultrasonography, if the physician is trained in this technique, should be obtained to rule out an abdominal aortic aneurysm. If the physician is untrained or there is evidence of aneurysm on ultrasonography, an abdominal CT should be obtained immediately.

✓ **Consider disk herniation when leg pain overshadows the back pain.** Back pain may subside as leg pain worsens. This pain tends to worsen with coughing, Valsalva maneuver, trunk flexion, and prolonged sitting or standing. Look for weakness of ankle or great-toe dorsiflexion (drooping of the big toe and inability to heel walk). Also look for decreased sensation to pinprick over the medial dorsal foot when there is compression of the fifth lumbar nerve root. Look for weak plantar flexion (inability to toe walk), diminished ankle reflex, and paresthesias or decreased sensation to pinprick of the lateral or plantar aspect of the foot when there is first sacral root compression **(L_5 and S_1 radiculopathy account for about 90% to 95% of all lumbar radiculopathies).** Raise each leg 30 to 60 degrees of elevation from the horizontal, and consider the test positive for nerve root compression if it produces pain down the leg below the knee along a nerve root distribution, rather than pain in the back. This leg pain is increased by dorsiflexion of the foot and relieved by plantar flexion. Pain generated at less than 30 degrees and greater than 70 degrees is nonspecific. Ipsilateral straight-leg raising is a moderately sensitive but not a specific test. A herniated intervertebral disk is more strongly indicated when contralateral radicular pain is reproduced in one leg by raising the opposite leg**. If nerve root compression is suspected, prescribe short-term bed rest and nonsteroidal anti-inflammatory drugs (NSAIDs). Arrange for general medical, orthopedic, or neurosurgical referral. Although controversial, some consultants recommend short-term corticosteroid treatment, such as prednisone, 50 mg qd $\times$ 5 days. It should be noted that the 2007 joint guidelines of the American College of Physicians and the American Pain Society recommend against using systemic steroids. This is because of a lack of proven benefit.** The patient should try at least 4 to 6 weeks of conservative treatment before submitting to an operation on the herniated disk. **Surgical treatment should be routinely avoided for patients with disk herniation and radiating pain in the absence of neurologic findings. Eighty percent of patients with sciatica recover with or without surgery. The presence of significant weakness in a myotome is perhaps the most important factor in the decision to perform a relatively early surgical procedure. If the weakness is profound or rapidly progressive, delaying surgery increases the risk for permanent deficit.** The rare cauda equina syndrome is the only complication of lumbar disk herniation that calls for emergent surgical referral. It occurs when a massive extrusion of disk nucleus compresses the caudal sac containing lumbar and sacral nerve roots. Bilateral radicular leg pain or weakness, bladder or bowel dysfunction, perineal or perianal anesthesia, decreased rectal sphincter tone in 60% to 80% of cases, and urinary retention in 90% of cases are common findings. An emergent MRI is the study of choice for confirming this diagnosis.

✓ **For patients who have nonspecific pain that can be treated in an outpatient setting, prescribe a short course of anti-inflammatory analgesics (ibuprofen, naproxen) for patients who do not have any contraindications for using them.** Because gastric bleeding and renal insufficiency are common with long-term use of NSAIDs, consider substituting acetaminophen (Tylenol), 1000 mg q4-6h (maximum four doses daily), especially in the older patient. (Give half this dose if the patient takes greater than or equal to three alcoholic drinks per day.) Also consider a short-term opiate, such as hydrocodone (Vicodin, Lorcet) or oxycodone (Percocet), if necessary. A brief course of a muscle relaxant, such as metaxalone (Skelaxin), 800 mg tid to qid (less drowsiness), cyclobenzaprine (Flexeril), 10 mg bid to qid (not recommended for the elderly), or lorazepam (Ativan) 0.5 to 1.0 mg qid (more sedating and care should also be taken in the elderly), may be effective. The potential benefits must be weighed against the increased rates of dizziness and drowsiness that accompany the use of muscle relaxants.

Recommend hot or cold packs (whichever the patient chooses) or alternate both hot and cold. Although not scientifically supported, these packs can often be comforting.

 At times sacroiliac dysfunction can cause incapacitating spasms of pain that are precipitated by minor movements or attempts to sit up. The patient will usually be able to localize the pain to the right or left side of the sacrum. Firmly palpating the dimple (sacral sulcus) with your thumb and eliciting pain may be the most reliable indication of SIJ pain. When the pain is significant and there are no neurologic findings to suggest nerve root compression or any red flags of underlying systemic disease, it can be quite rewarding to provide an intra-articular injection of a local anesthetic mixed with a corticosteroid. Improvement of pain is both diagnostic and therapeutic. Draw up 10 mL of 0.5% bupivacaine (Marcaine) mixed with 1 mL (40 mg) of methylprednisolone (Depo-Medrol) or 1 to 2 mL (6 to 12 mg) of betamethasone (Celestone Soluspan). Using a 1¼-inch, 22- to 27-gauge needle and sterile technique, inject deeply into the sacroiliac joint at the point of maximal tenderness or into the sacral sulcus immediately lateral to the sacrum (Figure 119-1). When the needle is in the joint, the needle should advance freely up to its hub without meeting resistance or bony obstruction. There should be a free flow of medication from the syringe without causing soft tissue swelling. If the needle meets any obstruction, reposition it with slight angulation of the needle tip out laterally until the needle advances easily. During the injection, fan upward into the superior fibrous tissue of the SIJ. The patient may feel a brief increase of pain, followed by dramatic relief in 5 to 20 minutes that is usually persistent. Pain is often relieved by 50% to 80%. Warn the patient that there may be a flare in pain when the anesthetic component wears off that could last for 24 to 48 hours. If the patient gets relief initially, any persistent symptoms should subside over the next 5 to 10 days. This should be performed in instances of acute pain, or an acute flare-up of chronic recurrent sacroiliac

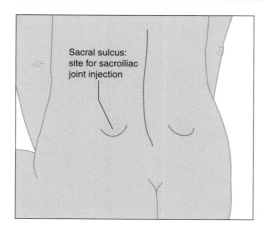

Sacral sulcus:
site for sacroiliac
joint injection

Figure 119-1 The dimple on either side of the sacrum (sacral sulcus) can serve as a landmark for injecting a painful sacroiliac joint.

pain. **Sacroiliac or SIJ belts can be used to provide compression, and, in some patients, stabilization and pain relief for SIJ dysfunction (samples can be found on the internet). The belt should be secured posteriorly across the sacral base and anteriorly, inferior to the anterior superior iliac spines** (Figure 119-2). This belt may be most helpful during walking and standing activities, but for some patients with significant pain and weakness, wearing it during sedentary activities may also be helpful in reducing symptoms.

✅ **For point tenderness of the lumbosacral muscles, substantial pain relief may also be obtained by injecting 10 to 20 mL of 0.25% to 0.5% bupivacaine (Marcaine) deeply into the points of maximal tenderness** of the erector spinae and quadratus lumborum muscles, using a 1¼-inch, 25- to 27-gauge needle. Quickly puncture the skin, drive the needle into the muscle belly, and inject the anesthetic, slowly advancing and withdrawing the needle and fanning out the medication in all directions. Often one fan block can reduce symptoms by 95% after injection and yield a 75% permanent reduction of painful spasms. Following injection, teach stretching exercises.

✅ **For severe pain that cannot be relieved by injections of local anesthetic,** it may be necessary to provide the patient with 1 to 2 days of bed rest, although most patients with acute low back pain recover more rapidly by continuing ordinary activities (within the limits permitted by their pain) than with bed rest or back-mobilizing exercises. Some patients with intractable excruciating pain (especially the elderly) require hospitalization.

✅ **Refer patients with uncomplicated back pain to their primary care provider for follow-up care in 3 to 7 days.** Reassure patients that back pain is seldom disabling and that it

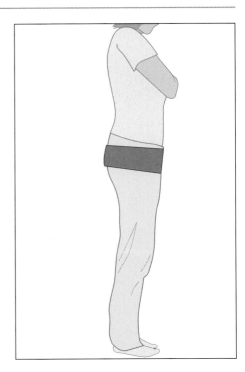

Figure 119-2 Sacroiliac joint (SIJ) belt.

usually resolves rapidly with their return to normal activity. Tell patients that the pain may be recurrent and that cigarette smoking, sedentary activity, and obesity are risk factors for back pain. Teach them to avoid twisting and bending when lifting, and show them how to lift with the back vertical, using thigh muscles and holding heavy objects close to the chest to avoid reinjury. **Encourage them to return to work or resume normal activities as soon as possible, with neither bed rest nor exercise in the acute phase, and to participate in an aerobic exercise program when the pain has subsided.** Heavy lifting, trunk twisting, and bodily vibration should be avoided in the acute phase.

What Not To Do:

(X) Do not be too eager to use antispasm medicines. Many have sedative or anticholinergic side effects.

(X) Do not apply lumbar traction. It has not been proven to be any better than a placebo for relieving back pain. Do not provide lumbar orthotics, back braces, or lumbar cushions. They have no proven benefit. Lumbar supports have not been proven to reduce the incidence of low back pain in industrial workers and should not be routinely recommended for the prevention of low back pain.

(X) Do not recommend bed rest for more than 2 days and only recommend it when the pain is severe. Bed rest does not increase the speed of recovery from acute low back pain and sometimes delays recovery.

Discussion

Low back pain affects men and women equally, with onset most often between the ages of 30 and 50 years. It is the most common and expensive cause of work-related disability in people who are younger than 45 years of age. A definitive diagnosis for **nonradiating low back pain** cannot be established in 85% of patients because of the weak associations between symptoms, pathologic changes, and imaging results. It can be generally assumed that much of this pain is secondary to musculoligamentous injury, degenerative changes in the spine, or a combination of the two. The approach discussed here is geared only to the management of acute injuries and flare-ups, from which most people recover on their own, which leaves only about 10% developing chronic problems. **With acute pain,** reassurance plus limited medication may be the most useful intervention. The 90% of back pain patients that become pain free are pain free within 3 months, and more than 90% of those patients recover spontaneously within 4 weeks. Even with diskogenic back pain or disk herniation with **radicular pain,** there are convincing data to support the nonoperative treatment of these patients in the absence of cauda equine syndrome or progressive neurologic deficit.

History and physical examination are essential to rule out **serious pathologic conditions** that can present as low back pain but require quite different treatment—aortic aneurysm, pyelonephritis, pancreatitis, abdominal tumors, pelvic inflammatory disease, ectopic pregnancy, and retroperitoneal or epidural abscess.

Older patients who experience radicular symptoms may have **spinal stenosis,** which may be accompanied by **neurogenic claudication,** a syndrome in which pain radiates down the legs, particularly when walking, and is often relieved by rest. This can be distinguished from vascular claudication, because the pain of neurogenic claudication starts even while the patient stands still. The pain is worsened by extension of the spine, which occurs with standing or walking, and improves with flexion, such as sitting or leaning forward.

(continued)

Discussion continued

The standard five-view radiograph study of the lumbosacral spine may entail 500 mrem of radiation, and yet, only 1 in 2500 lumbar spine plain films of adults below 50 years of age show an unexpected abnormality. In fact, many radiographic anomalies, such as spina bifida occulta, single-disk narrowing, spondylosis, facet joint abnormalities, and several congenital anomalies, are equally common in symptomatic and asymptomatic individuals. **It is estimated that the gonadal dose of radiation absorbed from a five-view lumbosacral series is equivalent to that from 6 years of daily anteroposterior (AP) and lateral chest films.** The World Health Organization now recommends that oblique views be reserved for problems remaining after review of AP and lateral films. For simple cases of low back pain, even with radicular findings, both CT scans and MRI are overly sensitive and often reveal anatomic abnormalities that have no clinical significance. In one study of MRI scans, only 36% of asymptomatic patients had normal disks at all levels, whereas 64% had demonstrable disease (52% with at least one bulging disk, 27% with disk protrusion, and 1% with frank herniation). CT and MRI should be reserved for patients for whom there is a strong clinical suggestion of underlying infection, cancer, or persistent neurologic deficit. These tests have similar accuracy in detecting herniated disks and spinal stenosis, but MRI is more sensitive for infections, metastatic cancer, and rare neural tumors.

Although adults are more apt to have disk abnormalities, muscle strain, and degenerative changes associated with low back pain, **athletically active adolescents** are more likely to have **posterior element derangements,** such as stress fractures of the pars interarticularis. Early recognition of this spondylolysis and treatment by bracing and limitation of activity may prevent nonunion, persistent pain, and disability.

Although the true prevalence of posterior pelvic pain is unknown, researchers estimate that 15% to 30% of patients with low back pain have SIJ dysfunction. Radiation of pain down one or both legs may occur, but usually not below the knee or accompanied by positive straight-leg raising or neurologic deficit. Imaging is often not helpful. Radiographs, MRI, bone scan, and CT scans do not differentiate symptomatic from asymptomatic patients. Often SIJ pain presents as a progressive problem with fluctuations in symptoms. There is no gold standard for treatment. The recommendations noted above are dependent on the clinician's experience and skills.

Malingering and drug-seeking are major psychological components to consider in patients who have frequent visits for back pain and whose responses seem overly dramatic or otherwise inappropriate. These patients may move around with little difficulty when they do not know they are being observed. They may complain of generalized superficial tenderness when you lightly pinch the skin over the affected lumbar area. When straight-leg raising is equivocally positive after testing the patient in a supine position, use distraction and reexamine the patient in the sitting position to see if the initial findings are reproduced. If there is suspicion that the patient's pain is psychosomatic or nonorganic, use the axial loading test, in which the head of the standing person is gently pressed down on. This should not cause significant musculoskeletal back pain. The rotation test can also be performed, in which the patient stands with his arms at his sides. Hold his wrists next to his hips and turn his body from side to side, passively rotating his shoulders, trunk, and pelvis as a unit. This maneuver creates the illusion that the spinal rotation is being tested, but, in fact, the spinal axis has not been altered, and any complaint of back pain should be suspect.

Another technique that is easier to perform is the heel tap test. With the patient supine and with the hips and knees flexed to 90 degrees, suggest to the patient that the next test may cause low back pain, and then lightly tap the patient's heel with the base of your hand. A complaint of sudden low back pain is an indication of malingering.

Suggested Readings

Anderson GBJ, Lucente T, Davis AM, et al: A comparison of osteopathic spinal manipulation with standard care for patients with low back pain, *N Engl J Med* 341:1426–1431, 1999.

Baker RJ, Patel D: Lower back pain in the athlete: common conditions and treatment, *Prim Care* 32:201–229, 2005.

Carey TS, Garrett J, Jackman A, et al: The outcomes and costs of care for acute low back pain among patients seen by primary care practitioners, chiropractors and orthopedic surgeons, *N Engl J Med* 333:913–917, 1995.

Deyo RA, Diehl AK, Rosenthal M: How many days of bed rest for acute low back pain? *N Engl J Med* 315:1064–1070, 1986.

Deyo RA, Rainville J, Kent DL: What can the history and physical examination tell us about low back pain? *JAMA* 268:760–765, 1992.

Deyo RA, Weinstein JN: Low back pain, *N Engl J Med* 344:363–370, 2001.

Devereaux MW: Low back pain, *Prim Care* 31:33–51, 2004.

Elam KC, Cherkin DC, Deyo RA: How emergency physicians approach low back pain: choosing costly options, *J Emerg Med* 13:143–150, 1995.

Frost H, et al: Randomised controlled trial of physiotherapy compared with advice for low back pain, *BMJ* 329:708, 2004.

Gross L: Metaxalone, *J Neurol Orthop Med Surg* 18:76–79, 1998.

Harwood MI, Smith BJ: Low back pain: a primary care approach, *Clin Fam Pract* 7:279–303, 2005.

Hurwitz EL, Morgenstern H, Harber P, et al: The effectiveness of physical modalities among patients with low back pain randomized to chiropractic care, *J Manipulative Physiol Ther* 25:10–20, 2002.

Jarvik JG, Hollingworth W, Martin B, et al: Rapid magnetic resonance imaging vs radiographs for patients with low back pain, *JAMA* 289:2810–2818, 2003.

Malmivaara A, Hakkinen U, Aro T, et al: The treatment of acute low back pain: bed rest, exercise, or ordinary activity? *N Engl J Med* 332:351–355, 1995.

Miller P, Kendrick D, Bentley E, et al: Cost-effectiveness of lumbar spine radiography in primary care patients with low back pain, *Spine* 27:2291–2297, 2002.

Prather H, Hunt D: Sacroiliac joint pain, *Dis Month* 50:670–683, 2004.

Small SA, Perron AD, Brady WJ: Orthopedic pitfalls: cauda equina syndrome, *Am J Emerg Med* 23:159–163, 2005.

Smeal WL, Tyburski M, Alleva J: Discogenic/radicular pain, *Dis Month* 50:636–669, 2004.

Suarez-Almazor ME, Belseck E, Russell AS, et al: Use of lumbar radiographs for the early diagnosis of low back pain: proposed guidelines would increase utilization, *JAMA* 277:1782–1786, 1997.

van Poppel MN, Koes BW, van der Ploeg T, et al: Lumbar supports and education for the prevention of low back pain in industry: a randomized controlled trial, *JAMA* 279:1789–1794, editorial 1826-1827, 1998.

van Tulder MW, Assendelft WJ, Koes BW, et al: Spinal radiographic findings and nonspecific low back pain. A systematic review of observational studies, *Spine* 22:427–434, 1997.

van Tulder MW, Koes BW, Bouter LM: Conservative treatment of acute and chronic nonspecific low back pain. A systematic review of randomized controlled trials of the most common interventions, *Spine* 22:2128–2156, 1997.

van Tulder MW, Koes BW, Bouter LM, et al: Management of chronic nonspecific low back pain in primary care: a descriptive study, *Spine* 22:76–82, 1997.

Wassell JT, Gardner LI, Landsittel DP, et al: A prospective study of back belts for prevention of back pain and injury, *JAMA* 284:2727–2732, 2000.

Monarticular Arthritis, Acute

Presentation

The patient complains of one joint that has become acutely red, swollen, hot, painful, and stiff, with pain on minimal range of motion. Rapid onset with fever and local warmth suggests the possibility of septic arthritis. A prominent monarticular synovitis with comparatively little pain, but where the joint is warm with a large effusion, especially of the knee, is typical of Lyme disease. A migratory tendonitis or arthritis often precedes gonococcal monarthritis. A history of similar attacks, especially of the first metatarsophalangeal joint, suggests the possibility of gouty arthritis. A history of recurrent knee swelling with minimal erythema and gradual onset after overuse or minor trauma is more likely associated with osteoarthritis and pseudogout.

A child between the ages of 3 and 10 years who presents with a limp or inability to walk may have a transient synovitis of the hip or a more serious septic arthritis.

What To Do:

✓ Ask about previous, similar episodes in this or other joints, as well as trauma, systemic illness, fever, tick bites (Lyme arthritis), sexual risk factors, IV drug use, skin infections, or rashes, and ask about any history of gout (see Chapter 114). Determine the rapidity of onset and the duration of symptoms. Remember that although a high-grade fever is especially concerning, the elderly or immunocompromised patient may fail to mount a fever in the face of infection. General malaise and rash can be associated with infection.

✓ Perform a thorough physical examination, looking for evidence of the above. Obtain cervical, anal, oral, or urethral swabs for culture and Gram stain or DNA probe when you suspect gonococcal arthritis. Cultures of synovial fluid are positive in no more than 50% of patients. Mucosal cultures are positive in 80% of cases.

✓ Examine the affected joint and document the extent of effusion, involvement of adjacent structures, and degree of erythema, tenderness, heat, and limitation of range of motion. True intra-articular problems cause restriction of active and passive range of motion, whereas periarticular problems (e.g., prepatellar bursitis, olecranon bursitis), which may mimic joint inflammation, restricting active range of motion more than passive range of motion. **Maximum pain at the limit of joint motion is characteristic of true arthritis.**

✓ Intra-articular fluid accumulation can often be detected by pressing on one side of the affected joint and, at the same time, palpating a wavelike fluctuance on the opposite side of the joint. In the knee, when the medial or lateral compartment is stroked, the fluid moves into the opposite compartment, resulting in a visible bulge. To detect effusion in the elbow joint, the triangular recess in the lateral aspect of the elbow, between the lateral epicondyle, radial head, and the olecranon process, should be palpated. To detect effusion in the ankle, the joint should be palpated anteriorly.

✅ **Although not always necessary, send a blood sample for complete blood count (CBC) and erythrocyte sedimentation rate (ESR), which may support a suspicion of an inflammatory or infectious process. When sepsis is suspected, obtain blood cultures.** Blood cultures are positive in about 50% of nongonococcal infections but are rarely positive (about 10%) in gonococcal infection. Serum uric acid measurement is not always helpful and may be misleading. Lyme antibodies may be appropriate as Lyme disease is becoming more and more prevalent, even in the absence of known tick bites. Most patients with Lyme arthritis have positive two-tier serologic tests for *B. burgdorferi* infection.

✅ **Consider obtaining radiographs of the affected joint** to detect possible unsuspected fractures or evidence of chronic disease, such as rheumatoid arthritis. The finding of crystal-induced chondrocalcinosis could support but not confirm the diagnosis of pseudogout arthritis or osteoarthritis. Occasionally, osteomyelitis or malignancy may be detected. **In most cases, radiographs are not helpful** in the diagnosis of the acute, nontraumatic, swollen, and painful joint, and they are not always a requirement during the initial evaluation.

✅ **Perform arthrocentesis to remove joint fluid for analysis, to relieve pain, and, in the case of septic or crystal-induced arthritis, to reduce the bacterial and crystal load within the joint.** Identify the joint line to be entered, make a pressure mark on the overlying skin with the closed end of a retractable pen to serve as a target. Then using sterile technique throughout, cleanse the skin over the most superficial area of the joint effusion with alcohol and povidone-iodine (Betadine), anesthetize the skin with 1% plain buffered lidocaine, and aspirate as much joint fluid as possible through a 16- to 18-gauge needle (smaller in small joints). The joint space of the knee (Figure 120-1, A) may be entered medially or laterally with the leg fully extended and the patient lying supine. Hold the needle parallel to the bed surface, and direct it just posterior to the patella into the subpatellar space. The elbow joint (Figure 120-1, B) is best entered at about 30 degrees of flexion, with the needle introduced proximal to the olecranon process of the ulna and just below the lateral epicondyle. Advance the needle medially into the joint space. The best site for needle entry of the wrist is on the dorsal radial aspect at the proximal end of the anatomic snuff box and the distal articulation of the radius. Place the wrist in about 20 degrees of flexion and introduce the needle perpendicular to the skin, advancing it toward the ulna into the joint space (Figure 120-1, C). The ankle joint (Figure 120-1, D) may be entered with the patient supine, the knee extended, and the foot plantarflexed. Find the small depression that is just medial to the extensor hallucis longus and tibialis anterior tendons, inferior to the distal tibia, then direct your needle into the tibiotalar articulation. For small joints, enter the midline on the dorsolateral aspect and advance a small needle into the joint space. Joints of the digits may have to be distracted by pulling on the end to enlarge the joint space. Fluoroscopy may be valuable in guiding needle placement for hip or shoulder joint aspiration.

✅ **Grossly examine the joint aspirate.** Clear, light-yellow fluid is characteristic of osteoarthritis or mild inflammatory or traumatic effusions. Grossly cloudy fluid is characteristic of more severe inflammation or bacterial infection. Blood in the joint is characteristic of trauma (a fracture or tear inside the synovial capsule) or bleeding from hemophilia or anticoagulants. A traumatic tap may cause the serous joint fluid to become bloody during aspiration and is not indicative of a previous hemarthrosis. This procedure can be performed safely in patients who are taking warfarin (Coumadin).

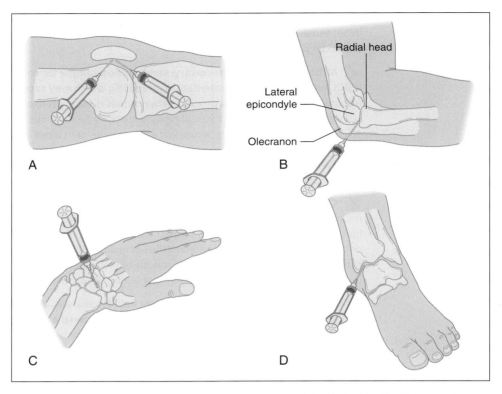

Figure 120-1 Entry sites for arthrocentesis. (A and D, Illustrations provided by Dr. D.H. Neustadt. B and C, Adapted from Akins CM: Aspiration and injection of joints, bursae and tendons. In Vander Salm TJ, Cutler BS, Brownell Wheeler H, editors: *Atlas of bedside procedures*, ed 2. Boston, 1988, Little Brown & Co.)

✓ **One drop of joint fluid may be used for a crude string or mucin clot test.** Wet the tips of two gloved fingers with joint fluid, repeatedly touch them together, and slowly draw them apart. As this maneuver is repeated 10 or 20 times, and the joint fluid dries, normal synovial fluid will form longer and longer strings, usually to 5 to 10 cm in length. Inflammation inhibits this string formation. This is a nonspecific test but may aid decision making at the bedside.

✓ If microscopic examinations are delayed, a tube with ethylenediaminetetraacetic acid should be used for anticoagulation, because anticoagulants (e.g., oxalate, lithium heparin) used in other tubes can confound crystal analysis.

✓ **The most important laboratory tests on joint fluid consist of a Gram stain and culture for possible septic arthritis.** Gram-positive bacteria can be seen in 80% of culture-positive synovial fluid, but gram-negative bacteria are seen less often; gram-negative diplococci are seen rarely. Polymerase chain reaction techniques can detect gonococcal DNA in the synovial fluid of some culture-negative cases of suspected gonococcal arthritis, but this test is not presently considered a standard evaluation.

✓ **A joint fluid total and differential leukocyte count is the next most useful test to order.** A count greater than 50,000 white blood cells (WBC)/mm^3 is characteristic of bacterial infection (especially when greater than 75% to 90% are polymorphonuclear neutrophils [PMNs]). In osteoarthritis, there are usually fewer than 2000 WBC/mm^3, and inflammatory arthritis (such as gout and rheumatoid arthritis) falls in the middle range of 2000 to 50,000 WBC/mm^3. One clinical study showed that 36% of patients with septic arthritis had a joint fluid WBC count of less than 50,000/mm^3. In a case review of 50 patients with septic arthritis, none had synovial fluid counts of less than 2500 WBC/mm^3. Therefore it is reasonable to conclude that when the clinical picture does not suggest infection, and the WBC count is less than 2000 WBC/mm^3, empirical antibiotic treatment is not necessary. Also, the presence of greater than 75% PMNs has a good positive predictive value for inflammation/infection and should be treated as infection.

✓ **There is no clear evidence to guide decision making when the count is between 2000 WBC/mm^3 and 50,000 WBC/mm^3.** Clinical judgment predominates in this range, with an emphasis on presumptive antibiotic treatment until a diagnosis is established. If possible, consult with an orthopedist before antibiotic treatment, because they may want to take the patient to the operating room (OR) prior to starting antibiotics.

✓ **Send a wet preparation to look for crystals.** Identification of crystals can establish a diagnosis of gout or pseudogout and avoid unnecessary hospitalization for suspected infectious arthritis.

✓ **If there is any suspicion of a bacterial infection (based on predisposing factors, fever, elevated ESR, cellulitis, lymphangitis, or the joint fluid results), always treat empirically and start the patient on appropriate intravenous antibiotics based on the results of the Gram stain or the presumptive organism.** Adequate treatment should include hospitalization for further IV antibiotics. In older patients, who are not at risk for sexually transmitted diseases (STDs), antibiotic coverage should be aimed at *Staphylococcus aureus*. Use vancomycin (Vancocin), 1.0 gm IV q12h, along with cefotaxime (Claforan), 1.0 g IV q12h, for uncomplicated infections, or alternatively, use vancomycin with either ceftriaxone (Rocephin), 1.0 or 2.0 g qd IV; ciprofloxacin (Cipro), 400 mg bid IV; or levofloxacin (Levaquin), 500 mg qd IV. For patients with suspected gonococcus, use ceftriaxone (Rocephin), 1.0 g qd IV, or cefotaxime (Claforan), 1.0 g q8h IV. If Gram stain shows gram-positive cocci in clusters, add vancomycin (Vancocin), 1.0 g q12h IV. Provide *Chlamydia* treatment with azithromycin (Zithromax), 1 g PO × 1, or doxycycline (Doryx), 100 mg bid × 7 days. For children older than 5 years of age, prescribe nafcillin (Unipen) or oxacillin (Prostaphlin), 150 to 200 mg/kg/day divided into 4 to 6 doses, plus ceftriaxone (Rocephin), 50 mg/kg/day (maximum 2 g) divided bid.

✓ **Inflammatory arthritis may be treated with nonsteroidal anti-inflammatory drugs (NSAIDs) (unless contraindicated), beginning with a loading dose, such as indomethacin (Indocin), 50 mg, or ibuprofen (Motrin), 800 mg, tapered to usual maintenance doses.**

✓ **If infection can be confidently excluded from the diagnosis, intra-articular injections of corticosteroids can be a useful adjunctive or alternative therapy.** Using aseptic technique, prepare the skin with povidone-iodine and alcohol. Using the techniques described above, with a 3- to 5-ml syringe and a 1¼-inch 27-gauge needle, inject 1 to 2 mL of 40 mg/mL methylprednisolone (Depo-Medrol) with 2 to 8 mL of bupivacaine (Marcaine), 0.25% to 0.5%, into the affected joint. For finger or toe joints, use a smaller volume (0.2 to 0.5 mL) of the more concentrated (80 mg/mL) methylprednisolone, along with a lesser volume of bupivacaine. Alternatively, triamcinolone hexacetonide (Aristospan Intra-articular), 20 to 40 mg/injection may be used. Warn patients of the 10% to 15% risk for postinjection flare or recurrent pain for 24 to 48 hours after the local anesthetic wears off.

✓ **When joint fluid cannot be obtained to rule out infection, it may be a good tactic to treat simultaneously for infectious and inflammatory arthritis.**

✓ **Splint and elevate the affected joint and arrange for admission or follow-up.**

✓ **Children complaining of acute hip pain** must be evaluated for the possibility of a septic arthritis versus a transient synovitis. Similar symptoms are present in these two diseases at the early stages, and differential diagnosis is difficult. To help differentiate between these two diseases, **obtain a CBC, ESR, C-reactive protein (CRP), and hip radiograph.**

✓ **Five reportedly independent predictors of septic arthritis are a temperature greater than 37° C (98.6° F), an ESR greater than 20 mm/h, a CRP greater than 1.0 mg/dL, a WBC greater than 11,000/mm^3, and a radiographic joint space difference between the affected and unaffected hips greater than 2 mm.** The likelihood of septic arthritis is 0.1% if none of the predictors is present, between 3% and 23% with two variables present, 24% to 77% with three, 82% to 97% with four, and 99.1% if all five predictors are present.

✓ **It may be reasonable to obtain an MRI or fluoroscopically directed joint aspiration in those children with three or four of these predictors.**

✓ When there is a low index of suspicion for a septic hip and there are no contraindications to NSAID use, place the child on ibuprofen (Motrin), 10 mg/kg tid for 5 days. In a small study, this was shown to shorten the duration of symptoms of transient synovitis by 2 days.

What Not To Do:

✗ Do not tap a joint through an area of obvious contamination, such as subcutaneous cellulitis. Synovial fluid may consequently be inoculated with bacteria. This is considered a relative contraindication to arthrocentesis.

✗ Do not send synovial fluid for chemistries, proteins, rheumatoid factor, or uric acid, because the results may be misleading. Synovial fluid glucose is not discriminatory for joint sepsis.

✗ Do not be misled by bursitis, tenosynovitis, or myositis without joint involvement. An infected or inflamed joint will have a reactive effusion, which may be evident as fullness, fluctuance, reduced range of motion, or joint fluid that can be drawn off with a needle. It is usually difficult to tap a joint in the absence of a joint effusion.

✗ Do not treat hyperuricemia with drugs that lower uric acid levels, such as allopurinol or probenecid, during an acute attack of gout (see Chapter 114).

✗ Do not inject corticosteroids into a joint until infection has been ruled out.

✗ Do not use NSAIDs when a patient has a history of active peptic ulcer disease with bleeding. Relative contraindications include renal insufficiency, volume depletion, gastritis, inflammatory bowel disease, asthma, hypertension, and congestive heart disease.

✗ Do not start maintenance NSAID doses for an acute inflammation. It will take 1 day or more to reach therapeutic levels and pain relief. When tolerated, always start with a loading dose.

Discussion

Monarticular joint disease (especially monarthritis) should be regarded as infectious until proven otherwise. Infectious arthritis requires prompt treatment to prevent joint destruction and spread of infection.

It should be kept in mind, however, that any polyarticular disease, such as rheumatoid arthritis or systemic lupus erythematosus, can initially present in a single joint and later be revealed to occur in other joints.

The acute, swollen/painful joint is most commonly caused by trauma, infection, or crystal-related disease. Trauma is the most common cause, followed by infection. Gout is the most common crystal-associated arthropathy.

Most acute bacterial arthritis is monarthritis, but polyarticular infectious arthritis occurs in approximately 12% to 20% of cases. The infectious cause varies according to patient factors, particularly age and sexual activity. *Staphylococcus aureus* is cited as the most common cause of infectious monarthritis in adults. *Neisseria gonorrhoeae* is the most common cause of acute monarthritis in young, sexually active adults. It is three to four times more common in women than in men. Neonates and children are at higher risk for group B streptococcus, *S. aureus, Escherichia coli,* and other gram-negative organisms.

Risk factors for septic joint include skin infection, prosthetic joint, joint surgery, rheumatoid arthritis, age older than 80 years, and diabetes. Also, intravenous drug abuse allows organisms to access joints, such as the sternoclavicular joint, which is uncommonly thought of in infectious arthritis.

Gout and pseudogout can present with abrupt onset of pain and effusion, raising suspicion of infection. When the history reveals longstanding symptoms in a joint, with exacerbations of preexisting disease (e.g., gout, or worsening of osteoarthritis with excessive use), this still should be differentiated from a new superimposed infection.

In patients with rheumatoid arthritis, pain in one joint out of proportion to pain in other joints always suggests infection.

Intra-articular trauma is more likely than extra-articular trauma to present as acute monarthritis; fracture, meniscal tears, and other internal derangements (e.g., ligament tears) are common forms of intra-articular trauma.

The history of trauma is a potential pitfall in the approach to the patient with acute monarthritis. Although some patients with a traumatic cause may be unable to recall the event, others falsely and inadvertently attribute their joint pain to a relatively minor injury. Clinically, the physical examination of a patient with traumatic acute monarthritis may be indistinguishable from crystal deposition and infectious disease. In fact, trauma can be the precipitant of crystal deposition and infection.

Synovial fluid aspiration is universally recommended in the patient with acute monarthritis. The urgent reason for tapping a joint effusion is to rule out a bacterial infection, which could destroy the joint cartilage in as little as 1 or 2 days. Beyond identifying an infection (with the Gram stain, culture, and WBC), further diagnosis of the cause of arthritis is not particularly accurate, nor is early definitive diagnosis necessary to decide on specific acute treatment.

Reducing the volume of the effusion may alleviate pain and stiffness, but this effect may be short lived, because the effusion may reaccumulate within hours.

Identification of crystals is essential for the diagnosis of gout or pseudogout, but one acute attack may be treated in the same manner as any other inflammatory arthritis. The workup for an exact diagnosis may, therefore, be deferred to follow-up after acute infection has been ruled out.

Infants and young children may present with fever and reluctance to walk from septic arthritis of the hip or knee, and arthrocentesis may require sedation or general anesthesia.

Acute arthritis in prosthetic joints is always of concern. Infections in prostheses are disastrous and require urgent consultation.

Suggested Readings

Arroll B, Goodyear-Smith F: Corticosteroid injections for osteoarthritis of the knee, *BMJ* 328:869, 2004.

Baker DG, Schumacher HR: Acute monoarthritis, *N Engl J Med* 329:1013–1020, 1993.

Fagan HB: Approach to the patient with acute swollen/painful joint, *Clin Fam Pract* 7:305, 2005.

Jung ST, Rowe SM, Moon ES, et al: Significance of laboratory and radiologic findings for differentiating between septic arthritis and transient synovitis of the hip, *J Pediatr Orthop* 23:368–372, 2003.

Kermond S, Fink M, Graham K, et al: A randomized clinical trial: should the child with transient synovitis of the hip be treated with nonsteroidal anti-inflammatory drugs, *Ann Emerg Med* 40:294–299, 2002.

Li SF, Henderson J, Dickman E, et al: Laboratory tests in adults with monoarticular arthritis: can they rule out a septic joint? *Acad Emerg Med* 11:276–280, 2004.

Siva C, Velazquez C, Mody A, et al: Diagnosing acute monoarthritis in adults: a practical approach for the family physician, *Am Fam Physician* 68:83–90, 2003.

Muscle Cramps

(Charley Horse)

Presentation

The patient complains of painful, visible, palpable muscle contractions, often affecting the gastrocnemius muscle or small muscles of the foot or hand. Ordinary cramps occur chiefly at rest during the night or after trivial movement but also can occur after forceful muscle contraction. Other muscle cramps are associated with exercise in the heat, occupations that cause overuse, pregnancy, and drug or alcohol use. Most cramps are transient in nature, but they are likely to recur after a severe episode. Following this, the muscles may be tender and painful for some time.

What To Do:

✓ **Look for a specific underlying cause.** Unaccustomed exercise and salt depletion from sweating are common precipitating causes (see Chapter 2). Drug-induced cramps can include those from alcohol, lithium, cimetidine, nifedipine, antipsychotic medications (see Chapter 1), clofibrate, and others. Hypothyroidism, hyperthyroidism, hyponatremia, hypokalemia, hyperkalemia, hypocalcemia, hypomagnesemia, and respiratory alkalosis (see Chapter 3) can all cause muscle cramping.

✓ **Address any specific cause. IV fluids with electrolyte replacement will help with heat cramps and alcohol-induced cramps.**

✓ **Ordinary muscle cramps can be treated immediately with passive or active stretching of the cramped muscle (dorsiflexing the foot for calf cramps).**

✓ **Nocturnal leg cramps have historically been treated with quinine sulfate tablets, 260 to 325 mg taken qhs.** Most studies show that quinine and its derivatives decrease the incidence, severity, and duration of night cramps. However, not all report favorable results, and their use has become somewhat controversial. Recently, the Food and Drug Administration (FDA) has warned against using quinine for non–FDA-approved symptoms of leg cramps and restless leg syndrome, because of reports of hematologic reactions. **A glass of tonic water (a source of quinine) before bed is a less toxic alternative worth trying.**

✓ **Oral magnesium (Slo-Mag, Mag 64), qd or bid, can be used to reduce leg cramps in pregnant women, without increasing serum concentrations.** Although one study failed to find a difference between magnesium and placebo in patients with nocturnal leg cramps, magnesium salts are commonly used to relieve nocturnal leg pain in Europe and Latin America.

✓ Provide appropriate follow-up to patients who have more than benign self-limited cramps.

What Not To Do:

Ⓧ Do not ignore muscle weakness, fasciculations, and wasting, which are signs of lower motor neuron disorders, including amyotrophic lateral sclerosis, polyneuropathy, peripheral nerve injury, and nerve root compression. Fasciculation and cramps without weakness or muscle atrophy are recognized as a benign syndrome. If there is any uncertainty, a normal electromyogram will rule out any serious disease processes.

Discussion

Most muscle cramps are thought to be caused by hyperactivity of the peripheral or central nervous system rather than the muscle itself. The pain results from a combination of ischemia, accumulation of metabolites, and possible damage to the muscle fibers. Electromyographic studies indicate that during ordinary muscle cramps, motor units fire at about 300 per second, far more rapidly than any voluntary contraction. This rapid firing rate causes the muscle tightness and pain.

The cramps occur when a muscle already in its most shortened natural position contracts further. True cramps, which by definition occur in the absence of fluid or electrolyte imbalance, are more prevalent in patients with well-developed muscles, in the latter stages of pregnancy, and in patients with cirrhosis. They are typically asymmetric, explosive in onset, and most frequently affect the gastrocnemius muscle and small muscles of the foot. The contraction, which is often visible, may leave soreness and even swelling. The most common type of true muscle cramp occurs at rest, usually during the night. **A small study showed that in elderly patients with nocturnal leg cramps that are unresponsive to quinine sulfate, verapamil provided relief to most.** There are reports that nitroglycerin paste applied to the overlying skin may relieve a muscle cramp rapidly, but the dose must be small to avoid hypotension, headache, and flushing.

Muscle cramps can also be a considerable source of discomfort in patients undergoing hemodialysis. There is limited evidence that nifedipine can also provide significant pain relief to this group of patients. In another study of hemodialysis muscle cramps, the combination of vitamin C and E supplements produced a 97% decrease in cramps.

Suggested Readings

Cohen SP, Mullings R, Abdi S: The pharmacologic treatment of muscle pain, *Anesthesiology* 101:495–526, 2004.

De Carvalho M, Swash M: Cramps, muscle pain, and fasciculations: not always benign? *Neurology* 63:721–723, 2004.

Schaefer TJ, Wolford RW: Disorders of potassium, *Emerg Med Clin North Am* 23:723–477, viii-ix, 2005.

Tews MC, Shah SM, Gossain VV: Hypothyroidism: mimicker of common complaints, *Emerg Med Clin North Am* 23:649–667, vii, 2005.

Muscle Strains and Tears

Presentation

Strains are acute injuries to muscle-tendon units that result from overstretching or overexerting. Strains may occur in the trapezius or paravertebral muscles during a motor vehicle collision, with a whiplash-type injury to the neck. A strain can also occur in the anterior thigh, hamstring group, groin, or gastrocnemius muscle while a person is accelerating, running, or playing in a sport such as tennis. There may be an insidious development of pain and tightness, which is worse with use and better with rest. With more severe injury, such as a bicep-tendon rupture, the pain may be immediate and disabling. Tears of the muscle belly tend to be partial, with sudden onset of pain and partial loss of function. Often a tear occurs with considerable bleeding, which can lead to remarkable hematomas, causing swelling at the site and dissecting along tissue planes to create ecchymoses at distant, uninvolved sites. Complete tears are more likely in the tendinous part of the muscle. They can produce immediate loss of function and retraction of the torn end, creating a deformity and bulge.

What To Do:

✅ Obtain a detailed history of the mechanism of injury. Elucidating an inciting event, determining the relieving and exacerbating factors, and timing of the pain can be the most important aspects of making an accurate diagnosis.

✅ For cervical strains, see Chapter 103.

✅ The anterior thigh (quadriceps) may be injured while the person is kicking, jumping, and sprinting. The hamstrings of the posterior thigh (biceps femoris, semitendinosus, semimembranosus, and adductor magnus) may tear during a powerful acceleration while a person is sprinting. Adductor strains of the groin occur during various sports activities, such as playing soccer or hockey. Calf muscle (gastrocnemius and soleus) strains are often seen with sudden accelerations from a dorsiflexed position. Upper arm (biceps) injury occurs with forceful lifting against resistance and with rupture of the long head of the biceps, usually presenting with anterior shoulder pain, possibly after hearing a "pop."

✅ Muscle strains may be classified as grade I (mild), grade II (moderate), or grade III (severe, in which the muscle is completely torn). Grade I strains are limited to local spasm and tenderness, and the patient may not notice the pain until the day after the injury. Grade II strains have a palpable area of tenderness and swelling. Passive stretching is usually painful. Grade III strains include tendinous rupture or midbelly tears that are usually accompanied by a visible and/or palpable defect or deformity.

✅ Perform a physical examination that defines the muscle that is involved and rules out bony involvement and other possible disease.

✅ Palpate the injured muscle, attempt active and passive range of motion, check for bony tenderness, and put proximal and distal joints through a range of motion in an attempt to elicit any joint pain (see Chapter 126 for specific evaluation of calf muscle strain).

✅ **Most strains can be easily diagnosed on physical examination, with pain on palpation of the involved muscle and pain on muscle contraction against resistance.**

✅ **Without signs of bony injury, plain radiographs are of little value. Ultrasonography can be useful for diagnosing muscle and tendon tears if the diagnosis is in question.**

✅ When there is a need to know the extent of injury for treatment and prognostic purposes, MRI can be used to confirm and delineate muscle strain or tears, and partial and complete tendon tears.

✅ **Acute treatment of grade I and II strains should include relative rest and possibly short-term use of acetaminophen or nonsteroidal anti-inflammatory drugs (NSAIDs). Cold packs with compressive soft splinting may be helpful when hemorrhage or swelling is present.** Short-term use of opiates may be required for particularly painful injuries.

✅ Even without hemorrhage or swelling, ice massage may be preferable to heat for providing comfort in the first 1 to 3 days. Freeze water in a small paper or Styrofoam cup, tear off the upper rim to expose the ice, and then massage the injured muscle with the ice, using slow, circular strokes for 5 to 20 minutes, using the cup as an insulator. It may be helpful to alternate heat and cold treatments and allow the patient to choose which is better for relieving pain or improving range of motion.

✅ **Severe grade II or grade III strains may require maximum immobilization with a rigid splint and/or with a sling or crutches.** Midbelly muscular tears are often treated conservatively, but complete tears of the tendon's insertion from the bone may require surgical repair.

✅ The more severe strains require orthopedic consultation and follow-up for treatment and rehabilitation.

✅ **Most minor grade I strains will resolve within 2 to 4 weeks. Healing time for all strains can be extremely variable and prone to reexacerbations** (especially hamstring injuries).

✅ The second stage of therapy for most strains begins when the patient's pain has subsided and should consist of gentle range-of-motion exercises, followed by progressive strengthening.

✅ Warn the patient that partial tears can become complete after rehabilitation and that potentially alarming ecchymosis may develop in the days following the injury. They will change color and percolate to the skin at distant sites that are dependent to the injury.

What Not To Do:

❌ Do not order radiographs when the injury is clearly isolated to a muscle or tendon and there is no bony involvement.

Ⓧ Do not prescribe muscle relaxants for acute muscular strain. One double-blind study demonstrated that adding cyclobenzaprine (Flexeril) to treatment with ibuprofen (Motrin) did not enhance pain relief but was associated with a higher rate of central nervous system (CNS) side effects.

Discussion

Groin injuries may result from a variety of causes. The most common groin injury in athletes is the abductor strain. Iliopsoas strain usually occurs during resisted hip flexion or hyperextension. Tenderness may be felt on deep palpation over the lateral aspect of the femoral triangle (adjacent to the femoral artery). This may be accentuated by having the patient raise his heel off the examining table to about 15 degrees.

High hamstring strains (partial avulsion of the muscle from its origin on the ischial tuberosity) occur when excessive stress is placed on the stretched hamstrings. Patients usually present with posterior thigh pain and can have radiation to the groin as well. The diagnosis is easily made when the examiner notes pain on palpation directly over the muscle insertion on the ischial tuberosity.

Sartorius strains lead to palpable tenderness over the anterior superior iliac spine.

Avulsion fractures and apophysitis should be considered in the skeletally immature pediatric age group.

The sports hernia presents as an insidious-onset, gradually worsening, deep groin pain that is diffuse in nature. It may radiate along the inguinal ligament, perineum, and rectus muscles. Coughing may increase the pain. Radiation of pain to the testicles is present in approximately 30% of afflicted men. On physical examination, no true hernia is palpable, because only the deep fascia is violated. MRI and bone scan might be helpful in ruling out other conditions (e.g., stress fractures), but not in making a definitive diagnosis of sports hernia. If symptoms persist after several weeks of conservative treatment, an athlete should undergo surgical exploration and repair.

Other potential causes of groin pain include the more common indirect and direct hernias; testicular disease, including torsion; hip disease, including avascular necrosis; and lumbar radiculopathy. Osteitis pubis, or pubic symphysitis, is a painful inflammatory condition involving the pubic symphysis and surrounding structures that is another possible cause for groin pain and is generally thought of as a self-limiting condition.

Potentially more serious intra-abdominal disease, including gastrointestinal (e.g., appendicitis), urologic (e.g., renal colic), and vascular (e.g., abdominal aortic aneurysm), can refer pain to the groin and should be considered when clinically compelling.

Rupture of the long head of the biceps is one of the most common musculotendinous tears. Proximal long-head tendon ruptures account for 96% of all biceps tendon ruptures. Rupture occurs more frequently in an aging population, specifically in patients who are older than 40 years, and generally occurs in tendinopathic tendons. Risk factors for biceps tendon ruptures include recurrent tendinitis, a history of rotator cuff tear, a history of contralateral biceps tendon rupture, age, poor conditioning, and rheumatoid arthritis.

The literature shows no clear consensus on the treatment of biceps-tendon rupture. Surgical repair tends to be favored in the younger and more athletic patient, whereas conservative, nonsurgical management is considered to be more appropriate in the middle-aged and older patient.

Overuse injuries affecting the medial aspect of the lower legs have traditionally been referred to as "**shin splints.**" This catchall diagnosis is gradually being replaced by that of **medial tibial stress syndrome (MTSS).** This condition predominantly affects running athletes. Patients who have MTSS typically present with shin pain that is related to running or jumping. Pain may be unilateral or bilateral. Examination of patients suffering from MTSS frequently reveals pain confined to the medial border of the tibia, although it can also be located laterally. Toe standing or resisted plantarflexion can exacerbate pain.

Rest is crucial for the treatment of MTSS. Ice, stretching, heel cups, NSAIDs, corticosteroid injection, and even crutches have been studied, but none has benefits that are greater than rest alone. Five to 7 days of rest are often enough to allow return to activity at a reduced intensity, gradually increasing loads to premorbid levels.

Suggested Readings

Glazer JL, Hosey RG: Soft-tissue injuries of the lower extremity, *Prim Care* 31:1005–1024, 2004.

Harwood MI, Smith CT: Superior labrum, anterior–posterior lesions and biceps injuries: diagnostic and treatment considerations, *Prim Care* 31:831–855, 2004.

Morelli V, Espinoza L: Groin injuries and groin pain in athletes: part 2, *Prim Care* 32:185–200, 2005.

Morelli V, Weaver V: Groin injuries and groin pain in athletes: part 1, *Prim Care* 32:163–183, 2005.

Naticchia J, Kapur E: New technology, new injuries in the hip/groin, *Clin Fam Pract* 7:267–278, 2005.

Turturro MA, Frater CR, D'Amico FJ: Cyclobenzaprine with ibuprofen versus ibuprofen alone in acute myofascial strain: a randomized, double-blind clinical trial, *Ann Emerg Med* 41:818–826, 2003.

Myofascial Pain Syndrome, Fibromyalgia

(Trigger Points)

Presentation

In myofascial pain syndrome, the patient, who is generally 25 to 50 years of age, will be troubled by the gradual onset of localized or regional unilateral fibromuscular pain that at times can be immobilizing. There may be a history of acute strain, or a history of predisposing activities, such as holding a telephone receiver between the ear and shoulder to free the arms, prolonged bending, poor postural habits, repetitive motions, and heavy lifting using poor body mechanics. The areas most commonly affected are the axial muscles, used to maintain posture, which include the posterior muscles of the neck and scapula and the soft tissues lateral to the thoracic and lumbar spine.

Careful examination of the painful region will reveal one or more "trigger points," which, when firmly pressed with an examining finger, will cause the patient to wince, cry out, or jump with pain. The underlying muscle may contain a small (2- to 5-mm) firm knot, nodule, or taut band of muscle fibers that produces the exquisitely tender trigger point and reproduces the pain of their chief complaint. Pain is often referred in a radicular pattern that may mimic the pain of cervical or lumbar disc herniation.

The patient with fibromyalgia, on the other hand, has widespread, bilateral symmetric musculoskeletal pain that is associated with multiple "tender points" on palpation and that do not cause any radiation of pain. This patient is often depressed or under emotional or physical stress and may have associated chronic fatigue with disturbed sleep, irritable bowel syndrome, cognitive difficulties, headache, morning stiffness, and sensations of numbness or swelling in the hands and feet. Other comorbid conditions might include irritable bladder symptoms, temporomandibular joint syndrome, myofascial pain syndrome, restless leg syndrome, and affective disorders. Cold or hot weather may be one of the precipitating causes of pain.

In both syndromes, most affected patients are women. Also, the pain is nonarticular, and there are no abnormal vital signs and no swelling, erythema, or heat over the painful areas.

What To Do:

✅ Obtain a careful history and perform a general physical examination with special attention to the painful area. Myofascial pain is local or referred regional muscular pain of short (days) or prolonged (months) duration, often causing head, neck, shoulder, upper and lower back, buttock, and leg pain and associated with trigger points, as described earlier. The patient can usually point to the pain with one finger (Figure 123-1).

✅ The pain of fibromyalgia is widespread (bilateral, above and below the waist), prolonged (>3 months), and associated with approximately 11 of 18 possible tender points (Figure 123-2).

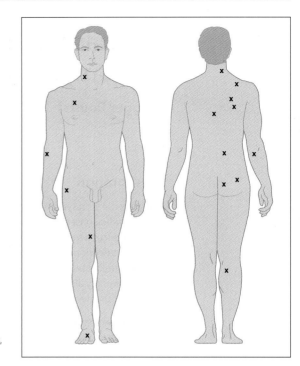

Figure 123-1 Most frequent locations of myofascial trigger points. (Adapted from Rachlin E, Rachlin I: *Myofascial pain and fibromyalgia: trigger point management,* ed 2. St Louis, 2002, Mosby.)

These tender points are predictable, and, unlike trigger points, they do not cause radiation of pain or have an underlying small tender muscular knot. The associated coexisting conditions mentioned earlier help to support this diagnosis.

✓ Other conditions should be considered, such as medication-induced myalgias (e.g., statins, colchicines, corticosteroids, antimalarial drugs), connective tissue diseases (e.g., dermatomyositis, polymyalgia rheumatica, systemic lupus erythematosus, rheumatoid arthritis), hypothyroidism and other endocrine disorders, and cancer. In addition, evaluate for true radicular pain with a neurologic examination, and, if indicated, straight-leg raising.

✓ With any suspicion that an underlying systemic illness exists, obtain appropriate radiographs and laboratory tests, such as an erythrocyte sedimentation rate, creatine phosphokinase (CPK) and thyroid-stimulating hormone. These and all other studies should be normal in both myofascial and fibromyalgia pain syndrome.

✓ **When a trigger point is found, have the patient maintain a comfortable, relaxed position. Map out its exact location (point of maximum tenderness) and place an "X" over the site with a marker or ballpoint pen.** If the trigger point is diffuse, there is no need to outline its location.

✓ When myofascial pain is suspected but trigger points are diffuse, unless contraindicated, prescribe a nonsteroidal anti-inflammatory drug (NSAID), such as naproxen sodium (Naprosyn), 250 mg, two tablets stat then one qid, or ibuprofen (Motrin), 800 mg stat then 600 mg qid × 5 days. A benzodiazepine such as lorazepam (Ativan), 1 mg qid, may also be helpful.

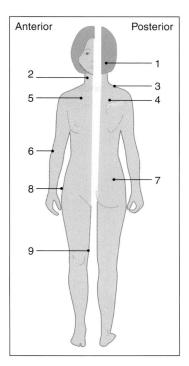

Figure 123-2 Location of nine bilateral (18) tender point sites for the American College of Rheumatology criteria for the classification of fibromyalgia. *1* = suboccipital muscle insertions; *2* = cervical, at the anterior aspects of the intransverse spaces at C5-7; *3* = trapezius, at the midpoint of the upper border; *4* = supraspinatus, at the origin, above the scapular spine near the medial border; *5* = second rib, at the costochondral junction; *6* = lateral epicondyle, 2 cm distal to the epicondyle; *7* = gluteal, in the upper outer quadrant of the buttock; *8* = greater trochanter, just posterior to the trochanteric prominence; *9* = knee, at the medial fat pad proximal to the joint line. (Adapted from Rachlin E, Rachlin I: *Myofascial pain and fibromyalgia: trigger point management,* ed 2. St Louis, 2002, Mosby.)

 ✓ **When a focal trigger point is present, suggest that the patient may get immediate relief with an injection. If the patient is willing, using proper aseptic technique and a 25- or 27-gauge, 1¼- to 1½-inch needle, inject through the mark you placed on the skin, directly into the painful site** (Figures 123-3 to 123-13). **Use 5 to 10 mL of 1% lidocaine (Xylocaine) or longer-acting 0.5% bupivacaine (Marcaine) with or without 20 to 40 mg of methylprednisolone (Depo-Medrol) or 2 to 5 mg of triamcinolone (Aristospan).** Attempt aspiration to be sure you are not in a blood vessel or pleural cavity and then "fan" the needle in all directions while injecting the trigger point. **Advise the patient before the procedure that there may be intensification of the pain before relief.** Intensification of the pain with or without radiation, while injecting slowly, is a good indicator that the needle is in the precise trigger point location. Inject most of the anesthetic into this most painful site. In addition, massage the area after the injection is complete to ensure total coverage. Within a few minutes the patient will often get complete or near-complete pain relief, which helps to confirm the diagnosis of myofascial pain syndrome. Inform the patient that there will be approximately 1 day of muscular soreness after the anesthetic wears off. The beneficial effect of this injection may last for weeks or months. A supplementary 5-day course of NSAIDs is optional.

✓ Secondary trigger points may develop in neighboring muscles as a result of stress and muscle spasm. It is common for patients to experience the pain of a secondary trigger point after a primary trigger point is eliminated. These trigger points can be treated in the same manner, either at the same visit or at an early follow-up visit if the symptoms persist.

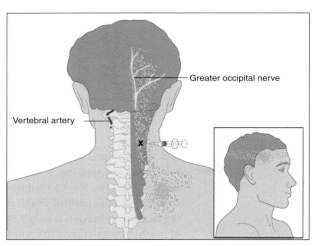

Figure 123-3 Suboccipital muscle. Injection of trigger point (*X*) in the obliquus capitis superior muscle with the patient in the prone position. Injection is localized directly over the trigger point and the superior portion of the occipital area to avoid the vertebral artery. The occipital triangle and vertebral artery are noted. The pain pattern is shown by *stippling*. (Adapted from Rachlin E, Rachlin I: *Myofascial pain and fibromyalgia: trigger point management*, ed 2. St Louis, 2002, Mosby.)

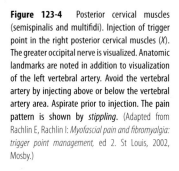

Figure 123-4 Posterior cervical muscles (semispinalis and multifidi). Injection of trigger point in the right posterior cervical muscles (*X*). The greater occipital nerve is visualized. Anatomic landmarks are noted in addition to visualization of the left vertebral artery. Avoid the vertebral artery by injecting above or below the vertebral artery area. Aspirate prior to injection. The pain pattern is shown by *stippling*. (Adapted from Rachlin E, Rachlin I: *Myofascial pain and fibromyalgia: trigger point management*, ed 2. St Louis, 2002, Mosby.)

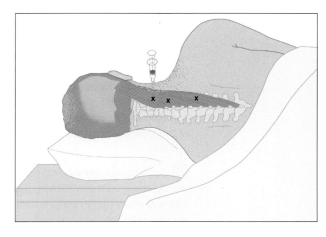

Figure 123-5 Splenius capitis and splenius cervicis. Injection of trigger points (*Xs*) in the right splenius capitis and cervicis with the patient lying on the uninvolved side. Avoid the vertebral artery. Aspirate prior to injection. Anatomic landmarks are noted. The trigger-point pattern is shown by *stippling*. (Adapted from Rachlin E, Rachlin I: *Myofascial pain and fibromyalgia: trigger point management*, ed 2. St Louis, 2002, Mosby.)

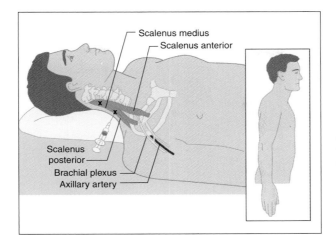

Figure 123-6 Scalene muscles. Injection of the scalenus medius muscle trigger points (*Xs*). The patient is supine, the head turned away from the area of pain. Anatomic landmarks are noted, including axillary artery and lateral chord. The referred pain pattern is shown by *stippling*. (Adapted from Rachlin E, Rachlin I: *Myofascial pain and fibromyalgia: trigger point management*, ed 2. St Louis, 2002, Mosby.)

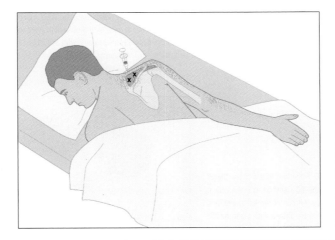

Figure 123-7 Supraspinatus. Injection of trigger points (*Xs*) in the right supraspinatus with the patient prone. The needle is directed directly over the supraspinous fossa of the scapula to avoid penetrating the rib cage. Anatomic landmarks are noted. The pain pattern is shown by *stippling*. (Adapted from Rachlin E, Rachlin I: *Myofascial pain and fibromyalgia: trigger point management*, ed 2. St Louis, 2002, Mosby.)

✅ **Moist, hot compresses and massage may also be comforting to the patient after discharge.**

✅ **Patients with the diffuse symptoms of fibromyalgia usually will not benefit from trigger point injection or NSAIDs. When other causes of such pain have been adequately ruled out, antidepressants, most commonly amitriptyline (Elavil), 10 to 50 mg qd, improve symptoms for up to several months. The muscle relaxant cyclobenzaprine (Flexeril), which is structurally similar to the tricyclic antidepressants, has also been found to be beneficial in doses of 15 to 45 mg/day divided tid. Tramadol (Ultram), 50 to 100 mg q4-6h (not to exceed 400 mg/day), is an analgesic that has also been found to benefit patients with fibromyalgia.**

✅ **Aerobic exercise and warm compresses improve function and reduce pain in persons with fibromyalgia.**

✅ Provide follow-up care for all patients in the event that their symptoms do not clear and they require further diagnostic evaluation and therapy.

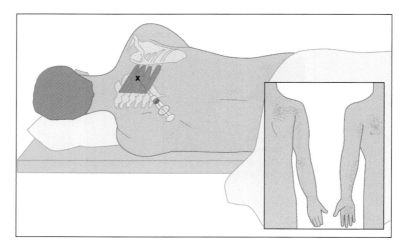

Figure 123-8 Serratus posterior superior. Injection of trigger point (*X*) in the right serratus posterior superior. Localize the trigger point by palpation and direct the needle in the direction of a rib and tangentially in relation to chest wall to avoid entering the intercostal space. Aspirate before injection. Trigger points in the region of muscle insertion are more easily palpated with abduction of the right scapula. Observe precautions to prevent pneumothorax. *Inset,* trigger-point pain pattern (*stippling*). (Adapted from Rachlin E, Rachlin I: *Myofascial pain and fibromyalgia: trigger point management,* ed 2. St Louis, 2002, Mosby.)

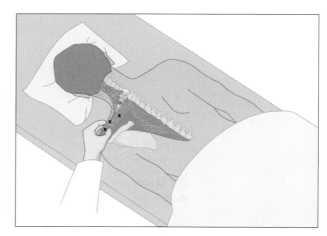

Figure 123-9 Trapezius. Injection for trigger points (*Xs*) in the left trapezius with the patient prone. The upper portion of the left trapezius is grasped between the thumb, index, and middle fingers and is elevated to avoid penetrating the apex of the lung. Several entries are usually necessary to treat all trigger points that are present. Aspirate prior to injection. The pain pattern is shown by stippling. (Adapted from Rachlin E, Rachlin I: *Myofascial pain and fibromyalgia: trigger point management,* ed 2. St Louis, 2002, Mosby.)

What Not To Do:

Ⓧ Do not order radiographs or laboratory tests for myofascial pain that is localized and relieved by trigger point injection.

Ⓧ Do not attempt to inject a very diffuse trigger point (more than 2 cm^2) or multiple scattered tender points as found in true fibromyalgia syndrome. Results are generally unsatisfactory.

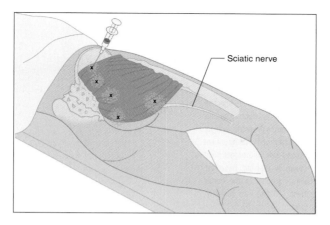

Figure 123-10 Gluteus maximus. Injection of trigger points (*Xs*) in the gluteus maximus. Anatomic landmarks are noted. Avoid the sciatic nerve. The pain pattern is shown by *stippling*. Injection may be performed with the patient in the prone or side-lying position. (Adapted from Rachlin E, Rachlin I: *Myofascial pain and fibromyalgia: trigger point management*, ed 2. St Louis, 2002, Mosby.)

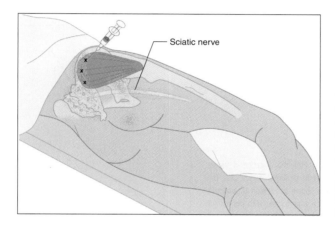

Figure 123-11 Gluteus medius. Injection of trigger points in the right gluteus medius. Multiple trigger points (*Xs*) are noted. Anatomic skeletal landmarks are shown together with the sciatic nerve. The patient is positioned lying on the uninvolved side. Injection may also be performed with the patient prone. The pain pattern is noted by *stippled area.* (Adapted from Rachlin E, Rachlin I: *Myofascial pain and fibromyalgia: trigger point management*, ed 2. St Louis, 2002, Mosby.)

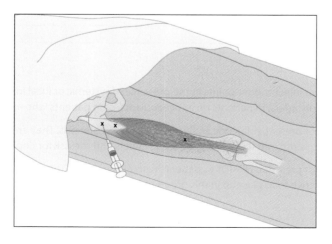

Figure 123-12 Rectus femoris. Injection of trigger points (*Xs*) in the right rectus femoris. Note trigger points in the area of origin and distally toward the area of insertion. The patient is supine. The trigger point pain pattern is shown by *stippling*. Anatomic landmarks are noted. (Adapted from Rachlin E, Rachlin I: *Myofascial pain and fibromyalgia: trigger point management*, ed 2. St Louis, 2002, Mosby.)

477

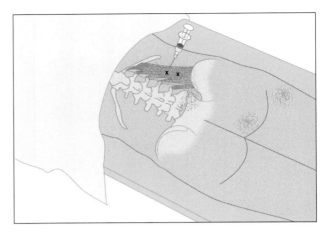

Figure 123-13 Quadratus lumborum. Injection of trigger points (*Xs*) in the right quadratus lumborum with the patient in the prone position. Injection may also be performed with the patient lying on the uninvolved side. The trigger point pain pattern is shown by *stippling*. Direct the needle tangentially or parallel to the frontal plane of the patient. (Adapted from Rachlin E, Rachlin I: *Myofascial pain and fibromyalgia: trigger point management,* ed 2. St Louis, 2002, Mosby.)

— Sciatic nerve

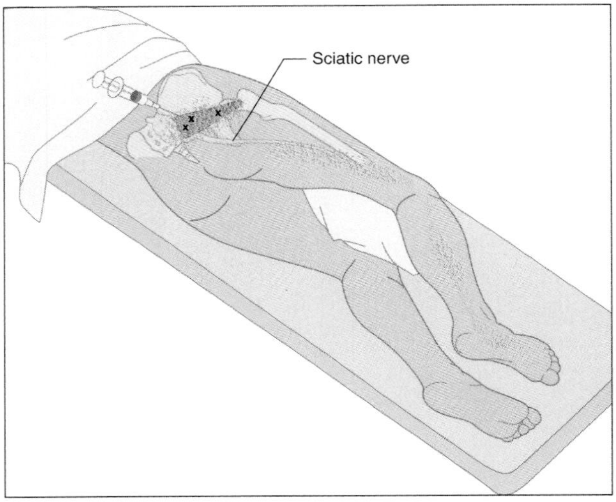

Figure 123-14 Piriformis. Injection of trigger points in the right piriformis muscle (*Xs*). The sciatic nerve is shown in addition to anatomic details. Injection is performed with the patient lying on the uninvolved side. A pillow is placed between the knees. The hip is flexed. The pain pattern is shown by *stippling.* (Adapted from Rachlin E, Rachlin I: *Myofascial pain and fibromyalgia: trigger point management,* ed 2. St Louis, 2002, Mosby.)

⊗ Do not inject trigger points in the presence of systemic or local infection, in patients with bleeding disorders, in patients on anticoagulants, or in patients who appear to be or feel ill.

⊗ Do not prescribe narcotic analgesics or systemic steroids. They are no more effective than the abovementioned therapy and add side effects and the risk for dependence.

⊗ Do not prescribe NSAIDs to patients with fibromyalgia. They have been found to be no more effective than placebo in this group of patients.

Discussion

Emergency physicians and other acute care clinicians often see patients with trigger points associated with simple self-limiting regional **myofascial pain syndromes,** which appear to arise from muscles, muscle–tendon junctions, or tendon–bone junctions. Myofascial disease can result in severe pain, but it is typically in a limited distribution, without the systemic feature of fatigue, and without the multiple somatic complaints of fibromyalgia. Trigger-point injection therapy, the treatment of choice for trigger points according to many, has gained widening acceptance in mainstream medicine. When symptoms recur or persist after this basic therapy or are accompanied by generalized complaints, acute care clinicians should refer these patients to a rheumatologist or primary care physician for follow-up and continued management.

When the quadratus lumborum muscle is involved (see Figure 123-13), **there is often confusion whether or not the patient has a renal, abdominal, or pulmonary ailment. The reason for this is the muscle's proximity to the flank and abdomen, as well as its attachment to the twelfth rib, which, when tender, can create pleuritic symptoms. A careful physical examination reproducing symptoms through palpation, active contraction, and passive stretching of this muscle can save this patient from a multitude of laboratory and radiograph studies.**

Another affected muscle that often confuses and misleads clinicians is the piriformis (Figure 123-14). **Piriformis syndrome is an uncommon and often undiagnosed cause of buttock and leg pain. It may be caused by anatomic abnormalities of the piriformis muscle and the sciatic nerve resulting in irritation of the sciatic nerve by the piriformis.**

The typical patient with piriformis syndrome **complains of buttock pain with or without radiation to the posterior thigh that sometimes extends below the knee to the calf, resembling typical sciatica and causes difficulty with walking. The cardinal characteristic of the syndrome is sitting intolerance secondary to intense buttock pain. Gluteal atrophy may occur.**

Buttock tenderness in the region of the greater sciatic foramen is present in almost all patients, and buttock pain is elicited when the patient lifts and holds the knee several inches off the examination table. There may be moderate relief of pain by applying traction on the affected extremity with the patient in the supine position. A tender sausage-shaped mass may be palpated over the piriformis muscle.

A complete neurologic examination should be performed to test motor power, sensory function, and reflexes of the lower extremities to help rule out spinal causes of sciatic pain. One should also consider intrapelvic diseases, such as tumors and endometriosis, as a possible cause of sciatic pain.

Conservative treatment of piriformis syndrome consists of prescribing NSAIDs, analgesics, and muscle relaxants and providing physical therapy, which includes stretching the piriformis muscle with internal rotation and hip adduction and flexion.

More aggressive therapy includes local injection of anesthetic and corticosteroids that may reconfirm the diagnosis through therapeutic success (see Figure 123-14). This may be repeated twice with recurrent pain. If this fails, surgery can be considered.

The most likely cause of chronic diffuse myalgia is **fibromyalgia.** Among adults who seek medical attention for fibromyalgia, less than one third recover within 10 years of onset. Symptoms tend to remain stable or improve over time.

Although fibromyalgia was long believed to be primarily a muscle disease, research has not found any significant pathologic or biochemical abnormalities in muscle tissue. Many researchers now believe that the disease is caused by abnormalities in central nervous system function. This would suggest that the pain of fibromyalgia is in part because of a decrease in the threshold for pain perception and tolerance experienced by these patients. Fibromyalgia patients also appear to experience pain amplification because of abnormal sensory processing in the central nervous system.

The diagnosis of fibromyalgia **is made by meeting the criteria of having widespread musculoskeletal pain for 3 months or longer and having 11 or more tender points among 18 potential sites defined by the American College of Rheumatology** (see Figure 123-2). **Some patients may not have an adequate number of tender points to make the diagnosis, but when typically associated symptoms are present, these patients should be treated for fibromyalgia.**

Education, reassurance, psychological support, and reminders to exercise regularly are important in all follow-up visits.

Suggested Readings

Abram SE: Does botulinum toxin have a role in the management of myofascial pain? *Anesthesiology* 103:223–224, 2005.

Benzon HT, Katz JA, Benzon HA, et al: Piriformis syndrome, *Anesthesiology* 98:1442–1448, 2003.

Gill JM, Quisel A: Fibromyalgia and diffuse myalgia, *Clin Fam Pract* 7:181–1990, 2005.

Nelson LS, Hoffman RS: Intrathecal injection: unusual complication of trigger-point injection therapy, *Ann Emerg Med* 32:506–508, 1998.

Papadopoulos EC, Khan SN: Piriformis syndrome and low back pain: a new classification and review of the literature, *Orthop Clin North Am* 35:65–71, 2004.

Rachlin E, Rachlin I: *Myofascial pain and fibromyalgia: trigger point management,* ed 2, St Louis, 2002, Mosby.

Patellar Dislocation

(Kneecap Dislocation)

Presentation

After a direct blow to the medial aspect of the patella or, more commonly, without contact and only after a sudden twisting motion to the opposite side of an outward-pointing planted foot (with a powerful contraction of the quadriceps while the thigh is turning inward), the patient's kneecap dislocates laterally. The patient, who is usually an adolescent, is brought in with the knee guarded and slightly flexed, in severe pain, with the patella situated lateral to the lateral femoral condyle, creating an obvious lateral deformity (Figure 124-1). Most often, there will have been a spontaneous reduction, and the patient reports that the knee or kneecap "gave way" or "gave out" with pain and then slipped back into place. A patient with recurrent, acute dislocation is usually able to relate an appropriate history and usually knows exactly what happened.

What To Do:

⊘ **For a persistent dislocation, provide immediate reduction. Pain medications and sedatives may be needed for reduction, but gaining the patient's confidence while holding and stabilizing the leg will minimize this need. Position the patient with a slight flexion of the hip to reduce strain on the quadriceps muscle (one way to do this is to have the patient sitting on the edge of the stretcher with legs down). Stand on the lateral side of the patient (for a medial dislocation, stand on the medial side of the patient). Slowly and gently extend the lower leg at the knee while holding the patella in place until the knee is fully extended. If needed, apply continuous gentle anteromedial force to the patella to lift it over the edge of the femoral condyle. Once reduced, apply a knee immobilizer and fit the patient with crutches.**

 ⊘ **Some practitioners have had luck with the following maneuver as well: gain the patient's confidence and cooperation while gently grasping the patella and stabilizing it by applying mild lateral traction and maintaining its position to prevent sudden motion. Place the patient in the semiprone position for relaxation. Then have the patient allow you to passively and very gradually extend the knee. When it is fully extended, slowly release traction on the patella while maintaining continuous control and gently let it slip into its normal anatomic position (medial force is generally not required). With experience, this technique rarely requires any analgesia or sedation, only a calm and reassuring approach.**

⊘ After the patella has been reduced and the patient is comfortable, **order knee radiographs, including patellar views,** to rule out an avulsion fracture of the superomedial pole of the patella, an osteochondral fracture of the lateral femoral condyle, or a fracture of the medial posterior patellar articular surface. There are associated fractures in 28% to 50% of

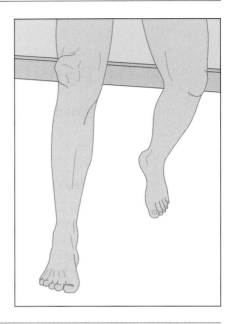

Figure 124-1 Patellar dislocation.

patellar dislocations, which can lead to degenerative arthritis. It must be appreciated that plain radiographs do not show a high percentage of osteochondral fractures occurring at the time of patellofemoral dislocation.

✅ If pain persists beyond early rehabilitation, new articular cartilage MRI techniques should be used to identify any undiagnosed osteochondral injuries. MRI also has a role in determining the extent and location of injury to the medial patellofemoral ligament.

✅ **A standard evaluation of the knee ligaments should be performed to rule out concurrent injury** (see Chapter 115).

✅ **Palpate for rents in the vastus medialis obliquus and the medial patellofemoral ligament or for a grossly dislocatable patella** (Figure 124-2). **Also note the presence of any swelling or effusion.**

✅ A hemarthrosis can develop from a capsular tear and/or an osteochondral fracture. Some authors suggest that when a tense and painful hemarthrosis is present, aspiration should be considered to reduce pain and check for fat droplets, indicating an occult osteochondral injury.

✅ **Fit the patient for crutches and a knee immobilizer that will keep the knee straight.**

✅ Provide analgesia as required, and instruct on the use of ice and elevation. Teach non–weight-bearing walking with crutches.

✅ Provide orthopedic follow-up in 1 to 3 days.

✅ Quadriceps isometrics, straight-leg raises, and single-plane motion exercises are begun early and progress as tolerated. Quadriceps strengthening is paramount and kept in balance with adequate extensor mechanism rehabilitation. **Repetition of the injury mechanism or mechanically similar activities must be avoided in the healing period.** Exercises should be

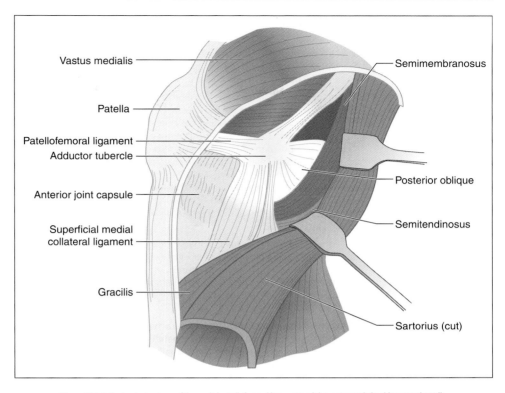

Figure 124-2 Anatomic structures of the medial patellofemoral ligament and the vastus medialis obliquus and patella.

done in a pain-free manner. Patellar pain may indicate unrecognized or progressive articular cartilage damage. As strength and symptoms allow, patients progress out of their brace in physical therapy to single plane walking, running, cutting, and finally sport-specific activity.

What Not To Do:

⊗ Do not try to force the patella to move medially. This may succeed in reduction but is unnecessarily painful and can cause harm.

Discussion

The patella is the largest sesamoid bone in the body, and it resides within the complex of the quadriceps and patellar tendons. It functions as both a lever and a pulley. As a lever, the patella magnifies the force exerted by the quadriceps on knee extension. As a pulley, the patella redirects the quadriceps force as it undergoes normal lateral tracking during flexion.

Most series on patellar dislocation report a greater incidence in women, although some series have reported equal numbers of men and women affected, and others have found a higher incidence in men. Depending on the study, 30% to 72% of dislocations can be expected to be sports related,

(continued)

Discussion continued

and 28% to 39% will have associated osteochondral fractures. Concurrent osteochondral injuries are a major contributor to adverse outcomes.

The most common sports involved are football, basketball, and baseball, but it is not unusual in gymnastics, simple falls, cheerleading, and dancing. This injury may occur when patients with normal anatomy are exposed to direct high-energy forces, but most studies find that it occurs more commonly when patients with abnormal anatomy are exposed to indirect forces. Some authors think that anatomic predispositions, such as patella alta, trochlear dysplasia, and ligamentous laxity, play greater roles in recurrent instability.

The average age of these patients is 16 to 20 years old; it is a rare injury for those older than age 30. The incidence of recurrent dislocation decreases with age. Fourteen-year-olds have a 60% incidence of redislocation, whereas 17- to 28-year-olds have an incidence of 30%.

Most patellar dislocations are of the lateral type. Horizontal, superior, and intracondylar patellar dislocations are very uncommon and usually require surgical reduction.

Relative indications for early operative intervention after an acute lateral patella dislocation are controversial, without clear supporting research, but include the following: (1) failure to improve with initial nonoperative care, (2) concurrent osteochondral injury, (3) continued gross patella instability, (4) palpable disruption of the medial patellofemoral ligament–vastus medialis obliquus–adductor mechanism, and (5) high-level athletic demands coupled with mechanical risk factors and an initial injury mechanism not related to contact.

One study suggests that most patients without anatomic abnormality do well whether they are treated conservatively or surgically, and that among patients with anatomic abnormality, half will do well if treated conservatively, whereas up to 80% will do well if treated surgically. Some studies show a trend toward increased osteoarthritis following surgical repair for patella dislocation.

Suggested Readings

Hinton RY, Sharma KM: Acute and recurrent patellar instability in the young athlete, *Orthop Clin North Am* 34: 385–396, 2003.

Morelli V, Rowe RH: Patellar tendonitis and patellar dislocations, *Prim Care* 31:909–924, viii-ix, 2004.

Plantar Fasciitis

("Heel Spur")

Presentation

Patients seek help because of gradually increasing inferior heel pain that has progressed to the point of inhibiting their normal daily activities. This fasciitis can develop in anyone who is ambulatory but appears to be more common in athletes (especially runners), those older than 30 years of age, those who stand for prolonged periods of time, and the overweight. There is no defining episode of trauma. The most distinctive clue is exquisite pain in the plantar aspect of the heel when taking the first step in the morning. There is gradual improvement with walking, but as the day progresses, the pain may insidiously increase. First-step pain is also present after the patient has been sitting. The heel is tender to palpation over the medial calcaneal tubercle and may be exacerbated by dorsiflexion of the ankle and toes, particularly the great toe, which creates tension on the plantar fascia. Often the midfascia is tender to palpation too. There is generally no swelling, heat, or discoloration.

What To Do:

✓ Obtain a general medical history in addition to details of the patient's current illness. Patients with systemic conditions and those with potential infection will have other areas of involvement or bilateral involvement. Other clues might include a history of diabetes, chemotherapy, retroviral infection, a rheumatologic disorder, or another similar chronic condition. A history of focal pain after localized trauma indicates a contusion to the heel (sometimes referred to as "fat pad syndrome").

✓ **Increased levels of activity or exercise may indicate that overuse is the cause of the pain.** Other potential precipitating factors include recent weight gain, a change in footwear, inappropriate or worn-out shoes, or working on cement floors. If the patient describes the sensation as "burning", "tingling," or "numbness," the cause may be peripheral nerve entrapment. Pain that develops in the evening after physical activity is often seen early in stress fracture.

✓ Perform a careful foot examination to determine the location of the point of maximal tenderness and to detect any signs of infection, atrophy of the heel pad, bony deformities, bruising, or breaks in the skin. **Diagnosis is made by eliciting pain with palpation in the region of the medial plantar tuberosity of the calcaneus (the origin of the plantar fascia). Pain may be worsened by passive dorsiflexion of the foot.**

✓ **Radiographs can be deferred and are not always required.** However, as clinical findings demand, they may be obtained to look for stress fractures of the metatarsals, tumors, osteomyelitis, calcifications, or spurs, which are located on the leading edge of the calcaneal inferior surface.

✓ **Unless contraindicated, prescribe nonsteroidal anti-inflammatory drugs (NSAIDs) for 2 to 3 weeks.**

✓ **Have the patient wear soft (viscoelastic) heel cushions, such as Bauerfeind Viscoheel (Bauerfeind USA, Kennesaw, Ga.), and a sports shoe with a firm, impact-resistant heel counter and longitudinal arch support. AirCast (DJO Global, Vista, Calif.) provides an alternative pneumatic compression dressing for the foot and ankle (AirHeel).**

✓ Use of dorsiflexion night splints may be particularly beneficial in preventing the severe pain that often comes with the first steps in the morning on awakening. However, compliance is low.

✓ **Ice massage can be helpful. The patient can roll his heel over a can of frozen juice concentrate, followed by stretching.**

✓ **Athletes should practice stretching the Achilles tendon before running by placing the sole flat, leaning forward against a counter or table, and slowly squatting while keeping the heel on the ground.** Others may stand, wearing tennis shoes, on the edge of a step, facing up stairs, slowly lowering their heels until they feel a pulling sensation in their upper calf. Hold for ½ to 1 minute or until there is pain. Repeat three times daily, increasing the stretch time to a maximum of 3 minutes per session. Although there may be a transient increase in pain after beginning this program, the heel pain usually begins to resolve within several weeks.

✓ **Have the patient reduce ambulatory activities and try to keep weight off the foot whenever possible.** Also, have female patients avoid thin-soled flats and high heels. Have runners decrease their mileage by 25% to 75% and avoid sprinting, running on hard surfaces, and running uphill. A program of cross training incorporating swimming and bicycling maintains cardiovascular fitness while decreasing stress on the feet.

✓ Although not often easily applied, recommend weight loss for those patients who are overweight.

✓ **When conservative measures have failed and there is an exquisitely tender area on the medial calcaneus, local corticosteroid injection may speed recovery.** Use with care because there may be increased risk of plantar fasciitis rupture. Palpate the heel pad to locate the point of maximum tenderness. Place the patient in the lateral recumbent position with the lateral aspect of the painful heel resting against the examination surface. Cleanse the skin with povidone-iodine, and using a 25-gauge, 1¼- to 1½-inch needle, inject the area with 2 mL of 0.25% or 0.5% of bupivacaine (Marcaine) along with betamethasone (Celestone Soluspan), 1 mL of 6 mg/mL, or methylprednisolone (Depo-Medrol), 1 mL of 40 mg/mL. Enter medially, perpendicular to the skin, and advance the needle directly down past the midline of the width of the foot to the plantar fascia until you can feel its thick and gritty substance. Inject the mixture slowly and evenly through the middle one third of the width of the foot while the needle is being withdrawn (Figure 125-1). Finish by putting the injected region through passive range of motion to spread the medication. Patients should be cautioned that they may experience worsening symptoms during the first 24 to 48 hours. This may be related to a possible steroid flare, which can be treated with ice and NSAIDs. Two or three injections at intervals of several weeks may be necessary.

✓ Studies are presently ongoing to evaluate the efficacy of injecting botulinum toxin into the foot. Initial studies have shown benefit; however, more investigation needs to be performed before suggesting this as a treatment.

✓ In all cases, orthopedic follow-up should be arranged.

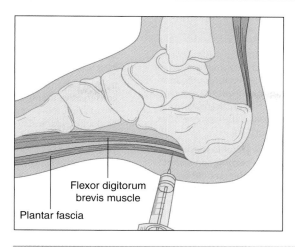

Flexor digitorum
brevis muscle

Plantar fascia

Figure 125-1 Proper location for injection.

What Not To Do:

 Do not inject into the heel pad itself, which may cause fat atrophy.

Discussion

The plantar fascia provides an intimate attachment to the overlying skin and functions to provide protection to the underlying muscles, tendons, arteries, and nerves. The fascia assists in the maintenance of the foot arch and keeps the foot in relative supination through the push-off phase of ambulation. During heel strike, the plantar fascia remains supple and allows the foot to adjust to the ground surface and absorb shock. Then, during the toe-off phase of ambulation, the plantar fascia becomes taut and thereby renders the foot a rigid lever, thus facilitating forward movement.

Plantar fasciitis, the most common cause of heel pain in adults, typically results from repetitive use or excessive load on the fascia. Persons who are overweight, female, or older than 40 years or who spend long hours on their feet are especially at risk for developing plantar fasciitis. Athletes, especially joggers and runners, also develop plantar fasciitis.

Tightness of the Achilles tendon contributes to increased tension on the plantar fascia during walking or running and is therefore an important contributor to plantar fasciitis. Stretching of the Achilles tendon can therefore alleviate some of the pain caused by plantar fasciitis. It should be relayed to the patient, however, that this can initially make the discomfort worse.

Mechanical causes of heel pain are generally synonymous with plantar fasciitis, but some cases are enigmatic in etiology and are deemed idiopathic. Although the word *fasciitis* implies inflammation, recent research indicates that it is more likely to be a noninflammatory, degenerative process that might be more appropriately called plantar fasciosis.

Acute onset of severe plantar heel pain after trauma or vigorous athletics may indicate rupture of the plantar fascia. The patient may have heard a "pop" or felt a tearing sensation. Findings suggestive of rupture include a palpable defect at the calcaneal tuberosity accompanied by localized swelling and ecchymosis.

If conservative treatment of plantar fasciitis fails to alleviate symptoms, radiographs are advisable to check for other causes of heel pain, such as stress fractures, arthritis, or skeletal abnormalities. Radiographs may show a spur on the leading edge of the calcaneal inferior surface, but this radiographic finding is not pathognomonic of the condition, nor is it necessary for the diagnosis. It is a common finding in the asymptomatic foot and is generally not the cause of a patient's heel pain.

(continued)

Discussion continued

If a patient with heel pain has persistent bilateral involvement, systemic disease may be the cause. Ankylosing spondylitis, Reiter disease, rheumatoid arthritis, systemic lupus erythematosus, and gouty arthritis all may cause medial calcaneal pain. Calcaneal bursitis and fat pad atrophy are other potential causes of heel pain.

The benefits of using injectable steroids for plantar fasciitis has become somewhat controversial; therefore they should be used only when conservative measures have failed. The main concern with the use of steroid injections is delayed rupture of the plantar fascia. Rupture is typically associated with resolution of plantar fasciitis symptoms, but a majority of these patients may go on to develop long-term sequelae, such as longitudinal arch strain, lateral plantar nerve dysfunction, stress fracture, and development of hammertoe deformity.

In most patients with plantar fasciitis, conservative therapy works best. Symptoms will usually resolve, but this may take many weeks or months. For the 10% or fewer with heel pain that persists for at least 1 year despite treatment, surgery should be considered, especially when the symptoms of plantar fasciitis are disabling. Determining the source of repetitive stress to the plantar fascia and addressing it as part of the treatment is crucial to both facilitating recovery and reducing the risk of recurrence. Chronic recurrences may indicate biomechanical imbalances in the foot, which may resolve with custom orthotics from a podiatrist.

Suggested Readings

Aldridge T: Diagnosing heel pain in adults, *Am Fam Physician* 70:332–338, 2004.

Sheon RP, Buchbinder R: Plantar fasciitis and other causes of heel and sole pain. [*UpToDate* website]. Available at http://www.uptodate.com. Accessed March 8, 2012.

Tallia AF, Cardone DA: Diagnostic and therapeutic injection of the ankle and foot, *Am Fam Physician* 68:1356–1362, 2003.

Torpy JM: Plantar fasciitis, *JAMA* 290:1542, 2003.

Williams SK, Brage M: Heel pain—plantar fasciitis and Achilles enthesopathy, *Clin Sports Med* 23:123–144, 2004.

"Plantaris Tendon" Rupture, Gastrocnemius Muscle Tear

(Calf Muscle Tear)

Presentation

The patient will come in limping, having suffered a whiplike sting in the calf while stepping off the foot hard or attempting a lunging shot during a game of tennis or similar activity. The patient may have actually heard or felt a "snap," described as being like the "pop" of a champagne cork, at the time of injury or may think someone actually kicked or shot him in the calf. The deep calf pain persists and may be accompanied by mild to moderate swelling and ecchymosis. Neurovascular function will be intact.

What To Do:

✓ Obtain a clear history of the mechanism of injury, either forceful ankle plantar flexion or knee extension while the foot is dorsiflexed, as is seen on the back leg during the "push off" of a lunging tennis shot. Pain may radiate to the knee or ankle.

✓ Perform a physical examination, which should reveal calf tenderness, especially along the medial musculotendinous junction of the medial gastrocnemius. There may be a defect in the muscle belly itself. Swelling will usually be asymmetric, and over time, any ecchymosis may be found spreading to a more dependent site over the ankle or foot. Dorsiflexion of the foot and resisted plantarflexion are typically painful. Peripheral pulses should be present and symmetric.

 ✓ **Rule out an Achilles tendon rupture, because this needs orthopedic evaluation for possible surgery. Palpate the Achilles tendon for a defect or deformity, which represents a torn segment. Squeeze the gastrocnemius muscle just distal to its widest girth, with the patient kneeling on a chair or lying prone on a stretcher with the legs overhanging the end** (Figure 126-1) **to examine for normal plantar flexion of the foot. Alternatively, the test may be performed with the patient's knees flexed and the feet up while he is supine. Always compare the affected leg with the contralateral limb. The resultant plantar flexion will be totally absent with a complete Achilles tendon tear.** A defect in the contour along the length of the Achilles tendon, pain distal to the body of the gastrocnemius, and lack of pain with palpation of the muscle belly are all typical of Achilles tendon rupture and not plantaris tendon rupture or a gastrocnemius tear.

✓ **When there is any uncertainty, a definitive diagnosis can be established with ultrasonography or MRI. With any Achilles tendon tear, orthopedic consultation is necessary.**

✓ If there is excruciating pain out of proportion to what would be expected with these injuries, the possibility of an acute compartment syndrome must be entertained, and immediate orthopedic consultation should be obtained.

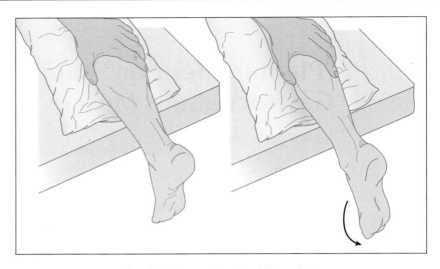

Figure 126-1 Thompson, Simmonds, or "calf squeeze" test.

✅ **When serious conditions have been ruled out, provide the patient with elastic support (e.g., Ace bandage, antiembolism stocking, Tubigrip) from the foot to the tibial tuberosity, with or without a posterior splint to provide additional comfort. Gravity equinus (allowing the toe to drop down naturally) is generally the most comfortable position.**

✅ **Patients with severe pain may require crutches for several days.** Some clinicians have begun using rocker-bottom postoperative boots for early ambulation.

✅ Have the patient keep the leg elevated above the level of his heart and at rest as much as possible for the next 24 to 48 hours, initially applying cold packs intermittently.

✅ An analgesic such as hydrocodone (e.g., Lorcet, Lortab) may be helpful initially, as well as nonsteroidal anti-inflammatory drugs (NSAIDs), if tolerated.

✅ **The temporary use of bilateral 1-inch heel wedges may also provide immediate comfort for ambulatory patients. Encourage patients to return to a heel-toe walking sequence as quickly as possible. When this is achieved, they can discontinue using the heel lift.**

✅ Gentle stretching may be initiated as soon as it can be accomplished without pain. Strengthening may begin as soon as 24 hours after the initial injury. Massage is helpful as an adjunct to a strengthening program.

✅ **Patients should be reassured about the generally benign nature of this injury and the excellent chance for a full recovery. They should also be warned about potentially alarming ecchymosis that may develop in the days following the injury and reassured that this is a benign phenomenon.**

✅ Athletes generally can return to training and competition in 4 to 6 weeks following the injury, although severe tears may take up to 12 weeks to heal. Sports-specific activities can be resumed once the athlete is pain free with full and symmetric range of motion (ROM) and full strength has been regained. Strengthening and stretching should continue for several months to overcome the increased risk for reinjury resulting from the deposition of scar tissue involved in the healing process.

What Not To Do:

(X) Do not bother getting radiographs of the area unless there is a suspected associated bony injury. This is a soft tissue injury that is not generally associated with fractures.

(X) Do not attempt to evaluate Achilles tendon function merely by asking the patient to plantarflex the foot. Achilles tendon function is only isolated with the calf squeeze test.

Discussion

The main function of the gastrocnemius muscle is to plantarflex the ankle. The plantaris muscle is a pencil-sized structure tapering down to a fine tendon that runs beneath the gastrocnemius and soleus muscles to attach to the Achilles tendon or to the medial side of the tubercle of the calcaneus. The function of the muscle is of little importance, and, with rupture of either the muscle or the tendon, the transient disability is due only to the pain of the torn fibers or swelling from the hemorrhage. Most instances of "tennis leg" are now thought to be the result of partial tears of the medial belly of the gastrocnemius muscle or to ruptures of blood vessels within that muscle. Throughout the belly of the muscle, the medial gastrocnemius has several origins of tendinous formation. Most strains or tears occur at this musculotendinous junction. The greater the initial pain and swelling, the longer one can expect the disability to last.

Tendon ruptures typically affect men in their third or fourth decade who are active in sports. The average occurrence of a gastrocnemius muscle tear is in the fourth to sixth decade. A tendon rupture is usually an indicator of intratendinous degenerative changes.

Achilles tendon injury can occur with the identical mechanism of a plantaris tendon or medial gastrocnemius rupture. Because the pain and debility may be similar, clinical differentiation is sometimes difficult.

The diagnosis of Achilles tendon rupture is missed by the initial examiner in up to 25% of patients. One misleading finding is that the patient is able to plantarflex the foot with no resistance, because several other muscles (toe flexors, peroneus) also perform this action. The expected defect in the tendon may also be obscured by edema or hemorrhage. The squeeze test (Thompson or Simmonds test) is usually an infallible sign of complete rupture, but a false negative might arise if the plantaris tendon is left intact. Imaging techniques—including real-time high-resolution ultrasonography and MRI—are now used to aid diagnosis. Ultrasonography usually costs less than MRI; however, when "limited MRI protocols" are available and only a few images of the suspected region of disease are obtained, pricing can be competitive and will give images superior to ultrasonography.

Other entities that can be confused with plantaris tendon and medial gastrocnemius rupture are Baker cyst rupture and deep venous thrombosis. When physical findings are dubious, the history along with Doppler ultrasonography will often help clarify the diagnosis.

Direct injection of steroids and administration of systemic corticosteroids and fluoroquinolone antibiotics are associated with an increase in the risk for Achilles tendon rupture. Other disease processes, such as rheumatoid arthritis, systemic lupus erythematosus, chronic renal failure, hyperuricemia, genetically determined collagen abnormalities, arteriosclerosis, and diabetes mellitus, have been implicated as risk factors for rupture. With age, tendons stiffen from the effects of reduced glycosaminoglycan content and increased collagen concentration. Blood and nutrient supply also are reduced with age.

Suggested Readings

Glazer JL, Hosey RG: Soft-tissue injuries of the lower extremity, *Prim Care* 31:1005–1024, 2004.

Legome E, Pancu D: Future applications for emergency ultrasound, *Emerg Med Clin North Am* 22:817–827, 2004.

Maffulli N, Wong J: Rupture of the Achilles and patellar tendons, *Clin Sports Med* 22:761–776, 2003.

van der Linden PD, Sturkenboom MC, Herings RM, et al: Increased risk of Achilles tendon rupture with quinolone antibacterial use, especially in elderly patients taking oral corticosteroids, *Arch Intern Med* 163:1801–1807, 2003.

Polymyalgia Rheumatica

Presentation

An elderly patient (more commonly female) complains of aching pain and stiffness of the proximal extremities. Shoulder pain and stiffness are most common, followed by the pain and stiffness in the hips, neck, and torso. The onset of symptoms is generally acute, but patients often do not seek professional help for more than a month. The pain and stiffness are characteristically worse in the morning, making it difficult to rise from bed, but improve throughout the day. Approximately one third of patients complain of constitutional "flulike" symptoms, including malaise, fatigue, anorexia, weight loss, and low-grade fever. A patient may ascribe her problem to muscle weakness or joint pains, but physical examination discloses that bilateral symmetric pain and tenderness of neck, shoulder, and hip muscles are the actual source of any "weakness." The patient may demonstrate limited active range of motion of the affected joints, but full passive range of motion and normal strength are typically present. There may be some mild arthritis of several peripheral joints, but the rest of the physical examination is negative, other than the finding of a patient who appears fatigued and uncomfortable.

What To Do:

✓ Perform a complete history and physical examination, particularly of the cervical and lumbar spine and nerve roots (strength, sensation, and deep tendon reflexes in the distal limbs should be intact with polymyalgia rheumatica [PMR]). Confirm the diagnosis of PMR by palpating tender shoulder muscles (perhaps also hips and, less commonly, neck).

✓ **Consider other diseases that can mimic PMR.** These include polymyositis, drug-induced myopathies (e.g., statins), hypothyroid myopathy, systemic lupus erythematosus, rheumatoid arthritis or other arthritides, bacterial endocarditis, fibromyalgia, depression, cervical or lumbar radiculopathies, and various malignancies or paraneoplastic syndromes.

✓ **Confirm the diagnosis by obtaining an erythrocyte sedimentation rate (ESR), which should be in the 40 to 100 mm/hr range.** (An especially high ESR, over 100 mm/hr, suggests more severe autoimmune disease or malignancy.) The classic laboratory finding in PMR is an ESR greater than 40 mm/hr. Elevation of the ESR is the only published laboratory criterion for diagnosing PMR.

✓ Two retrospective studies have found that as many as 20% of patients with PMR may present with a normal or only mildly elevated ESR (≥40 mm/hr). A normal ESR in the setting of a clinical diagnosis of PMR may indicate a milder form of the disease. With such patients, a C-reactive protein (CRP) level may be useful. CRP (normal value <0.5 mg/dL) is also typically elevated in PMR. One study has demonstrated that CRP is more sensitive than ESR in assessing disease activity in a diagnosis of PMR, but this test is not considered part of the published diagnostic criteria for PMR.

✓ **Diagnostic criteria for PMR include age older than 50 years; bilateral aching stiffness of the shoulders, neck, or pelvic girdle for more than 1 month; morning stiffness lasting longer than 1 hour; an ESR greater than 40 mm/hr; and the absence of any other disease— except giant cell arteritis (GCA) (also known as temporal arteritis)**—that may cause similar symptoms, such as polymyositis or rheumatoid arthritis. **An additional criterion: prompt response to daily treatment with at least 20 mg of prednisone.**

✓ **Always check for tenderness over the temporal arteries in patients with PMR to help rule out GCA.** Patients with PMR should be evaluated for clinical signs of GCA, and vice versa. New-onset headache or scalp pain in any patient older than 50 years of age must raise clinical suspicion of GCA. Jaw claudication, generally characterized as fatigue and pain of the muscles of mastication, is one of the most specific signs of GCA. Initial presentation may be of transient visual loss or amaurosis fugax. Diplopia may also be an early manifestation of GCA. Biopsy of the temporal artery remains the standard for diagnosis of GCA and should be performed in any patient with a high suspicion of GCA. Positive biopsy findings typically show granulomatous inflammation of the vessel wall with infiltration of multinucleated giant cells, macrophages, and T cells.

✓ **Corticosteroids are the cornerstone of treatment of PMR. The usual starting dose of prednisone is 10 to 20 mg daily. This is continued for 1 month and is carefully tapered by 1 to 2.5 mg monthly to a dosage of 10 mg daily, based on clinical response.** The dosage may be further tapered by 1 mg every 4 to 6 weeks to a maintenance dose of 5 to 7.5 mg daily.

✓ Failure to achieve a prompt and complete response to corticosteroid therapy should initiate a search by the clinician for a different cause of the symptoms, such as another rheumatic condition or an occult malignancy.

✓ Discontinuation of steroids may be attempted after 6 to 12 months if the ESR has normalized and the patient is symptom free. This is usually accomplished by continuing to taper the dosage by 1 mg every 6 to 8 weeks. Relapses are most common in the first 18 months of therapy.

✓ **The starting dose of glucocorticoids for GCA patients has not been definitively established. The current recommendation is to start these patients on 40 to 60 mg of prednisone daily.** The average GCA patient requires 24 or more months of corticosteroid treatment.

✓ Explain the syndrome to the patient and arrange for follow-up.

What Not To Do:

✗ Do not order diagnostic imaging methods such as MRI or ultrasonography to confirm the diagnosis of PMR. These studies are usually not indicated in the evaluation of PMR.

✗ Do not miss temporal arteritis (GCA), a common component of the PMR syndrome and a clue to the existence of ophthalmic and cerebral arteritis, which can have dire ophthalmologic and neurologic consequences. Palpate the temporal arteries for tenderness, swelling, or induration, and ask about transient visual or neurologic signs.

⊗ **Do not postpone diagnosis or treatment of temporal arteritis pending results of a temporal artery biopsy** showing giant cell arteritis. The lesion typically skips areas, making biopsy an insensitive diagnostic procedure. The progression to permanent visual loss has been found to occur in an average of 8.5 days after the onset of early symptoms (such as blurring, diplopia, or amaurosis fugax), and therefore immediate treatment may be critical. The accuracy of the biopsy will not be affected within a few weeks of initiating corticosteroid treatment.

Discussion

Polymyalgia rheumatica (PMR) is a systemic inflammatory disease that occurs in patients older than 50 years of age and is characterized by an elevated ESR, proximal extremity pain, morning stiffness, and rapid relief with the administration of corticosteroids. Giant cell arteritis, also known as temporal arteritis, is an inflammatory vasculitis of large and medium vessels primarily arising from the aortic arch. It occurs in adults older than 50 years of age and is characterized by headache, jaw claudication, and visual loss.

Many experts consider these two diseases to be points along a continuum of a specific systemic inflammatory disease syndrome, with PMR being the expression of a milder form of disease and GCA suggesting more severe disease. Both conditions are diseases of the elderly population, occurring exclusively in persons older than 50 years of age and peaking in incidence between 70 and 80 years of age. Women are affected twice as often as men, and whites of Northern European descent are most often predisposed to having these diseases. Various mechanisms have been postulated as causes of PMR, but the exact cause is unclear.

The disorder can generally be distinguished from other diseases on the basis of clinical presentation, laboratory evaluation, response to steroid therapy, or diagnostic imaging.

Stiffness, pain, and weakness are common complaints in many older patients, but polymyalgia rheumatica may respond dramatically to treatment. **Rheumatoid arthritis** produces morning stiffness but is usually present in more peripheral joints and without muscle tenderness. **Polymyositis** is usually characterized by increased serum muscle enzymes with a normal ESR and may include a skin rash (dermatomyositis). Often, a therapeutic trial of prednisone helps make the diagnosis. **Giant cell arteritis** can be a serious and, occasionally, fatal illness, with sudden irreversible visual loss, permanent hearing loss, or aortic dissection. Permanent visual loss occurs in approximately 15% of patients with GCA. Larger doses of corticosteroids are required than for polymyalgia rheumatica.

Suggested Readings

Donnelly JA, Torregiani S: Polymyalgia rheumatica and giant cell arteritis, *Clin Fam Pract* 7:225–247, 2005.

Evans JM, Vukov LF, Hunder GG: Polymyalgia rheumatica and giant cell arteritis in emergency department patients, *Ann Emerg Med* 22:1633–1635, 1993.

Radial Head Fracture

Presentation

A patient has fallen on an outstretched hand and has a normal, nonpainful shoulder, wrist, and hand, but, on careful examination, he has pain in the elbow joint. Swelling may be noted over the antecubital fossa, and the patient may be able to fully flex the elbow joint, but there is pain and decreased range of motion on extension, supination, and pronation. Tenderness is greatest on palpation over the radial head. Radiographs may show a fracture of the head of the radius. Often, however, no fracture is visible, and the only radiographic signs are of an elbow effusion or hemarthrosis pushing the posterior fat pad out of the olecranon fossa and the anterior fat pad out of its normal position on the lateral view (Figure 128-1). In all radiographic views, a line down the center of the radius should point to the capitellum of the lateral condyle, ruling out a dislocation.

What To Do:

✓ **Obtain a detailed history of the mechanism of injury and a physical examination, looking for the features described, and, when present, obtain radiographs of the elbow, looking for visible fat pads as well as fracture lines.** The evaluation should include an assessment of neurovascular status and a comparison with the uninjured elbow for baseline motion, strength, and stability. Examine the shoulder and wrist on the affected side to rule out an associated injury.

✓ **Radiographs are unnecessary if the patient can fully extend the elbow with the forearm in supination. It can be assumed that there is no elbow fracture,** and no further treatment is necessary other than reassurance and the possible use of acetaminophen or nonsteroidal anti-inflammatory drugs (NSAIDs).

✓ **For nondisplaced fractures, a sling is all that is necessary.** Refer these patients to an orthopedist within 3 to 5 days for definitive care. The patient should be instructed to not wait longer, because early mobilization is thought to be important for proper healing.

✓ **If there is a displaced or comminuted radial head fracture, immobilize the elbow in 90% of flexion and the forearm in full supination (preventing pronation and supination of the hand) with a gutter splint extending from proximal humerus to hand, and then place in a sling for comfort** (Figure 128-2). These patients should also receive early orthopedic consultation or follow-up, because with displacement of greater than 2 mm or comminution, surgical repair may be recommended.

✓ **Provide adequate analgesia,** especially during the first few days. NSAIDs alone or acetaminophen with hydrocodone (Vicodin) may be appropriate.

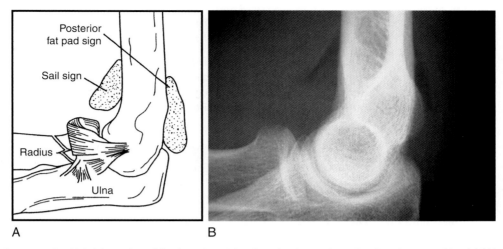

Figure 128-1 A and **B,** Radiologic evidence of elbow hemarthrosis. (Adapted from Raby N, Berman L, de Lacey G: *Accident and emergency radiology.* Philadelphia, 2005, Saunders.)

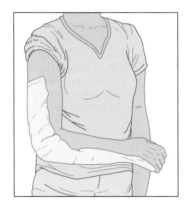 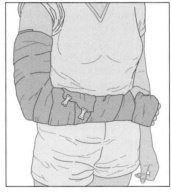

Figure 128-2 Long-arm gutter splint for complex radial head fractures.

✅ **When there is an inability to fully extend the elbow, along with a positive fat pad sign without a visible fracture, explain to the patient the probability of a fracture, despite radiographs that only demonstrate an effusion. Treat it as a nondisplaced fracture (see earlier) and arrange for follow-up.**

✅ **For uncomplicated fractures, range-of-motion exercises should begin within 3 to 7 days** to reduce the risk for developing permanent loss of motion because of elbow joint contractures.

What Not To Do:

❌ Do not obtain radiographs on all patients with minimal symptoms after a minor injury. The elbow extension test, as described earlier, can be used as a sensitive screening test for patients with acute injury to the elbow. Patients who can fully extend the affected elbow can be safely treated without radiography.

497

(X) Do not miss a dislocation of the radial head. Examine all radiographs; a line drawn through the radial head and shaft should always line up with the capitellum.

(X) Do not treat simple radial head fractures (minimal or no displacement without comminuted fragments) with prolonged immobilization. Joint motion is difficult to recover even with extensive physical therapy. Avoiding the problem by providing early mobilization is preferable to attempting to reverse an established joint contracture.

Discussion

The elbow is a hinge (ginglymus) joint between the distal humerus, the proximal ends of the radius and ulna, and the superior radioulnar joint. The lateral capitellum of the distal humerus articulates with the radial head, enabling flexion and extension as well as pronation and supination.

Radial head fractures are the result of trauma, usually from a fall on the outstretched arm. The force of impact is transmitted up the hand through the wrist and forearm to the radial head, which is forced into the capitellum, where it is fractured or deformed.

Small nondisplaced fractures of the radial head may show up on radiographs weeks later or never. Because pronation and supination of the hand are achieved by rotating the radial head on the capitellum of the humerus, very small imperfections in the healing of a radial head fracture that involves the joint may produce enormous impairment of hand function, which may be only partly improved by surgical excision of the radial head. Early orthopedic referral is essential, because treatment is controversial.

Management of complex radial head fractures depends on the severity of the fracture and associated injuries and includes early motion, open reduction and internal fixation with screws and wires, immediate and delayed excision, and the use of a prosthesis.

Most occult or small radial head fractures are treated symptomatically with early range-of-motion exercises and generally heal without functional loss.

Suggested Reading

Anderson SJ: Sports injuries, *Dis Month* 35:110–164, 2005.

Rosenblatt Y, Athwal GS, Faber KJ: Current recommendations for the treatment of radial head fractures, *Orthop Clin North Am* 39:173–185, 2008.

Radial Neuropathy

(Saturday Night Palsy)

Presentation

The patient has injured his upper arm, usually by sleeping with his arm over the back of a chair. He now presents holding the affected hand and wrist with his good hand and reports decreased or absent sensation on the radial and dorsal side of his hand and wrist and inability to extend his wrist (wrist drop), thumb, and finger joints. With the hand supinated (palm up) and the extensors aided by gravity, hand function may appear normal, but when the hand is pronated (palm down), the wrist and hand will drop (Figure 129-1).

What To Do:

✓ When there is a history of significant trauma, look for associated injuries. This sort of nerve injury may be associated with cervical spine fracture, injury to the brachial plexus in the axilla, or fracture of the humerus.

✓ **Document all motor and sensory impairment.** When practical, draw a diagram of the area of decreased sensation, and grade muscle strength of various groups (flexors, extensors, etc.) on a scale of 1 to 5. The triceps reflex should be preserved, but the brachioradialis reflex will be decreased or absent.

✓ Patients with radial palsy often appear to have weakness in addition to radial-innervated muscles. A study of volunteers found decreased strength of handgrip, key pinch, and thumb palmar adduction after radial nerve block. Patients have difficulty spreading the fingers, suggesting weakness of finger abduction, but this is correctable by supporting the fingers or extending the hand when the examiner holds the wrist level with the forearm.

✓ **If there is complete paralysis or complete anesthesia, arrange for early neurologic consultation and treatment. Incomplete lesions may be satisfactorily referred for delayed follow-up evaluation and physical therapy.**

✓ **Construct a splint, extending from proximal forearm to just beyond the metacarpophalangeal joint (leaving the thumb free), which holds the wrist in 90-degree extension** (Figure 129-2). This and a sling will help protect the hand, also preventing edema and distortion of tendons, ligaments, and joint capsules, which can result in loss of hand function after strength returns.

✓ Explain to the patient the nature of his peripheral nerve injury; if minor, recovery may take place over a few hours; if more significant, there may be a slow rate of regeneration (about 1 mm per day or approximately 1 inch per month). Stress the importance of splinting and physical therapy for preservation of the eventual return of function. **Arrange for follow-up.**

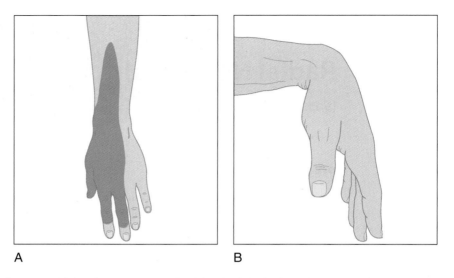

A   B

Figure 129-1 A, Decreased or absent sensation on the radial and dorsal sides of the hand and wrist. **B,** Hand will drop when positioned palm down.

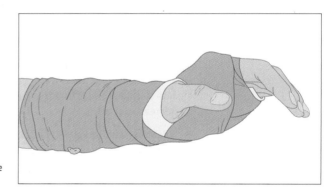

Figure 129-2 Construct a splint that holds the wrist in 90-degree extension.

What Not To Do:

(X) Do not be misled by the patient's ability to extend the interphalangeal joints of the fingers, which may be accomplished by the ulnar-innervated interosseous muscles.

Discussion

Usually, there is no difficulty in establishing the diagnosis of radial palsy. This neuropathy is produced by compression of the radial nerve as it wraps around the humerus at the spiral groove, where its proximity to the bone makes it susceptible to injury. Most commonly, it occurs when a person falls into a deep sleep, either drug-induced or a result of intoxication, and is held up by his arm thrown over the back of a chair or compressed in some other similar fashion. Because depressant drugs and alcohol predispose a person to prolonged sleep in one position (without the movement typical of normal sleep), the weight of the body may exert pressure on the arm for enough time (usually a period of several hours) to produce wallerian degeneration of nerve fibers. Less severe forms may befall the swain who keeps his arm on his date's chair back for an entire double feature, ignoring the growing pain and paresis.

If the injury to the radial nerve is in the forearm, sensation typically is spared, despite the wrist drop. The deficient groups will be the wrist ulnar extensors as well as the metacarpophalangeal extensors. A high radial palsy in the axilla (e.g., from leaning on crutches) will involve all of the radial nerve innervations, including the triceps.

In many circumstances, this condition gives rise to a temporary neuropathy or plexopathy, which generally resolves within hours or days. In most cases, the moderate to severe Saturday night palsy resolves spontaneously and completely over the course of a few months. Pain control, a wrist splint, and passive range-of-motion exercises are usually sufficient treatment.

It should be kept in mind though, that **if the compression is severe and prolonged,** a more grave form of this condition known as "crush syndrome" may occur. Skeletal muscle injury, brought about by protracted immobilization, leads to muscle decay, causing rhabdomyolysis, which may in turn precipitate acute renal failure. This condition is potentially fatal and has an extremely high morbidity.

Suggested Reading

Devitt BM, Baker JF, Ahmed M, et al: Saturday night palsy or Sunday morning hangover? A case report of alcohol-induced Crush Syndrome, *Arch Orthop Trauma Surg* 131:39–43, 2011.

Scaphoid Fracture

Presentation

The patient (usually 14 to 40 years of age) fell on an outstretched hand (FOOSH) with the wrist held rigid and extended and now complains of decreased range of motion and a deep full pain in the wrist, particularly on the dorsal radial side. Physical examination discloses no deformity or ecchymosis but shows pain with motion and palpation and often swelling. Swelling may be seen, especially in the anatomic snuff box, the hollow seen on the radial aspect of the wrist when the thumb is in full extension (between the tendon of the extensor pollicis longus and the tendons of the abductor pollicis longus and extensor pollicis brevis) (Figure 130-1). The pain, which may be mild, is worsened by gripping or squeezing.

What To Do:

✅ For comfort, apply a cold pack and a temporary splint or sling and administer any necessary analgesic.

✅ A thorough history and well-performed physical examination, along with a high index of suspicion, are necessary to make the diagnosis.

✅ **The classic hallmark of anatomic snuff box tenderness on examination is a highly sensitive (90%) indication of scaphoid fracture, but it is nonspecific (specificity, 40%). Other physical examination maneuvers should be performed. Tenderness of the scaphoid tubercle (i.e., extend the patient's wrist with one hand and apply pressure to the tuberosity at the proximal wrist crease with the opposite hand [Figure 130-2]) has a sensitivity of 87% but is more specific than snuff box tenderness (57%). Absence of tenderness with these two maneuvers makes a scaphoid fracture highly unlikely.**

✅ **Pain with the scaphoid compression test (applying a longitudinal axial load to the scaphoid via the proximal phalanx of the thumb through to the first metacarpal [Figure 130-3]) may also be helpful in identifying an underlying scaphoid fracture. Another maneuver that suggests fracture of the scaphoid is pain in the snuff box with pronation of the wrist, followed by ulnar deviation (52% positive predictive value, 100% negative predictive value) (Figure 130-4).**

✅ Be vigilant for associated injuries, such as fractures of the distal radius, lunate, or radial head at the elbow, scapholunate dissociation, or median nerve injury.

✅ **When any clinical suspicion for a scaphoid fracture is raised, obtain radiographs of the wrist that include a scaphoid view (a posteroanterior view in ulnar deviation). Conservative estimates suggest that 10% to 20% of scaphoid fractures are not visible on any view in**

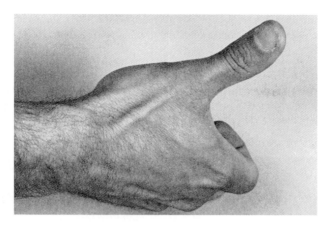

Figure 130-1 Examine for swelling or tenderness within the anatomic snuff box.

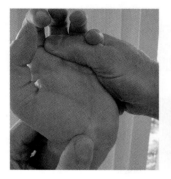

Figure 130-2 Palpating the scaphoid tubercle while extending the wrist.

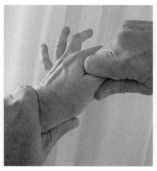

Figure 130-3 The scaphoid compression test.

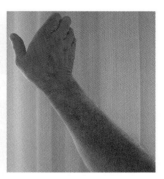

Figure 130-4 Pronation of the wrist, followed by ulnar deviation.

the acute setting (Figure 130-5). An abnormal scaphoid "fat stripe" or "stripe sign" may appear as an outward bulging radiolucent line in the soft tissue adjacent to the scaphoid, representing bleeding within the joint space, and may indicate the presence of an occult fracture.

✅ **When there is scaphoid tenderness or pain elicited by any of the aforementioned diagnostic maneuvers but radiographs are negative, the wrist should still be immobilized in a short-arm thumb-spica splint with the wrist in mild extension and the thumb interphalangeal joint free** (Figure 130-6). Follow-up radiographs at 2 weeks may reveal bone resorption adjacent to a fracture site or early callus formation if an occult fracture was present; otherwise, all splinting can be removed. Arrange for follow-up within 5 to 7 days.

✅ **When occult fractures are suspected in athletes, individuals opposed to wearing a splint for 2 weeks, or workers who require a more urgent diagnosis, a bone scan, CT, or MRI may be considered for additional imaging.** A bone scan may be positive 24 hours after the injury; however, it can take 4 days for abnormal uptake to appear at the fracture site. A normal bone scan 4 days after injury is accurate in excluding scaphoid fracture. MRI is very sensitive and will have an abnormal bone marrow signal 48 hours postfracture; however, it may not clarify fracture displacement. A CT scan gives clearer fracture visualization and is more accurate for determination of displacement.

✅ **When initial radiographs demonstrate a scaphoid fracture, the treatment is dictated by the degree of injury.** For nondisplaced fractures (<1 mm of fracture separation without any visible step-off on any radiographic view), the treatment of choice is a long-arm thumb-spica splint, with follow-up with a hand surgeon or orthopedist arranged for 5 to 7 days after treatment.

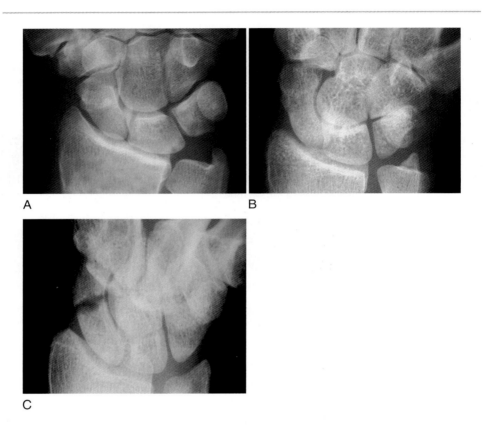

A

B

C

Figure 130-5 A, B, and **C,** Radiograph of the wrist demonstrating a scaphoid fracture—identified (with certainty) on one projection only. (Adapted from Raby N, Berman L, de Lacey G: *Accident and emergency radiology.* Philadelphia, 2005, Saunders.)

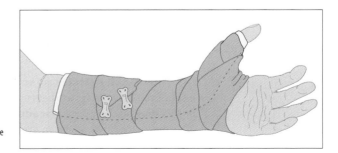

Figure 130-6 Splint or cast the wrist in mild extension, including the thumb but leaving the interphalangeal (IP) joint free.

✓ **For fractures with significant displacement, angulation, or comminution or for fractures involving the proximal pole of the scaphoid, immediate orthopedic or hand surgeon consultation should be made.**

✓ Patients who are placed in a splint should be given standard cast instructions.

✓ It is very important to explain to the patient the common difficulty of visualizing scaphoid fractures on radiographs, the common difficulty in healing of scaphoid fractures because of variable blood supply, and the resultant necessity of keeping this splint or cast in place until reevaluated by a specialist.

✓ **Provide a sling to keep the elbow flexed at 90 degrees, and prescribe acetaminophen or nonsteroidal anti-inflammatory drugs (NSAIDs), adding narcotics when necessary.**

✓ As with any acute injury, have the patient apply ice for 15 to 20 minutes three or four times per day if this provides comfort, and maintain elevation above the level of the heart as much as possible.

What Not To Do:

✗ Do not assume a wrist injury is "just a sprain" when radiographs are negative. Any wrist injury with significant tenderness, pain on range of motion, and swelling should be splinted and referred for further evaluation.

Discussion

Of all the wrist injuries encountered in the emergency department, fracture of the scaphoid is one of the most commonly missed. Radiographic findings can be subtle or even absent. Accurate early diagnosis of scaphoid fracture is critical, however, because the morbidity associated with a missed or delayed diagnosis is significant and can result in long-term pain, loss of mobility, decreased function, and litigation.

The scaphoid bone is unique for two reasons. First, it spans both the proximal and distal carpal row, making an intact scaphoid imperative for carpal stability. Second, the scaphoid relies on an interosseous blood supply that enters distal to its middle third and provides the sole blood supply to its proximal pole. Therefore fractures through the proximal third disrupt the blood supply and are prone to osteonecrosis and nonunion.

The location of the scaphoid fracture (proximal, middle, or distal third) depends mostly on the position of the forearm at the time of the injury. Fracture of the middle third is most common (80%), followed by fractures of the proximal third (15%), fractures of the distal third (4%), and fractures of the distal tubercle (1%).

In general, the more proximal, oblique, or displaced the fracture, the greater the risk of interrupting the blood supply. Distal fractures heal most rapidly, often within 6 weeks. In contrast, proximal fractures, because of the tenuous blood supply, may take 6 months. Nonunion complicates up to 20% to 30% of proximal-third fractures and 10% to 20% of middle-third fractures. Nonunion of distal-third fractures is relatively rare. In addition to nonunion, patients are also at risk for the development of avascular necrosis of the scaphoid. This outcome occurs in approximately 10% of proximal-pole fractures and 5% of middle-third fractures.

Open reduction and internal fixation has now become standard for all proximal-pole fractures and is required for unstable fractures. Also consider surgical referral for any athlete or manual laborer, because many surgeons offer percutaneous screw fixation techniques to these patients to decrease the time of cast immobilization.

Distal radius fractures also occur with FOOSH injuries. The patient presents with pain, swelling, ecchymosis, and tenderness about the wrist. A Colles fracture, the most common distal radius

(continued)

Discussion continued

fracture, is a closed fracture of the distal radial metaphysis in which the hand and wrist are dorsally displaced.

Stable distal radius fractures may be managed in a short-arm splint or short-arm cast. All others should be referred for reduction and fixation. A stable distal radius fracture is extra-articular, without comminution, and with minimal or no displacement. Certainly, fractures must be referred for orthopedic consultation if there is greater than 20 degrees of dorsal tilt, loss of radial inclination (20 to 30 degrees need to be maintained), articular step-off greater than 2 mm, or radial shortening greater than 5 mm.

Stable distal radius fractures in children (e.g., torus or "buckle" fractures, Salter I or II fractures) may be treated with a short-arm cast for 4 to 6 weeks. One study demonstrated that children with buckle fractures had a good or excellent outcome, regardless of whether they were treated with a cast or splint.

Suggested Readings

Breederveld RS, Tuinebreijer WE: Investigation of computed tomographic scan concurrent criterion validity in doubtful scaphoid fracture of the wrist, *J Trauma* 57:851–854, 2004.

Brydie A, Raby N: Early MRI in the management of clinical scaphoid fracture, *Br J Rad* 76:296–300, 2003.

Davidson JS, Brown DJ, Barnes SN, Bruce CE: Simple treatments for torus fractures of the distal radius, *J Bone Joint Surg Br* 83:1731–1735, 2001.

Kaneshiro SA, Failla JM, Tashman S: Scaphoid fracture displacement with forearm rotation in a short-arm thumb spica cast, *J Hand Surg Am* 24:984–991, 1999.

Murphy DG, Eisenhauer MA, Powe J, et al: Can a 4-day bone scan accurately determine the presence or absence of scaphoid fracture? *Ann Emerg Med* 26:434–438, 1995.

Parmelee-Peters K, Eathorne SW: The wrist: common injuries and management, *Prim Care* 32:35–70, 2005.

Perron AD, Brady WJ: Evaluation and management of the high-risk orthopedic emergency, *Emerg Med Clin North Am* 21:159–204, 2003.

Phillips TG, Reibach AM, Slomiany WP: Diagnosis and management of scaphoid fractures, *Am Fam Physician* 70:879–884, 2004.

Plint AC, Perry JJ, Tsang JL: Pediatric wrist buckle fractures: should we just splint and go? *Can J Emerg Med* 6:397–401, 2004.

Stoffelen D, Broos P: Minimally displaced distal radius fractures: do they need plaster treatment? *J Trauma* 44:503–505, 1998.

Waeckerle JF: A prospective study identifying the sensitivity of radiographic findings and the efficacy of clinical findings in carpal navicular fractures, *Ann Emerg Med* 16:733–737, 1987.

Shoulder Dislocation

Presentation

The patient arrives holding one arm with the opposite hand, complaining of severe pain, stating that his "shoulder is out," unable to move it without increasing the pain. Often, the patient had had the arm lifted horizontally to the side ("quarterback position") when it was leveraged posteriorly, causing the dislocation. Recurrent dislocations may be the result of relatively minor forces, such as those produced when reaching into the back seat of a car from the driver's seat or rolling over while asleep.

The deltopectoral groove may show a bulge (caused by the dislocated head of the humerus), and the acromion appears to be prominent laterally, with an emptiness beneath the acromion where the humeral head should be (Figure 131-1).

Ninety percent of shoulder dislocations are anterior, as just described. Most of the others are posterior and are usually caused by a seizure, with patients complaining only of shoulder pain. Inferior dislocations (luxatio erecta) are rare and occur with the arm above the head at the time of injury. The patient presents with the forearm elevated to the level of the forehead and reports, "I can't put my arm down." Neurovascular injury and fracture often accompany these unusual dislocations.

What To Do:

✓ Quickly examine the patient to rule out neurologic or vascular deficits. **Test and record the sensation over the deltoid to establish whether there is an injury to the axillary nerve (approximately 1% incidence).**

✓ **Provide analgesia when necessary;** IV narcotics may be needed.

✓ An alternative is the use of intra-articular lidocaine. After preparing the skin with povidone-iodine, using a 1½-inch, 20-gauge needle, inject 20 mL of 1% lidocaine 2 cm inferiorly and directly lateral to the acromion, in the lateral sulcus left by the absent humeral head.

✓ **Often, analgesics are not needed. If the clinician can gain the patient's trust, apply gentle, stabilizing traction to the patient's affected arm.**

✓ **Reduction should be performed promptly. Obtaining radiographs may be unnecessary and may serve only to delay this procedure. There is no need to obtain radiographs when you feel confident about your clinical diagnosis and there was a relatively atraumatic mechanism of injury (especially when there is a history of a previous shoulder dislocation).**

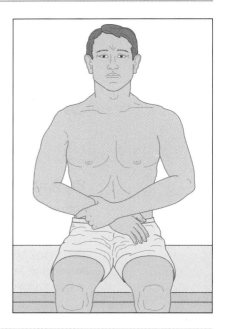

Figure 131-1 Shoulder dislocation with loss of the normal deltoid bulge. (Adapted from Ruiz E, Cicero JJ: *Emergency management of skeletal injuries*. St Louis, 1995, Mosby.)

✅ **Radiographs should be obtained in patients older than 40 years of age and when significant trauma is involved, such as from a fall from a height or a motor vehicle collision.**

✅ Keep in mind that with the exception of proximal humeral fractures, fractures are not contraindications to reduction.

✅ **If the patient is relatively comfortable and cooperative, you can begin reducing the shoulder without first starting an IV for administering analgesics. Muscle spasm is the main obstacle, and gentle and gradual maneuvers are always more likely to be successful than high-force rapid movement techniques, which are more likely to cause complications.**

✅ **Patients who cannot relax because of pain should be given either intra-articular lidocaine or procedural sedation and analgesia (PSA)** (see Appendix E).

✅ Positioning is more important than strength for relocation. Several techniques can be employed successfully. If one does not work, try another.

✅ **With all techniques, gain the patient's confidence by holding the arm securely, asking him to relax. Tell him that there will not be any sudden movements and that if any pain occurs, you will stop and let him get comfortable before starting again. Then, in a very calm and gentle manner, ask the patient to let his muscles go loose so that his shoulder can stretch out "like taffy." This may need to be said repeatedly.**

 ✅ **Using a modified Hennepin technique** with the elbow flexed at 90 degrees, apply steady traction at the distal humerus. Pull inferiorly and, at the same time, externally rotate the forearm very, very slowly. If the patient complains of pain, stop rotating, allow him to relax, and let the shoulder muscles stretch while traction is maintained along the humerus. Resume external rotation when he is comfortable again. Using this method, full external rotation alone will reduce most anterior shoulder dislocations (Figure 131-2, *A*).

✓ If the shoulder joint is not felt or seen to reduce, slowly and gently adduct the humerus while maintaining traction and external rotation until the humerus is against the anterior chest wall, and then very slowly internally rotate the forearm until it meets the anterior chest. Most shoulder dislocations can be reduced comfortably this way, often without the use of any analgesics (Figure 131-2, *B*).

✓ **Scapular rotation** is an alternative technique that can be used when the lateral border of the scapula can be palpated. Reduction is accomplished by scapular manipulation. With the patient sitting up, have an assistant face the patient and gently lift the outstretched wrist of the affected arm until it is horizontal. The assistant then places the palm of his free hand against the midclavicular area of the injured shoulder as counterbalance and then gently but firmly pulls the patient's arm toward himself while applying slight external rotation to the humerus. At the same time, manipulate the scapula by pushing the inferior tip medially and dorsally using both thumbs, while stabilizing the superior aspect of the scapula with the upper hand (Figure 131-3).

✓ This technique can be modified by placing the patient in the prone position with the affected arm hanging dependent over the side of the examination table. Downward traction is applied to the arm with the same slight external rotation of the humerus, and scapular rotation is performed in the same manner as noted earlier.

✓ **The Spaso technique** for reducing anterior shoulder dislocations is simple, requires minimal force, and can be performed by a single clinician. With the patient supine, the clinician grasps the wrist or distal forearm of the affected extremity, very slowly lifts the arm vertically, and, with application of gentle traction, rotates the humerus slightly externally until a "clunk" is felt, indicating a successful reduction.

✓ **The Cunningham technique** is reported to be painless and fast, using only proper positioning and massage to accomplish reduction. Seat the patient comfortably, as upright as possible, with shoulders relaxed. Supporting the affected arm, slowly and gently move the humerus into full adduction. Gently massage the trapezius and deltoids; this helps to relax the patient and reassures that the doctor is not going to do anything painful.

✓ Then, move on to gently massaging the biceps at the midhumeral level. Ask the patient to shrug his shoulders, continuing the biceps massage. Wait for the patient to relax fully, and the humeral head will slip back into place. (Warn the patient that it may feel strange as this happens and not to fight against the movement [Figures 131-4 and 131-5].) If the patient cannot relax enough to cooperate, or the arm cannot be adducted, this approach will not work. Videos and detailed instructions can be found at **www.shoulderdislocation.net**.

✓ **For difficult reductions where PSA is being used,** the traditional traction against countertraction method can be employed. In this method, while the patient lies supine, the clinician grasps the patient's affected arm by the wrist and applies traction at a 45-degree angle of abduction while an assistant provides countertraction by wrapping a sheet around the patient's torso and pulls on it in the opposite direction.

✓ **Reexamine the shoulder after it is reduced.** Neurovascular status should again be rechecked.

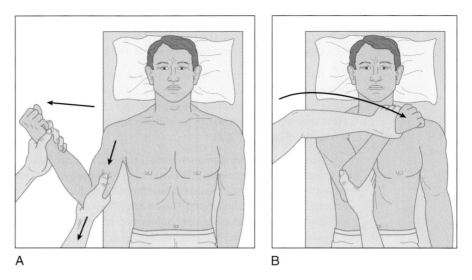

Figure 131-2 A, Slow and gentle external rotation technique. **B,** Slow and gentle adduction followed by gradual internal rotation will reduce the majority of dislocations that do not respond to external rotation alone. (Adapted from Ruiz E, Cicero JJ: *Emergency management of skeletal injuries.* St Louis, 1995, Mosby.)

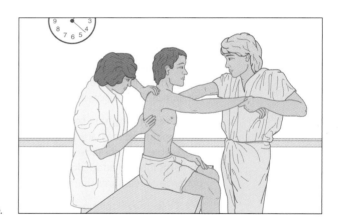

Figure 131-3 Scapular rotation technique.

✅ **Postreduction films are only required if there is uncertainty regarding reduction or if fractures were noted on prereduction radiographs. No studies to date have shown a single postreduction fracture, given the use of more modern, gentler techniques of reduction.**

✅ **When the patient is comfortable and limited range of motion has been restored, secure the reduction in a sling and a swathe around the arm and chest.** (Although this represents standard postreduction treatment, a recent study suggests that no immobilization at all may actually be the treatment of choice.)

✅ Discharge the patient once he is alert, with a prescription for analgesics as needed and an appointment for orthopedic follow-up in 1 week (sooner if any problem).

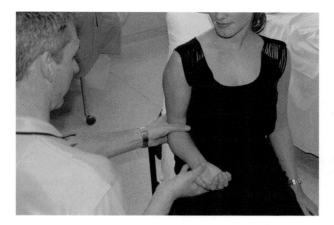

Figure 131-4 Dr. Neil Cunningham demonstrates his technique for reducing shoulder dislocations. Seat the patient comfortably, as upright as possible, with shoulders relaxed. Supporting the affected arm, slowly and gently move the humerus into full adduction. Then gently massage the trapezius and deltoids. (Adapted from Shaw G: Breaking news: believe it or not: painless reduction of dislocated shoulders. *Emerg Med News* 33:1, 28, 2011.)

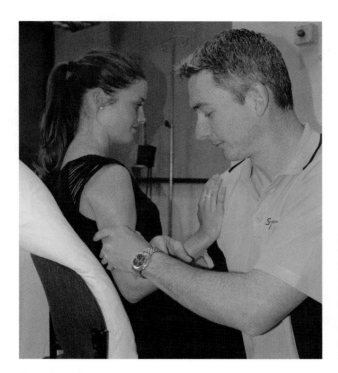

Figure 131-5 In the second part of the technique, Dr. Cunningham demonstrates how to gently massage the biceps at the midhumeral level. The next step is to ask the patient to shrug her shoulders, continuing the biceps massage. Wait for the patient to fully relax, and the humeral head will slip back into place. (Adapted from Shaw G: Breaking news: believe it or not: painless reduction of dislocated shoulders. *Emerg Med News* 33:1, 28, 2011.)

What Not To Do:

⊗ Do not perform any reduction technique using high-force or rapid movements.

⊗ Do not use the forearm as a lever to force reduction and possibly fracture the neck of the humerus.

⊗ Do not redislocate the shoulder by repeating the motions of the mechanism of injury.

Discussion

The shoulder is the most mobile joint in the human body. It allows the upper extremity to rotate up to 180 degrees in three different planes, enabling the arm to perform a versatile range of activities. This mobility comes at a cost: it leaves the shoulder prone to dislocation.

In younger patients, most shoulder dislocations are caused by direct trauma and sports injuries. **In elderly persons, falls are the predominant cause, and the dislocation often is accompanied by a fracture.**

An excessive external rotation or abduction force usually causes anterior dislocations, whereas posterior dislocations usually occur when the humeral head is driven posteriorly with great force and internal rotation, as during a seizure. Posterior dislocations can be subtle and more difficult to diagnose.

The strategy is to relocate the shoulder with minimal damage to the joint capsule and anterior labrum of the glenoid fossa, hoping the patient does not become a chronic dislocator with an unstable shoulder. Chronic dislocators are easier to reduce and come less often to the emergency department, because they learn how to relocate their own shoulders. Of patients whose first shoulder dislocation occurs before 20 years of age, 90% will have a recurrent dislocation. Only 14% of first dislocations after 40 years of age recur.

Posterior dislocations can be reduced using traditional in-line traction on the dislocated arm, along with countertraction using a sheet. Posterior pressure on the humeral head may help.

Inferior dislocations can also be reduced using traction/countertraction, but with scapular rotation as an adjunct.

Numerous studies have shown that early surgical intervention, rather than conservative treatment (especially in the younger athletic population), provides a reduced incidence of recurrent dislocation.

Treatment after reduction traditionally includes immobilization of the shoulder for 4 weeks, followed by rehabilitation. One Australian study suggests that putting the arm in internal rotation (the normal sling position) results in more pronounced labral detachment, inhibiting healing of the underlying injury. Additionally, for patients with anterior shoulder dislocation, sling immobilization (internal rotation) provides no benefit, and positioning in external rotation, using an Ultrasling or similar device, might be more effective.

It might be preferable not to immobilize the shoulder at all, and total immobilization may actually cause worse problems, such as a frozen shoulder, but this remains unproven. After 1 or 2 days, the patient with the uncomplicated shoulder, dislocation should be instructed to start gentle range of motion exercises to help prevent this complication. It should be stressed to the patient that they should not reproduce the position that originally caused the dislocation.

Suggested Readings

Baykal B, Sener S, Turkan H: Scapular manipulation technique for reduction of traumatic anterior shoulder dislocations: experience of an academic emergency department, *Emerg Med J* 22:336–338, 2005.

Burton JH, Bock AJ, Strout TD, et al: Etomidate and midazolam for reduction of anterior shoulder dislocation, *Ann Emerg Med* 40:496–504, 2002.

Garnavos C: Technical note: modifications and improvements of the Milch technique for the reduction of anterior dislocation of the shoulder without premedication, *J Trauma* 32:801–803, 1992.

Hendey GW: Necessity of radiography in the emergency department management of shoulder dislocations, *Ann Emerg Med* 36:108–113, 2000.

Hendey GW, Kinlaw K: Clinically significant abnormalities in postreduction radiographs after anterior shoulder dislocation, *Ann Emerg Med* 28:399–402, 1996.

Kosnick J, Raphael E, Malachias Z, et al: Anesthetic methods for reduction of acute shoulder dislocations: a prospective randomized study comparing intra-articular lidocaine with intravenous analgesia and sedation, *Am J Emerg Med* 17:566–570, 1999.

Matthews DE: Intra-articular lidocaine versus intravenous analgesic for reduction of acute anterior shoulder dislocation: a prospective randomized study, *Am J Sports Med* 23:54–58, 1995.

McNamara RM: Reduction of anterior shoulder dislocation by scapular manipulation, *Ann Emerg Med* 22:1140–1144, 1993.

Miller SL, Cleeman E, Auerbach J, Flatow EL: Comparison of intra-articular lidocaine and intravenous sedation for reduction of shoulder dislocations: a randomized prospective study, *J Bone Joint Surg Am* 84:2135–2139, 2002.

Murrell GAC: Treatment of shoulder dislocation: is a sling appropriate? *Med J Aust* 179:370–371, 2003.

Quillen DM, Wuchner M, Hatch RL: Acute shoulder injuries, *Am Fam Physician* 70:1947–1954, 2004.

Riebel GD, McCabe JB: Anterior shoulder dislocation: a review of reduction techniques, *Am J Emerg Med* 9:180–188, 1991.

Shaw G: Breaking news: believe it or not: painless reduction of dislocated shoulders, *Emerg Med News* 33(1):28, 2011.

Shuster M, Abu-Laban RB, Boyd J, et al: Prospective evaluation of a guideline for the selective elimination of prereduction radiographs in clinically obvious anterior shoulder dislocation, *Can J Emerg Med* 4:257–262, 2002.

Shuster M, Abu-Laban RB, Boyd J: Prereduction radiographs in clinically evident anterior shoulder dislocation, *Am J Emerg Med* 17:653–658, 1999.

Westin CD, Gill EA, Noyes ME, et al: Anterior shoulder dislocation: a simple and rapid method for reduction, *Am J Sports Med* 23:369–371, 1995.

Yuen MC, Yap PG, Chan YT, Tung WK: An easy method to reduce anterior shoulder dislocation: the Spaso technique, *Emerg Med J* 18:370–372, 2001.

Tendinopathy: Tendinosis, Paratenonitis

(Tendinitis)

Presentation

There is pain along an involved tendon, often poorly localized, that worsens with motion, resisted contraction, or passive stretching. A vibratory crepitus may be felt on palpation during tendon movement. Common sites include the posterior heel, the inferior aspect of the patella, the greater tuberosity of the shoulder, the thumb side of the wrist (de Quervain disease, see Chapter 107) and the lateral elbow (tennis elbow, see Chapter 116). There may be a history of repetitive overuse of the tendon or of a single sudden pull. Older patients participating in occasional sports are particularly prone to tendon injuries.

What To Do:

✓ Obtain a history that includes details of pain onset and potential precipitating factors. Include questions about general health that may reveal sources of a secondary tendinopathy, such as psoriasis, a sexually transmitted disease, a puncture wound, gout, or the use of a fluoroquinolone within the past 3 months.

✓ Perform a physical examination that includes inspection and careful palpation while gently putting the tendon through its range of motion (as much as comfort allows). Palpation should reveal focal tenderness that essentially reproduces the patient's pain. At the Achilles tendon, this may be 3 to 5 cm above the calcaneal insertion (classic midportion tendinopathy) or, less commonly, at the insertion (insertional tendinopathy) itself. The tenderness of patellar tendinopathy (jumper's knee) is generally found on the inferior patellar pole of the proximal attachment of the patellar tendon and is best palpated when the knee is in about 30 degrees of flexion and the quadriceps muscle is totally relaxed. Calcific tendinitis in or around the rotator cuff tendons of the shoulder usually exhibits specific tenderness over the greater tuberosity of the proximal humerus. This tendinopathy usually has an abrupt onset of pain and can severely limit shoulder movement secondary to the severe pain. The cardinal signs of lateral and medial elbow tendinopathy are tenderness at the origins of the elbow extensors and flexors, respectively. To help rule out cervical disorders, the neck should be examined carefully in all cases of shoulder and elbow tendinopathy.

✓ **If there is swelling, erythema, fever, puncture of the skin, gonorrhea, or marked pain, you must first rule out infection. Send blood for complete blood count (CBC) and erythrocyte sedimentation rate (ESR) and request consultation. Consider gonococcal tenosynovitis and obtain a sexual history, recognizing that females can often have nonsymptomatic infections. If this is being considered in sexually active women, obtain appropriate cervical cultures** (see Chapter 83).

✓ **Radiographs are usually of little diagnostic value. They may reveal calcifications, osteochondritis, or osteophytes that suggest chronic inflammation but do not necessarily correlate with symptoms.** However, radiographic evidence of calcification within the shoulder, along with the clinical history and physical examination, can help to make the diagnosis of calcific tendinitis. The most common site of calcium deposition is within the supraspinatus tendon.

✓ **In most other cases of tendinopathy, many expert clinicians believe that a confident diagnosis can be made clinically, thus obviating the need for any imaging studies.** In cases in which the history and examination may not be typical, both ultrasonography and magnetic resonance imaging provide additional information that may be helpful. The clinician must bear in mind that there are many cases in which abnormal tendon morphology does not parallel pain when interpreting imaging findings.

✓ **Instruct the patient to avoid the precipitating activity, and prescribe a nonsteroidal anti-inflammatory drug (NSAID) unless it is contraindicated by allergy, bleeding, gastritis, or renal insufficiency.** The role of anti-inflammatory therapy, such as oral NSAIDs or steroids, remains controversial. Although no inflammatory infiltrates have been documented in histologic analyses of tendinopathic samples, **anti-inflammatory medications do help to diminish pain and facilitate rehabilitation in cases of chronic tendinopathy and most certainly have a place in the management of insertional tendinitis and calcific tendinitis of the shoulder. One recent trial suggests that a 7-day treatment course with a once-daily dose of a 100-mg ketoprofen topical patch can provide pain relief without the adverse events associated with systemic delivery of a NSAID.** (Keep in mind that this is more expensive than oral NSAIDs.)

✓ Cryotherapy (ice) has also been shown to be useful to help facilitate therapy in tendinopathy.

✓ **With overuse injuries, occasionally complete rest or cessation of the training that caused the symptoms may be required for a short time to settle severe symptoms. Even splinting with use of a sling or providing crutches may help to prevent or minimize painful motion.**

✓ Because repair and remodelling of collagen fibers are stimulated by loading of the tendon, **only very short courses of complete rest should be prescribed.**

✓ **The AirCast AirHeel (DJO Global, Vista, Calif.) pneumatic compression dressing for the foot and ankle can provide pain relief with Achilles tendinopathy.**

✓ **A patellofemoral brace with a patellar cutout and lateral stabilizer may improve patellar tracking and help in the recovery of jumper's knee.**

✓ More time than expected is required for collagen turnover, repair, and remodelling; therefore **patients and clinicians must understand that these conditions may take months, rather than weeks, to resolve.**

✓ **Appropriate and progressive exercises represent the gold standard for tendon rehabilitation.**

✓ Operative treatment is recommended for patients who do not respond adequately to an extended trial of conservative treatment. Surgery for overuse tendinopathies usually involves excision of fibrotic adhesions and degenerated nodules, or decompression of the tendon by longitudinal tenotomies.

What Not To Do:

❌ Do not inject corticosteroids directly into the tendon or provide repeat steroid injections, which may potentiate infection, lead to tendon atrophy, weaken the tendon, or cause it to rupture. Repeated subfascial or subcutaneous injections can result in atrophy of the skin and subcutaneous tissue and loss of pigmentation. Because overuse tendinosis is not an inflammatory condition, the rationale for using corticosteroids may need reassessment. Corticosteroids, however, provide short-term pain reduction by mechanisms that are poorly understood.

❌ Do not confuse the Haglund deformity (pump bump), a superficial bursitis that forms a bony enlargement of the calcaneus where a low-cut shoe rubs over the heel, with Achilles tendinopathy. This is most often seen in adolescent females and is treated with changes in footwear, shoe padding, or, when necessary, orthotics.

Discussion

Under the light microscope, normal tendon consists of dense, clearly defined, parallel, and slightly wavy collagen bundles. Histopathologic examination of symptomatic Achilles tendons reveals degeneration and disordered arrangement of collagen fibers.

Until recently, if a patient presented with a history of exercise-related pain and tenderness at one of the common sites of tendinopathy (the Achilles, patellar, rotator cuff, or elbow tendons), and if history and examination features suggested that pain was emanating from the tendon, the patient would most likely have been diagnosed as having "tendinitis," an inflammatory condition of the tendon. Most of these conditions are truly tendinoses.

As long ago as 1976, Giancarlo Puddu of Rome examined the Achilles tendons of symptomatic runners and showed that inflammatory cells are absent. Others have shown that the major lesion in chronic Achilles **tendinopathy** "is a degenerative process characterized by a curious absence of inflammatory cells and a poor healing response."

New nomenclature is reflective of the underlying histopathologic changes in patients with overuse tendon disorders and favors use of the term "tendinopathy" as a generic descriptor of clinical conditions. These include **tendinosis** (chronic degeneration), **tendinitis** (acute inflammation of the tendon), **paratenonitis** (inflammation of the outer layer of the tendon [paratenon] alone, whether or not the paratenon is lined by synovium), **tenosynovitis** (inflammation of the synovial tendon sheath), and partial and complete **tendon ruptures** (see Chapter 122).

Tendinosis can be associated with paratenonitis. The majority of overuse tendinopathies in athletes are the result of tendinosis, with collagen degeneration and fiber disorientation, increased mucoid ground substance, and an absence of inflammatory cells.

The etiology of Achilles tendon overuse injuries is multifactorial. Excessive repetitive overload of the tendon is, however, regarded as the main pathologic stimulus that leads to its tendinopathy. Whereas paratenonitis is characterized by **"squeaky" crepitus**, exquisite tenderness, and swelling that does not move with tendon action, chronic Achilles tendinopathy is notable for absence of crepitation and swelling, with focal tender nodules that move as the ankle is dorsiflexed and plantarflexed.

Another cause of posterior heel pain in the setting of overuse injury is **retrocalcaneal bursitis,** in which there is inflammation of the commonly afflicted bursa anterior to the insertion of the Achilles tendon on the calcaneus.

Achilles tendon disorders occur most often in athletes involved in running sports.

Patients suffering from jumper's knee are usually tall athletes.

In children and adolescents, tendons are relatively stronger than the bones into which they insert. Osgood-Schlatter lesions are traction apophysitis of the tibial tubercle. The condition presents as localized tenderness and radiographic fragmentation in athletic adolescents between the ages of 8 to 13 (in girls) and 10 to 15 (in boys). These lesions are typically self-limiting.

Discussion continued

It is thought that calcific tendinitis of the shoulder becomes acutely painful only when the calcium is undergoing resorption. This is one form of tendinopathy for which steroid injection may be beneficial. Gentle exercises with a physical therapist can help maintain range of motion.

Fluoroquinolone-induced tendinopathy can occur weeks to months following completion of a course of these antibiotics. This tendinitis is similar to the overuse injuries described. The Achilles tendon is most frequently affected, but any tendon complaint warrants inquiry regarding recent or distant fluoroquinolone use. Treatment is the same as it is for overuse tendinopathy, but subsequent fluoroquinolone use should be avoided. When any patient has **tenosynovitis of more than one tendon,** consider quinolone tendinopathy as well as gonococcal infection as possible causes.

Suggested Readings

Hurt G, Baker CL: Calcific tendinitis of the shoulder, *Orthop Clin North Am* 34:567–575, 2003.

Khan KM, Cook JL, Kannus P, et al: Time to abandon the "tendinitis" myth, *BMJ* 324:626–627, 2002.

Khan K, Cook J: The painful nonruptured tendon: clinical aspects, *Clin Sports Med* 22:711–725, 2003.

Wilder RP, Sethi S: Overuse injuries: tendinopathies, stress fractures, compartment syndrome, and shin splints, *Clin Sports Med* 23:55–81, vi, 2004.

Toe Fracture

(Broken Toe)

Presentation

The patient has stubbed, hyperflexed, hyperextended, hyperabducted, or dropped a weight on a toe. He presents with pain, swelling, ecchymosis, and decreased range of motion (ROM) or point tenderness. There may or may not be any deformity. Often, after stubbing the toe, there is little discomfort and no deformity, but the toe appears purple, and the patient wants to be sure that the "toe is not broken."

What To Do:

✓ Examine the toe, particularly for lacerations that could become infected, subungual hematoma that may require drainage, prolonged capillary filling time in the injured or other toes that could indicate poor circulation, or decreased sensation in the injured or other toes that could indicate peripheral neuropathy and may interfere with healing. When a fracture exists, most patients have point tenderness at the fracture site or pain with gentle axial loading of the digit (i.e., compressing the distal phalanx toward the foot). Most displaced or angulated fractures and dislocations present with a visible deformity.

✓ **Radiographs often are not essential but may be necessary to provide patient satisfaction and to detect open fractures, angulated fractures, and fractures of the great toe.** They may have little effect on the initial treatment of closed nonangulated lesser toe injuries but may help predict the duration of pain and disability (e.g., fractures entering the joint space or Salter-Harris fractures greater than type I or II).

✓ **Adult patients who are simply worried about their "purple" toe, when there is little or no pain or swelling and there is no angulation, should be encouraged to forgo the unnecessary irradiation of their foot, because the treatment will be essentially the same whether or not a fracture is present. You can still give the autonomy of decision making to the patient by stating, "I'd be glad to order an x-ray if you still want it."**

✓ With or without a radiograph, **a bruise or a stable, nondisplaced fracture of one of the lesser toes should be treated with comfortable footwear,** usually consisting of a semirigid-sole shoe to limit joint movement. They can use whatever footwear provides them with the greatest comfort and protection. Buddy taping (described next) can be offered to the patient if it provides any improvement in comfort; otherwise, it is an unnecessary inconvenience. If helpful, the patient may also take acetaminophen or over-the-counter nonsteroidal anti-inflammatory drugs (NSAIDs), unless contraindicated.

✓ Uncomplicated fractures of the great toe can be managed in the same manner as "turf toe," described in this chapter under the Discussion.

✓ **Displaced or angulated phalangeal fractures must be reduced with linear traction after a digital block** (see Appendix B) **or injection of the fracture hematoma. Angulation can be further corrected by using a finger as a fulcrum to reverse the direction of the distal fragment. The broken toe should fall into its normal position when it is released after reduction.** The nail bed of the fractured toe should lie in the same plane as the nail bed of the corresponding toe on the opposite foot. If it does not, rotational deformity should be suspected and corrected by further manipulation. If any deformity persists, specialty referral is indicated.

 ✓ **Postreduction, splint the broken toe by taping it to an adjacent, nonaffected toe (buddy taping).** Slide one thickness of gauze or Webril cotton pads between the two toes, and, using half-inch tape, bind the toes together. Give the patient additional padding and tape so that he may revise the splinting, and (if there is a fracture) advise him that he will require such immobilization for approximately 1 week, by which time there should be good callus formation around the fracture and less pain with motion. Inform the patient that he must keep the padding dry between his toes while they are taped together or the skin will become macerated and break down. If the toe required reduction, warn him not to separate his toes when replacing the padding.

✓ **Also recommend rest, elevation, and mild analgesic medication. A cane, crutches, or hard-soled shoe that minimizes toe flexion may also provide greater comfort.** Let the patient know that, in many cases, a soft slipper or an old sneaker with the toe cut out may be more comfortable.

✓ If the fracture is not of a phalanx but of the metatarsal, buddy taping is not effective.

✓ Arrange for follow-up if the toe is not much better within 1 week. **Orthopedic or podiatric referral is indicated in patients with circulatory compromise, open fractures, significant soft tissue injury, fracture-dislocations, displaced intra-articular fractures, or fractures of the first toe that are unstable or involve more than 25% of the joint surface.**

✓ **Because of the first toe's role in weight bearing, balance, and pedal motion, fractures of this toe require referral much more often than other toe fractures.** Deformity, decreased range of motion, and degenerative joint disease in this toe can impair a patient's functional ability.

What Not To Do:

✗ Do not tape toes together without padding between them, unless the tape is changed frequently and the skin is dried thoroughly if it becomes wet. (A hair dryer works well.) Friction and wetness will otherwise macerate the interdigital skin.

✗ Do not let the patient overdo ice, which should not be applied directly to skin and should not be used for more than 10 to 20 minutes per hour. It is questionable whether or not cryotherapy provides any benefit, and it should be used only if it reduces discomfort.

✗ Do not overlook the possibility of acute gouty arthritis (severe pain in the first metatarsophalangeal [MTP] joint), which sometimes follows minor trauma after a delay of a few hours (see Chapter 114).

Discussion

The first toe has only two phalanges; the second through the fifth toes generally have three, but the fifth toe sometimes can have only two. Sesamoid bones generally are present within flexor tendons in the first toe. In children, a physis (i.e., cartilaginous growth center) is present in the proximal part of each phalanx.

The same mechanisms that produce toe fractures may cause a ligament sprain, contusion, dislocation, tendon injury, or other soft tissue injury. With a clinically significant injury, radiographs are often required to distinguish these injuries from toe fractures. Tendon injuries are uncommon in closed injuries of the toes.

If there is no toe fracture, the treatment is the same, but the pain, swelling, and ability to walk may improve in 3 days rather than 1 to 2 weeks.

Although patients call the emergency department or clinic wanting to know whether or not their toe may be broken, if there is no deformity, they can usually be managed adequately over the telephone and seen the next day.

Stress fractures can occur in toes. They typically involve the medial base of the proximal phalanx and usually occur in athletes. Stress fractures have a more insidious onset and may not be visible on radiographs for the first 2 to 4 weeks after the injury.

Turf toe is a hyperextension sprain of the first metatarsophalangeal (MTP) joint with resulting subluxation and damage to the joint capsule. Hyperflexion, valgus, and varus stress can also cause MTP injury. Classic signs and symptoms include pain located over the plantar and medial aspect of the first MTP joint with associated swelling and ecchymosis. More severe injuries will exhibit marked swelling, limited range of motion, and an antalgic gait. **Radiographs should be obtained to rule out associated fractures and possible degenerative arthritis.** Treatment should be individualized, depending on the severity of the injury. **Mild sprains respond to supportive care, including elevation, compression, and acetaminophen or NSAIDs. Further hyperextension can be limited with stiff, solid footwear. Moderate sprains require additional immobilization with cast padding, Ace wrap, and use of a stiff cast boot. Early ROM and strengthening exercises should be advanced as symptoms permit. Severe injuries warrant complete immobilization, crutches, and NSAIDs (if tolerated), as well as narcotic analgesics (if needed) and specialist consultation.**

Suggested Readings

Hatch RL, Hacking S: Evaluation and management of toe fractures, *Am Fam Physician* 68:2413–2418, 2003.

Pommering TL, Kluchurosky L, Hall SL: Ankle and foot injuries in pediatric and adult athletes, *Prim Care* 32:133–161, 2005.

Torticollis

(Wryneck)

Presentation

The patient, usually a young or middle-aged adult, complains of neck pain and is unable to turn his head, usually holding it twisted to one side, with involuntary spasm of the neck muscles and the chin pointing to the other side. These symptoms may have developed gradually, after minor turning of the head, after vigorous exercise, or overnight during sleep. Spasm in the occipitalis, sternocleidomastoid, trapezius, splenius cervicis, or levator scapulae may be visible and/or palpable (Figure 134-1).

What To Do:

✅ Ask the patient about precipitating factors, and perform a thorough physical examination, looking for muscle spasm, point tenderness, signs of injury, nerve root compression, masses, or infection. Include a careful nasopharyngeal examination as well as a basic neurologic examination.

✅ When forceful trauma is involved and fracture, dislocation, or subluxation is possible, obtain lateral, anteroposterior, and odontoid radiographic views of the cervical spine. If there are neurologic deficits, a CT scan or MRI may be better to visualize nerve involvement (as well as herniated disk, hematoma, or epidural abscess).

✅ With signs and symptoms of infection (e.g., fever, toxic appearance, lymphadenopathy, tonsillar swelling, trismus, pharyngitis, or dysphagia), especially in the pediatric patient, obtain a contrast-enhanced CT scan and consider obtaining a complete blood count and erythrocyte sedimentation rate (ESR) to help rule out retropharyngeal abscess formation. Arrange for specialty consultation as needed.

✅ **When there is no suspicion of a serious illness or injury, carefully examine the side of the neck in spasm for tender trigger points.** Press your examining finger firmly and deeply into the neck muscles along muscular borders and their origins and insertions, searching for one or two spots approximately the size of your fingertip that cause the patient to wince in pain. **If a localized trigger point is discovered, you may consider treating this as for any other source of myofascial pain and thus inject these areas with 5 to 10 mL of bupivacaine (Marcaine) 0.25% to 0.5%, with or without a corticosteroid** (see Chapter 123). Trigger-point injection can often partially or completely relieve the symptoms of the acute and painful form of torticollis.

✅ **After trigger-point injection or when a trigger point cannot be found (or the patient elects not to have the injection), have the patient apply ice to decrease inflammation and spasm for the first 48 hours; then switch to heat. If not contraindicated, give**

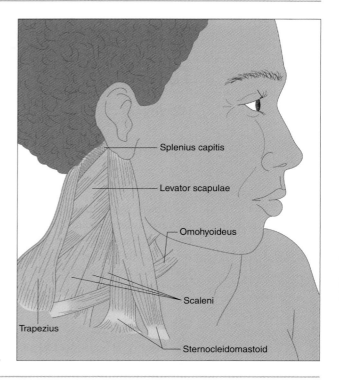

Figure 134-1 Wryneck.

acetaminophen or anti-inflammatory analgesics (e.g., ibuprofen, naproxen) and a muscle relaxant—consider metaxalone (Skelaxin), cyclobenzaprine (Flexeril), or diazepam (Valium).

Alternating heat with ice massages may also be helpful, as well as gentle range-of-motion exercises and friction massage.

A soft cervical collar can be provided if it affords comfort. This should be worn for as short a period as tolerated. Position the wider segment of the collar on the side that produces the greatest comfort for the patient.

Inform the patient that with successful trigger-point injection, there may be mild soreness the next day and complete resolution of discomfort over the next week. Symptoms usually resolve spontaneously within 2 weeks without treatment. If symptoms persist beyond this period, further evaluation is warranted.

What Not To Do:

Do not overlook infectious causes presenting as torticollis, especially the pharyngotonsillitis of young children, which can soften the atlantoaxial ligaments and allow subluxation.

Do not fail to consider the unusual disk herniation or bony subluxation that, on occasion, can present as acute wryneck or torticollis.

Ⓧ Do not undertake violent spinal manipulations in the emergency department, which can make acute torticollis worse and potentially cause other problems.

Ⓧ Do not confuse torticollis with a dystonic drug reaction (see Chapter 1) from phenothiazines or butyrophenones.

Discussion

Torticollis is an involuntary twisting of the neck to one side, secondary to spasm and contraction of the neck muscles. The ear is pulled toward the contracted muscle while the chin is facing in the opposite direction. The term *torticollis* is derived from the Latin words *tortus* ("twisted") and *collum* ("collar" or "neck"). Twisting of the neck may also be accompanied by the elevation of one shoulder up toward the contracted neck muscles.

Although torticollis may signal an underlying disorder, in the acute care setting, it is usually a local musculoskeletal problem—only more frightening and noticeable because of the apparent deformity of the neck—and need not always be worked up comprehensively when it first presents to the clinician.

Torticollis can be a symptom as well as a disease, with a host of underlying disorders. Abnormalities of the cervical spine can range from fracture, subluxation, and osteomyelitis to tumor. Infectious causes include retropharyngeal abscess, cervical adenitis, tonsillitis, and mastoiditis. Head tilting can occur to compensate for an essential head tremor, and idiopathic spasmodic torticollis and cervical dystonia should be suspected when symptoms are prolonged.

Suggested Readings

Cersosimo MG, Koller WC: Movement disorders, *Med Clin North Am* 87:133–161, 2003.

Roberson DW: Pediatric retropharyngeal abscesses, *Clin Pediatr Emerg Med* 5:1413–1422, 2004.

Ulnar Collateral Ligament Tear of the Thumb

(Ski Pole or Gamekeeper's Thumb)

Presentation

The patient fell while holding onto a ski pole, banister, or other fixed object, forcing his thumb radially into abduction and causing pain at the base of thumb. The metacarpophalangeal (MCP) joint of the thumb is swollen and tender and may be ecchymotic. When tested for stability, it may show varying degrees of joint widening toward the radial (or palmar) aspect more than the metacarpophalangeal joint of the other thumb. The patient's power pinch between the thumb and index finger, if possible at all, is less strong than with the other hand (Figure 135-1).

What To Do:

✅ Obtain a history of the mechanism of injury, and examine the thumb, hand, and wrist thoroughly. Tenderness to palpation should be greatest along the ulnar border of the proximal thumb.

✅ **Stress testing of the first metacarpophalangeal joint should be performed while the joint is in 30 degrees of flexion and the thumb is held in full extension.** The patient may not be able to tolerate this part of the examination because of pain, and it can consequently be deferred until specialist follow-up.

✅ A complete ulnar collateral ligament (UCL) tear induces the appearance of a palpable mass in the ulnar aspect of the joint and instability to radial stress, reaching an angle of 30 degrees or higher when compared with the contralateral thumb.

✅ **Obtain radiographs, which may be negative or show a small avulsion fracture of the proximal phalanx at the insertion of the ulnar collateral ligament.**

✅ Treat with ice, elevation, rest, acetaminophen, or anti-inflammatory medications, for comfort.

✅ **A soft dressing with an immobilizing elastic bandage that incorporates the thumb may be adequate for sprains or mild partial tears.**

✅ **A thumb spica provides support to the wrist and thumb for the more significant ligament injuries.** The patient's thumb should be positioned in a comfortable neutral position, and a 2-inch padded splint, which can be molded around the thumb, should be applied (Figures 135-2 and 135-3).

✅ **Explain to the patient with a significant partial or a complete ligament tear that this particular injury may not heal with closed immobilization and sometimes requires operative repair. Complete tears that require surgical repair** should be done 1 to 3 weeks after the injury.

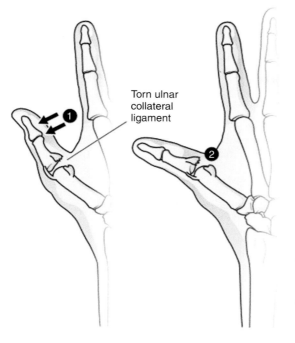

Torn ulnar
collateral
ligament

Figure 135-1 Rupture of the ulnar collateral ligament (gamekeeper's thumb). *1,* This injury is caused by forcible abduction. If unrecognized and untreated, progressive MCP subluxation may occur (*2*) with interference during grasp, causing significant permanent disability. Suspect this injury when there is a complaint of pain in this region. Look for tenderness on the medial side of the MCP joint. (From Roberts JR, Hedges JR: *Clinical procedures in emergency medicine,* ed 5. St Louis, Saunders, 2009. Adapted from McRae R: *Practical fracture treatment.* Edinburgh, 1981, Churchill Livingstone. Reproduced by permission.)

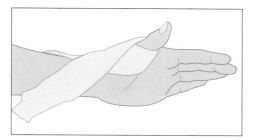

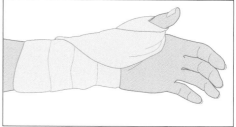

Figure 135-2 Apply the splint in a cross fashion around the dorsum of the thumb incorporating the MCP joint. (Adapted from Hart RG, Kleinert HE, Lyons K: A modified thumb spica splint for thumb injuries in the ED. *Am J Emerg Med* 23:777-781, 2005.)

Figure 135-3 After the thumb and wrist have been positioned comfortably, an elastic bandage can be applied. (Adapted from Hart RG, Kleinert HE, Lyons K: A modified thumb spica splint for thumb injuries in the ED. *Am J Emerg Med* 23:777-781, 2005.)

✓ Arrange for reexamination and hand specialist or orthopedic referral after a few days, when the swelling has decreased.

Discussion

This same lesion was once produced by the repeated breaking of the necks of rabbits by Scottish hunters or gamekeepers—hence the name.

Injury to the UCL is a frequent lesion that occurs from a radially directed force on the abducted thumb. Rupture of the UCL may be total or partial and usually takes place at its phalangeal point of insertion. The rupture of the thumb UCL can be an isolated lesion or can occur in combination with other joint structures, such as the volar plate or dorsal capsule. When the ligament ruptures distally, retraction may be associated with the interposition of the adductor pollicis aponeurosis, with the torn

UCL lying superficially at the proximal end of the aponeurosis. This injury, called a Stener lesion, can inhibit proper healing of the ligament. MRI can detect the torn ligament and reveal displacement, if present.

Nondisplaced UCL tears are usually treated conservatively. Surgical intervention is usually reserved for Stener lesions and complete undisplaced tears with laterolateral instability, because conservative treatment leads to chronic instability and arthrosis.

Avulsion fractures involving more than 20% of the articular surface may require pinning.

Suggested Readings

Cerezal L, Abascal F, Garcíía-Valtuille R, et al: Wrist MR arthrography: how, why, when?, *Radiol Clin North Am* 43:709–731, 2005. viii.

Hart RG, Kleinert HE, Lyons K: A modified thumb spica splint for thumb injuries in the ED, *Am J Emerg Med* 23:777–781, 2005.

PART 10

Soft Tissue Emergencies

■ Philip Buttaravoli ■ Michael Sheeser ■ Kevin Wyne

Bicycle Spoke Injury and Other Crush Injuries

Presentation

A small child, riding on the back of a friend's bicycle, gets her foot caught between the spinning spokes and the frame or fender supports. The skin over the lateral or medial aspect of the foot or ankle is crushed and abraded with underlying soft tissue swelling (Figure 136-1).

What To Do:

✓ Obtain a detailed history, perform a general examination to rule out any possible associated injuries, and then perform a focal examination of the foot and ankle. Note any darkened areas of skin crush, and examine for underlying areas of bony tenderness by applying indirect stress and/or axial loading to the metatarsals and malleoli.

✓ Cleanse the area with a gentle scrub (ShurClens, Betadine).

✓ **Provide any tetanus prophylaxis required** (see Appendix H), and apply a temporary normal saline/povidone-iodine dressing.

✓ **Perform radiographic studies to rule out any fracture. Apply ice to the affected area to reduce pain and swelling while awaiting radiographs.**

✓ **Dress the wound with a nonadherent cover, such as oil emulsion (Adaptic) gauze. Incorporate a bulky compressive dressing consisting of gauze fluffs, knitted cotton roller gauze (Kerlix), and a mildly compressive Ace wrap (or equivalent dressing material).**

✓ Have the patient keep the foot strictly elevated above the level of her heart over the next 24 hours, and then schedule her for a wound check within 48 hours.

✓ **Inform the parents that the crushed skin is not a simple abrasion. There is a greater risk for infection, and any darkened area may not survive.** They should understand that a slow-healing sore might result or skin grafting might be required, and therefore close follow-up is necessary with surgical referral if warranted.

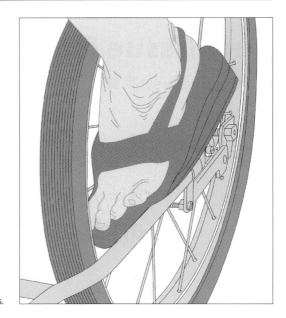

Figure 136-1 Foot caught in bicycle spokes.

✓ Encourage the patient and the parents to wear proper closed-toe footwear when riding a bicycle to minimize the chance of future injuries.

✓ Consider modifications to the bicycle to minimize the chance of injury, including bicycle chain and spoke guards.

✓ Take advantage of time with parents to emphasize the importance of wearing a helmet whenever riding a bicycle.

What Not To Do:

✗ Do not assume that the injury is merely a simple abrasion because the radiographs are negative.

Discussion

Bicycle spoke injuries are similar to but not as serious as historic wringer injuries. Fractures are not commonly associated with these injuries, but often there is severe soft tissue injury. Consequences of a crush injury can be minimized by the use of compression dressings, elevation, and early follow-up.

Suggested Readings

D'Souza LG, Hynes DE, McManus F, et al: The bicycle spoke injury: an avoidable accident? *Foot Ankle Int* 17:170–173, 1996.

Griffiths DM, MacKellar A: Bicycle-spoke and "doubling" injuries, *Med J Aust* 149:618–619, 1988.

Hostetler SG, Schwartz L, Shields BJ, Xiang H, Smith GA: Characteristics of pediatric traumatic amputations treated in hospital emergency departments: United States, 1990-2002, *Pediatrics* 116:e667–e674, 2005.

Roffman M, Moshel M, Mendes DG: Bicycle spoke injuries, *J Trauma* 20:325–326, 1980.

Contusion

(Bruise)

Presentation

The patient has fallen, has been thrown against an object, or has been struck on his or her body. Though the initial pain has subsided, there continues to be point tenderness, swelling, ecchymosis, hematoma, or pain with use. On physical examination, there is minimal or no loss of function of muscles and tendons (beyond mild splinting because of pain), no instability of bones and ligaments, and no crepitus or tenderness produced by remote stress (such as weight bearing or axial compression on the leg or manual flexing of a rib) (Figure 137-1).

Common sites of painful bruising are the shin, iliac crest ("hip pointer"), and anterior thigh (quadriceps). Contusions are often sports related. Patients often seek medical attention for trivial injuries after being struck by an object because of initial severe pain, growing discoloration of the skin, worsening swelling, fear of an underlying fracture, or secondary gain after an altercation.

What To Do:

✓ Take a thorough history to ascertain the mechanism of injury, and perform a complete examination to document structural integrity and intact function. Determine if there is a history of bleeding problems or if the patient is taking any medications that increase the risk for hemorrhage (e.g., aspirin, warfarin).

✓ Document neurovascular status and range of motion of an injured extremity. Examine surrounding areas to identify other possible injuries.

✓ **Ecchymosis and/or swelling out of proportion to the mechanism of injury warrant an investigation of possible bleeding disorders (e.g., hemophilia, idiopathic thrombocytopenia, leukemia) as well as abuse.** Bruises in the shape of an instrument (e.g., belt, extension cord) generally are diagnostic of abuse. Patterned bruises can also be caused by coining and cupping, which are innocent cultural remedies employed by traditional Asian families.

✓ **Suspected domestic, elder, or child abuse should be reported immediately to the appropriate authorities.**

✓ With an extensive muscle contusion, consider looking for secondary rhabdomyolysis.

✓ **Pain out of proportion to the injury of a muscle or severe pain increasing over time within a muscle compartment warrants prompt measurement of the compartment pressure to rule out the ischemic pain of compartment syndrome.** Pain on passive range

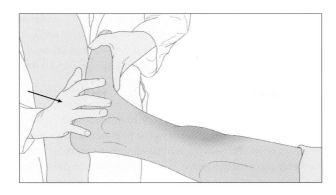

Figure 137-1 Foot percussion provides indirect stress of tibia to rule out fracture.

of motion with stretching of the affected muscle group is the most sensitive finding with acute compartment syndrome. One reliable intracompartmental pressure monitoring device is the Stryker Intra-Compartmental Pressure Monitor System (Stryker Surgical, Kalamazoo, Mich.).

Reserve radiographs for possible foreign bodies and bony injury. Fractures are uncommon after a direct blow but are suggested by pain with remote percussion, stressing of bone (i.e., applying torsion), or an underlying deformity or crepitus. **The yield is very low when radiographs are ordered on the basis of pain and swelling alone.**

Explain to the patient that swelling will peak in 1 day and then resolve gradually. Also inform him that swelling, stiffness, and pain may be reduced by good treatment during the first 1 to 2 days. Continued swelling, especially after a thigh contusion, should be investigated for a possible enlarging hematoma.

Recent controversial data on the use of ice and nonsteroidal anti-inflammatory drugs (NSAIDs) for the treatment of contusions may lead a clinician to assume that there is no proven dogma when it comes to treating this mostly self-limited condition. RICE therapy remains a reasonable and still generally accepted approach to managing contusions.

- *R*est the affected part. Restrict movement to prevent further damage—use an Ace wrap or splint as needed.
- *I*ce (usually an ice bag, wrapped in a towel and applied to site of injury for 10 to 20 minutes every 1 to 3 hours for the first 24 hours). Ice should not be applied directly to the skin.
- *C*ompress, if possible (using an Ace wrap), by adding light pressure to reduce swelling. Compression should not be too tight, because this may cause numbness or increased pain.
- *E*levate the affected part—ideally, above the level of the heart to reduce swelling by allowing fluid to drain from the affected area.

Provide appropriate analgesia. (Acetaminophen with or without hydrocodone may be the best choice; NSAIDs are not likely to cause any problem if used only for the first 2 to 3 days.)

Elderly patients with pretibial hematomas who are on drugs that promote bleeding (e.g., warfarin, aspirin) can develop pressure necrosis of the overlying skin. With surgical consultation, large hematomas should be evacuated. One technique is to perform a hematoma block with lidocaine, after which a sterile Yankauer suction cannula is inserted through a stab incision overlying the hematoma. The hematoma is then evacuated by wall suction, using a to-and-fro movement of the cannula. The cavity is irrigated with normal saline, the incision is left open or repaired with a tape closure, and then a compression dressing is applied to the lower leg. Follow-up should be arranged within 2 days.

✅ **If a significant hematoma is present with a hip pointer** (iliac crest contusion), patients will present with pain over the iliac crest and may have difficulty ambulating and may have a fluctuant mass over the area, resulting from the hematoma. Aspiration of this hematoma can provide some pain relief and help prevent development of myositis ossificans or compression of the lateral femoral cutaneous nerve. This should be accompanied by surgical consultation, radiographs to rule out an iliac fracture, and follow-up. Injection of a long-acting local anesthetic (e.g., bupivacaine) may provide short-term pain relief. Plain radiographs are essential to rule out fracture or apophyseal avulsion in the skeletally immature patient. If left untreated, this condition can lead to periostitis or the formation of bone exostosis. Crutches can be used if weight bearing on the affected leg is painful.

✅ **For a quadriceps contusion,** immediately putting the knee in 120 degrees of flexion tamponades further hemorrhage and limits muscle spasm. This hyperflexion can be maintained by wrapping the knee in this position using 6-inch Ace bandages. A figure-eight pattern will be most effective. Crutches will be required, because the wrapping should be kept in place for 24 hours. Myositis ossificans traumatica (ossification in muscle with fibrosis, causing pain and swelling) occurs in approximately 9% of patients with quadriceps contusions 3 or more months after initial injury. Therefore **large intramuscular hematomas or the inability to passively flex the knee more than 70 to 80 degrees, or both, requires orthopedic consultation to consider surgical evacuation.** MRI has the highest sensitivity and specificity for a suspected soft tissue hematoma.

✅ Other issues that should be considered in the patient with multiple ecchymoses are conditions that result from frequent falls, such as substance abuse and neurologic, metabolic, and infectious abnormalities often seen in the elderly.

✅ **Patients with minor contusions not requiring radiographs can be reassured and informed that you do not want to expose them to any unnecessary radiation.**

✅ Explain to the patient about gravitational migration and possible color changes of ecchymosis. Do this so that when green, purple, or yellow discoloration appears farther down the limb in the days following the injury, the patient is not frightened into thinking that he has another injury or complication.

✅ Arrange for reevaluation and follow-up if there is continued or increasing discomfort or swelling. Large muscular contusions may require physical or occupational therapy until full function has returned.

What Not To Do:

Ⓧ Do not apply an elastic bandage to the middle of a limb, where it may act as a venous tourniquet. Include the entire distal limb in the wrapping if a compression dressing is necessary.

Ⓧ Do not recommend the use of heat. During the first 24 to 48 hours, this may lead to increased hemorrhage and edema. After 48 hours, the literature shows it to be of limited benefit.

⊗ Do not use corticosteroids to help decrease inflammation, because these medications have been associated with unwanted atrophy of both affected and unaffected muscles.

⊗ Do not take for granted that all patients understand what is meant by RICE therapy. Make sure that patients understand the treatment regimen to avoid prolonging or worsening their conditions. For example, prolonged, direct application of ice packs can lead to frostbite-type injuries.

Discussion

Contusions are caused by blunt trauma to the skin and underlying soft tissues, resulting in tissue and cellular damage and bleeding within the various tissue planes. Bruising or ecchymosis consists of visible blood that is infiltrating into the subcutaneous interstitial tissues.

Resultant tissue necrosis and hematoma lead to inflammation. This inflammatory response is often thought to be detrimental; however, some literature indicates a worsened long-term outcome of muscle contusions in patients placed on anti-inflammatory medications. Controversy also surrounds cryotherapy, with some literature touting its benefits and others questioning its usefulness.

The acute therapy of contusions concentrates on reduction of the acute edema; all other components of rehabilitative treatment are postponed until the pain, inflammation, and edema are reduced. Patients need to know this course and must understand that the more the swelling can be reduced, the sooner the injuries can heal, the function can return, and the pain will decrease. Edema of hands and feet is especially slow to resolve, because these structures usually hang in a dependent position and require much modification of activity to rest and elevate. Early mobilization with minor contusions assists in a speedy recovery.

Abuse of children and the elderly is common and must be considered in any patient

presenting with a contusion. Rates of abuse are generally underreported, but are noted to be higher in minority children, especially with risk factors such as young or single parents, unstable family situations, and lower levels of education. Although accidental bruising tends to occur in a predictable distribution (shins, chin, forehead, lower arms, hips), bruising associated with abuse may be clustered and often involves the face, ears, head and neck, trunk, buttocks, and arms. The distribution may suggest defensive injuries (ulnar aspect of arms and lateral aspect of the thighs). Handprints, oval finger marks, belt marks (long, broad bands of ecchymosis that may end in a horseshoe-shaped mark caused by the buckle) or loop marks (from doubled-up wire, rope, or extension cords) should raise suspicion for abuse-related injuries and merit a more detailed evaluation and physical examination. Bite marks (intercanine distance of 2.5 to 3 cm suggests adult teeth) or multiple bruises in various stages of healing also merit more detailed evaluation.

Bear in mind that injuries in domestic violence are usually central and in areas covered by clothing (e.g., chest, breast, abdomen). The face, neck, throat, and genitals are also frequently the site of injury. Defensive injuries are also commonly observed.

Suggested Readings

Beiner JM, Jokl P: Muscle contusion injuries: current treatment options, *J Am Acad Orthop Surg* 9:227–237, 2001.

DeLee JC, Drez D, Miller MD, et al: *DeLee and Drez's orthopaedic sports medicine*, ed 3, Philadelphia, 2009, Saunders Elsevier.

Endom E: *Physical abuse in children: epidemiology and clinical manifestations.* Available at http://www.uptodate.com/online/content/topic.do?topicKey=peds_soc/5402. Accessed December 15, 2011.

Herbenick M, Omori MS, Fenton P: *Contusions: treatment and medication.* Available at http://emedicine.medscape.com/article/88153-treatment. Accessed December 15, 2011.

Jain AM: Emergency department evaluation of child abuse, *Emerg Med Clin North Am* 17:575–593, v, 1999.

Karthikeyan GS, Vadodaria S, Stanley PR, et al: Simple and safe treatment of pretibial haematoma in elderly patients, *Emerg Med J* 21:69–70, 2004.

MacAuley D: Do textbooks agree on their advice on ice? *Clin J Sports Med* 11:67–72, 2001.

Maguire S, Mann MK, Sibert J, Kemp A: Are there patterns of bruising in childhood which are diagnostic or suggestive of abuse? A systematic review, *Arch Dis Child* 90:182–186, 2005.

Fingernail or Toenail Avulsion

Presentation

These injuries may result from a variety of causes: The patient may have had a blow to the nail, such as its being caught in a closing car door; the nail may have been torn away by a fan blade or other piece of machinery; or a long, hard toenail may have been caught on a fixed object and been pulled off of the nail bed. The nail may be completely avulsed, partially held in place by the nail folds, or adhering only to the proximal nail bed (Figures 138-1). On occasion, an exposed nail bed will have a pearly appearance, with minimal bleeding, making it seem as if the nail is still in place when, actually, it has been completely avulsed. See the anatomy of the fingernail in Figure 138-2.

What To Do:

✓ After taking a standard history, examine the finger for sensory and motor function, giving special attention to a possible avulsion of the extensor tendon (see Chapter 108).

✓ **Obtain radiographs if there was any crushing or high-velocity shearing force involved.** Radiographs are otherwise unnecessary.

✓ Complicated crush injuries, especially where there is severe damage or tissue loss of the germinal matrix, require specialty consultation.

✓ **Perform a digital block** (see Appendix B) **to anesthetize the entire nail bed.**

✓ **Cleanse the nail bed with normal saline, and remove any loose cuticular debris. Whenever possible, salvage the nail or any remaining fragment for replacement over the nail bed.** This will provide the most comfortable dressing (with the most accurate anatomic and physiologic match) for the patient.

✓ **If the partially avulsed nail is still tenuously attached, it can be left in place, or, to make it easier to clean, you can remove it** by separating it from the nail fold using a straight hemostat and/or fine scissors. **Cleanse the nail thoroughly** with normal saline, cut away any contaminated portions of the distal free edge of the nail, and remove only loose cuticular debris from the remainder of the nail. **Do not excise any of the proximal nail root.**

✓ If bleeding interferes with inspection and wound management, a finger tourniquet can be applied to provide a bloodless field. If a commercial tourniquet is not available for a finger injury, place a tight surgical glove onto the patient's hand, cut a small opening at the tip of the glove finger, and then roll up the glove finger over the injured digit until it forms a tight band around the base of the finger. Place a hemostat on this tourniquet so that you do not forget to remove it at the end of the procedure.

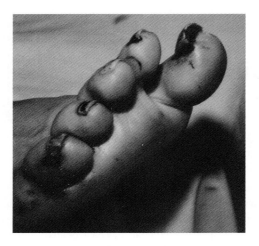

Figure 138-1 Partially avulsed toenail of the great toe.

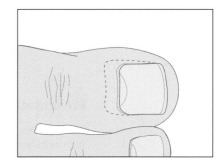

Figure 138-2 Avulsed nail reinserted under the eponychium.

✓ **Reduce any displaced or angulated fractures of the distal phalanx.** If a stable reduction cannot be obtained, consult an orthopedic, hand, or podiatric surgeon for possible pinning.

✓ **Inspect the nail bed for lacerations, and, if large or displaced wounds are present, carefully reapproximate with fine (6-0 or 7-0) absorbable sutures. Small and well-approximated nail bed lacerations need not be primarily repaired** (see Chapter 146).

✓ **Reinsert the nail root under the eponychium** (Figure 138-3), **and apply a fingertip-type dressing** (see Appendix C).

✓ If the nail does not fit tightly under the eponychium, it can be sutured in place at its base (see Chapter 147) or just held in place with a conforming gauze dressing.

✓ **A loose-fitting nail can also be glued in place using cyanoacrylate topical skin adhesive (Dermabond).** Place several drops of tissue adhesive onto a clean, dry nail bed. Insert the clean, dry nail root first under the eponychium. Lower the rest of the nail onto the nail bed and hold it in place using a swab to apply gentle pressure for 1 minute. Apply a simple protective dressing. Do not apply bacitracin or other antibiotic ointment, because this may dissolve the adhesive.

✓ **If the nail is missing, badly damaged, or severely contaminated, replace it with a substitute.** An artificial nail can be cut out of the sterile aluminum foil found in a suture pack or can be cut from a sheet of fine-mesh Vaseline gauze. Cut this substitute nail into the shape and size of the original nail, including the nail root, so that it can completely cover the nail bed, including the germinal matrix. Insert this stent under the eponychium in place of the nail and apply a fingertip dressing after it is in place. The aluminum stent can be secured in place using tissue adhesive as previously described.

✓ **Leave the replaced nail or these stents in place until the underlying nail bed hardens and the original nail or stent separates spontaneously.**

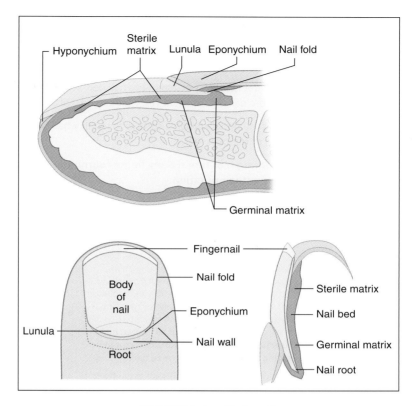

Figure 138-3 Anatomy of the fingernail.

✅ If the wound was contaminated, the tissue crushed, or the patient immunocompromised, it is acceptable to prescribe 3 to 4 days of a first-generation cephalosporin as prophylaxis. However, even fractures of the distal phalanx do not usually require antibiotics.

✅ Provide appropriate tetanus prophylaxis (see Appendix H).

✅ Along with a soft fingertip dressing, a protective fingertip splint can be applied (see Chapter 111).

✅ The patient should be given standard wound instructions, and elevation of the injured digit above the level of the heart should be stressed.

✅ Initially, the dressing should be changed every 3 to 5 days, but the nail (or artificial substitute) should always be left in place.

What Not To Do:

❌ Do not dress an exposed nail bed (where the nail has not been replaced) with an ordinary gauze dressing or any supposedly nonadherent dressing. These dressings will adhere to the nail bed, require lengthy soaks, and usually will cause an extremely painful removal.

(X) Do not ignore wide or displaced nail bed lacerations or fractures of the distal phalanx. The new nail can become deformed or ingrown wherever the bed is not smooth and straight. The best method for preserving the original anatomic alignment of the soft tissues is to replace the avulsed nail back into its original position and hold it there.

(X) Do not débride any portion of the nail bed, sterile matrix, or germinal matrix to help prevent future nail deformity. Severely damaged nail bed tissue will usually survive.

(X) Do not use nonabsorbable sutures to repair a nail bed. These would be extremely difficult and painful to remove.

(X) **Do not forget to remove any finger tourniquet that had been applied. This may result in ischemic autoamputation.**

Discussion

The eponychium is unlikely to scar to the nail bed; however, unless there is infection, inflammation, or considerable tissue damage, separating the eponychium from the nail matrix by reinserting the nail or inserting an artificial stent helps to prevent the development of adhesions and future nail deformities. **Proper alignment of all injured nail bed structures is the most important factor in preventing a subsequent deformed nail.**

Antibiotic prophylaxis for fingertip injuries has been evaluated in several studies, but there is no data that demonstrates any benefit. Before discharge,

patients should be counseled on the importance of monitoring carefully for signs of infection, including worsening pain or redness, purulent drainage, red streaking, and fever.

Minimally traumatized avulsed nails can actually re-adhere and grow normally if carefully replaced in their proper anatomic positions.

A fine mesh Vaseline gauze stent left in the nail sulcus will be pushed out as the new nail grows.

Complete regrowth of an avulsed nail usually requires 4 to 5 months at 1 mm per week.

Suggested Readings

Fiel EL: Management of nail bed lacerations, *Am Fam Physician* 65:1997–1998, 2002.

Strauss EJ, Weil WM, Jordan C, Paksima N: A prospective, randomized, controlled trial of 2-octylcyanoacrylate versus suture repair for nail bed injuries, *J Hand Surg Am* 33:250–253, 2008.

Van Beek AL, Kasson MA, Adson MH, Dale V: Management of acute fingernail injuries, *Hand Clinic* 6:23–35, 1990; discussion 37–38.

Wang QC, Johnson BA: Fingertip injuries, *Am Fam Physician* 63:1961–1966, 2001.

Fingertip Avulsion, Superficial

Presentation

The mechanisms of injury can be diverse: a knife, a meat slicer, a closing door, broken glass, spinning fan blades, or turning gears. Depending on the angle of the amputation, varying degrees of tissue loss will occur from the volar pad or the fingertip.

What To Do:

Determine the exact mechanism of injury and inquire as to the patient's hand dominance, age and skeletal maturity, occupation and hobbies, length of time since the injury, prior hand injuries or surgery, and tetanus immunization status.

Examine the injury to determine whether it is a crush versus a sharp injury, whether there is an associated nail or nail bed injury (see Chapter 146), or whether there is bone involvement.

Obtain a radiograph of any crush injury or an injury caused by a high-speed mechanical instrument, such as a hedge trimmer or lawn mower.

Provide tetanus prophylaxis when indicated (see Appendix H).

Wounds that are infected; associated with tendon injuries; associated with fractures (other than tuft fractures); show exposed bone, accompanied by digit dislocations; as well as wounds greater than 1 cm with absent, destroyed, or heavily contaminated tissue, require specialty consultation with a hand surgeon.

With larger wounds that do not require specialty consultation, **perform a digital block to obtain complete anesthesia** (see Appendix B).

Thoroughly débride and irrigate the wound. Uncontaminated wounds secondary to sharp amputations require only a gentle cleansing with saline or an equivalent agent.

When active bleeding is present, provide a bloodless field by wrapping the finger from the tip proximally with a Penrose drain. Secure the proximal portion of this wrap with a hemostat and unwrap the tip of the finger. Alternatively, cut the tip off a small-sized surgical glove finger; place the glove over the hand, then roll the cut end down over the injured finger, forming a constricting band. A commercial digital tourniquet (Turnicot) may also be used.

For wounds with less than 1 sq cm of full-thickness tissue loss, you may allow the injury to granulate. A small patch of hemostatic gauze (Surgicel, ActCel, GuardaCare) or foam (Gelfoam) can be applied (following thorough irrigation) to reduce further bleeding. A simple nonadherent dressing (see Appendix C) **with some gentle compression can then be applied.**

✅ **If there is greater than 1 sq cm of full-thickness skin loss and there is no exposed bone, there are three options** that may be followed after surgical consultation.

○ Simply apply the same nonadherent dressing used for a smaller wound. (Use the hemostatic gauze or foam only at the discretion of the hand surgeon.)

○ If the avulsed piece of tissue is available and is not severely crushed or contaminated, convert it into a modified full-thickness graft and suture it in place. Any adherent fat and as much cornified epithelium as possible must be cut and scraped away using a scalpel blade. This will produce a thinner, more pliable graft that will have much less tendency to lift off its underlying granulation bed as the cornified epithelium dries and contracts. Leaving long ends on the sutures will allow a compressive pad of an overlying moistened cotton bolus to be tied on and will help prevent fluid accumulation under the graft (Figure 139-1). A simple fingertip compression dressing (e.g., Tubegauze) can serve the same purpose.

○ When there is a large area of tissue loss that has been thoroughly cleaned and débrided, and the avulsed portion has been lost or destroyed and there is no exposed bone, consider a thin split-thickness skin graft on the site. This option should only be pursued after consultation with a hand specialist. Using buffered 1% lidocaine (Xylocaine) containing 1:100,000 epinephrine, raise an intradermal wheal on the volar aspect of the patient's wrist or hypothenar eminence until it is the size of a quarter. Then, using a No. 10 scalpel blade, slice off a very thin graft from this site. Apply the graft in the same manner as the full-thickness one (described earlier) with a compression dressing.

✅ **In infants and young children (younger than 2 years), fingertip amputations can be sutured back on in their entirety as a composite graft (i.e., containing more than one type of tissue). If the amputated tissue is contaminated or not available, the wound can usually be dressed and allowed to granulate.**

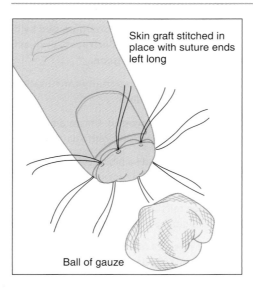
Skin graft stitched in place with suture ends left long

Ball of gauze

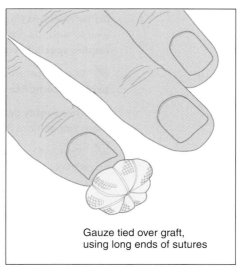
Gauze tied over graft, using long ends of sutures

Figure 139-1 Simple fingertip compression dressing.

✓ In older children and adults, composite grafts will usually fail, and therefore it is important to consult your hand surgeon before any repair is attempted.

✓ **When the loss of soft tissue has been sufficient to expose bone,** simple grafting will be unsuccessful, and surgical consultation is required.

✓ **Schedule a wound check in 2 days.** During that time, the patient should be instructed to keep his finger elevated to the level of his heart or above, and maintained at rest.

✓ **Apply a protective aluminum splint for comfort** (see Chapter 111).

✓ Unless the bandage gets wet, a dressing change need not be done for 5 to 7 days, at which time the cotton bolster dressing can be removed and active range of motion begun.

✓ **Always have the patient return immediately if there is increasing pain, purulent drainage, red streaking extending from wound, or other signs of infection**.

✓ If the wound is contaminated, a 3- to 5-day course of an antibiotic, such as cephalexin (Keflex), 500 mg qid, may be effective prophylaxis, but antibiotics are not routinely required, even for an uncomplicated, open phalanx-tip fracture.

✓ Recommend an analgesic, such as acetaminophen, and, if needed, prescribe a narcotic, such as hydrocodone with acetaminophen (Lorcet, Vicodin), 5 to 10 mg q4h prn for pain.

What Not To Do:

✗ Do not apply a graft directly over bone or over a potentially devitalized or contaminated bed.

✗ Do not attempt to stop wound bleeding by cautery or ligature, measures that are likely to increase tissue damage and are probably unnecessary.

✗ **Do not forget to remove any constricting tourniquet used to obtain a bloodless field. This may lead to ischemic autoamputation.**

Discussion

The fingertip, the most distal portion of the hand, is the most susceptible to injury and thus the most often injured part. Treating small- and medium-sized fingertip amputations without grafting is appropriate in most cases. Allowing repair by wound contracture may leave the patient with as good a result and likely better sensation, without the discomfort or minor disfigurement of a split-thickness graft. This open technique is not recommended for wounds greater than 1 cm, because healing time will exceed 3 to 4 weeks, and it will significantly delay return to work. A potential complication of this technique includes loss of volume and fingertip pulp.

Skin grafting may allow the patient more use of his or her finger and less sensitivity at the injury site. This technique should only be undertaken by experienced providers after discussion with a hand specialist. The full-thickness graft will give an early tough cover that is insensitive but is more durable and has a more normal appearance. Unlike the full-thickness graft, a thin split-thickness graft will allow wound contracture and thereby allow skin with normal sensitivity to be drawn over the end of the finger, resulting in a smaller defect.

The nature of the wound, the preferences of the follow-up physician, and the special occupational and emotional needs of the patient should determine the technique followed. Explain the options to the patient, who can help decide the course of action.

Suggested Reading

Saladino R, Antevy P: *Management of fingertip injuries*. [*UpToDate* website]. Available at http://www.uptodate.com. Accessed August, 2011.

Fishhook Removal

Presentation

The patient has been snagged with a fishhook and arrives with it embedded in the skin (Figure 140-1). This most commonly occurs on the hand, face, scalp, or upper extremity but can involve any body part. Structures deep to the skin and subcutaneous tissue are usually not involved.

What To Do:

⊘ Inquire about or examine to see the type of hook involved. Is it a single or treble (multiple) hook, and does it have a single barb or multiple barbs (Figure 140-2)?

⊘ All items attached to the hook (i.e., fishing line, bait, and the body of any lure) should be removed.

⊘ Radiographs are generally not required or helpful but may aid in determining the type of fishhook and depth of penetration in difficult cases or if patient is unsure of the type of hook.

⊘ Any fishhook injury that may involve deeper structures, such as bone tendons, vessels, nerves, or joints, may benefit from a specialist consultation.

⊘ Patients with fishhooks that are imbedded in the eye or in a location in which removal may injure the eye should have the eye covered with a protective metal shield. With an eye injury, an ophthalmologist should be immediately consulted.

⊘ **For uncomplicated cases, cleanse the hook and wound with povidone-iodine or another antiseptic solution.**

⊘ Provide tetanus prophylaxis as needed (see Appendix H).

⊘ **Most patients will benefit from slowly administered local infiltration of 1% buffered lidocaine using a 27-gauge needle inserted through the same puncture created by the fishhook.**

⊘ After local anesthesia, children can usually be successfully treated by using verbal distraction and hiding the procedure from their view. When cooperation cannot be obtained, consider procedural sedation and analgesia (see Appendix E).

 ⊘ **Fishhooks with more than one point (e.g., treble fishhooks) should have the uninvolved points taped or cut off to avoid embedding these during removal. If more than one point of a treble hook is embedded in the skin, use an orthopedic pin cutter to snap** the shaft of the treble hook, thereby separating it into multiple single hooks. The following standard techniques can then be used.

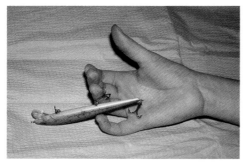

Figure 140-1 Fishhook impalement.

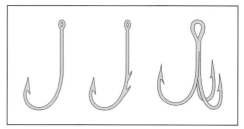

Figure 140-2 Examples of various hooks and barbs.

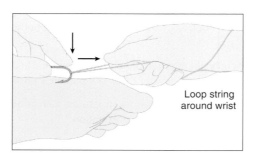

Loop string
around wrist

Figure 140-3 "String" technique.

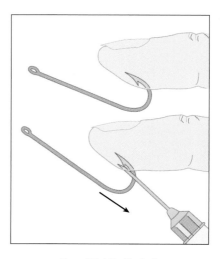

Figure 140-4 Needling hook.

 For hooks lodged superficially, first try the simple "retrograde" technique. Push the hook back along the entrance pathway while applying gentle downward pressure on the shank (like the "string" technique, without the string) (Figure 140-3).

If the hook does not come out, an 18-gauge needle may be inserted into the puncture hole and used as a miniature scalpel blade. A No. 11 scalpel blade can then be used to slightly enlarge the puncture wound for easier removal, if needed. Manipulate the hook into such a position that you can cut the bands of connective tissue caught over the barb and release it.

 For more deeply embedded hooks, "needling" the hook is an alternative technique that requires somewhat greater skill but allows work on an unstable skin surface, such as a finger or ear (Figure 140-4). Slide a large-gauge (No. 20 or 18) hypodermic needle through the puncture wound alongside the hook. Now blindly slide the needle opening over the barb of the hook and, holding the hook firmly, lock the two together. With the barb covered, remove the hook and needle as one unit. Because the needle does not cut through the dermis, there is often

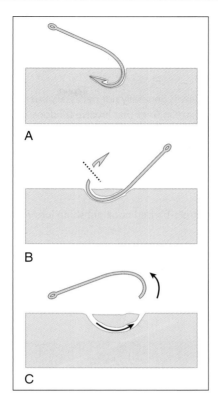

Figure 140-5 Advance and cut method: single-barbed fishhook.

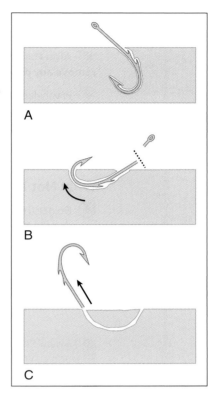

Figure 140-6 Advance and cut method: multiple-barbed fishhook.

no need for local anesthesia, although when available, most patients still appreciate getting it. **When anesthesia is used, this technique can be made easier by slightly enlarging the entrance wound with a No. 11 scalpel blade.**

 ✅ **When a single hook is embedded in a stable skin surface, such as the back, scalp, or arm, the best way to remove it is by using a simple "string" or "string-yank" technique** (see Figure 140-3). Align the shaft of the hook so that it is parallel to the skin surface. Press down on the hook with the index finger to disengage the barb. Place a loop of string (fishing line or 1-0 silk) over the wrist and around the hook, and with a quick jerk opposite from the direction in which the shaft of the hook is running, pop the hook out. When done properly, this procedure is painless and does not require anesthesia. The hook may shoot out in the direction that the string is being pulled; so, be careful that no one is standing in the path of the fishhook, and use protective eyewear.

✅ **When the hook is deeply embedded, the barbed end of the hook is protruding through the skin, or the previous techniques cannot be used, proceed with the "push through" maneuver.** Locally infiltrate the area with 1% buffered lidocaine. Then, using pliers or a needle holder, push the point of the hook along with its barb up through the skin. **When dealing with a single-barbed hook, use an orthopedic pin cutter or metal snip to cut off the tip of the hook and remove the shaft** (Figure 140-5); **with a multiple-barbed hook, cut off the shaft of the hook and pull the tip through** (Figure 140-6). To help push the tip of the hook up through the skin when the skin is tenting, you can place the open end of a 3- or 5-mL syringe barrel (with the plunger removed) over the tenting skin to provide downward countertraction.

✓ **After the hook is removed, cleanse the wound with povidone-iodine solution and remove any debris (e.g., bait).**

✓ Prophylactic antibiotic therapy is generally not necessary but may be considered for persons who are immunosuppressed or have injuries that involve tendons, cartilage, joints, or bone.

✓ Provide follow-up in 2 days for high-risk patients. Provide immediate follow-up care for any patient who develops signs or symptoms of infection (rare).

What Not To Do:

✗ Do not try to remove a multiple-barbed hook or fishing lure without first removing or covering the free hooks.

✗ Do not attempt to use the "string" technique if the hook is near the patient's eye.

✗ Do not routinely prescribe prophylactic antibiotics. Even hooks that have been contaminated by fish rarely cause secondary infection.

Discussion

In places with crowded fishing conditions, and especially in areas where fly fishing is popular, fishhook injuries are not uncommon because of the volume of anglers.

Most embedded fishhooks can be removed with minimal surgical intervention. In general, the retrograde and string-yank methods should be the first techniques attempted, because they result in the least amount of tissue trauma. The more invasive procedures, such as the advance and cut techniques, usually are reserved for more difficult cases. Sometimes multiple techniques must be attempted before the fishhook is successfully removed.

With the string, retrograde, and needling techniques, there is no lengthening of the puncture track or creation of an additional puncture wound. The quickest and easiest method for removing a fishhook is the string technique. Use it in the field with no special equipment or anesthesia. It is not recommended, however, when the hook is positioned on a skin surface that is likely to move when the string is pulled. The skin movement may cause the vector forces to change, and therefore the barb may not release.

Suggested Readings

Bothner J: *Fish-hook removal techniques.* [*UptoDate* website]. Available at http://www.uptodate.com. Accessed August, 2011.

Gammons M, Jackson E: Fishhook removal, *Am Fam Physician* 63:2231–2237, 2001.

Foreign Body Beneath Nail

Presentation

The patient complains of a paint chip or wooden sliver under the nail. There may be only mild discomfort, but frequently there is severe throbbing pain. Most subungual foreign bodies are completely visible and are lodged under the distal portion of the nail. Occasionally, a wooden sliver will be large and deeply embedded over the proximal germinal matrix.

Often the patient has unsuccessfully attempted to remove the foreign body, which has broken off and could not be grabbed using household tweezers.

What To Do:

Paint Chip

- ○ **Without anesthesia, remove the overlying nail by shaving it with a No. 15 scalpel blade** (Figure 141-1). This is done by using light strokes in a proximal to distal direction. This technique gradually creates a U-shaped defect in the nail, exposing most of the paint chip and releasing it from beneath the nail.
- ○ Cleanse remaining debris with normal saline, and trim the nail edges smooth with scissors.
- ○ Provide tetanus prophylaxis if necessary (see Appendix H), and then dress the area with antibiotic ointment and a bandage strip.

Sliver

- ○ **For small slivers, it may be possible to take a 23- or 25-gauge needle and push it into the exposed end of the splinter, angling the needle up toward the distal nail plate. Then, when the needle is firmly lodged in the splinter (while maintaining the same angle), the sliver can be pulled out by using the needle tip for traction** (Figure 141-2).
- ○ **When presented with a large or friable splinter, a more extensive excision of an overlying nail wedge is required.** Therefore you will need to perform a digital block (see Appendix B).
- ○ **Slide a small (but strong) straight iris scissors between the nail and nail bed on both sides of the sliver and cut out the overlying V-shaped wedge of nail** (Figure 141-3). The point of the V should be at or near the proximal tip of the splinter. The wedge of nail plate will fall away, and the exposed sliver can be easily picked away.

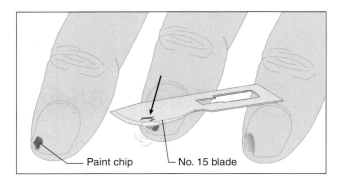

Figure 141-1 Paint chip removal. This technique creates a U-shaped defect that releases the paint chip foreign body.

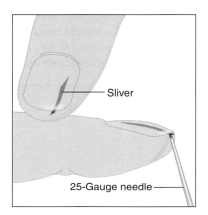

Figure 141-2 Sliver removal. Angle the tip of the scissors blade up into the nail plate, not down and into the nail bed.

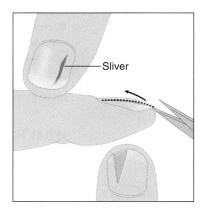

Figure 141-3 Sliver removal. Push a 23- or 25-gauge needle into the exposed end of the splinter, angling the needle up toward the distal nail plate. Then, when the needle is firmly lodged in the splinter (while maintaining the same angle), the sliver can then be pulled out by using the needle tip for traction.

○ **Cleanse any remaining debris with normal saline, and trim the fingernail until the corners are smooth.**

○ Provide tetanus prophylaxis (see Appendix H) if needed.

○ Dress with antibiotic ointment and a bandage. Have the patient redress the area two to three times daily until healed and keep the fingernail trimmed close.

What Not To Do:

❌ Do not run the tip of the scissors into the nail bed while sliding it under the fingernail (instead angle the tip up into the undersurface of the nail). Damage to the germinal matrix could potentially lead to a permanent nail plate deformity.

❌ Do not routinely prescribe antibiotics. When the foreign body has been removed, there is little risk for infection.

Discussion

It is usually not possible to remove a long sliver from beneath the fingernail using the "shaving" technique with a scalpel blade without injuring the surrounding proximal nail bed and causing the patient considerable discomfort.

After providing a digital block, it is sometimes possible to remove the sliver by surrounding it with the tips of a hemostat that have been slipped between the nail and nail bed. Then, by grasping it, the entire sliver can be withdrawn. If any significant debris remains visible, however, the overlying nail wedge probably should be removed to help prevent a nail bed infection.

Very small and minimally painful subungual foreign bodies, particularly the ones composed of nonreactive materials, may not need to be removed at all and can be managed conservatively. Some clinicians will only provide analgesics and allow uninfected slivers to grow out with the nail. The sliver can be removed more easily in 10 to 14 days. These patients should be informed of the possible increased risk for infection, and they require easy access to follow-up care with any increased pain or swelling or subungual purulence.

A large foreign body made of reactive material, or one that results in significant discomfort, should always be promptly and completely removed.

Suggested Readings

Chan C, Salam GA: Splinter removal, *Am Fam Physician* 67:2557–2562, 2003.

Kaye R: Subungual slivers may be treated conservatively (letter), *Am Fam Physician* 69:2525, 2004.

Salam GA: Removing splinters should be a very simple procedure (letter), *Am Fam Physician* 69:2525, 2004.

Impalement Injuries, Minor

Presentation

A sharp metal object, such as a needle, heavy wire, nail, or fork, is driven into or through a patient's extremity. In some instances, often because prehospital care providers have been trained to leave impaled objects in place, the patient may arrive with an additional large object attached; for instance, a child who has stepped on a nail going through a board (Figure 142-1). As minor as most of these injuries are, they tend to create a spectacle and draw a crowd; this is especially true when the impaled objects are two TASER darts lodged in a handcuffed prisoner.

What To Do:

✓ **If the patient arrives with an impaled object attached to something that is acting like a lever and causing pain with any movement, either quickly cut off this lever or, when the object is known to be smooth and straight, immediately pull the patient's extremity off the sharp object. (An exposed nail or metal spike can usually be cut with an orthopedic pin cutter** [Figure 142-2].)

✓ **Obtain radiographs when pain and further damage from a leveraged object are not problems and when there is suspicion of an underlying fracture (as might occur with a nail gun) or fragmentation or hooking of the impaled object (as might occur with a heavy wire that has been thrown from under a lawnmower).** When radiographs are necessary in the face of a painful mobile impaled object, fully immobilize and secure the object before moving the patient, thereby preventing further pain or injury. Administer analgesics as appropriate for pain, especially for pain anticipated during evaluation of the object during radiography.

✓ **It is not necessary to radiograph a penetrating nail, fork, or other nonmalleable, nonfragile object that will remain intact under the skin and is easily removed, regardless of its radiographic appearance.** Radiographs offer little useful information regarding joint or tendon involvement, nor do they, in most instances, give any additional information that is not evident on clinical examination. If a puncture-type fracture is suspected, a radiograph will be more revealing if it is taken after the foreign body has been removed.

✓ Examine the extremity for possible neurovascular or tendon injury.

✓ Cleanse the object and puncture wounds with a povidone-iodine solution or equivalent antiseptic.

 ✓ **Rapid removal using sudden forceful traction on firmly embedded smooth, straight objects (e.g., fork, nail, or letter spike) is generally the most appropriate method for taking out these objects.**

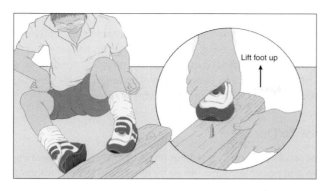

Figure 142-1 Foot stuck to nail with rapid removal.

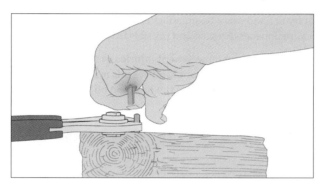

Figure 142-2 Cut an exposed nail with an orthopedic pin cutter.

✓ **If surgical débridement is anticipated after removal of the object, infiltration of an anesthetic should be provided before removal.** Otherwise, patient preference should determine whether or not a local anesthetic is used. Local anesthesia will usually not give complete pain relief when a deeply embedded object is removed; inform the patient of this.

✓ Contaminated objects that track superficially under the dermis may be released using the same techniques described in Chapter 153.

✓ **Objects with small barbs, such as crochet needles, fish spines, and TASER darts, can be removed by first anesthetizing the area and then applying firm traction until the barb is revealed through the puncture wound. The fibrils of connective tissue caught over the barb can then be cut with a No. 11 scalpel blade or fine scissors. To provide better exposure, the entrance wound can be enlarged using the No. 11 blade.**

✓ Most prehospital care services have protocols for removing low-risk TASER darts in the field, because the longest No. 9 barb is less than ¼ inch in length. Use caution and appropriate consultation, however, when confronted with TASER darts lodged in the eye, ear, mouth, neck, groin/perineum, and female breast, and with any injury associated with apparent vascular or neurologic injury.

✓ **After removal of the impaled object, the wound should be appropriately débrided and irrigated as described for puncture wounds** (see Chapter 151). Tetanus prophylaxis should be provided (see Appendix H), and, except for contaminated wounds, such as a fish spine, prophylactic antibiotics should not routinely be prescribed. The decision to use antimicrobials should be individualized for each patient based on his general health and the nature of the impaled object (e.g., clean vs. grossly contaminated) as well as the location of the injury (e.g., deep vs. superficial, possible joint or tendon involvement, and highly contaminated punctures of the foot). A 3- to 5-day course of an antibiotic effective against *Staphylococcus* and *Streptococcus* species should be provided when appropriate.

What Not To Do:

(X) Do not send a patient for a radiograph with a leveraged object impaled, thus creating further pain and possible injury with every movement. When radiographs are necessary, fully immobilize these objects.

(X) Do not try to hand saw a board attached to an impaled object. The resultant movement will obviously cause unnecessary pain and possibly harm.

(X) **Do not confuse minor impalement injuries of the distal extremities with major impalement injuries where major blood vessels may be involved. Patients can rapidly exsanguinate from these wounds if the impaled object is removed prematurely.**

Discussion

Simple impalement injuries of the distal extremities should not be confused with major impalement injuries of the neck and trunk, groin, or buttock, from which the foreign object should not be precipitously removed. With major impalement injuries, careful localization with radiographs is required, and full exposure and vascular control in the operating room are also necessary to prevent rapid exsanguination when the impaled object is removed from the heart or a great vessel. Large impalement injuries of the extremities (especially of the groin, thigh, and axilla) also require immediate surgical consultation and thorough consideration of potential neurovascular and musculoskeletal injuries.

Suggested Reading

American College of Emergency Physicians: Clinical policy for the initial approach to patients presenting with penetrating extremity trauma, *Ann Emerg Med* 33:612–636, 1999.

Laceration, Simple

Presentation

The patient may have been accidently cut by a knife, glass shard, or other sharp object, which resulted in a clean, straight wound (Figure 143-1). Impact with a hard object at an angle to the skin may tear up a flap of skin. Crush injury from a direct blow may produce an irregular or stellate laceration with a variable degree of devitalized tissue, abrasion, and visible contamination. Wounds may involve vascular areas of the face and scalp, where the risk for infection is low, or the extremities where infection becomes a greater risk, along with the possibility of tendon and nerve damage. The elderly and patients on chronic steroid therapy may present with "wet tissue paper" skin tears following relatively minor trauma.

What To Do:

A history should establish the approximate time of injury. Risk for infection increases as the length of time from wounding to repair increases. A report of a sensation of "something in the wound" should be taken seriously. Frequently, the patient's perception is correct.

Determine the exact mechanism of injury, which should alert you to the possibility of an underlying fracture, retained foreign body, wound contamination, or tendon or nerve injury. Chin lacerations are associated with mandibular fractures. A fall onto gravel, glass fragments

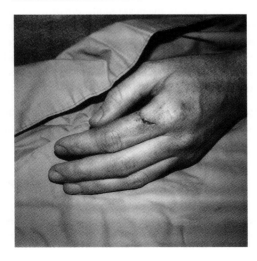

Figure 143-1 Simple laceration.

from automobile windshields, lacerating glass shards, or sharp wooden or plastic fragments may produce buried foreign bodies. Wounds occurring in natural bodies of water will be contaminated. Forceful injuries caused by a sharp metal or glass edge are most likely to cause tendon or nerve lacerations.

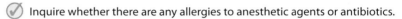 **Investigate for any underlying factors associated with the patient that may increase the risk of wound infection**. These include conditions such as diabetes, peripheral vascular disease, malnutrition or morbid obesity, acquired immunodeficiency syndrome (AIDS), alcoholism, and renal failure. Patients on chemotherapy or who are taking chronic immunosuppressive doses of corticosteroids are also at increased risk. **When these risk factors are present or there is a high degree of bacterial contamination, especially with soil or other debris, early administration of prophylactic antibiotics should be considered.** Open fractures and exposed joints or tendons are other instances for which antibiotics should be used. In general, decontamination is far more important than antibiotics. **Most simple lacerations should not receive prophylactic antibiotics. Antibiotics are justified for infected wounds or when foreign body removal must be postponed.**

Inquire whether there are any allergies to anesthetic agents or antibiotics.

Ask about tetanus immunization status and provide prophylaxis where indicated (see Appendix H). **The elderly, immigrants, and people with limited formal education are more likely than the general population to have low tetanus protection.**

Wound examination should always be conducted under optimal lighting conditions and with minimal bleeding. Place the patient in a comfortable supine position and stabilize the injured part. The treating clinician should be seated in a comfortable position.

Inspect and palpate for embedded foreign bodies, and check for sensation and motor function distal to the laceration. When lacerations continue to bleed despite reasonable direct pressure, a sphygmomanometer can be placed proximal to the injury and inflated to a pressure greater than the patient's systolic blood pressure. This will allow proper examination in a bloodless field.

Test tendon function against resistance. If function is weak or intact but there is pain, suspect a partial tendon laceration. Inspect the tendon through a full range of motion. For injuries to the hand, test the function of the flexor digitorum profundus and superficial tendons separately. Test skin sensation distal to the laceration and note any diminished sensitivity. **Tendon and nerve lacerations deserve specialty consultation. The following also require surgical consultation: joint capsule disruptions; repair of specialized structures, such as the parotid or lacrimal duct, eyelid margin, or tarsal plate; extensive injuries; or those involving significant tissue loss.**

Consider imaging studies if there might be a retained foreign body. Most glass fragments will be revealed on ordinary radiographs. CT scanning can detect more types of foreign material than plain film radiography, and high-resolution ultrasonography has been very successful in detecting various types of soft tissue foreign objects.

Consider procedural sedation and analgesia for children. Follow your hospital protocol (see Appendix E).

Children may also benefit from a topical anesthetic agent, especially for scalp and facial lacerations. Lidocaine 4% plus epinephrine 1:1000 (0.1%) plus tetracaine 0.5%

(LET) is safe, effective, and inexpensive. Put 3 mL on a cotton ball and press firmly into the wound for 20 to 30 minutes, either with tape or with the parent's gloved hand. After removing the cotton, test the effectiveness of the anesthesia by touching with a sterile needle. If any sensitivity remains, infiltrate the area with buffered lidocaine, as described later. Adding 150 mg of methylcellulose to the 3 mL of LET will convert this solution into a gel that can be applied directly into the wound, and it does not require cotton to hold it in place. Either preparation can be applied when the patient first arrives.

✅ **When a local anesthetic is required for cleansing, inspecting, and/or repairing a wound, buffer plain lidocaine 1% (Xylocaine) solution by adding 1 mL of sodium bicarbonate solution to every 9 to 10 mL of lidocaine and allow it to approximate body temperature in a pocket.** Buffering and warming reduce the pain of injection. The maximum safe dose of lidocaine is 4.5 mg/kg (up to 300 mg). Bupivacaine (Marcaine) is slightly slower in onset but has a much longer duration of action and may be useful for crush injuries and fractures where pain is expected to be prolonged beyond closure of the laceration. Bupivacaine cannot be buffered with as much bicarbonate as lidocaine, because it precipitates in alkaline solution. Only 0.1 mL of bicarbonate should be used per 10 mL of bupivacaine. Epinephrine is sometimes added to lidocaine on the face for its short-lived help with hemostasis and duration of anesthesia, but its benefits should be weighed against the disadvantage of increased pain on injection and its potential for possible slower healing and subsequent increased infection rate. Bicarbonate inactivates epinephrine.

✅ To further reduce pain, inject subdermally very slowly. Begin inside the cut margin of the wound, avoid piercing intact skin, work from the area already anesthetized, and use a 27- or 30-gauge needle on a 5- or 10-mL syringe. Also, repetitive pinching of the skin during lidocaine infiltration reduces patient discomfort (Figure 143-2).

✅ Use regional blocks to avoid distorting tissue or where there is no loose areolar tissue to infiltrate, such as the fingertip (see Appendix B). Some data suggest that percutaneous facial regional nerve blocks were more painful and less effective than local infiltration.

✅ **Clean the wound after anesthesia is complete. Superficial lacerations with little or no visible contamination, facial lacerations, and scalp lacerations may be cleaned by gentle scrubbing with a gauze sponge soaked in normal saline or a 1% solution of povidone-iodine.** (Dilute the stock 10% Betadine 10-fold with 0.9% NaCl.) **Deeper contaminated lacerations may require pressure irrigation with a syringe and splash**

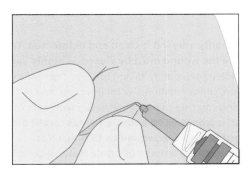

Figure 143-2 Demonstration of the pinching of the skin with the thumb and forefinger, just behind the area of injection with the anesthetic. Note the perpendicular relationship of the needle to the thumb and forefinger. (Adapted from Fosko SW, Gibney MD, Harrison B: Repetitive pinching of the skin during lidocaine infiltration reduces patient discomfort. *J Am Acad Dermatol* 39:74-78, 1998.)

shield, such as ZeroWet or Splashield, using the same 1% povidone-iodine solution or plain saline. A 35-mL syringe attached to a 19-gauge needle or plastic catheter (Angiocath) will also be effective. **Heavily contaminated wounds can first be cleaned using a gauze sponge and a nonionic surfactant cleanser (Shur-Clens).** Studies have shown that there is no greater risk for infection when a wound is irrigated with tap water. **A constant high-pressure flow from a faucet is a cheap alternative to jet lavage and eliminates the need for syringes, splash guards, and basins.** Warm or lukewarm water should be used for patient comfort.

✓ **All remaining visible debris, foreign bodies, and devitalized tissue must be removed, either by using forceps, by scraping with the edge of a scalpel blade, or by excision with scalpel or scissors. Cosmetic considerations will influence the degree to which facial lacerations are débrided**. Excision of contaminated nonviable wound edges should be kept to a minimum on the face, with tissue preservation being of primary concern.

✓ **Hair generally does not need to be removed.** When necessary, shorten hair with scissors rather than shaving with a razor.

✓ **Simple lacerations seldom require special techniques for hemostasis.** Direct pressure for 10 minutes, elevating the affected extremity, correct wound closure, and a compression dressing should almost always stop the bleeding.

✓ **Examine the wound again,** free of blood and with good lighting. Examine any deep structures, such as tendons, by direct visualization through their full range of motion, looking for partial tendon lacerations. Remember that the extensor tendons of the hand are very superficial and are highly susceptible to laceration. If there is any question about a partial tendon laceration, splint the wound and obtain orthopedic consultation.

✓ **If the wound has been heavily contaminated** with debris, is crushed with devitalized tissue, or has been exposed to pus, feces, saliva, or vaginal discharge, consider excising the entire wound and closing the fresh surgical incision, if practical. Otherwise, **provide for open management by loosely packing with sterile fine-mesh gauze covered with multiple layers of coarse absorptive gauze, after soaking them in normal saline or, in highly contaminated wounds, a 1% solution of povidone-iodine.** Unless the patient develops a fever or has increasing pain or purulent discharge from the wound, leave the dressing undisturbed for 3 to 5 days, when the risk for infection decreases. Have the patient begin cleaning the wound with mild soap and water in 24 to 48 hours. If there are no signs of infection, the granulating wound edges may then be approximated as a **delayed primary closure.**

✓ **Close the wound primarily only if it is clean and uninfected. The maximum "golden period," within which time the wound must be closed, is highly variable.** Each individual laceration should be considered separately, taking the time from injury to presentation into account along with location, contamination, risk for infection, and importance of cosmetic appearance, before deciding whether to perform primary wound closure. **The generally accepted "golden period" is from 6 to 10 hours, whereas recent data indicate that for clean wounds, this period might safely be extended to 19 hours.** Facial wounds may be closed up to 36 hours after injury. Minimize the amount of suture material buried inside the wound: the less suture used, the less chance of infection.

Wound Closure Options

Steri-Strips

○ **Wound closure tapes (Steri-Strips) and tissue adhesives offer the lowest risk for infection and are most successfully used on simple superficial lacerations with minimal tension. Tape strips are the closure material of choice for "wet tissue paper" skin tears.** Before application, degrease the skin with alcohol wipes, being careful not to get any alcohol into the wound. An adhesive agent such as tincture of benzoin may then be thinly applied to the skin surrounding the laceration (again, avoiding the open wound). Push the wound edges together and apply the tape to maintain approximation (Figure 143-3). An alternative to Steri-Strips alone for "wet tissue paper skin" repair is to use Mepitel (Mölnlycke Healthcare, Dunstable, UK), either in combination with Steri-Strips or alone as a porous semitransparent dressing. This material is coated with soft silicone that creates a gentle adhesion between the dressing and the intact skin. Mepitel is placed over the wound after the wound edges have been approximated and is then covered with a standard absorbent dressing. The Mepitel is left in place until wound healing has occurred.

Topical Skin Adhesive

○ **Cyanoacrylate topical skin adhesive (Dermabond, Indermil, Epiglu) can be used with small wounds in a location that does not allow the application of a length of wound closure tape. These adhesives can also be used in combination with the tape strips** (Figure 143-4). Tissue glues, like tape closures, are rapid and relatively painless to apply; therefore they generally do not require the use of a painful local anesthetic. There is also no need for suture removal. In addition, cyanoacrylate tissue adhesives have a barrier function against microbial penetration and serve as an optimal wound dressing that creates a moist environment, thus enhancing wound healing.

○ With the wound edges completely dry and meticulously approximated, the adhesive is carefully expressed through the tip of the applicator and gently brushed over the wound surface, covering 5 to 10 mm on either side of the wound edges (Figure 143-5). Initially, only a thin layer should be applied, because thicker layers may result in release of unpleasant heat as the glue polymerizes. After allowing the first layer of the adhesive to polymerize for 30 to 45 seconds, two to three additional layers should be applied, waiting 5 to 10 seconds between successive layers. **Usually reserved for low-tension wounds, tape closure strips and tissue adhesives can be used over areas of moderate skin tension if an appropriate immobilizing dressing or splint is applied.** Otherwise, simple wound coverings are optional. Ointments should not be used, because they will loosen the adhesive. The patient's wound is allowed to get wet briefly each day during showering or bathing.

Staples

○ **Most scalp lacerations and many trunk and proximal extremity lacerations that are straight, without edges that curl under (invert), can be most easily and rapidly repaired using skin staples.** However, staples do not allow meticulous repairs and should not be used in areas of cosmetic concern. Push wound edges together and staple so that edges evert slightly. Hair does not interfere with this technique and does not cause a problem if caught under a staple.

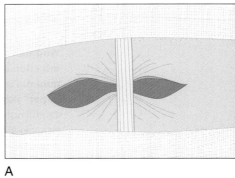

A

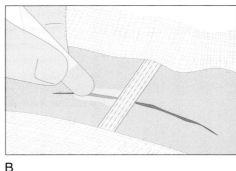

B

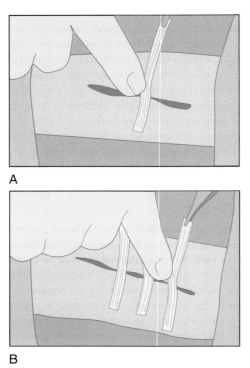

A

B

Figure 143-3 A, The tape is placed on one side of the wound at its midpoint while the clinician grasps it with forceps in the dominant hand. The opposite wound edge is then gently apposed by pushing with a finger of the nondominant hand. **B,** The remaining open sections of the wound are bisected by additional tape strips until the strips are within 2 to 5 mm of each other. (Adapted from Singer AJ, Hollander JE: *Lacerations and acute wounds.* Philadelphia, 2002, FA Davis, 2002.)

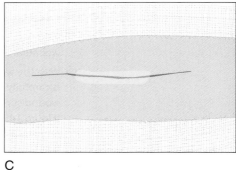

C

Figure 143-4 Closing a long or complex wound. **A,** The wound is bisected with a strip of surgical tape. **B,** The wound limbs on either side of the tape are glued. **C,** The strip is removed, and the central portion of the wound is glued. Some practitioners prefer to leave the tape strip and apply the adhesive over it. (Adapted from Singer AJ, Hollander JE: *Lacerations and acute wounds.* Philadelphia, 2002, FA Davis.)

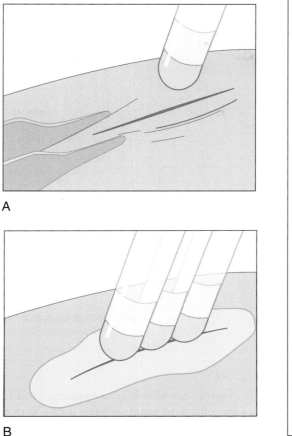

A

B

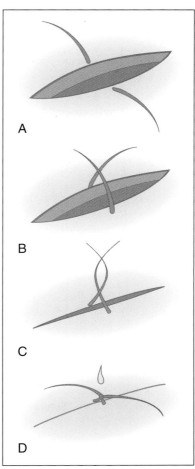

A

B

C

D

Figure 143-5 A, To prevent inadvertent runoff of the Dermabond adhesive, position the wound in a horizontal plane. Manually approximate the wound edges with forceps or gloved fingers. Use gentle brushing strokes to apply a thin film of liquid to the approximated wound edges, and maintain proper eversion of skin edges as you apply Dermabond adhesive. The adhesive should extend at least ½ centimeter on each side of the apposed wound edges. Apply Dermabond adhesive from above the wound. **B,** Gradually build up three or four thin layers of adhesive. Ensure that the adhesive is evenly distributed over the wound. Maintain approximation of the wound edges until the adhesive sets and forms a flexible film. This should occur about 1 minute after applying the last layer. (Adapted from Singer AJ, Hollander JE: *Lacerations and acute wounds.* Philadelphia, 2002, FA Davis.)

Figure 143-6 Hair apposition technique. **A,** Choose four to five strands of hair in a bundle on either side of the scalp laceration. **B,** Using artery forceps, cross the strands. **C,** Make a single twist to appose wound. **D,** Secure with a single drop of glue. (Adapted from Ong ME, Coyle D, Lim SH, Stiell I: Cost-effectiveness of hair apposition techniques for suturing. *Ann Emerg Med* 46:237-242, 2005.)

Hair Approximation Technique

○ With simple linear scalp lacerations, where the hair is at least 3 cm long and there is no active hemorrhage, closure can be obtained without using any anesthesia by using the hair apposition technique with tissue glue (Figure 143-6). Patients are able to wash their hair 3 days after repair.

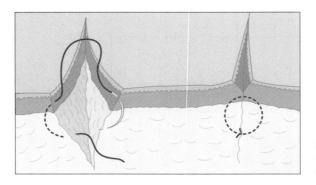

Figure 143-7 Absorbable intradermal sutures. (Adapted from Singer AJ, Hollander JE: *Lacerations and acute wounds*. Philadelphia, 2002, FA Davis.)

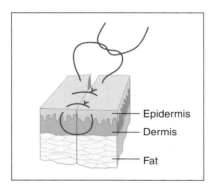

Epidermis
Dermis
Fat

Figure 143-8 Simple sutures. (Adapted from Singer AJ, Hollander JE: *Lacerations and acute wounds*. Philadelphia, 2002, FA Davis.)

Suture

○ **For deep or irregular lacerations, or lacerations on hands, feet, and skin over joints, use a monofilament nonabsorbable suture, such as nylon (Ethilon) or polypropylene (Prolene) (either 4-0, 5-0, or 6-0), using the smallest diameter with sufficient strength. Deep absorbable sutures (Vicryl, Vicryl Rapide) assist in approximating wound edges by decreasing tension and lessening dead space in which transudate and blood could accumulate** (Figure 143-7). Because of an increased risk for infection, one relative contraindication to deep suture placement is contamination of the laceration.

○ A good strategy to realign skin and minimize sutures is to begin by approximating the midpoint of the wound and then bisecting the remaining gaps with subsequent sutures. Put known landmarks together first (e.g., vermilion border, flexion creases, wrinkles). Simple interrupted stitches in most body sites should be about 0.5 cm apart, 0.5 cm deep, and 0.5 cm back from the wound edge (Figure 143-8). Make each dimension 0.25 cm for cosmetic closure on the face. Angle the needle going in and coming out so that it grasps more subcutaneous tissue than skin. The wound edges should evert so that the dermis is aligned level on both sides, thereby minimizing visible scar. Tie each stitch with only enough tension to approximate the edges. A continuous running suture (Figure 143-9) is a more rapid technique of closing a fairly straight laceration. When there is wound edge inversion (where the wound edge curls under), the length of the wound edge can be completely excised, or

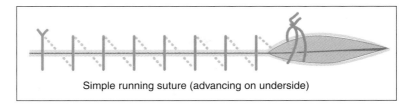

Simple running suture (advancing on underside)

Figure 143-9 Simple running suture. (Adapted from Singer AJ, Hollander JE: *Lacerations and acute wounds*. Philadelphia, 2002, FA Davis.)

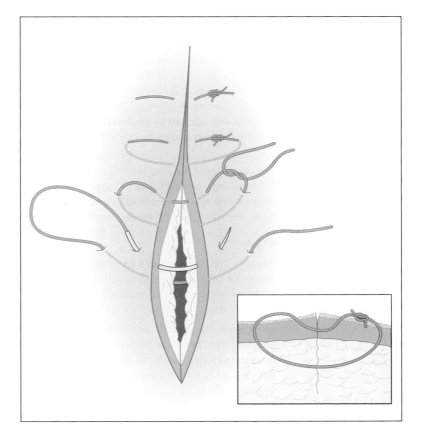

Figure 143-10 Vertical mattress suture. (Adapted from Singer AJ, Hollander JE: *Lacerations and acute wounds*. Philadelphia, 2002, FA Davis.)

vertical mattress sutures can be placed between simple interrupted stitches (Figure 143-10).

- ○ **When small children require sutures in a location that will make suture removal very difficult, use polyglactin (Vicryl Rapide) absorbable suture material.** Standard polyglactin (Vicryl) is more slowly absorbed and is more likely to cause discomfort or suture abscess.

- ○ **After closing the wound with sutures, apply bacitracin antibiotic ointment and a sterile protective nonadherent dressing, which will protect the wound from gross**

contamination and provide absorption, compression, and immobilization. Splint lacerations over joints. Scalp lacerations do not require messy ointment and may need a temporary compression dressing only if there is excessive bleeding or swelling. **Facial wounds generally do not require special dressings but should be cleaned twice a day with half-strength hydrogen peroxide on a cotton-tipped applicator to prevent crusting between wound edges.** This cleaning should be followed by reapplication of antibiotic ointment.

○ **Give patients clear, specific discharge instructions** that explain the potential complications of their injuries, and tell them when and where to go for reevaluation and follow-up care.

○ **Schedule a wound check in 2 days if the patient is likely to develop any problems with infection, require dressing changes, or need continued wound care.** Always recheck for sensory and tendon function distal to the healing wound after repair. Instruct patients to return at any time if there is bleeding, loss of function, or signs of infection (increasing pain, pus, fever, swelling, redness or heat). **After 48 hours, most sutured wounds can be re-dressed with a simple bandage that can be easily removed and replaced by the patient, allowing a shower each day.**

○ Wound closure strips can be left in place until they fall off on their own. Additional tape can be applied if the original closure strips fall off prematurely. A transparent polyvinyl film dressing, such as OpSite or Tegaderm, can be applied over the closure strips when they are first applied to provide a waterproof cover. This must be removed if water gets under the transparent film dressing. Mepitel is an alternative dressing described above.

Suture Removal

○ **Remove facial sutures in 3 to 5 days to reduce the risk for visible stitch marks.** The epidermis should have resealed by this time, but the dermis will not have developed much tensile strength; so, reinforce the wound edges with wound closure strips for a few more days.

○ **Most scalp, chin, trunk, and limb stitches should be removed in 7 days. Sutures may be left in for 10 to 14 days where there is tension across wound edges, as over the extensor surfaces of large joints.** Sutures are easily and painlessly cut with the tip of a No. 11 or 12 scalpel blade or fine scissors and removed with simple smooth forceps (Figure 143-11). Cut alternate loops of running sutures when these are ready to be removed.

What Not To Do:

(X) Do not prescribe prophylactic antibiotics for simple lacerations. Antibiotics do not reduce infection rates and only select for resistant organisms. Several clinical studies and a meta-analysis have found that there is no benefit to prophylactic antibiotics for routine laceration repair. Most infections can be easily treated when they occur. Limit prophylactic antibiotics to high-risk wounds.

(X) Do not close a laceration if there is visible or suspected contamination, debris, or nonviable tissue that cannot be adequately removed or if there are any signs of infection. Dress it open for delayed primary closure.

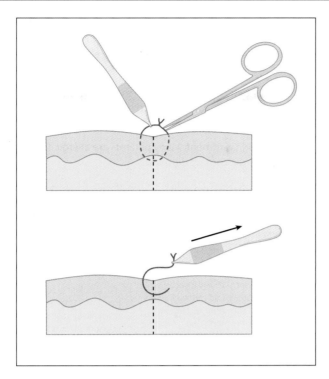

Figure 143-11 Simple suture removal. (Adapted from Singer AJ, Hollander JE: *Lacerations and acute wounds.* Philadelphia, 2002, FA Davis.)

✖ Do not substitute antibiotics for wound cleansing and débridement.

✖ Do not rely only on direct wound examination when a foreign body is suspected by history. Obtain a radiograph, ultrasonogram, or CT scan to ensure that the wound is free of any foreign material.

✖ Do not use high-pressure irrigation with noncontaminated wounds. It is unnecessary and may even increase the risk for infection in clean wounds.

✖ Do not use undiluted skin cleansing solution, such as 10% povidone-iodine or any skin scrub containing detergents or soap, in an open wound. They kill tissue and can even increase the infection rate.

✖ Do not miss a hidden human bite. Any laceration over the knuckles of the hand should be considered a human bite until proven otherwise (see Chapter 144).

✖ Do not shave an eyebrow. The hair is a useful marker for reapproximating the skin edges and can take months to years to grow back.

✖ Do not remove too much skin or underlying tissue when débriding the face and scalp.

✖ Do not place tissue adhesives within a wound or between wound margins.

✖ Do not allow tissue glue to drip into the patient's eye. When working near the eye, cover the lid with moistened gauze for protection. When available, high-viscosity Dermabond should be used. It is six times thicker than the original formulation and significantly reduces runoff.

(X) Do not use buried absorbable sutures in a wound with a high risk for infection.

(X) Do not insert drains in simple lacerations. They are more likely to introduce infection than prevent it.

(X) Do not apply ointments or petroleum jelly to wounds closed with tissue adhesives or sterile tape closures. This will cause these products to loosen prematurely and may lead to early wound dehiscence.

(X) Do not use Neosporin ointment. Many patients are allergic to the neomycin and develop a very uncomfortable allergic contact dermatitis.

Discussion

The most important goal of early wound care is preventing infection while attaining a functional closure with minimal scarring. Patients have these same concerns, along with the desire for the least painful repair. Development of wound infections, failure to detect foreign bodies, and missed injuries of tendons and nerves are common sources of litigation associated with lacerations. Careful history and wound examination, thorough cleansing, and débridement, as well as liberal use of delayed primary closure, all reduce these risks. One must strike a balance at times between excising enough tissue to prevent infection and not excising so much that a deformity will be created or limiting future options for elective scar revision. Always inform patients about your concern about possible wound infection, small hidden foreign bodies, or the delayed discovery of nerve or tendon injury. Always examine for these possibilities when rechecking a wound, and give patients realistic expectations about future scarring.

It is interesting to note that there is probably no clinically important difference in infection rates between using clean nonsterile gloves and sterile gloves during the repair of uncomplicated traumatic lacerations.

Nonabsorbable suture material is the standard for percutaneous use, because nylon and polypropylene are low-reactive materials with good tensile strength. This, of course, is also true for stainless steel staples. Staples should not be used in anyone who may need an MRI before removal. Their use should also be delayed if CT scanning is planned, because of the possible scatter artifacts the staples can cause.

Buried absorbable sutures are more reactive and, in animal studies of contaminated wounds, have been shown to increase the risk for infection. The

placement of these sutures, however, has not been shown to increase infection in clean wounds.

Tissue glue is nonreactive and has the added advantage over sutures of being quickly applied and painless (a special benefit when children are involved). The clinician using these tissue adhesives must always use the same care in providing adequate wound cleansing as with sutured wounds. The limitations of the adhesive's tensile strength and tendency toward wound dehiscence must also be taken into consideration. If cyanoacrylates get into undesirable areas, such as the eye, the glue can be removed with a petroleum-based product (e.g., ophthalmic bacitracin or erythromycin).

Surgical tapes are the least reactive of all closure techniques. They cannot be used in hairy areas, however, and they lose significant holding ability when wet.

Primary closure is the closure of a wound at the time of presentation. Delayed primary closure is the closure of a wound 3 to 4 days after the injury. Delayed primary closure should be used for heavily contaminated wounds or contaminated wounds in a host predisposed to infection. Wounds that are grossly contaminated or infected can be treated with wet to dry dressing or packing changes as often as two to three times per day to provide automatic cleansing and débridement. When the wound appears clean, without signs of infection, it can be closed typically within 3 to 5 days.

Healing by secondary intention is simply allowing a wound to heal without formal closure, other than in some instances applying a protective dressing. The primary advantage to this technique is its ease of use. The disadvantage is the associated delay in wound closure and possible increased scar size.

Discussion continued

For some small wounds, this nonclosure technique may be most appropriate. Simple hand lacerations, less than 2 cm in length and without deep structure involvement (distal to the distal volar wrist crease), that have been left open without repair have been shown to heal without cosmetic or functional difference compared with primary closure.

Suturing, therefore, may not offer any advantages over simple cleansing and dressing of small hand lacerations. Healing by secondary intention may produce superior aesthetic results on concave surfaces of the face and ears (e.g., the medial canthal area, nasal alar crease, nasolabial area, and concave fossa and concha of the auricle). Where practical, those wounds may be covered with moistened cotton or gauze and held in place with a dressing to provide better wound edge alignment.

Patients will sometimes report a previous allergic reaction to a local anesthetic. True allergy to local anesthetics is extremely rare and usually involves the anesthetic's preservative. Most often, an anesthetic from another class (amide or ester) can be substituted. Procaine or benzocaine (esters) can be substituted for lidocaine or bupivacaine (amides). These patients are often really allergic to methylparaben, the preservative used in multidose vials of lidocaine. When the type of anesthetic that caused the reaction is unknown, an alternative is to use an anesthetic agent that is unrelated to both esters and amides. Diphenhydramine diluted to a 1% solution is effective but painful to inject. Benzyl alcohol (a preservative in normal saline vials) in a 0.9% solution with epinephrine 1:100,000 is less painful to inject and is longer acting than diphenhydramine.

Ointments probably facilitate healing and reduce infection by their occlusive, rather than antibiotic, properties. White petrolatum may be as good as antibiotic ointment and avoids the risk for allergic reaction. When an antibiotic ointment is selected, neomycin-containing products (e.g., Neosporin) should be avoided because of their propensity for producing contact dermatitis. Options for dressings over the ointment have become numerous. It is unclear whether any one dressing is superior to the others; therefore personal preference and patient convenience should help determine which dressing material to use. In general, a dressing that protects a wound from contamination and, when necessary, provides mild compression and immobilization, along with absorption, while providing a warm moist environment is best to promote healing.

Permanent hyperpigmentation was observed in some wounds, caused by dermabrasion after excessive exposure to sunlight for the 6 months following injury. It is unclear whether this should be extrapolated to simple skin lacerations, but some clinicians recommend that sunscreens be used for several months to prevent hyperpigmentation.

Suggested Readings

Achar S, Kundu S: Principles of office anesthesia: part I. Infiltrative anesthesia, *Am Fam Physician* 66:91–95, 2002.

Al-Nammari SS, Reid AJ: Prophylactic antibiotics are not indicated in uncomplicated hand lacerations, *Emerg Med J* 24:218, 2007.

Al-Qattan MM: Vicryl Rapide versus Vicryl suture in skin closure of the hand in children, *J Hand Surg Br* 30:90–91, 2005.

Bartfield JM, Sokaris SJ, Raccio-Robak N: Local anesthesia for lacerations: pain of infiltration inside vs outside the wound, *Acad Emerg Med* 5:100–104, 1998.

Bruns TB, Worthington JM: Using tissue adhesive for wound repair: a practical guide to dermabond, *Am Fam Physician* 61:1383–1388, 2000.

Capellan O, Hollander JE: Management of lacerations in the emergency department, *Emerg Med Clin North Am* 21:205–231, 2003.

deLemos D: *Closure of skin wounds with sutures*. [*UptoDate* website]. Available at http://www.uptodate.com. Accessed August, 2011.

Ernst AA, Marvez-Valls E, Nick TG, et al: Topical lidocaine adrenaline tetracaine (LAT gel) versus injectable buffered lidocaine for local anesthesia in laceration repair, *West J Med* 167:79–81, 1997.

Fernandez R, Griffiths R, Ussia C: Water for wound cleansing, *Cochrane Database Syst Rev* 4:CD003861, 2002.

Forsch RT: Essentials of skin laceration repair, *Am Fam Physician* 78:945–951, 2008.

Fosko SW, Gibney MD, Harrison B: Repetitive pinching of the skin during lidocaine infiltration reduces patient discomfort, *J Am Acad Dermatol* 39:74–78, 1998.

Hock MOE, Ooi SBS, Saw SM, et al: A randomized controlled trial comparing the hair apposition technique with tissue glue to standard suturing in scalp lacerations (HAT study), *Ann Emerg Med* 40:19–26, 2002.

Hollander JE, Singer AJ: Laceration management, *Ann Emerg Med* 23:356–367, 1999.

Karounis H, Gouin S, Eisman H, et al: A randomized, controlled trial comparing long-term cosmetic outcomes of traumatic pediatric lacerations repaired with absorbable plain gut versus nonabsorbable nylon sutures, *Acad Emerg Med* 11:730–735, 2004.

Mehta PH, Dun KA, Bradfield JF, et al: Contaminated wounds: infection rates with subcutaneous sutures, *Ann Emerg Med* 27:43–48, 1996.

Moscati RM, Mayrose J, Reardon RF, et al: A multicenter comparison of tap water versus sterile saline for wound irrigation, *Acad Emerg Med* 13:404–409, 2007.

Perelman VS, Francis GJ, Rutledge T, et al: Sterile versus nonsterile gloves for repair of uncomplicated lacerations in the emergency department, *Ann Emerg Med* 43:362–370, 2004.

Priestley S, Kelly AM, Chow L, et al: Application of topical local anesthetic at triage reduces treatment time for children with lacerations, *Ann Emerg Med* 42:34–40, 2003.

Quinn J, Wells G, Sutcliffe T, et al: A randomized trial comparing octylcyanoacrylate tissue adhesive and sutures in the management of lacerations, *JAMA* 277:1527–1530, 1997.

Scarfone RJ, Jasani M, Gracely EJ: Pain of local anesthetics: rate of administration and buffering, *Ann Emerg Med* 31:36–40, 1998.

Smack DP, Harrington AC, Dun C, et al: Infection and allergy incidence in ambulatory surgery patients using white petrolatum vs bacitracin ointment: a randomized controlled trial, *JAMA* 276:972–977, 1996.

Stamou SC, Maltezou HC, Psaltopoulou T, et al: Wound infections after minor limb lacerations: risk factors and the role of antimicrobial agents, *J Trauma* 46:1078–1081, 1999.

Talen DA, Abrahamian FM, Moran GJ, et al: Tetanus immunity and physician compliance with tetanus prophylaxis practices among emergency department patients presenting with wounds, *Ann Emerg Med* 43:305–314, 2004.

Tarsia V, Singer AJ, Cassara GA, Hein MT: Percutaneous regional compared with local anaesthesia for facial lacerations: a randomised controlled trail. *Emerg Med J* 22:37–40, 2005.

Valente JH, Forti RJ, L16F Freundlich, et al: Wound irrigation in children: saline solution or tap water? *Ann Emerg Med* 41:609–616, 2003.

Whittaker JP, Nancarrow JD, Stemme GD: The role of antibiotic prophylaxis in clean incised hand injuries, *J Hand Surg Br* 30:162–167, 2005.

Wilson L, Martin S: Benzyl alcohol as an alternative local anesthetic, *Ann Emerg Med* 33:495–499, 1999.

Mammalian Bites

Presentation

Histories of animal bites are usually volunteered, but the history of a human bite, such as one obtained over the knuckle during a fight, is more likely to be denied or explained only after direct questioning. Mammalian animal bites generally consist of either domesticated animal bites, most commonly dog or cat bites, or wild animal bites, such as those from rodents, lagomorphs (rabbits and hares), skunks, raccoons, and bats. Human bites are either purposeful, occlusional, crushing injuries, or inadvertent clenched-fist injuries, as previously mentioned, which are also known as "fight bites."

A single bite may contain various types of injury, including abrasions, puncture wounds, avulsions, lacerations, and crush injuries, as well as underlying fractures, foreign bodies, and tendon and nerve injuries, not all of which are immediately apparent.

Patients either will present with a fresh wound soon after the injury or will delay and only seek help after developing painful signs of infection.

What To Do:

⊘ All bite wounds require a detailed history that includes the exact mechanism of injury and the approximate time that it took place. General health questions should include discussions regarding underlying illness (diabetes, transplanted organs, asplenia, immunosuppression) or medications (steroids, chemotherapy) that would increase the patient's risk for infection. The status of previous tetanus immunization should also be determined. Determine the type of animal that bit, whether the attack was provoked (a rabid animal is more likely to make an unprovoked attack), what time the injury occurred, and, when available, the current health status and vaccination record of the animal. Also find out if the animal has been captured and is being held for observation.

⊘ Examination should determine the extent and nature of all skin and soft tissue injuries, with special attention given to any possible tendon, nerve, joint, or vascular injury. Fight bite injuries (which are typically over the dorsal metacarpophalangeal joints) should be examined meticulously through a full range of motion with the hand in full flexion and extension to ensure that tendon injuries are not missed. **A tendon injury sustained with the fingers flexed will be missed if the hand is only examined in extension. Bony tenderness, pain on range of motion of a joint, swelling, and/or a forceful mechanism (e.g., a large biting animal) may indicate a need for radiographs or special imaging studies to rule out underlying fractures.** (Dog bites have caused open depressed skull and facial fractures in small children.) **Radiographs of hands injured by human teeth are also recommended.**

✅ **Report the bite to the police or appropriate local authorities.**

✅ **Simple abrasions and contusions that do not break through the dermis require only cleansing with 1% povidone-iodine (Betadine) solution or even just soap and water, as well as tetanus prophylaxis when required. (Potential rabies exposure also requires prophylaxis; see later in this chapter.)**

✅ **Small puncture wounds cannot be successfully irrigated, but large puncture wounds and lacerations should be anesthetized with lidocaine (Xylocaine) 1% and thoroughly cleansed and irrigated with a dilute 1% povidone-iodine solution** (10% povidone-iodine solution, diluted 1:10 in normal saline). Puncture wounds can be enlarged with a stab wound from a No. 15 scalpel blade to permit fluid to escape and then *slowly* irrigated at lower than optimal pressure (to prevent inadvertent soft tissue infiltration with the irrigation solution). This can be accomplished using a large gauge plastic catheter (Angiocath) with a 10-mL syringe. **Open lacerations can be cleansed with a high-jet lavage using an irrigation shield (Zerowet or Splashield) with a 10-mL syringe.** Devitalized tissue should be sharply débrided and the wound fully explored in a bloodless and well-lit field, looking for foreign bodies or tendon or joint involvement.

✅ **Most uninfected facial lacerations should be closed using sutures or tape closures to provide the most effective cosmetic repair.** A plastic surgeon or otorhinolaryngologist should be consulted about significant injuries to the special structures of the face and about wounds involving significant tissue loss.

✅ **Nonhuman animal bite wounds of the scalp, neck, trunk, and proximal extremities that are clean, uninfected, open lacerations may also be closed using tape closures, staples, or nonabsorbable suture material.** Buried sutures should be avoided, because they increase the risk for infection.

✅ **Wounds of the hand, foot, or wrist; puncture wounds; wounds with much devitalized tissue or those more than 6 hours old; or wounds that appear to be infected should be left open. Other wounds that should not be closed, except when on the face, include human, cat, monkey, pig, and wild carnivore bites, which result in infection-prone injuries.**

✅ Patients who have a high risk for infection, such as those with diabetes, immunosuppressed conditions, and renal failure, should have their wounds left open. These wounds can be loosely packed with saline-soaked fine-mesh gauze for delayed primary closure after approximately 72 hours.

✅ **Prophylactic antibiotics are indicated for bites of the hand, wrist, or foot or for a bite over a joint. They are also advised for punctures that are difficult or impossible to irrigate adequately or where there is significant tissue crushing that cannot be débrided. Antibiotics should also be prescribed for** patients who are older than 50 years or for those who are asplenic, alcoholic, or diabetic; with altered immune status or peripheral vascular insufficiency; or who have a prosthetic or diseased cardiac valve or a prosthetic or seriously diseased joint.

✅ **Human, cat, pig, wild carnivore, and monkey bites that are other than abrasions and superficial split-thickness lacerations also require prophylactic antibiotics.** Cats' teeth are slender, very sharp, and can easily penetrate the soft tissues and joints. Domestic pigs can also inflict deep injuries.

✅ **Face, scalp, ear, and mouth injuries do not require prophylactic antibiotics. Rodent and lagomorph bites also do not need antibiotic treatment.**

✅ **When a prophylactic antibiotic is indicated, prescribe amoxicillin/clavulanic acid (Augmentin), 875/125 mg × 5 days for adults. For children, 45 mg amoxicillin/kg/day, divided bid (80 to 90 mg/kg/day if drug-resistant** *S. pneumoniae* **is suspected). Oral solutions 200, 400, 600 mg amoxicillin/5 mL. Initiate the first dose as soon as possible.**

✅ **If penicillin allergic, prescribe the following:**

Dog Bite

○ Clindamycin (Cleocin), 300 mg qid, + levofloxacin (Levaquin), 500 mg qd × 5 days, for adults, or

○ Clindamycin, 10 mg/kg tid (oral solution: 75 mg/5 mL) + trimethoprim-sulfamethoxazole (TMP/SMX) (Bactrim, Septra), 8 to 12 mg TMP/kg/day divided bid (oral solution: 40 mg TMP/5 mL) for children

Cat Bite

○ Cefuroxime axetil (Ceftin), 500 mg bid × 5 days (for children, 15 to 30 mg/kg/day divided bid; oral solution 125 or 250 mg/5 mL) or

○ Doxycycline (Vibramycin), 100 mg bid × 5 days

Raccoon or Skunk Bite

○ Doxycycline (Vibramycin), 100 mg bid × 5 days

Human Bite

○ Clindamycin (Cleocin), 300 mg qid, + ciprofloxacin (Cipro), 500 mg bid (or TMP/SMX [Bactrim, Septra] DS bid) × 5 days

✅ **With early signs of infection, the same antibiotic coverage can be used, but it should be continued for a full 10 to 14 days.** Before antibiotics are started, obtain aerobic and anaerobic cultures from deep within the wound and then irrigate and débride as described.

✅ **Hand infections, joint infections, and moderate to severe soft tissue infections require specialty consultation and consideration for hospitalization, IV antibiotics, and possible surgical intervention.** Other indications for admission or specialty consultation after a bite injury include injury or probable injury to deep structures (bones, joints, tendons, arteries, or nerves). **A cat bite over a joint may require IV antibiotics.** Always consult the appropriate specialist in a timely manner when confronted with any situation that you are uncomfortable treating yourself.

✅ **All bite wounds require appropriate tetanus prophylaxis** (see Appendix H).

✅ **Rabies postexposure prophylaxis (PEP) is required for all bite wounds from animals suspected of being rabid as well as for situations involving contact of mucous membranes with rabid saliva or a scratch from a potentially rabid animal.** With potential human exposures involving bats, prophylaxis might be appropriate even if a bite, scratch, or mucous membrane exposure is not apparent when there is reasonable probability that such exposure might have occurred. This would include persons who were in the same room as the bat and who might be unaware that a bite or direct contact had occurred (e.g., a sleeping person awakens to find a bat in the room, or an adult witnesses a bat in a room with a previously unattended child, mentally disabled person, or intoxicated person) and rabies cannot be ruled out by testing the bat (see Appendix F).

✓ Because of local variations in animal vectors and endemics, consultation with a state or local health department is prudent before a decision is made to initiate antirabies postexposure prophylaxis (PEP).

✓ **In the United States, urban dogs and cats, domestic ferrets, small rodents (e.g., squirrels, hamsters, guinea pigs, gerbils, chipmunks, rats, and mice) and lagomorphs (including rabbits and hares)** are at low risk for being rabies carriers. The animal's behavior is sometimes helpful and is easily evaluated in wild animals, because most tend to shun humans. The urban appearance of a skunk, fox, or bat in broad daylight showing no fear of humans is abnormal and should greatly raise one's index of suspicion. An unprovoked bite from such an animal would be considered a bite with a high risk for rabies and requires PEP.

✓ If a biting animal with normal behavior has been captured, it should be quarantined with a veterinarian or reliable owner for 10 days. If the animal displays no signs of illness during this time, PEP is not indicated.

✓ If a person is bitten by an animal that cannot be observed or tested for rabies (e.g., one that has escaped), the decision to initiate PEP is based on the local epidemiology of rabies.

✓ **When the decision has been made to provide postexposure prophylaxis** *(note that the 2010 CDC guidelines have reduced the total number of human diploid cell [rabies] vaccine [HDCV] vaccine to four),* **give:**

○ 20 U/kg of human rabies immune globulin (Hyperab, Imogam, RIG) injected into or around the bite. If unable to give the full dose in this manner, inject the remainder IM in the gluteal muscle.

○ One mL of vaccine, human diploid cell culture (HDCV, Imovax), or 1 mL of either of the two other available rabies vaccines given IM in the deltoid area in adults, or into the lateral thigh in young children. Repeat doses of the vaccine are given on days 3, 7 and 14.

○ For patients previously immunized (usually veterinarians or animal handlers), rabies immune globulin is not given, and only 1 mL of the vaccine is given IM with a single repeat dose on day 3.

✓ **For human bites,** while the presence of HIV inhibitors in saliva renders the virus noninfective in most cases (the risk of infection is one twentieth the risk for transmission through a needle stick), there are case reports of human immunodeficiency virus (HIV) transmission by human bites. **Centers for Disease Control and Prevention (CDC) guidelines recommend postexposure prophylaxis for both the bite victim and the bite source if either party is known to be HIV positive or at high risk and if any blood exposure has occurred. When prophylaxis is indicated,** offer zidovudine (Retrovir), 200 mg tid, + lamivudine (3TC), 150 mg bid, +/− indinavir (Crixivan), 800 mg qd, all PO, × 4 weeks. These patients require follow-up testing and counseling. The chance for hepatitis B transmission from a bite appears to be greater than that for HIV. Unlike HIV prophylaxis, it is reasonable to delay treatment of potential hepatitis B exposure for 48 to 72 hours pending serologic results from bite victim and source. Provide hepatitis prophylaxis for patients who have been bitten by known carriers of hepatitis B. Administer hepatitis B immune globulin, 0.06 mL/kg IM, at the time of injury, and schedule a second dose in 30 days.

✓ **For hand injuries or crushing injuries and contusions, apply an immobilizing splint with a mild compressive dressing and have the patient keep the extremity elevated above the level of the heart.**

✓ After 24 hours, the patient should begin cleansing the wound once daily with gentle soap and water, followed by reapplication of a new dressing. Hand injuries should remain immobilized for 2 to 3 days until edema and pain have mostly resolved.

✓ **Have the patient return for a wound check in 2 days, or 1 day for cat bites and bites of the hand and any time there is any sign of infection.** Explain the potential for a serious complication, such as septic arthritis, osteomyelitis, and tenosynovitis, which will require specialty consultation. **Preparing patients for the worst while initiating aggressive treatment is the best defense against any potential future litigation.** Always provide patients with clear, specific, written discharge instructions.

What Not To Do:

✗ Do not overlook a puncture wound.

✗ Do not infiltrate irrigant solution into tissue planes in puncture wounds.

✗ Do not suture debris, nonviable tissue, or a bacterial inoculum into a wound.

✗ Do not use buried absorbable sutures, which act as a foreign body and a nidus for infection.

✗ Do not attempt to treat bite wounds using monotherapy with penicillin, clarithromycin, amoxicillin, or a first-generation cephalosporin. These antibiotics will not provide the coverage necessary for the mixed aerobic and anaerobic floras that are commonly cultured from these wounds.

✗ Do not waste time and money obtaining cultures and Gram stains of fresh wounds. The results of these tests do not correlate well with the organisms that subsequently cause infection.

✗ Do not provide rabies prophylaxis for incidental contact, such as petting a rabid animal or contact with blood, urine, or feces (e.g., guano) of a rabid animal. These experiences do not constitute an exposure, according to the Centers for Disease Control and Prevention.

Discussion

Animal bites are often brought promptly to the attention of medical personnel, if only because of a legal requirement to report the bite or because of fear of rabies. Bite wounds account for 1% of all emergency department visits in the United States, most caused by dogs and cats. Most dog bites are from household pets rather than strays. Dog bites account for 80% to 90% of all animal bites requiring medical care. A disproportionate number of these dog bites are from German Shepherd dogs.

Children are especially prone to animal bites, especially of the face. Bites occur most commonly among children who disturb the animals while they are sleeping or feeding, separate them during a fight, try to hug or kiss an unfamiliar animal, or accidentally frighten an animal. Women are more often bitten by cats, and young men are commonly bitten by dogs. Dog bites tend to be avulsion

(continued)

Discussion continued

injuries with a component of crush. Cat bites more commonly are puncture wounds. Because most cat bites are inflicted by the patient's own animal, cat bite victims tend to delay care until signs of infection develop. Malpractice claims and other civil lawsuits often follow bite injuries.

Although these wounds may look innocuous initially, they frequently lead to serious infection with a potential for serious complications. A single bite may contain various types of injury, including abrasions, contusions, avulsions, lacerations, crush injuries, or puncture wounds. Less readily apparent are injuries to deeper tissues (including vascular structures, tendons, nerves, and bone), as well as potential foreign bodies. Both dog and cat bites show high rates of infection with *Staphylococcus* and *Streptococcus* species, as well as *Pasteurella multocida* and many different gram-negative and anaerobic bacteria. Infecting organisms generally result from the aerobic and anaerobic microbial flora of the oral cavity of the biting animal, rather than the victim's own skin flora. In addition to these organisms, 10% to 30% of all human bites are infected with *Eikenella corrodens*, which sometimes shows resistance to the semisynthetic penicillins but sensitivity to penicillin. Most infections are polymicrobial. A number of risk factors that identify the likelihood of wound infection and define the patient likely to develop this complication have been identified. An important risk factor is delay of more than 24 hours in seeking treatment. Puncture wounds are much more likely than other types to become infected. Facial wounds show an infection rate of only 4%, regardless of treatment, whereas hand wounds have an infection rate of 28%. Septicemia mainly occurs in compromised hosts.

Human bites generally are more severe than animal bites, particularly in clenched-fist injuries. The teeth may cause a deep laceration that implants oral organisms into the joint capsules or dorsal tendons, causing devastating complications that include cellulitis, septic arthritis, tenosynovitis, and osteomyelitis.

Adequate débridement and irrigation are clearly more effective than prophylactic antibiotics and are often all that is required to prevent animal bite infections. Not all bites cause infection. Approximately 2% to 5% of all typical dog bite wounds seen in emergency departments become infected. This figure includes, however, many trivial surface abrasions. Wounds that have fully penetrated the skin have an infection rate of 6% to 13%, depending on location. In comparison, the infection rate of clean lacerations of all types repaired in the emergency department is approximately 3% to 5%.

Less than 0.1% of all animal bites in the United States result in rabies. The incubation period for humans depends on the distance from the bite to the brain, with an average of 1 to 3 months. Given this relatively long incubation period, **postexposure prophylaxis for rabies is considered a medical urgency, not a medical emergency.** For questions on local rabies risk, local public health services may be available and provide valuable support. In the United States, only Hawaii remains consistently rabies free. Since 1980, a total of 21 (50%) of the 36 human cases of rabies diagnosed in the United States have been associated with bat variants.

Signs of rabies among all forms of wildlife cannot be interpreted reliably; therefore any wild animal that bites and is captured should be euthanized at once (without unnecessary damage to the head) and the brain submitted for rabies testing. If the results of testing are negative by immunofluorescence testing, the saliva can be assumed to contain no virus, and the person bitten does not require postexposure prophylaxis; if it has been started, it can be discontinued.

In the continental United States, rabies among dogs is reported most commonly along the United States–Mexico border and sporadically in areas with enzootic wildlife rabies. During most of the 1990s, more cats than dogs were reported to be rabid in the United States. Most of these cases were associated with the epizootic of rabies among raccoons in the eastern United States.

When consultation is necessary for managing a case of potential rabies exposure and local or state health departments are not available, help can be obtained through the Division of Viral and Rickettsial Diseases of the Centers for Disease Control and Prevention (CDCP). During work hours, phone (404) 639-1050; after hours and on weekends and holidays, call (770) 488-7100. Help is also available at http://www.rabies.com.

In most other countries—including most of Asia, Africa, and Latin America—dogs remain the major species with rabies and the most common source of rabies among humans.

Monkey bites must be given special consideration. In addition to being highly prone to severe infection, they may cause an inoculum of the herpes B virus and require antiviral therapy with acyclovir, valacyclovir, or famciclovir.

Suggested Readings

Broder J, Jerrard D, Olshaker J, et al: Low risk of infection in selected human bites treated without antibiotics, *Am J Emerg Med* 22:10–13, 2004.

Brook I: Microbiology and management of human and animal bite wound infections, *Prim Care* 30:25–39, 2003.

Centers for Disease Control and Prevention: Updated rabies postexposure prophylaxis guidelines, *MMWR* 48:1–21, 1999.

Dire DJ, Hogan DE, Riggs MW: A prospective evaluation of risk factors for infections from dog bite wounds, *Acad Emerg Med* 1:258–266, 1994.

Donkor P, Bankas DO: A study of primary closure of human bite injuries to the face, *J Oral Maxillofac Surg* 55:479–781, 1997.

Elenbaas RM, McNabney WK, Robinson WA: Evaluation of prophylactic oxacillin in cat bite wounds, *Ann Emerg Med* 13:155–157, 1984.

Freer L: North American wild mammalian injuries, *Emerg Med Clin N Am* 22:445–473, 2004.

Gibbons RV: Cryptogenic rabies, bats, and the question of aerosol transmission, *Ann Emerg Med* 39:528–536, 2002.

Moran GJ: Dogs, cats, raccoons, and bats: where is the real risk for rabies? *Ann Emerg Med* 39:541–543, 2002.

Moran GJ, Talan DA, Mower W, et al: Appropriateness of rabies postexposure prophylaxis treatment for animal exposures, *JAMA* 284:1001–1007, 2000.

Rosen RA: The use of antibiotics in the initial management of recent dog bite wounds, *Am J Emerg Med* 3:19–23, 1985.

Rupprecht CE, Briggs D, Brown CM, et al: Use of a reduced (4-dose) vaccine schedule for postexposure prophylaxis to prevent human rabies. Recommendations of the Advisory Committee on Immunization Practices. Centers for Disease Control and Prevention, *MMWR Recomm Rep* 59:1–19, 2010.

Talan DA, Abrahamian FM, Moran GJ, et al: Clinical presentation and bacteriologic analysis of infected human bites in patients presenting to emergency departments, *Clin Infect Dis* 37:1481–1489, 2003.

Talan DA, Citron DM, Abrahamian FM, et al: Bacteriologic analysis of infected dog and cat bites, *N Engl J Med* 340:85–92, 1999.

Tu AH, Girotto JA, Singh N, et al: Facial fractures from dog bite injuries, *Plast Reconstr Surg* 109:1259–1265, 2002.

Turner TWS: Do mammalian bites require antibiotic prophylaxis? *Ann Emerg Med* 44:274–276, 2004.

Marine Envenomations

Presentation

After swimming in the ocean and coming into contact with marine life, the patient may seek medical attention because of local pain, swelling, or skin discoloration. Marine animal envenomations can be divided into two major categories: puncture wounds and focal rashes. Severe envenomations can be accompanied by systemic symptoms, such as vomiting, paralysis, seizures, respiratory distress, and hypotension. This review is limited to the more common injuries with minor local reactions.

Puncture Wounds

A laceration or puncture wound of the leg with blue edges suggests a stingray attack. There is immediate local intense pain, edema of soft tissue, and a variable amount of bleeding. The pain is excruciating and seems out of proportion to what might be expected based on the wound appearance alone. The pain usually peaks after 60 to 90 minutes, may radiate centrally, generally resolves over several hours, and may last as long as 48 hours. Retained fragments of the stingray's barb may be present in the wound.

A single small ischemic (e.g., pallor and cyanosis) puncture wound with a red halo and rapid swelling suggests a lionfish or scorpion fish envenomation. The pain is immediate, intense, and radiating. Untreated, the pain peaks 60 to 90 minutes after the sting, persists for at least 6 to 12 hours, and sometimes lasts for days. The severity of envenomations seems to be mild for lionfish, more severe for scorpion fish, and most severe or even life-threatening for stonefish, which is another member of the Scorpaenidae.

The dorsal or pectoral fin spines of the catfish can often inflict an envenomation when puncturing the skin. Symptoms include intense pain, paresthesias, and numbness that may last 30 minutes to 48 hours. Erythema, hemorrhage, edema, cyanosis, and lymphangitis also are common localized findings. Catfish have retroussé barbs (tip turned up) and can produce significant damage and be difficult to remove (Figure 145-1).

Multiple small punctures in an erratic pattern, with or without purple discoloration, or retained fragments are typical of sea urchin envenomations. The venomous spines can inflict burning pain that is initially minor but intensifies over 30 minutes and lasts several hours. The area surrounding the puncture wounds may be red and swollen. Some spines contain a blue-black dye that stains the wound or causes temporary tattooing.

Focal Rashes

An intense red, itchy rash follows contact with a bristle worm.

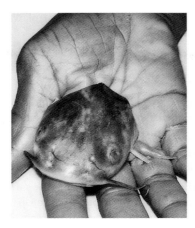

Figure 145-1 Catfish spine impalement.

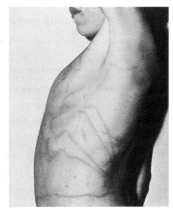

Figure 145-2 "Tentacle prints" from the Atlantic Portuguese man-of-war.

Contact with feather hydroids and sea anemones induces a mild reaction, consisting of instantaneous burning, itching, and urticaria. Envenomation may result in a lesion with a pale center and an erythematous or petechial ring; this is followed by increasing edema and ecchymosis. Although most lesions resolve in 48 hours, more severe envenomations may result in vesicle formation, which can lead to an abscess, eschar, or hyperpigmentation.

The sting of the fire coral induces intense burning pain, redness, itching, and painful pruritus with large wheals, with central radiation and reactive regional lymphadenopathy. Fire coral (not a true coral) has a razor-sharp lime carbonate exoskeleton that can cause skin lacerations containing exoskeleton debris.

Envenomation from a jellyfish causes immediate pain that may be described as mild to moderate stinging or burning. Pain is followed by the development of an erythematous rash.

Most jellyfish with suspended tentacles create "tentacle prints" or a whiplike pattern of darkened reddish-brown, purple, or frosted and crosshatched stripes in the precise areas of skin contact (Figure 145-2). Vesiculation and skin necrosis may follow and can last 24 hours or longer. Occasionally, there will be residual hyperpigmentation. Tentacles still may be adherent on patient presentation.

What To Do:

Puncture Wounds

○ **To most effectively relieve pain and attenuate some of the thermolabile protein components of the venom, soak the wound in hot (not scalding) water (approximately 45° C [113° F]) for 30 to 90 minutes or longer for pain control.** Have the patient use an unaffected limb as a control to test the water temperature and thereby avoid scalding.

○ **During hot water treatment or while waiting for it to be available, infiltrate in or around the wound with 0.5% bupivacaine or 1% or 2% lidocaine without**

epinephrine to provide further pain control. When necessary, be generous and add narcotic analgesics.

○ Irrigate larger wounds as soon as possible with a jet lavage of normal saline or dilute 1% povidone-iodine solution (add 10% Betadine to 0.9% NaCl in a 1:10 ratio), and remove visible pieces of spine or debris.

○ **Obtain radiographs to detect any hidden radiopaque fragments of retained stingray, catfish, or sea urchin spines. Ultrasonography may also be used to locate any remaining pieces.**

○ When anesthesia is complete and pain has been controlled, thoroughly explore, débride, and irrigate open wounds.

○ **Remove fragile sea urchin spines using the same technique as for a superficial sliver** (see Chapter 153). Care should be taken in removal of these spines, because they are brittle and may crumble in the wounds. Thin retained spines without symptoms generally are absorbed or extruded; therefore, if difficult or impractical to remove, they can be left in place. Every effort should be made to remove spines adjacent to a tendon or joint. If left in place, treatment should include a 7- to 14-day course of nonsteroidal anti-inflammatories (NSAIDs) (if not contraindicated), and, if a severe secondary reaction occurs, prednisone should be prescribed (unless infection is suspected).

○ Lightly pack larger wounds open for delayed primary closure (see Chapter 143).

○ Ensure current tetanus prophylaxis (see Appendix H).

○ **Prophylactic antibiotics are not required for minor abrasions, superficial punctures, and superficial lacerations. Injuries with potential for serious infection include large lacerations, deep puncture wounds (particularly near joints), and wounds with retained foreign material.**

○ **These infection-prone wounds, and any wound in an immunocompromised individual of any type, require antibiotic treatment. Ciprofloxacin (Cipro), 500 mg bid, or doxycycline (Vibramycin), 100 mg bid for adults, and trimethoprim-sulfamethoxazole (Bactrim/Septra), 8 to 12 mg TMP/kg/day divided bid for children, all prescribed for 3 to 5 days, are the most appropriate regimens for coverage of pathogenic marine microbes.** The genus *Vibrio* is particularly common in the ocean and poses a serious risk for immunosuppressed patients. Rapidly progressive cellulitis or myositis indicates *Vibrio parahaemolyticus* or *Vibrio vulnificus*. Also known to inoculate marine wounds are *Erysipelothrix rhusiopathiae* and *Mycobacterium marinarum*. In the more severe wounds, the recommended initial parenteral antibiotics include cefoperazone (Cefobid), ceftazidime (Fortaz), gentamicin (Garamycin), ciprofloxacin, ceftriaxone (Rocephin), and cefuroxime (Zinacef).

○ **For infected wounds, obtain both aerobic and anaerobic cultures, and alert the clinical microbiology laboratory that standard antimicrobial susceptibility testing media may need to be supplemented with NaCl to permit growth of marine bacteria. Institute the above-mentioned antibiotics, except for minor wound infections with the classic appearance of erysipelas, which can be treated with erythromycin or cephalexin. Prescribe antibiotics for 7 to 14 days.** Hospitalization may be required for severe infections and in those individuals who are immunosuppressed.

○ Provide pain control with NSAIDs and narcotic analgesics as required.

○ Follow up all wounds in 1 to 2 days with periodic revisits until healing is complete.

Focal Rashes

○ **For fire coral, jellyfish, hydroid, or sea anemone stings, decontaminate the area with a liberal soaking of 5% acetic acid (vinegar). Less effective alternatives include baking soda or a solution of a dilute (¼ strength) household ammonia.** Vinegar and ammonia may be applied continuously by applying soaked compresses until the pain is relieved or for 30 minutes.

○ **The most effective way to control pain is by using hot water (45° C [113° F]) immersion to inactivate the heat-labile protein toxins.** Application of vinegar will stabilize any undischarged stinger cells (nematocysts) and prevent further injury.

○ Any lacerations from fire coral must be anesthetized, explored, and cleansed. Any retained foreign debris must be removed; then the wound should be lightly packed with moist, fine-mesh gauze for delayed primary closure in 3 to 5 days.

○ **After decontamination with vinegar, remove any visible large jellyfish tentacles with forceps or double-gloved hands. Remove small particles by applying shaving foam, or some equivalent, and gently shaving the area with a safety razor, dull knife, tongue blade, or plastic card; then clean with an antibacterial soap and flush with water or saline solution.**

○ Treat any generalized allergic or systemic reactions with antihistamines, corticosteroids, epinephrine, and IV fluids as indicated.

○ **When irritation from sponges, bristle worms, or other marine creatures causes erythematous or urticarial eruptions, it usually means that tiny spicules and spinules are embedded in the skin.** Apply vinegar compresses to help neutralize toxins and relieve pain. Dry the skin, apply the sticky side of a piece of adhesive tape to the affected area, and peel the tape back to remove these particles. Cosmetic deep-cleansing strips for skin pores (Bioré Pore Perfect) can also be effective if available. Gauze soaked with glue, applied to the area and allowed to dry, is another method of removing embedded particles when the gauze is peeled away.

○ **Residual inflammation can be treated with topical corticosteroids, such as triamcinolone (Aristocort A) 0.1% or 0.5% cream or desoximetasone (Topicort) emollient cream or ointment 0.25% (dispense 15 g and apply tid to qid). A topical steroid in combination with a topical anesthetic can be additionally soothing (e.g., Pramosone cream, lotion, or ointment 2.5% tid to qid). Systemic antihistamines will also be helpful for pruritus, and, on occasion, systemic corticosteroids will be required.**

○ Tetanus prophylaxis should be administered if indicated.

○ Provide pain control with NSAIDs and narcotic analgesics as required.

○ **Advise the patient about sun avoidance and the use of sun blocks to prevent possible postinflammatory hyperpigmentation.** Hydroquinone (Eldoquin-Forte) 4% skin bleaching cream can be prescribed to be rubbed in bid when hyperpigmentation occurs.

○ Check wounds for infection in 2 and 7 days.

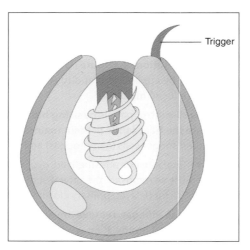

Figure 145-3 Nematocyst prior to discharging. (Adapted from Stauffer AR, Auerbach PS: Marine envenomations: common Florida injuries. *EMpulse* 8:12, 2003.)

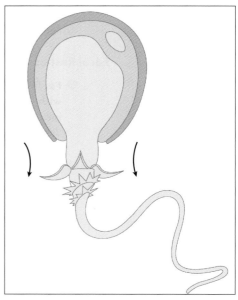

Figure 145-4 Nematocyst after discharge occurs. (Adapted from Stauffer AR, Auerbach PS: Marine envenomations: common Florida injuries. *EMpulse* 8:12, 2003.)

What Not To Do:

(X) Do not use fresh water or isopropyl (rubbing) alcohol to decontaminate jellyfish stings. It may cause any remaining nematocysts to rupture and trigger additional stinging.

(X) Do not use full-strength ammonia as a substitute for vinegar compresses. It is a powerful skin irritant.

(X) Do not constrict limbs tightly.

Discussion

Many marine animals have developed systems for attack and defense that on accidental exposure to humans result in envenomation. Most envenomations are not life threatening, often presenting only as minor contact dermatitis or a small puncture wound. Venomous marine organisms can be difficult to identify or may not be seen at the time of envenomation.

Marine animals responsible for envenomation can be broken into two large groups—vertebrates and invertebrates. Venomous vertebrate marine animals include stingrays, lionfish, scorpion fish, stonefish,

and catfish, whereas venomous invertebrates include jellyfish, anemones, and fire coral.

Treatment can be based on the nature and appearance of the wound when the specific sea creature cannot be identified.

Although one should always be wary of the possibility for anaphylaxis and cardiopulmonary collapse, particularly in elderly victims with previous sensitization to venom antigens, these complications are rarely seen with stings from creatures found in North American waters.

Discussion continued

Any wound acquired in the marine environment can become infected, and this is particularly likely if the wound is large, is a puncture, or is contaminated with bottom sediment or organic matter.

Stingray victims are generally innocent beach walkers who step on the back of the ray, which reflexively strikes upward with its tail, inflicting a penetrating wound along the upper foot, ankle, or lower leg. Injuries also are sustained to the hand or arm in the process of trying to remove a stingray that has been caught while fishing. The anatomic structure of the stingray's spine causes a deep, jagged painful wound that may contain fragments of the barb. This barb is located on the dorsum of the proximal portion of the tail. Submersion of the affected area in hot water (43° to 46° C) may help mitigate the pain: in one retrospective review, 65 (67%) of 97 patients with stingray wounds had complete analgesia with hot water immersion alone. Other remedies, including applying the cut half of an onion (Australian), or urinating on the wound are unproven.

Scorpion fish, lionfish, and stonefish stings occur in divers and fisherman, and sometimes in keepers of marine aquariums or those involved in illegal tropical fish trade. (Intravenous stonefish antivenin is indicated in cases of severe systemic reactions to stonefish.) Catfish stings are common when the fish are handled or kicked. Certain catfish species produce venom in glands at the base of the dorsal spine, but most do not, and catfish venom causes only mild local pain, redness, and swelling. Of more concern is the wound caused by the spine and the likelihood of infection that may take months to resolve.

Sea urchin victims are stung when they step on, handle, or brush up against these sessile creatures. The sea urchin secretes a toxin on the surface of its spines that is transferred into the wound when they penetrate the skin. The brittle spines also tend to break off and remain in the wound.

Jellyfish, sea anemones, and fire coral envenomate their prey through nematocysts (Figures 145-3 and 145-4). Nematocysts are venom-containing stinging organelles located in specialized epithelial cells called cnidocytes. Jellyfish tentacles vary in length from a few millimeters to more than 40 meters. Tentacles that have separated from the jellyfish are still capable of stinging for weeks or months after becoming detached, even if dried.

Although not as effective as heat or vinegar, papain (unseasoned meat tenderizer or papaya latex [juice]) also have been reported to relieve the pain associated with jellyfish stings. If either is used, it should be applied for no longer than 15 minutes. Isopropyl alcohol (which some suggest may worsen the pain), dilute ammonium hydroxide, sodium bicarbonate, olive oil, urine, and sugar are also described in marine medical literature as potentially effective.

"Safe Sea" sunscreen with jellyfish sting protective lotion (Nidaria Technology, Boca Raton, Fla.) is a commercial product that shows promise as an effective "sting inhibitor" when applied to human skin before jellyfish tentacle contact. This product has been studied in two trials involving human volunteers and has demonstrated a clinically important benefit.

The sea wasp, or box jellyfish, which inhabits the Indo-Pacific Ocean, is the most venomous sea creature and can induce death in 30 seconds. If a patient who is stung by this member of the Scyphozoa survives long enough to receive medical care, sheep antivenom is available.

True and soft corals can cause lacerations secondary to mechanical trauma. There is no envenomation, but wounds often become infected, having poor healing and a persistent exudate. These wounds should be carefully cleaned and débrided and treated with daily wet-to-dry dressings until clean.

Minor bites from octopi, sharks, moray eels, and barracudas are usually the result of the marine creature's instinct to protect itself against a perceived danger. Treatment is symptomatic; local cleansing and topical dressing usually are adequate. If the wound becomes infected, antibiotics as previously described should be initiated.

Suggested Readings

Auerbach PS: Marine envenomations, *N Engl J Med* 325:486–493, 1991.

Auerbach PS: Envenomation by aquatic invertebrates. In Auerbach PS, editor: *Wilderness medicine*, ed 5, Philadelphia, 2007, Mosby Elsevier, p 1691.

Auerbach PS: Envenomation by aquatic vertebrates. In Auerbach PS, editor: *Wilderness medicine*, ed 5, Philadelphia, 2007, Mosby Elsevier, p 1730.

Clark RF, Girard RH, Rao D, et al: Stingray envenomation: a retrospective review of clinical presentation and treatment in 119 cases, *J Emerg Med* 33:33–37, 2007.

Meyer PK: Stingray injuries, *Wild Environ Med* 8:24–28, 1997.

Perkins RA, Morgan SS: Poisoning, envenomation, and trauma from marine creatures, *Am Fam Physician* 69:885–890, 2004.

Schwartz S, Meinking T: Venomous marine animals of Florida: morphology, behavior, health hazards, *J Florida Med Assoc* 84:433–440, 1997.

Singletary EM, Rochman AS, Bodmer JCA, Holstege CP: Envenomations, *Med Clin North Am* 89:1195–1224, 2005.

Nail Bed Laceration

Presentation

The patient has either cut into his nail with a sharp edge or crushed his finger (commonly in a door). With shearing forces, the nail may be avulsed from the nail bed to varying degrees, and there may be an underlying bony injury.

What To Do:

✓ Provide appropriate **tetanus prophylaxis** (see Appendix H).

✓ **Obtain radiographs** of any crush injury. Distal tuft fractures are common with these injuries.

✓ Complex crush injuries or injuries resulting in significant tissue loss or deformity require specialty consultation with a hand surgeon.

✓ **A small, stable laceration through the nail, with minimal wound separation, can simply be cleansed and sealed with tissue adhesive (Dermabond).**

✓ **With a larger or more complicated laceration through the nail, remove the entire nail to allow suturing of the nail as follows:**

  ○ **Perform a digital block for anesthesia** (see Appendix B).
  ○ A bloodless field may need to be established using a **finger tourniquet.**
  ○ **Use a straight hemostat or periosteal elevator to separate the nail from the nail bed** (Figure 146-1). Keep instrument pointed toward the nail plate and not toward the nail bed, to prevent further injury.
  ○ Cleanse the wound thoroughly with saline.
  ○ **Suture with a fine absorbable material** (6-0 or 7-0 Vicryl or Dexon) (Figure 146-2).
  ○ **Replace the nail back into its normal anatomic position, as noted below.**

✓ **When a crush injury results in open hemorrhage from under the fingernail, manage as follows:**

  ○ **Perform a digital block for anesthesia** (see Appendix B).
  ○ **The nail must then be completely elevated to allow proper inspection of the damaged nail bed.**
  ○ A bloodless field may need to be established with a finger tourniquet to help visualization.

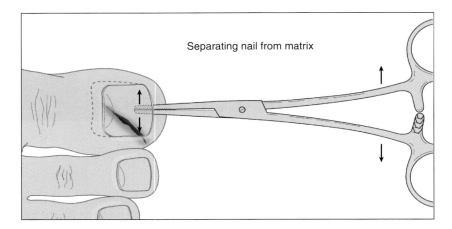

Figure 146-1 Separate nail from nail bed using a straight hemostat.

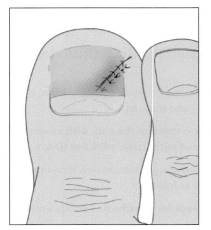

Figure 146-2 The nail bed can be repaired after it has been fully exposed.

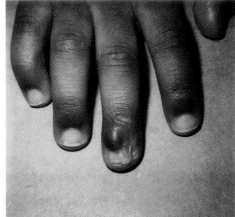

Figure 146-3 Improper nail bed repair will increase the risk for future fingernail or toenail deformity.

○ **Angulated fractures need to be reduced** (see Chapter 111).

○ **Large nail bed lacerations should be sutured with a fine absorbable suture** (6-0 or 7-0 Vicryl or Dexon). Small lacerations with minimal wound edge separation do not require suturing.

○ **An intact nail should be cleaned and reinserted for protection and proper tissue alignment, or an alternative nail bed dressing can be applied** (see Chapter 138).

○ **Tissue adhesive can be used to bond the nail to the nail bed and seal open spaces or defects in the nail** (see Chapter 138). Cover with an appropriate fingertip dressing.

✓ Inform the patient that a new nail will slowly push off the replaced nail or artificial stent.

What Not To Do:

✗ Do not use nonabsorbable sutures to repair the nail bed. The patient will be put through unnecessary suffering when the sutures are removed.

✗ Do not place a dressing that requires removal onto an exposed nail bed. Any such dressing will adhere tenaciously to the nail bed and will be extremely painful to remove (even after a short period of time).

Discussion

The objective of a nail bed repair is to provide a flat, smooth surface on which the new nail will grow. It is crucial that the provider is attentive while addressing these injuries, because mismanagement can lead to further complications. If a wound is inadequately repaired or if a wound is allowed to heal by secondary intention, additional scar tissue may cause the nail to split or become nonadherent.

It is also necessary to provide separation of the eponychium from the germinal matrix to prevent potential adhesions from forming. Replacement of the original nail into its normal anatomic position,

with the nail root under the eponychium, is the best method of preserving future nail integrity. When the nail has been severely damaged or is missing, an artificial stent can be provided (see Chapter 138).

Significant nail bed injuries can be hidden by hemorrhage and a partially avulsed overlying nail. These injuries must be repaired to help prevent future deformity of the nail (Figure 146-3). Surgical consultation should be obtained when nail bed lacerations involve the germinal matrix under the base of the nail.

Suggested Reading

Wang QC, Johnson BA: Fingertip injuries, *Am Fam Physician* 63:1961–1966, 2001.

Nail Root Dislocation

Presentation

The patient has caught his finger in a car door or dropped a heavy object on his exposed toe, causing a painful deformity. The base of the nail will be found resting above the eponychium instead of in its normal anatomic position beneath. The cuticular line that had joined the eponychium at the nail fold will remain attached to the nail at its original position (Figures 147-1 to 147-3).

What To Do:

✓ Perform a thorough evaluation to ensure that neurovascular status is intact.

✓ **Obtain a radiograph to rule out an underlying fracture (which may require reduction as well as protective splinting).**

✓ Anesthetize the area using a digital block (see Appendix B).

✓ **Lift the base of the nail off the eponychium and thoroughly cleanse and inspect the nail bed.** Minimally débride loose cuticular tissue, and test for a possible avulsion of the extensor tendon (see Chapter 109).

✓ If there are significant nail bed lacerations, the entire nail will need to be removed and lacerations repaired using a fine absorbable suture, such as 6-0 Vicryl or chromic gut (see Chapter 146). **Just replacing the nail root into its normal position will correct most small and simple nail bed lacerations.**

✓ **Using a hemostat, reinsert the root of the nail under the eponychium.**

✓ Reduce any underlying angulated fractures by grabbing the distal phalanx and firmly bending it back into normal alignment. (This will help to stabilize and hold the nail root under the eponychium.) Unstable fractures may require fixations and consultation with a specialist.

✓ **If the nail still tends to drift out from under the eponychium, it can be sutured in place using two 4-0 or 5-0 nylon or Prolene stitches in the proximal corners** (see Figure 147-1).

✓ Any nonabsorbable sutures should be removed after 1 week.

✓ Cover the area with a fingertip dressing (see Appendix C), and splint any underlying fracture (see Chapter 111).

✓ **Provide tetanus prophylaxis (see Appendix H).**

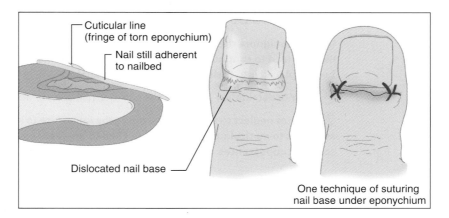

Cuticular line
(fringe of torn eponychium)

Nail still adherent
to nailbed

Dislocated nail base

One technique of suturing
nail base under eponychium

Figure 147-1 Dislocated nail root.

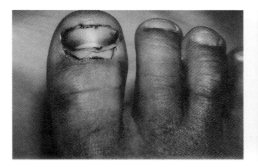

Figure 147-2 The subtle appearance of a dislocated nail root can be inadvertently overlooked by the clinician.

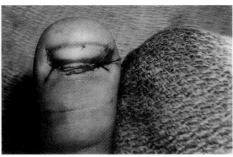

Figure 147-3 Appearance of the same toenail as shown in Figure 147-2 after a thorough cleansing, reinsertion of the nail root under the eponychium, and being sutured in place.

✓ Follow-up should be provided in 3 to 5 days. Patients should be advised to leave the dressing and splint (if applicable) in place until his or her follow-up evaluation. If the dressing becomes wet or soiled, the patient should return immediately for redressing of the wound.

✓ Instruct patients to return immediately if there is increasing pain or any other sign of infection (redness, swelling, purulent drainage, or red streaking). The patient should be advised that it is normal to have blood continue to ooze from beneath nail in the first 1 to 2 days following his or her injury.

✓ **Prescribe appropriate pain management,** including Tylenol and anti-inflammatories such as ibuprofen, as well as narcotic medications if indicated. Instruct the patient to keep the extremity elevated above the level of the heart as much as possible for further comfort.

✓ **Prophylactic antibiotics are not routinely required, even with associated fractures of the distal phalanx,** except in immunocompromised patients. Significantly contaminated wounds should receive 3 to 5 days of cephalexin (Keflex), 500 mg qid.

What Not To Do:

(X) **Do not ignore the nail root dislocation and simply provide a fingertip dressing. This is likely to lead to continued bleeding or to a later infection, because tissue planes have not been replaced into their natural anatomic position.**

(X) Do not débride any portion of the nail root, nail bed, sterile matrix, or germinal matrix.

(X) **Do not neglect to thoroughly irrigate the injury site to minimize the risks of infection, as well as to meticulously repair the nail bed to prevent complications and to maximize cosmetic appearances.**

Discussion

The germinal matrix lies protected under the eponychium, forming the area from which the nail is produced. Growth takes place in the nail root, or lunula. The lunula is the pale crescent-shaped structure under the proximal portion of the nail.

Because the nail is not as firmly attached at the lunula and root as it is to the distal nail bed, impact injuries can avulse only the base (nail root), leaving the nail lying on top of the eponychium.

It may be surprising that this injury is often missed, but at first glance, a dislocated nail can appear to be in place, and without careful inspection, a patient can return from radiology with negative radiographs and be treated as if he only had an abrasion or a contusion. The attachment of the cuticle from the nail fold of the eponychium to the base of the nail forms a constant landmark on the nail. If any nail is showing proximal to this landmark, it indicates that the nail is not in its normal position beneath the eponychium.

Suggested Readings

Altergott C, Garcia FJ, Nager AL: Pediatric fingertip injuries: do prophylactic antibiotics alter infection rates? *Pediatr Emerg Care* 24:148–152, 2008.

Saladeno RA, Atevy P: *Management of fingertip injuries.* [*UpToDate* website]. Available at http://www.uptodate.com. Accessed December 15, 2011.

Wang QC, Johnson BA: Fingertip injuries, *Am Fam Physician* 63:1961–1966, 2001.

Needle (Foreign Body) in Foot

Presentation

Although a needle could be embedded under any skin surface, most commonly a patient will have stepped on one while running or sliding barefoot on a carpeted floor. In general, but not invariably, the patient will complain of a foreign body sensation with weight bearing. A very small puncture wound will be found at the point of entry, and frequently, a portion of the needle will be palpable. Occasionally, the needle goes in eye first, and a thread is hanging out of the puncture.

What To Do:

✓ **Tape a partially opened paper clip as a skin marker to the plantar surface of the foot, with the tip of the opened paper clip over the entrance wound.** Instruct the patient not to allow anyone to remove the paper clip until after the needle is removed (Figure 148-1, *A*).

✓ **Send the patient for anteroposterior and lateral radiographs of the foot with the skin marker in place** (Figure 148-1, *B*).

 ✓ Evaluate the radiographs. If the needle appears to be very deep, you may want to call in a consultant who can remove the needle under fluoroscopy. **If the needle is relatively superficial, inform the patient that removing a needle is not as easy as it appears.** Let him know that a simple technique will be used to locate and remove the needle but that sometimes the needle is hidden within the tissue of the foot ("like a needle in a haystack"). If the needle cannot be located within 10 to 15 minutes, to avoid further damage to the foot, a consultant will be called in to arrange for removal under fluoroscopy.

✓ **Establish a bloodless field** by elevating the leg above the level of the heart, tightly wrapping an Ace bandage around the foot up to the calf. Finally, inflate and clamp off a sphygmomanometer calf cuff at approximately 50 to 75 mm Hg above the patient's systolic pressure. This will become uncomfortable within 10 to 15 minutes and thereby serve as an automatic timer for the procedure. Do not leave the tourniquet inflated for more than 15 to 30 minutes, regardless of the patient's symptoms.

✓ Remove the Ace wrap, clean, and then paint the area with povidone-iodine solution. **Depending on the location of the foreign body, consider performing a posterior tibial or a sural nerve block. Augment this as needed with locally infiltrated buffered 1% lidocaine (Xylocaine).**

✓ The radiographs should reveal an approximate location of the needle relative to the paper clip skin marker.

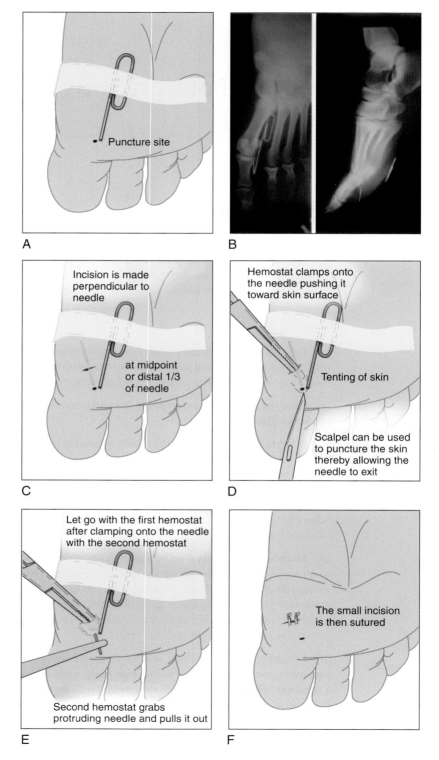

A

B

Incision is made perpendicular to needle

at midpoint or distal 1/3 of needle

Puncture site

C

Hemostat clamps onto the needle pushing it toward skin surface

Tenting of skin

Scalpel can be used to puncture the skin thereby allowing the needle to exit

D

Let go with the first hemostat after clamping onto the needle with the second hemostat

Second hemostat grabs protruding needle and pulls it out

E

The small incision is then sutured

F

Figure 148-1 Procedure for removing a needle from the foot.

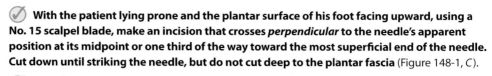

✓ **With the patient lying prone and the plantar surface of his foot facing upward, using a No. 15 scalpel blade, make an incision that crosses *perpendicular* to the needle's apparent position at its midpoint or one third of the way toward the most superficial end of the needle. Cut down until striking the needle, but do not cut deep to the plantar fascia** (Figure 148-1, *C*).

✓ **As the needle is cut across, there will be an audible clicking sound. Spread the incision apart, visualize the needle, and grasp it firmly with a hemostat or small Kelly clamp.**

✓ **Now push the needle out in the direction from which it entered. Even the eye or back end of a broken needle is sharp enough to be pushed to the skin surface.**

✓ **If the needle tents up the skin and will not push through, nick the overlying skin surface with a scalpel blade until the needle exits** (Figure 148-1, *D*). **Grab this end with another clamp, let go of the first clamp, and remove the needle** (Figure 148-1, *E*).

✓ Let the thigh cuff down, and suture the incision closed. Apply an appropriate dressing (Figure 148-1, *F*).

✓ Provide tetanus prophylaxis as indicated (see Appendix H).

What Not To Do:

✗ Do not pull on a thread that is hanging out of a puncture wound. It could potentially break off, leaving an infection-prone foreign body behind. The thread will come out with the needle if the described technique is used.

✗ Do not ignore the patient who thinks he stepped on a needle but in whom a puncture wound cannot be found. Obtain a radiograph anyway, because the puncture wound is probably hidden.

✗ Do not give the patient the impression that the removal will be quick and easy.

✗ Do not make the incision near the tip of the needle or directly over and parallel to the needle. The needle will not be exactly where it is thought to be, and the incision will very likely miss exposing the needle.

✗ **Do not persist in extensively undermining or extending the incision if the needle is not located within approximately 10 minutes of beginning the procedure. This is unlikely to be productive and may do the patient harm.**

✗ Do not routinely place the patient on prophylactic antibiotics.

Discussion

Many a young doctor has been found sweating away at the foot of an emergency department stretcher, unable to locate a needle foreign body. The secret for improving the chances of success is in realizing that the radiograph gives you only an approximate location of the needle and that the incision must be made in a direction and location best suited for locating the needle, not removing it.

There are three additional principles to keep in mind. First, the position of the needle on radiographs

(continued)

Discussion continued

needs to be correlated with the anatomy of the skin surface rather than the bony anatomy of the foot. Second is the simple geometric principle that the surest way to intersect a line (the needle) is to bisect it in the plane perpendicular to its midpoint. Third, the only structures of importance in the forefoot or heel that lie plantar to the bones are the flexor tendons, and they lie close to the bones.

Let the patient know how difficult it sometimes is to locate the needle and remove it; this can create a win-win situation: the clinician looks good if it is found and still looks experienced and well-informed if it is not found.

If the patient is taken to fluoroscopy, the clinician or radiologist can place a hemostat around the needle under a real time radiographic image. It can then be pushed out using the same technique described earlier. **Ultrasonography may be an alternative modality for localizing an underlying needle, but it is thought to be technically demanding and requires practice.**

Using the simple technique described, linear foreign bodies, such as needles, can be removed from the sole of the foot without extensive dissection, complex or cumbersome equipment, or repeated radiographic studies.

Suggested Readings

Blankenship RB, Baker T: Imaging modalities in wounds and superficial skin infections, *Emerg Med Clin North Am* 25:223–234, 2007.

Gilsdorf JR: A needle in the sole of the foot, *Surg Gynecol Obstet* 163:573–574, 1986.

Hegenbarth MA: Bedside ultrasound in the pediatric emergency department: basic skill or passing fancy? *Clin Pediatr Emerg Med* 5:201–216, 2004.

Lammers RL, Magill T: Detection and management of foreign bodies in soft tissue, *Emerg Med Clin North Am* 10:767–781, 1992.

Leidelmeyer R: The embedded broken-off needle, *JACEP* 5:362–363, 1976.

Paronychia

Presentation

The patient presents with finger or toe pain that has developed rapidly, either over the past several hours or over a few days. This pain is accompanied by a very red, tender swelling of the nail fold, or this swelling may be less red and tender and appear chronic in nature. There are three distinct varieties.

- Acute paronychia almost always involves fingers and usually quickly becomes very painful. It is caused by the introduction of pyogenic bacteria, either spontaneously or as a result of minor trauma, and results in acute inflammation and abscess formation within the thin subcutaneous layer between the skin of the eponychial fold and the germinal layer of the eponychial cul-de-sac (Figure 149-1, *A*). In its earliest form, there may only be cellulitis with no collection of pus. Fluctuance that may be difficult to detect, along with local purulence at the nail margin, may occur, and infection may extend beneath the nail margin to involve the nail bed.

- Chronic paronychia (Figure 149-1, *B*) is most commonly seen with an ingrown toenail, with chronic inflammation, thickening and purulence of the eponychial fold, and loss of the cuticle. The toenail edge may be embedded in the lateral nail fold. There may or may not be granulation tissue. This also occurs with individuals whose hands are frequently exposed to moisture and minor trauma.

- The third variety of paronychia is a subungual abscess, which occurs in the same location as a subungual hematoma and presents with pain and entrapped pus that is visible between the nail plate and the nail bed (Figure 149-1, *C*).

What To Do:

Acute Paronychia

 When there is minimal swelling and there appears to be only cellulitis, gently slide an 18-gauge needle parallel to and along the surface of the nail plate (with the bevel up) to separate and lift up the cuticle of the swollen lateral nail fold from the nail. Alternatively, use a large-gauge needle with the bevel down to elevate the lateral nail fold. When this separation or puncture of the cuticle occurs, pus will often unexpectedly drain from the eponychial cul-de-sac. (Digital block anesthesia may not be required, because you are only puncturing or separating epithelial cuticular tissue.) Instruct the patient to then soak the finger in warm antibacterial soap and water for 10 to 15 minutes at least four times per day. The patient can remain quite mobile if he uses a disposable cup to soak his finger while performing his daily routine.

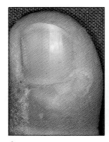

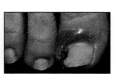

A Acute paronychia   B

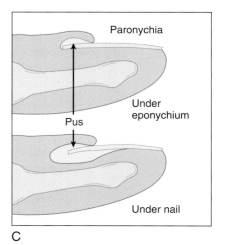

C

Figure 149-1 A, Acute paronychia of finger with red, hot, tender nail fold showing pus beneath the cuticle. **B,** Chronic paronychia with an ingrown toenail. **C,** Subungual extension of pus.

✓ **If no pus was obtained,** provide close follow-up and consider prescribing an antibiotic:

○ In uncomplicated cases, without likely oral flora exposure: cephalexin 250 to 500 mg qid × 7 days or dicloxacillin 250 to 500 mg qid × 7 days.

○ In cases involving more significant disease, or immunosuppression: amoxicillin/ clavulanate (Augmentin), 875 mg/125 mg bid or clindamycin (Cleocin), 300 mg qid × 7 days.

○ **In cases with suspected community-acquired methicillin-resistant *Staphylococcus aureus* (CA-MRSA):** trimethoprim-sulfamethoxazole, 1 to 2 double-strength tablet(s) bid × 7 days or clindamycin (Cleocin), 300 mg qid × 7 days.

✓ **When there is significant pain and swelling of the nail fold** (there may or may not be a visible overlying pustule), consider performing a digital block to prevent potential manipulative discomfort (see Appendix B). **Then, as above, slide an 18-gauge needle or a No. 15 scalpel blade along the surface of the nail plate (keep the blade flat against the nail) under the nail fold, separating or incising the cuticle and thereby opening the eponychial cul-de-sac and draining the pus** (Figure 149-2, *A*).

✓ There should be no deliberate invasion into the dermis (although there may be an inadvertent stick); therefore it may still be unnecessary to perform a digital block.

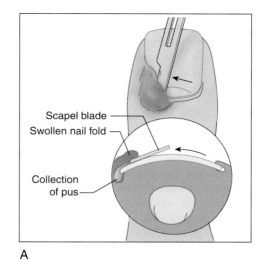

A

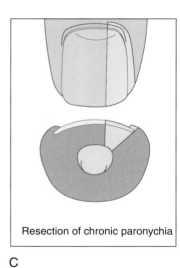

B   C

Figure 149-2 A, Draining acute paronychia without invasion of skin. **B,** A gauze wick may help to ensure continued drainage. **C,** Extensive excision of chronic paronychia.

✅ Although not necessary, a tiny wick (1 cm of ¼-inch plain gauze or a thin strip of nonadherent dressing) may be slid into the opening to help promote continued drainage (Figure 149-2, *B*).

✅ **Unroof and débride any periungual pustule.**

✅ **Most important, instruct the patient (as described above) to perform warm soaks for 10 to 15 minutes at least qid for 1 to 2 days.** He may apply ointment covered by a simple bandage between soaks.

✅ **When drainage has been provided, antibiotics are not routinely required, and cultures will not benefit the patient or change management, with several notable exceptions.** Exceptions include marked cellulitis, a condition of immunosuppression, possible CA-MRSA, and suspicion of unusual infections (*Pseudomonas* spp., fungal infections). In these special cases, prescribe antibiotics as discussed above. Follow-up should be provided within 2 to 3 days.

Chronic Paronychia

✅ **When symptoms and findings are minimal, consider conservative treatment or temporizing the condition by sliding a cotton wedge or waxed dental floss under the corner of an ingrown nail to lift the nail edge from its embedded position. (Anesthesia is usually not required.)** Instruct the patient to use warm soaks at least four times per day. When candidiasis is suspected, the area should be kept dry and treated with local applications of nystatin or a topical antifungal medication combined with a topical steroid (e.g., betamethasone 0.05% + clotrimazole 1% [Lotrisone] cream).

✅ **Follow-up with a podiatrist is important for ingrown toenails. Instruct the patient to cut toenails straight across to prevent recurrences. Recommend loose-fitting stockings and shoes with a roomy toe box.** Also, instruct the patient to decrease activities such as running or other sports that put pressure on the toes. **Inform him that it may take 3 months for an embedded toenail to grow beyond the lateral nail fold and that a cotton wedge must be repeatedly replaced until this occurs.**

✅ **When symptoms and findings are more extensive, a more aggressive approach— and one more likely to be successful—that requires a unilateral or bilateral digital block** (see Appendix B) **and a bloodless field (use a rubber tourniquet) is to sharply excise the affected portion of the nail, nail bed, and matrix down to the periosteum of the distal phalanx** (Figure 149-2, *C*). First cleanse the toe with an iodine-povidone solution, and then elevate the outer edge of the nail plate by inserting a fine straight hemostat under the nail. Excise approximately one quarter to one third of the nail plate with strong fine scissors to make a longitudinal cut; then pull it out from under the eponychium with the hemostat (Figure 149-3).

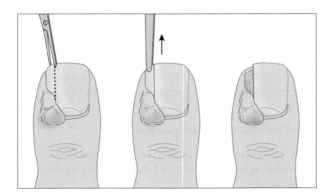

Figure 149-3 For more severe acute and chronic infections, removing a portion of the nail helps to prevent recurrence.

✓ **When only a small amount of granulation tissue is present after the nail plate is excised, the nail bed may be left in place and only the granulation tissue excised. The remaining granulation tissue can be cauterized using silver nitrate.** The patient is instructed to soak the toe in warm water for 20 minutes twice per day and arrange for multiple follow-up visits.

Subungual Abscess (When Pus Is Visible beneath the Nail)

✓ **Consider conservative treatment not requiring a digital block. Merely perform a trephination using the same "hot paper clip" technique used for a subungual hematoma** (see Chapter 156). **The patient must perform frequent warm soaks over the next 36 hours to prevent recurrence.**

✓ **A more aggressive approach, requiring digital block, is to excise a portion of the nail. Unlike the more extensive procedure used with chronic paronychia, only a portion of the nail plate need be removed** (see Figure 149-3). After performing a digital block, cleansing with iodine-povidone and performing a bloodless field, insert a fine straight hemostat between the nail and the nail bed, and push and spread until you enter the eponychial cul-de-sac. Often it is at this point that pus is discovered and released. Using a pair of strong fine scissors, cut away the one quarter to one third of the nail plate bordering the paronychia. Separate the cuticle using the hemostat, and pull this unwanted fragment away. **A nonadherent dressing is required over the exposed nail bed, as well as an early dressing change (within 24 hours). Frequent soaks are also required. Inform the patient that extensive damage to the germinal matrix by the infection may preclude healthy nail regrowth.**

✓ **When there is a distal collection of pus under the nail plate,** a simple excision of an overlying wedge of nail using scissors should provide complete drainage.

What Not To Do:

✗ Do not order cultures or radiographs for uncomplicated cases. However, remember that CA-MRSA is increasingly prevalent and may affect antibiotic choice if antibiotic therapy is indicated.

✗ Do not make an actual skin incision while treating acute paronychia. The cuticle needs only to be separated from the nail to release any collection of pus.

✗ Do not remove an entire fingernail or toenail to drain simple paronychia. The patient will be left with a very sensitive exposed nail bed unnecessarily.

✗ Do not attempt to drain a herpetic whitlow. When coalescing vesicles with surrounding erythema are present, assume that the infection is caused by herpes simplex virus. Treatment involves inhibition of viral replication with acyclovir (Zovirax), valacyclovir (Valtrex), or famciclovir (Famvir) (see Chapter 54).

✗ Do not confuse a felon (with a tense tender fingerpad) with a paronychia. Felons will require more extensive surgical treatment.

Discussion

Acute paronychia most commonly results from nail biting, finger sucking, aggressive manicuring, a hang nail, or penetrating trauma. **Most infections are minor and can be treated easily with conservative methods.** The more extensive the infection is, the more aggressive the surgical approach must be. Patients who have been adequately treated should be relatively asymptomatic within 3 to 5 days.

Ingrown toenails (onychocryptosis) occur most frequently in the early to midadolescent period. They tend to occur during periods of rapid foot growth when shoes get too tight. A precipitating event is usually cutting the nail at an angle to the sulcus. Subsequent growth causes a spicule of the nail, usually in the lateral sulcus, to penetrate the skin. This spicule introduces bacteria and infection into the surrounding tissue with formation of pus and granulation tissue.

Whenever conservative therapy is instituted, the patient should be advised of the advantages and disadvantages of that approach. If the patient is not willing or reliable enough to perform the required aftercare or cannot accept the potential treatment failure, it would seem prudent to begin with the more aggressive treatment modes.

No single antibiotic will provide complete coverage for the array of bacterial and fungal pathogens cultured from paronychias. In theory, amoxicillin/clavulanate clindamycin should be the most appropriate antibiotics, but because most paronychias are easily cured with simple drainage, systemic antibiotics are usually not indicated. **In immunocompromised patients, those with peripheral vascular disease, and those in whom unusual pathogens are suspected, cultures and antibiotics are indeed warranted.**

Remain alert to the possible complications of neglected paronychia, such as osteomyelitis, septic tenosynovitis of the flexor tendon, or a closed-space infection of the distal fingerpad (felon). Recurrent infections may be caused by a herpes simplex infection (herpetic whitlow) or fungus (onychomycosis). Tumors such as squamous cell carcinoma or melanoma, cysts, syphilitic chancres, warts, or foreign body granulomas can occasionally mimic paronychia.

Failure to cure paronychia within 4 or 5 days should prompt specialized culture techniques, biopsy, or referral.

Suggested Readings

Brook I: Paronychia: a mixed infection. Microbiology and management, *J Hand Surg Br* 18:358–959, 1993.

Clark DC: Common acute hand infections, *Am Fam Physician* 68:2167–2176, 2003.

Goldstein B, Goldstein A: *Paronychia and ingrown toenails.* [*UpToDate* website]. Available at http://www.uptodate.com. Accessed October, 2010.

Golladay ES: Outpatient adolescent surgical problems, *Adolesc Med Clin* 15:503–520, 2004.

Moran GJ, Talan DA: Hand Infections, *Emerg Med Clin North Am* 11:601–619, 1993.

Reyzelman AM, Trombello KA, Vayser DJ, et al: Are antibiotics necessary in the treatment of locally infected ingrown toenails? *Arch Fam Med* 9:930–932, 2000.

Rockwell PG: Acute and chronic paronychia, *Am Fam Physician* 63:1113–1116, 2001.

Rounding C, Hulm S: Surgical treatments for ingrowing toenails, *Cochrane Database Syst Rev* 2:CD001541, 2000.

Shaw J, Body R: Best evidence topic report. Incision and drainage preferable to oral antibiotics in acute paronychial infection? *Emerg Med J* 22:813–814, 2005.

Wilson R, Truesdell AG, Villines TC: Inflammatory lesions on every finger, *Am Fam Physician* 72:317–318, 2005.

Pencil Point Puncture

Presentation

The patient presents after being stabbed or stuck with a sharp pencil point. He may be openly or unconsciously worried about lead poisoning. A small puncture wound lined with graphite tattooing will be present (Figure 150-1). The pencil tip may or may not be present, visible, or palpable. If the puncture wound is palpated, an underlying pencil point may give the patient a foreign body sensation.

What To Do:

✔ **Reassure the patient or parent that there is no danger of lead poisoning. Pencil "leads" are made of clay and graphite, which is primarily carbon and nontoxic.**

✔ Conduct a full examination, including sensory and motor function of the affected area.

✔ Obtain a thorough history relating to the injury, and assess the patient's risk of developing complications, which are rare.

✔ **Palpate and inspect for a foreign body. If uncertain, obtain a radiograph or ultrasonogram to rule out the presence of a foreign body. Most often, there is no foreign body; there are only the embedded black graphite particles.**

✔ Administer local anesthesia if necessary; then thoroughly scrub the wound.

 ✔ **To reduce the amount of tattooing, the wound may be scraped (dermabraded) with the tip of a scalpel blade** (Figure 150-2). Always administer local anesthesia using lidocaine (1% with or without epinephrine) before scraping wound.

✔ **Warn the patient or family about signs of infection (increasing pain, redness, swelling, red streaking,) and inform them that there may be a permanent black tattoo that can be removed later if the resulting mark is cosmetically unacceptable** (Figure 150-3).

✔ **Administer tetanus prophylaxis, if necessary** (see Appendix H).

What Not To Do:

✘ Do not excise the entire wound on the initial visit.

✘ Do not prescribe prophylactic antibiotics, because these are not necessary.

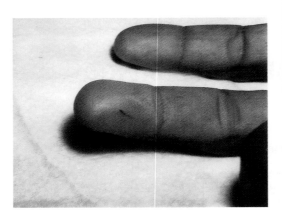

Figure 150-1 Acute pencil point puncture.

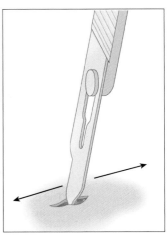

Figure 150-2 Dermabrade to reduce tattooing.

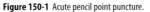

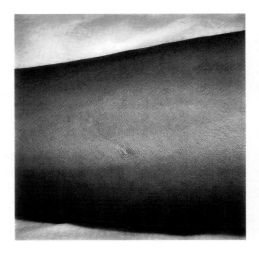

Figure 150-3 Residual tattoo from old pencil point puncture.

Discussion

It is unwise to excise the entire wound, because the resultant scar might be more unsightly than the tattoo. **If a superficial pencil tip foreign body exists,** see Chapter 154 for an easy removal technique. **Most of these wounds do not contain a foreign body but only the appearance of one. Tattoo prevention should be the clinician's primary concern.** If tattooing is present and of cosmetic concern, the patient may benefit from a referral to a dermatologist for removal.

Rarely, deep punctures or foreign bodies may require exploratory surgery in the operating room.

Suggested Reading

Baddour LM: *Overview of puncture wounds.* [*UpToDate* website]. Available at http://www.uptodate.com. Accessed August 2011.

Puncture Wounds

Presentation

Most commonly, the patient will have stepped or jumped onto a nail. There may be pain and swelling, but often the patient is only asking for a tetanus shot. He can usually be found in the emergency department with his foot soaking in a basin of povidone-iodine (Betadine) solution. The wound entrance usually appears as a linear or stellate tear in the cornified epithelium on the plantar surface of the foot.

What To Do:

✅ Obtain a detailed history to ascertain the time interval since injury, the force involved in creating the puncture (if possible), the estimated depth of penetration, and the relative cleanliness of the penetrating object. Also ascertain whether there was believed to be complete or partial removal of the object and if there is any residual foreign body sensation in the wound. Note the type of footwear (tennis or rubber-soled shoes) and the potential for foreign body retention. Also ask about tetanus immunization status and underlying health problems that may potentially diminish host defenses. (In multiple studies, diabetes has been associated with an increased incidence of infectious complications from plantar puncture wounds.)

✅ **Have the patient lie prone, backward on the gurney, so that raising the head of the bed flexes his knee and brings the sole of the foot into clear view.** Place the foot on a pillow. Clean the surrounding skin, and carefully inspect the wound. Provide good lighting, and take your time. Examine the foot for signs of deep injury, such as swelling and pain with passive motion of the toes. Although the occurrence is unlikely, test for loss of sensory or motor function.

✅ **If the puncture was created by a slender object, such as a sewing needle or thumb tack that is verified to have been removed intact, no further treatment is necessary. If there is any question that a piece may have broken off in the tissue, obtain radiographs** (see Chapter 148).

✅ Most metal and glass foreign bodies are visualized on plain films, whereas plastic, aluminum, rubber fragments, thorns, spines, and wood are more radiolucent and may require ultrasonography, a CT scan, or MRI for visualization. Retained foreign bodies increase the potential for infection and should be suspected in patients who present with infection, who are not responding to treatment for infection, who have inordinate pain, who believe that there is a foreign body in their wound, or who have a foreign body sensation when the puncture wound is palpated. These foreign bodies must be removed (see Chapter 154).

✅ With deep, highly contaminated wounds, orthopedic or podiatric consultation should be sought. With the most serious of these wounds, consideration should be given to providing a wide débridement in the operating room. This is done to prevent the catastrophic complication of osteomyelitis. Although controversial, deep wounds such as these may be considered for treatment with a prophylactic antibiotic.

✅ **If there was a deep puncture through a rubber-soled sport shoe, it may be reasonable (although not proven) to use a quinolone, such as levofloxacin (Levaquin), for 3 to 4 days, or, in children, cefuroxime axetil (Ceftin, Zinacef) to cover for** *Pseudomonas.*

✅ **Most superficial puncture wounds require only simple débridement, possibly with irrigation. In these wounds, prophylactic antibiotics are not indicated.**

✅ The plantar surface of the foot is exceedingly well innervated, and even simple débridement is likely to be painful. In appropriate circumstances and depending on the location of the injury/foreign body, consider performing a posterior tibial or a sural nerve block.

✅ **Saucerize (shave) the puncture wound using a No. 10 scalpel blade to remove the surrounding cornified epithelium and any debris that has collected beneath its surface** (Figure 151-1, *A* and *B*). Alternatively, the jagged cornified epidermal skin edges overlying the puncture tract may be painlessly trimmed using a scalpel or scissors.

✅ **If debris is found, remove what is visible and then gently slide a large-gauge blunt needle or an over-the-needle (Angiocath) catheter down the wound track and slowly irrigate with a physiologic saline solution, moving the catheter in and out until debris no longer flows from the wound** (Figure 151-1, *C* and *D*). If the puncture wound is small and there is little room for effluent to exit, make a stab wound with a No. 15 blade through the dermis to enlarge the opening and allow the effluent to more easily escape.

✅ **Provide tetanus prophylaxis** (see Appendix H).

✅ Cover the wound with a Band-Aid and instruct the patient regarding the warning signs of infection.

✅ Arrange for follow-up at 48 hours. Spend some time on documentation and patient education. **Talk about delayed osteomyelitis and the importance of medical attention if there is continued aching or discomfort 1 to 2 weeks postinjury. Explain that even with proper care, foreign material may be embedded deeply in the wound, and infection could occur. Explain that in most cases, prophylactic antibiotics do not prevent these infections and that the best practice is close observation and aggressive therapy if infection occurs.**

✅ **Patients presenting 24 hours postinjury will often have an established wound infection. In addition to the débridement procedures described, patients who have an early infection usually respond quickly to an oral antistaphylococcal antibiotic, such as clindamycin (Cleocin), if they do not have a retained foreign body. Always suspect retained foreign bodies, and strongly consider imaging studies for all infected wounds that do not respond to antibiotics.**

✅ Provide patients with crutches for non–weight bearing, and encourage them to soak the infected foot.

✅ Consider hospitalization for patients with severe infection or who have risk factors for serious complications (e.g., diabetes, peripheral vascular disease, immune suppression).

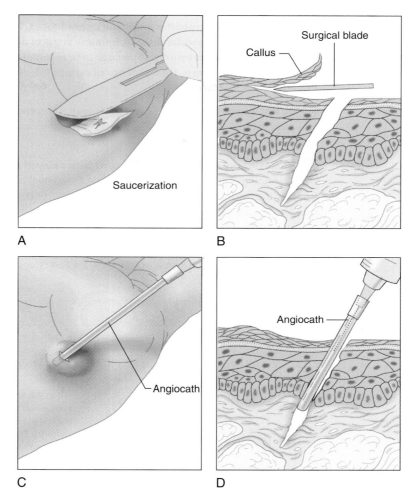

Figure 151-1 Simple débridement and irrigation for puncture wounds.

What Not To Do:

Ⓧ Do not be falsely reassured by having the patient soak in Betadine. This does not provide any significant protection from infection and is not a substitute for débridement and irrigation.

Ⓧ Do not attempt a jet lavage within a puncture wound. This will only lead to subcutaneous infiltration of irrigant and the possible spread of foreign material and bacteria.

Ⓧ Do not perform blind probing of a deep puncture wound. This is not likely to be of any value and may do harm.

Ⓧ Do not obtain radiographs for simple nail punctures, except for the unusual case in which large radiopaque particulate debris is suspected to be deeply embedded within the wound or the physical examination suggests bony injury.

(X) **Do not routinely prescribe prophylactic antibiotics. Reserve them for patients with diabetes, peripheral vascular disease, immune suppression, or deep, highly contaminated wounds. In fact, there is insufficient evidence to recommend the use of prophylactic antimicrobials to decrease the incidence of serious infections in any of these puncture wounds.**

(X) **Do not ignore the patient who returns with a recurrent infection.** If antibiotics fail to cure an initial wound infection, suspect a retained foreign body; obtain an ultrasonogram, CT scan, or MRI; and consult an appropriate foot surgeon.

(X) **Do not ignore the patient who returns with delayed foot pain,** even if there are minimal physical findings and radiographs are negative. Osteomyelitis may present weeks or even months after the initial injury. These patients demand special imaging to rule out a retained foreign body, and an erythrocyte sedimentation rate (ESR) and C-reactive protein (CRP) should be obtained. These patients should then be referred to a surgical foot specialist for a bone scan or MRI and, if there is evidence of bone infection, surgical débridement.

(X) Do not begin soaks at home, unless there are early signs of developing infection.

Discussion

The most common sites for puncture wounds are the feet. The complication rate from plantar puncture wounds is higher than the rate for puncture wounds elsewhere in the body (with the exception of the hands). One reason is the small distance from the plantar skin surface to bones and joints of the feet. Another is the force with which puncture wounds are inflicted when the weight of the body pushes against a sharp object. Additionally, penetration of a shoe and stocking by a nail (or other sharp object) can push foreign bodies into the deepest recesses of the wound. These foreign bodies are rarely seen on plain radiographs.

Small, clean, superficial puncture wounds uniformly do well. The pathophysiology and management of a puncture wound, therefore, depend on the material that punctured the foot, the location of the wound, the depth of penetration, the time to presentation, the footwear penetrated, whether there is an indoor versus a more infection-prone outdoor injury, and the underlying health status of the victim. Punctures in the metatarsophalangeal joint area may also be of higher risk for serious wound complications because of the greater likelihood of penetration of joint, tendon, or bone. Early presenters tend to be children or adults seeking tetanus prophylaxis. These patients tend to have a low incidence of infection. Patients who present late usually have increasing pain, swelling, or drainage as evidence of an early or established infection. Unsuspected retained foreign bodies, often pieces of a tennis shoe or sock, are a source of serious infection. Other common foreign bodies include rust, gravel, grass, straw, and dirt.

When the foot is punctured, the cornified epithelium acts as a spatula, cleaning off any loose material from the penetrating object as it slides by. This debris often collects just beneath this cornified layer, which then acts like a trap door, holding it in. Left in place, this debris may lead to early abscess formation, cellulitis, and lymphangitis. Saucerization allows the removal of debris and the unroofing of superficial small foreign bodies or abscesses found beneath the thickly cornified skin surfaces.

There are many different ways to manage plantar puncture wounds. There are very few scientific data to support any one universal standard of care. Some physicians are very conservative in their approach, whereas others advocate liberal use of radiographs, prophylactic antibiotics, and aggressive débridement procedures that include removing a core of tissue the length of the puncture wound. Some believe that irrigation of deep puncture wounds is futile because the irrigant solution does not completely drain out of the wound. The approach presented here is reasonable and rational, given the data that are available at this time. **Because there is no clear evidence supporting either a conservative or**

Discussion continued

an aggressive approach, it is wise to get your patient involved in the decision-making process, and to ensure close follow-up, regardless of the approach.

Puncture wounds of the foot reportedly have an overall infection rate as high as 15%. The probability of wound infection is increased with deeper penetrating injuries, delayed presentation (>24 hours), gross contamination, penetration through a rubber-soled shoe, outdoor injuries, injuries that occur from the neck of the metatarsals to the web space of the toes, and decreased resistance to infection. **Specifically, diabetic patients typically present for care later and have higher rates of osteomyelitis (up to 35%). In one study, they were also 5 times more likely to require multiple operations and 46 times more likely to have a lower extremity amputation as a result of a plantar puncture wound.**

Joint puncture wounds have the potential to penetrate the joint capsule and produce septic arthritis. Penetration of bone and periosteum can produce osteomyelitis.

Osteomyelitis caused by *Pseudomonas aeruginosa* remains the most devastating of puncture wound complications. The exact incidence of osteomyelitis remains uncertain and is estimated to be between 0.04% and 0.5% in plantar puncture wounds. The metatarsal heads are most at risk for osteomyelitis. A nail through the sole of a tennis or sport shoe is known to inoculate *Pseudomonas* organisms. Any patient who is considered to have penetration of the bone, joint space, or plantar fascia, particularly over the metatarsal heads, should be warned of the potential for serious infection and then referred to an orthopedic surgeon or podiatrist for early follow-up evaluation.

Suggested Readings

Armstrong DG, Lavery LA, Quebedeaux TL, Walker SC: Surgical morbidity and the risk of amputation due to infected puncture wounds in diabetic versus nondiabetic adults, *South Med J* 90:384–389, 1997.

Chisholm CD, Schlesser JF: Plantar puncture wounds: controversies and treatment recommendations, *Ann Emerg Med* 18:1352–1357, 1989.

Chudnofsky CR, Sebastian S: Special wounds. Nail bed, plantar puncture, and cartilage, *Emerg Med Clin North Am* 10:801–822, 1992.

Fitzgerald RH, Cowan JDE: Puncture wounds of the foot, *Orthop Clin North Am* 6:965–972, 1975.

Patzakis MJ, Wilkins J, Brien WW, et al: Wound site as a predictor of complications following deep nail punctures to the foot, *West J Med* 150:545–547, 1989.

Pennycook A, Makower R, O'Donnell AM: Puncture wounds of the foot: can infective complications be avoided? *J Roy Soc Med* 87:581–583, 1994.

Raz R, Miron D: Oral ciprofloxacin for treatment of infection following nail puncture wounds of the foot, *Clin Infect Dis* 21:194–195, 1995.

Schwab RA, Powers RD: Conservative therapy of plantar puncture wounds, *J Emerg Med* 13:291–295, 1995.

Verdile VP, Freed HA, Gerard J: Puncture wounds to the foot, *J Emerg Med* 7:193–199, 1987.

Ring Removal

Presentation

A ring has become tight on the patient's finger after an injury (usually a sprain of the proximal interphalangeal [PIP] joint) or after some other cause of swelling, such as a local reaction to a bee sting. Sometimes, chronic tight-fitting rings begin to obstruct lymphatic drainage, causing swelling and further constriction (Figure 152-1). The patient usually wants the ring removed even if it requires cutting the ring off, but occasionally, a patient has a very personal attachment to the ring and objects to its cutting or removal.

What To Do:

✅ Immediately recognize vascular insufficiency, amputation, motor or sensory compromise, and other important injuries distal to the ring.

✅ Limit further swelling by applying ice and elevating the extremity.

✅ **When a fracture is suspected, order appropriate radiographs, either before or after removing the ring.**

✅ With substantial injuries, a digital or, preferably, a metacarpal block might be necessary to allow comfortable removal of the ring.

 ✅ **In most cases, lubrication with soap and water or a water-soluble lubricant, along with proximal traction on the skin (thereby drawing the skin taut beneath the ring), is enough to help the ring twist off the finger** (Figure 152-2). Grasping the ring after covering it with a gauze sponge may give you greater traction. **A large, threaded metal nut can simply be unscrewed after lubricating the finger.**

✅ **If this simple method is not successful, consider several other techniques that preserve the ring. (With rare exceptions, these techniques can be performed with 2.0 to 3.0 silk, umbilical tape, Penrose drains, phlebotomy tourniquets, or other similar available items.)**

 ○ **Exsanguination of the digit: Exsanguinate the finger by applying a tightly wrapped spiral of Penrose drain or flat rubber phlebotomy tourniquet tape around the exposed portion of the finger, elevate the hand above the head, wait 15 minutes, and then inflate a blood pressure cuff to 50 to 75 mm Hg above the patient's systolic pressure as a tourniquet around the upper arm above the exsanguinated finger** (Figure 152-3). Wrap the cuff with cotton cast padding to keep the Velcro connection from separating, and clamp the tubing to prevent a slow air leak. **Remove the tight rubber wrapping from the finger, and, leaving the**

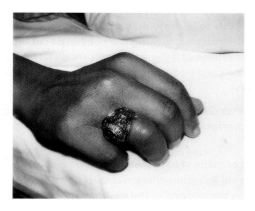

Figure 152-1 Tight-fitting ring with secondary lymphatic obstruction and swelling.

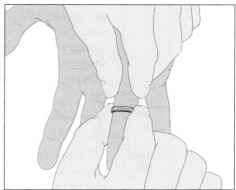

Figure 152-2 Pull skin taut and twist ring off.

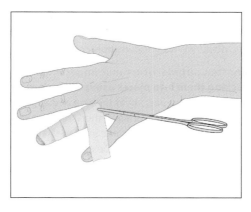

Figure 152-3 Tourniquet technique.

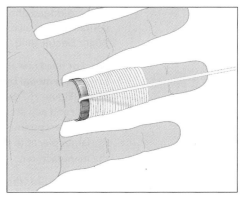

Figure 152-4 String technique.

arm tourniquet in place and inflated, again attempt to twist the ring off using lubrication. If necessary, this procedure may be repeated several times until the swelling is adequately reduced.

○ **String wrap or string pull technique:** A technique that tends to be rather time consuming and only moderately effective (but one that can be readily attempted in the field) is the **string wrap or coiled-string technique.** Slip the end of a string (kite string is good) under the ring and wind a tight single-layer coil down the finger, compressing the swelling as you go. Pull up on the end of the string under the ring; then slide and wiggle the ring down over the coil (see Figure 152-4).

○ **Another associated technique is to pull a length of string under the ring using a hemostat and then tie it into a large loop that can be placed around the clinician's wrist.** This will allow traction to be applied, and the string will slide around and around the circumference of the ring as it is pulled, using lubricant, as mentioned previously. A small lubricated Penrose drain may be substituted for string (see Figure 152-5).

✅ **If the ring is still unable to be removed with these techniques, and there is the potential for vascular compromise, the ring will need to be cut off. (Also, cut the ring if the patient endorses this approach or if there is significant distal injury or too much pain with the other techniques.)** Inform the patient that a jeweller should be able to repair the band after removal.

✅ **A standard ring cutter can be used to cut through a narrow ring band. Bend the ring apart with pliers or hemostats placed on either side of this "saw cut" to allow removal** (Figure 152-6).

✅ **If the band is wide or made of hard metal, it will be much easier to cut out a 5-mm wedge from the ring using an orthopedic pin cutter** (Figure 152-7, *A*). **Take a cast spreader, place it in the slot left by the removal of the wedge, and spread the ring open** (Figure 152-7, *B*). Alternatively, two cuts may be made on opposite sides of the ring, allowing it to be removed in halves.

✅ Another useful device for removing constricting metal bands is the Dremel Moto-Tool, with its sharp-edged grinder attachment. Protect the underlying skin with a heat-resistant shield. If a dental drill is available, it can also cut steel. Motorized commercial ring cutters are also available (Vigor Electric Ring Cutter, http://www.rainbowsupply.com).

✅ **For hard metal (tungsten carbide) or ceramic finger rings that cannot be twisted off, attempt removal by cracking them into pieces using a standard vice grip–style locking pliers** (Figure 152-8). Place the locking pliers over the ring and adjust the jaws to clamp lightly. Release and adjust the tightener one-third turn and then clamp again. Repeat until a crack is heard; then continue clamping in different positions until the hard material breaks away. Return the larger pieces to the patient, because they may be able to receive a replacement ring from the manufacturer.

✅ **For a child who sticks a finger into a round hole in a plastic toy, sports helmet, or other plastic product and becomes entrapped, release the finger by first cutting around the hole using a standard orthopedic cast cutter.** This will allow the patient's finger to be released from the large plastic object, leaving a plastic ring around the patient's freed finger. This smaller object can now be removed using any of the earlier techniques or by just protecting the underlying skin and using the cast cutter to cut this plastic ring in half.

What Not To Do:

❌ Do not insist that a ring must be cut off when a patient requests that the ring not be removed, if the patient is expected to have only transient swelling of the hand or finger and there is no evidence of any vascular compromise of the affected finger. If the patient is vigilant and reliable, he can be warned of the signs of vascular compromise (pallor, cyanosis, pain, and/or increased finger swelling) and instructed to keep his hand elevated above the level of his heart and to apply cool compresses. He should then be made to understand that he is to return for further care if the circulation becomes compromised, because of the possible risk of losing his finger. Be understanding, and document the patient's requests and the directions given to him.

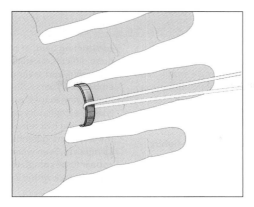

Figure 152-5 String-loop technique.

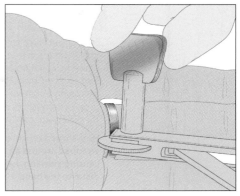

Figure 152-6 Ring-cutter technique.

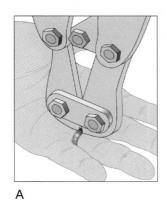

A

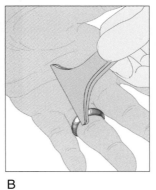

B

Figure 152-7 A and **B,** Orthopedic pin-cutter technique.

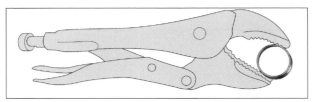

A

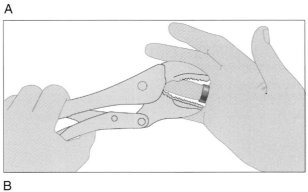

B

Figure 152-8 A and **B,** Vice grip–style locking pliers are used to crack tungsten carbide or ceramic rings. (Adapted from Hajduk SV: Letter to the editor: emergency removal of hard metal or ceramic finger rings. *Ann Emerg Med* 37:736, 2001.)

Discussion

The constricting effects of a circumferential foreign body can lead to obstruction of lymphatic drainage, which, in turn, leads to more swelling and further constriction. Eventually, venous and arterial circulation is compromised. If it is believed that these consequences are inevitable, be direct with the patient about having the ring removed.

Hair-thread tourniquets can become tightly wrapped around an infant's finger, toe, or penis, causing swelling, ischemia, or discoloration distal to the band (Figure 152-9). **Removing this** constricting band of one or more fibers can be quite difficult. It usually requires local anesthesia, dissection, and severing of the deeply embedded fibers with a large-gauge needle and magnifying loupes. Another technique is to use lysis by a depilatory agent, such as Nair or Neet. By applying hair remover to the hair tourniquet, the constricting bands may be lysed within 10 to 15 minutes. Even when the constricting bands appear to be completely released, provide for a wound check within 24 hours.

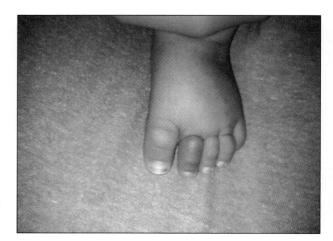

Figure 152-9 Hair tourniquet with distal venous and lymphatic engorgement on the second toe of a toddler.

Suggested Readings

Bothner J: *Ring removal techniques*. [*UpToDate* website]. Available at http://www.uptodate.com. Accessed October 2010.

Chiu TF, Chu SJ, Chen SG, et al: Use of a Penrose drain to remove an entrapped ring from a finger under emergent conditions, *Am J Emerg Med* 25:722–723, 2007.

Cresap CR: Removal of a hardened steel ring from an extremely swollen finger, *Am J Emerg Med* 13:318–320, 1995.

Greenspan L: Tourniquet syndrome caused by metallic bands: a new tool for removal, *Ann Emerg Med* 11:375–378, 1982.

Stone DB, Levine MR: Foreign body removal. In Roberts JR, Hedges JR, editors: *Roberts and Hedges clinical procedures in emergency medicine*, ed 5, Philadelphia, 2010, WB Saunders, pp 648–652.

Sliver, Superficial

(Splinter)

Presentation

The patient has caught himself on a sharp splinter (usually wooden) and either cannot grasp it, has broken it trying to remove it, or has found that it is too large and painful to remove. The history may be somewhat obscure. On examination, a puncture wound should be found with a tightly embedded sliver that may or may not be palpable over its entire length (Figure 153-1, *A*). There may only be a puncture wound without a clearly visible or palpable foreign body.

What To Do:

✓ Obtain a careful history. Find out if the patient has any foreign body sensation. Be suspicious of all puncture wounds (especially on the foot) that have been caused by a wooden object.

✓ **If it is unclear whether a wooden foreign body is beneath the skin, order a high-resolution ultrasound (US) study using a linear array transducer that focuses in the near field-of-view. A 7.5- or 10-MHz probe is used to search for small superficial objects, whereas a 5.0-MHz probe is recommended for larger, deeper objects** (Figure 153-2). Most of the literature regarding US detection of foreign bodies involves superficial objects, and there is a concern that sensitivity is reduced with deeper foreign bodies, as well as with lower frequency probes. CT scanning can be used to detect deep wooden foreign bodies that are less than 24 hours old when ultrasonography has failed; radiation and cost are considerable with this modality. MRI is the most costly imaging study, but it is the most sensitive.

✓ **If the sliver is visible or easily palpated, locally infiltrate with 1% lidocaine (Xylocaine) with epinephrine, and clean the skin with povidone-iodine solution. (Inserting the needle through the entrance wound will avoid the pain of a needle stick through the dermis.) With proper lighting, and using a No. 15 scalpel blade, cut down over the entire length of the sliver, completely exposing it. The sliver can now be easily lifted out and completely removed. Cleanse the open track with normal saline or 1% povidone-iodine on a gauze sponge** (Figure 153-3). Débride contaminated tissue if necessary. This superficial wound (see Figure 153-1, *B*) can now be easily closed using wound-closure strips or tissue adhesive. Avoid sutures when possible, especially absorbable, buried sutures, because of the increased risk for infection.

✓ **A more vertical splinter should be approached in the same manner, but the incision will be straight down along the length of the sliver as deep as possible, thereby releasing the entire foreign body from the surrounding tissue. Be careful not to incise any important anatomic structures, such as nerves, vessels, or tendons.**

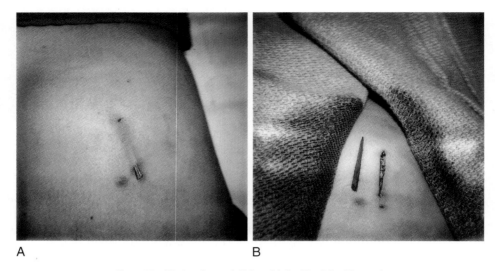

Figure 153-1 Wooden splinter in child's buttock before **(A)** and after **(B)** removal.

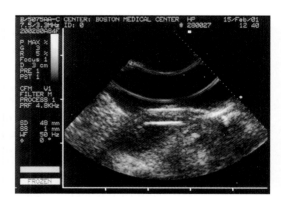

Figure 153-2 Ultrasonogram of the hand with a wooden toothpick in the superficial soft tissue. (Courtesy A. Dewitz, MD, Boston Medical Center, Boston.)

✓ **When a sliver is lost under the dermis but is still palpable, anesthetize the skin in the usual manner, but first establish a bloodless field. Inform the patient that it is often difficult to find such a splinter under the skin ("like a needle in a haystack") and that you will limit your search to about 10 to 15 minutes because further exploration may cause harm.**

✓ **Attempt to stabilize the palpable foreign body with the fingers of your nondominant hand while you cut down on the most superficial point of the sliver with a No. 15 scalpel blade until it is exposed.** Always be cognizant of potential anatomic structures that must be avoided. When the splinter is exposed, grab it with plain forceps and release it from the surrounding tissue by cutting down on as much of its length as necessary to free it up.

✓ **When a sliver is lost under the dermis and cannot be palpated or located using this technique, it can be managed in one of two ways. Small organic foreign bodies that are not embedded in the deep tissues of the hand or foot (or any other high-risk**

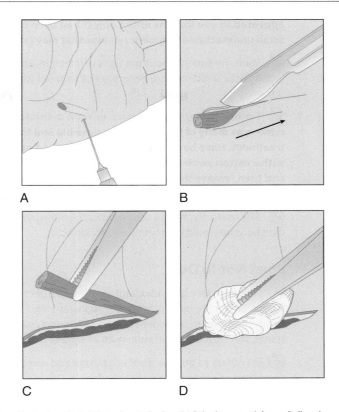

Figure 153-3 A, Inject with a local anesthetic. **B,** Incise down to the sliver. **C,** Lift the sliver out with forceps. **D,** Clean the wound track with a wet gauze sponge.

location) and clean inert foreign bodies (such as small metallic fragments) can be left in place and treated expectantly. They will either heal over without consequence or, as with most organic foreign bodies, form an abscess that can be drained, thereby releasing the foreign body. These patients should initially be placed on an antibiotic, such as cephalexin (Keflex), and fully informed of the risks, as well as being included in the decision-making process.

✅ **Alternatively, these patients can have the foreign body removed by a clinician who is skilled in ultrasound-guided techniques.**

✅ Patients who have larger organic foreign bodies or foreign bodies located in high-risk areas or patients who are at high risk for infectious complications (e.g., diabetes, peripheral vascular disease, other immunocompromised condition) must have these foreign bodies removed as soon as possible using the ultrasound-guided technique.

✅ Give tetanus prophylaxis, if necessary (see Appendix H).

✅ **Even after the foreign body has been found and removed, be cautious about telling the patient that the splinter has been entirely removed. Inform him that although it**

appeared to you that the entire object had been removed, there is always a chance that a small undetectable fragment remains that may later cause infection.

✓ Warn the patient about the signs of infection, and schedule a 48-hour wound check. Prophylactic antibiotics are generally not required when the sliver is thought to be completely removed.

✓ **For fine cactus spines, briars, or even multiple small splinters, use fine forceps to remove as many of these slivers as possible and then send the patient home to complete treatment. Have him apply nontoxic household glue (such as Elmer's Glue, not Krazy Glue) with a cotton swab and top it with a single layer of gauze. Instruct him to let the glue dry and then remove the gauze and glue. The spines or briars will usually come out with the gauze.**

✓ **Alternatively,** he can use blackhead removal strips (e.g., Bioré) following the same directions he would use to remove blackheads.

What Not To Do:

✗ Do not order plain radiographs unless a suspected sliver is made of glass or metal. Wooden foreign bodies are radiolucent. After approximately 1 day of absorbing water from adjacent tissue, they tend to be isodense on CT scanning as well. In addition, cactus and sea urchin spines, thorns, plastic, and aluminum all tend to be difficult to visualize on plain radiographs.

✗ Do not try to pull the sliver out by one end unless you feel confident that the material it is composed of will not fragment or be friable. Otherwise, it is likely to break and leave a fragment behind or leave a trail of debris.

✗ Do not try to locate a foreign body in a bloody field.

✗ Do not make an incision across a neurovascular bundle, tendon, or other important structure.

✗ Do not attempt to remove a deep, poorly localized foreign body. Those cases may require referral to a surgeon for removal in the operating room (OR), perhaps with fluoroscopic or ultrasound guidance.

✗ Do not rely entirely on ultrasonography to rule out the possibility of a retained foreign body. There can be false-negative examinations. When there is a high index of suspicion that a foreign body is present, MRI is the most sensitive imaging study.

✗ Do not be lulled into a false sense of security because the patient thinks the entire sliver has already been removed. Although a foreign body sensation is moderately specific, it is not sensitive enough to be definitive.

Discussion

Wood, glass, and metallic splinters are among the most common retained foreign bodies. Most superficial splinters may be removed by the patients themselves, leaving to physicians and other clinicians only the deeper and larger splinters or retained splinters that have broken off during an attempt at removal.

The most common error in the management of soft tissue foreign bodies is failure to detect their presence. Signs and symptoms of a hidden foreign body might include sharp pain or a foreign body sensation with palpation over the puncture wound, dark discoloration beneath the skin, a palpable mass beneath the skin, or a patient's suspicion that a foreign body is present. An organic foreign body is almost certain to create an inflammatory response and become infected if any part of it is left beneath the skin. It is for this reason, along with the fact that wooden slivers tend to be friable and may break apart during removal, that complete exposure is generally necessary before the sliver can be taken out.

There are no controlled studies that clearly identify which splinter removal technique works best under which conditions. Therefore, under certain circumstances, it may be perfectly reasonable to simply pull out a sliver without exposing it fully, as demonstrated. Of course, very small and superficial slivers can be removed by loosening them and picking them out with a No. 18-gauge needle, again avoiding the more elaborate techniques previously described.

When only the outer skin layers are involved, reassuring the patient, gently manipulating the wound, and incising the overlying epidermis with the needle can usually obviate the need for anesthesia.

If the foreign body is thought to be relatively superficial but cannot be located, explain to the patient that more harm may be caused by exploring and excising further. The splinter will be watched until it forms a "pus pocket," thus making it more easily removed at a later time. If this procedure is followed, it should always be coordinated with a follow-up clinician. The patient should be placed on an antibiotic, such as cephalexin (Keflex), and provided with follow-up care within 48 hours. These retained foreign bodies may also become encapsulated within granulation tissue and can be removed at a much later date. The patient should be so informed.

When making an incision over a foreign body, always take the underlying anatomic structures into consideration. Never make an incision if there is any chance that a neurovascular bundle, tendon, or other important structure may be severed or incised.

When a patient returns after being treated for a puncture wound, and there is evidence of nonhealing or recurrent exacerbations of inflammation, infection, or drainage, assume that the wound still contains a foreign body, begin antibiotics, get appropriate imaging studies, and refer him for surgical consultation.

Suggested Readings

Blankenship RB, Baker T: Imaging modalities in wounds and superficial skin infections, *Emerg Med Clin North Am* 25:223–234, 2007.

Chan C, Salam GA: Splinter removal, *Am Fam Physician* 67:2557–2562, 2003.

Lammers RL, Magill T: Detection and management of foreign bodies in soft tissue, *Emerg Med Clin North Am* 10:767–781, 1992.

Reynolds RD: Letter to the editor: removing splinters should be a very simple procedure, *Am Fam Physician* 69:2525, 2004.

Salam GA: Letter to the editor: removing splinters should be a very simple procedure, *Am Fam Physician* 69:2528, 2004.

Tibbles CD, Porcaro W: Procedural applications of ultrasound, *Emerg Med Clin North Am* 22:797–815, 2004.

Subcutaneous Foreign Bodies

(Metal, Dental Fragments, Glass, Gravel, and Hard Plastic)

CHAPTER 154

Presentation

Small, moderate-velocity metal fragments can be released when a hammer strikes a second piece of metal, such as a chisel. The patient has noticed a stinging sensation and a small puncture wound or bleeding site and is worried that there might be something inside. A BB projectile will produce a more obvious but very similar problem. Another mechanism for producing hard radiopaque foreign bodies is puncturing with glass shards, especially by stepping on glass fragments or receiving them in a motor vehicle collision. Falling onto gravel can also force sharp fragments under the skin through a small puncture wound. Physical findings will show a puncture wound and may show an underlying dark discoloration or a palpable foreign body (FB).

What To Do:

✓ **Be suspicious of a retained foreign body in all wounds produced by a high-velocity missile or sharp fragile object. The most common error in the management of soft tissue foreign bodies is failure to detect their presence.** (Retained foreign bodies are responsible for 14% of lawsuits and 5% of legal settlements.)

✓ Obtain a thorough mechanism of injury history, and determine if the patient suspects that there is a foreign body in the wound or has a foreign body sensation. A high index of suspicion for occult foreign bodies is advised in cases of seizure, syncope, abuse, and assault, as well as in self-inflicted wounds.

✓ Examine the wound, inspecting it and palpating over any puncture, looking for discoloration, inordinate pain, or the sensation of an underlying object (by either the patient or the examiner).

✓ **When there is any suspicion of an underlying FB, obtain radiographs of the wound to document its presence and location. If there is any possibility that the FB may be radiolucent (such as wood, plastic, aluminum, plant thorns, or spines), ultrasonography or CT scanning must be used to rule out an underlying object** (see Chapter 153). CT should also be used to locate or rule out FBs located in potentially dangerous sites (such as intraorbital or intraocular).

✓ **Clearly visible and palpable embedded objects, such as windshield glass in the forehead or gravel in a knee, can usually be grasped with fine, smooth forceps and simply picked out of the puncture wound.**

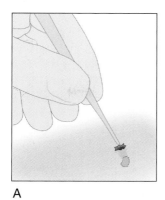
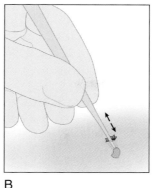

A   B

Figure 154-1 A, Puncture wound. **B,** Fan probe until foreign body is struck.

✓ **When the FB is lost down a narrow tract and is not visible, a different approach is required.**

✓ Explain to the patient how difficult it often is to remove a small metal fleck that is stuck in or under the skin. Inform him that often these are left in without any problem (like shrapnel injuries).

✓ **For all small, hard, inert FBs, inform the patient that a simple technique will be attempted but that to avoid more damage, the search will not extend beyond 10 to 15 minutes.**

 ✓ If the FB is in an extremity, it is preferable, and sometimes essential, to establish a bloodless field. For all cases, provide optimal lighting conditions and arrange comfortable positioning of both the patient and the clinician.

✓ **Anesthetize the area with a *small* infiltration of 1% or 20% lidocaine (Xylocaine) with epinephrine (to avoid tissue swelling).**

 ✓ **Take a blunt stiff metal probe (not a needle), and gently slide it down the apparent track of the puncture wound. Move the probe back and forth, fanning it in all directions, until a clicking contact between the probe and the foreign body can be felt and heard. This should be repeated several times, until it is certain that contact is being made with the foreign body** (Figure 154-1).

✓ **After contact is made, fix the probe in place by resting the hand that is holding the probe against a firm surface. Then, with the other hand, cut down along the probe with a No. 15 scalpel blade until the foreign body is reached. Do not remove the probe** (Figure 154-2).

✓ **Reach into the incision with a pair of forceps, using the opposite hand, and remove the foreign body (located at the end of the probe)** (Figure 154-3).

✓ Close the wound loosely with strip closures or tissue adhesive.

✓ If the foreign body is very superficial and easily palpable beneath the skin, it may be advantageous to eliminate the probe and just cut down directly over the foreign body while stabilizing it between the fingers of your nondominant hand.

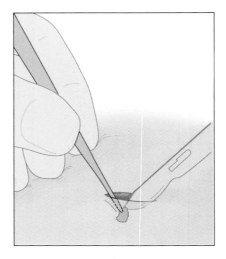

Figure 154-2 Cut down probe to foreign body.

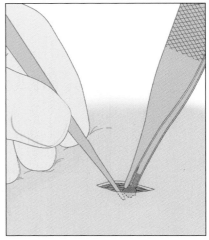

Figure 154-3 Foreign body removed with forceps while probe remains in contact with it.

✓ **If the entrance wound is large, the probe may not be required. Instead, a hemostat may be inserted using a spreading technique to search for and then remove the foreign body. A small puncture may be enlarged** by using a No. 15 blade to make a stab wound into the opening of the puncture.

✓ Provide tetanus prophylaxis (see Appendix H).

✓ **Warn the patient about the signs of a developing infection.**

✓ If the foreign body cannot be located in approximately 15 minutes, inform the patient of the various possibilities: in the case of a nonimmunogenic, small FB (like a metal fleck), the wound will probably heal without complications. Alternately, a more immunogenic or larger foreign body may migrate to the skin surface over a period of months or years, at which time it can be more easily removed. If an abscess should form, this may make removal of the FB easier with drainage of the abscess cavity. Should the wound or surrounding structures become infected, antibiotics may be helpful, but definitive treatment remains the removal of the object.

✓ **Patients with glass, sea shell fragments, gravel, or other potentially harmful objects embedded subcutaneously should have them removed as soon as possible and will require ultrasound guidance, surgical consultation, or referral if they cannot be easily located and removed.**

✓ If the wound is in a complex area, such as the palm of the hand or periorbital region, consultation for removal in the operating room, on an immediate or delayed basis, may be appropriate. Always inform the patient, and document when a retained foreign body is suspected.

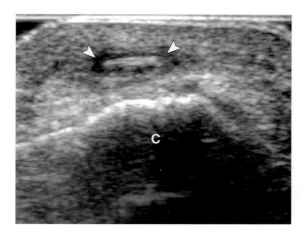

Figures 154-4 A 47-year-old woman with rose-thorn foreign body. Ultrasound image shows linear hyperechoic foreign body *(arrowheads)* with surrounding hypoechoic halo of inflammation. *C*, calcaneus. (From Jacobson JA: Musculoskeletal ultrasound: focused impact on MRI, *AJR Am J Roentgenol* 193:619–627, 2009.)

✓ **Ultrasonography is the most reliable method for detecting superficial radiolucent foreign bodies and may be used for guidance in their retrieval.** Note that a negative ultrasonogram does not reliably rule out the possibility of a retained subcutaneous FB.

✓ When ultrasonography is available and the clinician is familiar with its use, the following technique can be used when the simple techniques described above have been nonproductive.

✓ A high-frequency linear transducer (7.5 to 10 MHz) is placed over the location of the suspected foreign body (with or without the use of a stand-off pad). Use of a "stand-off pad" can elevate the transducer several millimeters above the area of interest. This allows better sound transmission and an improved view of the underlying soft tissues. A glove filled with ultrasound gel can serve as a stand-off pad. Foreign bodies will usually appear hyperechoic to the surrounding soft tissue. Material such as wood or plastic tends to produce shadowing (Figure 154-4). Metal objects tend to produce reverberation or comet-tail artifact. The body part can also be placed in a water bath to enhance visualization of the structure of interest. The area is scanned throughout its entirety in search for a hyperechoic object in both the sagittal and transverse planes. Once found, the depth down from the skin can be measured as well as the size of the object. Survey the area surrounding the object for vessels. Vessels and other sensitive structures in close proximity to the foreign body should discourage all but the highly skilled practitioner from attempting to remove the object.

✓ Center the transducer over the foreign body, and mark the skin to identify the optimal incision site. After anesthetizing the skin and making a lateral incision, image the foreign body in the long axis, and insert a forceps or hemostat under ultrasound vision and guide it toward the object. If you are unable to remove the foreign body under long-axis view, attempt this in a short-axis view. In general, the technique works better for linear-shaped objects. Remember, bone and articular surfaces may appear hyperechoic and cast shadows similar to those of a foreign body. Scar tissue may also appear hyperechoic.

✅ Antibiotics are not routinely prescribed but may be justified when FB removal must be postponed; when there is suspected penetration of bones, joints, or tendons; or in patients who are highly susceptible to infection.

✅ Always provide the patient with the name of a clinician who can perform the necessary follow-up care.

✅ **Schedule a wound check within 48 hours, and warn the patient about signs of infection.**

What Not To Do:

❌ Do not disregard a patient's suspicion that an FB may be present, especially when glass or wood may be involved.

❌ Do not cut down on the metal probe if there is any possibility of cutting across a neurovascular bundle, tendon, or other important structure.

❌ Do not attempt to cut down to the FB unless it is very superficial or there is a probe in place and in contact with the FB. Often a blind incision will be unproductive and may only extend the injury.

❌ Do not blindly grab for something in a wound with a hemostat. An important anatomic structure may be damaged.

Discussion

Every effort should be made to identify the presence of a FB during the initial visit. When a FB is discovered in a wound, the clinician must weigh the risk of leaving the FB in place against the potential harm of attempting to remove it. Small, inert, deeply embedded objects that cause no symptoms can usually be left in place. Vegetative FBs cause intense inflammation and should be removed immediately. Foreign bodies that are heavily contaminated should be removed as soon as possible. Glass, metal, and plastic are relatively inert, and removal can be postponed if necessary.

Any patient who complains of an FB sensation should be assumed to have one, even if nothing can be seen radiographically.

Almost all glass is visible on plain radiographs, but small fragments, between 0.5 and 2.0 mm, may not be visible, even when left and right oblique projections are added to the standard anteroposterior and lateral views.

Radiographs are usually of little value in accurately locating metallic flecks. Even when skin markers are used, because of variances in the angle of the x-ray beam, the apparent location of the FB is often significantly different from the real location. An incision made over the apparent location therefore usually produces no FB. Needle localization under fluoroscopy or ultrasound guidance may be required for those objects that must be removed, if the simple probe technique described (or alternative technique) fails to deliver the FB.

If removal of a metallic object is attempted and a strong eye magnet is available, it can be substituted for the probe described earlier. First, enlarge the entrance wound; then, after contact with the magnet, the object can be dissected out or even pulled out with the magnet.

Moderate-velocity metallic FBs rarely travel deeply into the subcutaneous tissue, but a potentially serious injury must be considered when these objects strike the eye. A specialized orbital CT scan may be obtained in these cases. MRI is better at detecting nonmetallic FBs within the orbit or globe of the eye, but before MRI is attempted, a simple

Discussion continued

radiograph should be obtained to ensure that a metal fragment is not present. MRI is more sensitive than CT or ultrasonography for identifying all nonmetallic soft tissue FBs.

The benefit of prophylactic antibiotics for retained FBs has not been studied. Clinical experience

suggests that wound infections associated with a retained FB are resistant to antibiotics. These wound infections often resolve spontaneously once the FBs are removed.

Suggested Readings

American College of Emergency Physicians: Emergency ultrasound guidelines, *Ann Emerg Med* 53:550–570, 2009.

Blankenship RB, Baker T: Imaging modalities in wounds and superficial skin infections, *Emerg Med Clin North Am* 25:223–234, 2007.

Blankstein A, Cohen I, Heiman Z, et al: Ultrasonography as a diagnostic modality and therapeutic adjuvant in the management of soft tissue foreign bodies in the lower extremities, *Isr Med Assoc J* 3:411–413, 2001.

Capellan O, Hollander JE: Management of lacerations in the emergency department, *Emerg Med Clin North Am* 21:205–231, 2003.

Chisholm CD, Wood CO, Chua G, et al: Radiographic detection of gravel in soft tissue, *Ann Emerg Med* 29:725–730, 1997.

Courter BJ: Radiographic screening for glass foreign bodies—what does a "negative" foreign body series really mean? *Ann Emerg Med* 19:997–1000, 1990.

Crawford R, Matheson AB: Clinical value of ultrasonography in the detection and removal of radiolucent foreign bodies, *Injury* 20:341–343, 1989.

DeBoard RH, Rondeau DF, Kang CS, et al: Principles of basic wound evaluation and management in the emergency department, *Emerg Med Clin North Am* 25:23–39, 2007.

Ginsburg MJ, Ellis GL, Flom LL: Detection of soft tissue foreign bodies by plain radiography, xerography, computed tomography and ultrasonography, *Ann Emerg Med* 19:701–703, 1990.

Lammers RL, Magill T: Detection and management of foreign bodies in soft tissue, *Emerg Med Clin North Am* 10:767–781, 1992.

Levine MR, Gorman SM, Young CF, Courtney DM: Clinical characteristics and management of wound foreign bodies in the ED, *Am J Emerg Med* 26:918–922, 2008.

Lyon M, Brannam L, Johnson D, Blaivas M, Duggal S: Detection of soft tissue foreign bodies in the presence of soft tissue gas, *J Ultrasound Med* 23:677–681, 2004.

Manthey DE, Storrow AB, Milburn JM, et al: Ultrasound versus radiography in the detection of soft tissue foreign bodies, *Ann Emerg Med* 28:7–9, 1996.

Montano JB, Steele MT, Watson WA: Foreign body retention in glass-caused wounds, *Ann Emerg Med* 21:1360–1363, 1992.

Pfaff JA, Moore GP: Reducing risk in emergency department wound management, *Emerg Med Clin North Am* 25:189–201, 2007.

Rajesh G: *Ultrasound-guided procedures. V. Foreign body localization. Ultrasound guide for emergency physicians.* Available at http://www.sonoguide.com/foreign_bodies.html. Accessed December 2011.

Schlager D, Sanders AB, Wiggins D, et al: Ultrasound for the detection of foreign bodies, *Ann Emerg Med* 20:189–191, 1991.

Steele MT, Tran LV, Watson WA, et al: Retained glass foreign bodies in wounds: predictive value of wound characteristics, patient perception, and wound exploration, *Am J Emerg Med* 16:627–630, 1998.

Turkcuer I, Atilla R, Topacoglu H, et al: Do we really need plain and soft-tissue radiographies to detect radiolucent foreign bodies in the ED? *Am J Emerg Med* 24:763–768, 2006.

Turner J, Wilde CH, Hughes KC, et al: Ultrasound-guided retrieval of small foreign objects in subcutaneous tissue, *Ann Emerg Med* 29:731–734, 1997.

Subungual Ecchymosis
(Tennis Toe)

Presentation

The patient had a crushing injury over the fingernail after getting it caught between two heavy objects (i.e., car door or door jamb) or striking it with a heavy object, such as a hammer. The pain is initially intense but rapidly subsides over the first half hour. By the time the patient is examined, only mild pain and sensitivity remains. There is a light brown or light blue-brown discoloration beneath the nail (Figure 155-1). A similar but painless condition can occur with repeated minor trauma to a toenail, which can occur inside a sport shoe when rapid thrusting of the athlete's toes into the toe box occurs as a result of abrupt stops, such as on a tennis or basketball court ("tennis toe") (Figure 155-2).

What To Do:

✓ With any significant trauma, obtain a radiograph to rule out a possible fracture of the distal phalangeal tuft.

✓ **With traumatic ecchymosis, if there is continued painful sensitivity, apply a protective fingertip splint.**

✓ **Many patients are expecting nail trephination after experiencing a previous subungual hematoma** (see Chapter 156). **Therefore it is often helpful to explain to the patient that you are not drilling a hole in the nail.** Tell him that there is not enough blood under the nail for the procedure to improve discomfort and that it could actually do harm and might even be very painful.

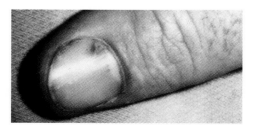

Figure 155-1 Subungual ecchymosis.

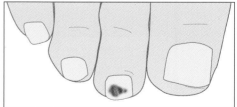

Figure 155-2 Transverse black-brown discoloration of second toenail. (Adapted from Adams BB: Jogger's toenail. *J Am Acad Dermatol* 48[Suppl 5]:S58-S59, 2003.)

✅ Inform the patient with a larger injury that, in time, he may lose the fingernail (or toenail) but that a new nail will replace it.

✅ **Tennis or "jogger's" toe resolves with or without treatment. Tennis players and runners need to wear properly fitting sport shoes that have an adequate toe box that does not allow the most distal toe to slam into the end of the shoe.** The patient should also be informed that improperly cut nails can allow the same type of trauma to occur.

What Not To Do:

❌ Do not perform trephination of the nail.

Discussion

Unlike the painful space-occupying subungual hematoma, the subungual ecchymosis represents only a thin extravasation of blood beneath the nail or a mild separation of the nail plate from the nail bed. Trephination will not relieve any pressure or pain and may indeed cause excruciating pain, as well as opening this space to possible infection. The patient's familiarity with nail trephination (as noted) may give him the erroneous expectation that he should have his nail drilled.

Bear in mind that **not all dark patches under the nail are subungual hematomas.** Diagnoses such as malignant melanoma, Kaposi sarcoma, and splinter hemorrhages (often associated with infective endocarditis) should be considered when the history of trauma and the physical examination are not consistent with a simple subungual hemorrhage.

Suggested Readings

Adams BB: Jogger's toenail, *J Am Acad Dermatol* 48(Suppl 5):S58–S59, 2003.

Kastle RK, Bothner J: *Subungual hematomas*. [*UpToDate* website]. Available at http://www.uptodate.com. Accessed August 2011.

Wang QC, Johnson BA: Fingertip injuries, *Am Fam Physician* 63:1961-1966, 2001.

Subungual Hematoma

Presentation

After a blow or crushing injury to the fingernail or toenail (i.e., stubbing one's toe or having one's finger closed in a door), the patient experiences severe throbbing pain that persists for hours. The fingertip is very sensitive, and the fingernail has an underlying deep blue-black discoloration, which may be localized to the proximal portion of the nail or extend beneath its entire surface (Figure 156-1, *A* and *B*). The nail margins should be completely intact without any free blood visible.

What To Do:

✓ Evaluate for possible extensor tendon avulsion (baseball finger) by having the patient fully extend the distal interphalangeal (DIP) joint (see Chapter 108).

✓ **If there is a concern for an underlying fracture, radiographs may be obtained.** Comminuted tuft fractures commonly underlie larger subungual hematomas and are helpful in determining the patient's expected length of pain and possible disability. If the mechanism of injury is clear, it is not necessary to delay nail trephination (see below) before obtaining radiographs.

✓ **Keep in mind that not all dark patches under the nail are subungual hematomas.** Consider the diagnosis of a simple ecchymosis (see Chapter 155), melanoma, Kaposi sarcoma, splinter hemorrhages (often associated with infective endocarditis), and other tumors when the history of trauma and the physical examination are not consistent with a simple subungual hematoma.

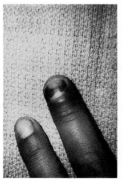
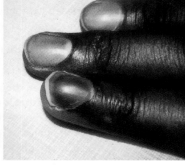

A   B

Figure 156-1 A and **B,** Subungual hematomas.

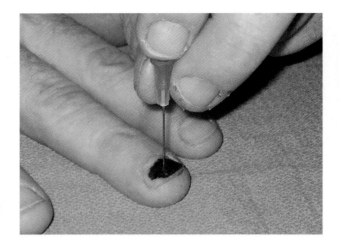

Figure 156-2 Trephination with a sterile, disposable, 23-gauge, double-bevel, 1-inch needle. (From Bonisteel PS: Practice tips. Trephining subungual hematomas. *Can Fam Physician* 54:693, 2008.)

✅ **If significant pain is present, paint the nail with 10% providone-iodine (Betadine) solution (or equivalent antiseptic) and perform trephination at the base of the nail with an electric cauterizing lance or carbon laser. A single-bevel 18-gauge needle or 23-gauge double bevel may also be used with a boring technique** (Figure 156-2).

✅ **When trephination is performed quickly with a hot cauterizing lance or paperclip, patients do not feel the heat before the relief of pressure. Tap rapidly a few times with the cautery or drill in the same spot at the base of the hematoma until the hole is through the nail.** When resistance from the nail gives way, stop further downward pressure to avoid damaging the underlying nail bed.

✅ **Persistent bleeding from this opening can be controlled by simply having the patient hold a folded 4 × 4 gauze pad firmly over the trephination site while holding his hands over his head.**

✅ Apply an antibacterial ointment, such as Betadine, and cover the trephination site with a Band-Aid.

✅ **To prevent infection, instruct the patient to keep his finger protected from soaking in contaminated water for approximately 1 week.**

✅ The patient should be instructed to monitor for signs of infection (worsening pain, redness, swelling, red streaking, fevers) and to return immediately if these occur.

✅ **A protective aluminum fingertip splint may also be comforting, especially if the bone is fractured** (see Chapter 111).

✅ **If little discomfort is present, when the patient initially seeks care, protective splinting and an analgesic may be all that is required.** Be sure to explain to the patient that you are not drilling a hole in his nail to reduce the possibility of infection and that putting a hole in his nail will not provide him with significantly more pain relief. That being said, always allow the patient to select his choice of method(s) for pain relief.

✅ Inform the patient that he will eventually lose his fingernail, and a new nail will grow out after 3 to 6 months.

What Not To Do:

✖ Do not perform trephination on a subungual ecchymosis (see Chapter 155).

✖ Do not perform a digital block. Anesthesia should not be necessary under most circumstances.

✖ Do not perform trephination on a patient who is no longer experiencing any significant pain at rest. A mild analgesic and protective splint will usually suffice.

✖ Do not make such a small opening that free drainage does not occur. A slender electrocautery tip may have to be bent to the side or spread apart for it to produce a wide enough hole.

✖ Do not hold a cautery wire on the surface of the nail without applying enough slight pressure to melt through the nail. Just holding the hot tip adjacent to the nail can heat up the hematoma and increase the pain without making a hole to relieve the pressure.

✖ Do not send a patient home to soak his finger after trephination. This is unnecessary (there is never reaccumulation of blood), and it may break down the protective fibrin clot and introduce bacteria into this previously sterile space.

✖ Do not routinely prescribe antibiotics. Even when opening a subungual hematoma with an underlying fracture of the distal phalanx, antibiotics have not been shown to be of any value in preventing infection. A brief course of cephalexin (Keflex) may be justified when treating patients with diabetes and peripheral vascular disease or those who are immunocompromised.

✖ Do not remove the nail, even with a large subungual hematoma, as long as the nail and nail margins are intact. It is not necessary to inspect for nail bed lacerations or repair them with a closed injury.

Discussion

The subungual hematoma is a space-occupying mass that produces pain secondary to increased pressure against the very sensitive nail bed and matrix. Given time, the tissues surrounding this collection of blood will stretch and deform until the pressure within this mass equilibrates. Within 24 to 48 hours, the pain therefore subsides. Although the patient may continue to complain of pain with activity, performing trephination at this time may not improve his discomfort to any significant extent and will potentially expose him to a small risk for infection. If trephination is not performed, explain this to the patient, who may be requesting trephination too late. The patient is often the best judge whether the pain is sufficient to warrant taking on this very small risk for infection.

Though many clinicians use a heated paper clip as a cautery device, it may be contraindicated in many settings, because it involves the use of an open flame to heat the material. Many paper clips are also made of metals that do not heat sufficiently to penetrate the nail. However, if it is the only device available, it is usually sufficiently effective (Figure 156-3). An alcohol wipe that is partially pulled from its foil package, when lit with a match, can serve as a readily available flame for heating up a paper clip.

There is some controversy in the literature about whether the nail should be removed if the hematoma occupies greater than 25% to 50% of the nail, because there may be an underlying nail bed laceration. It appears that trephination alone is safe and effective for treating these closed injuries, without apparent risk for infection or significant secondary nail deformity. There is some risk for missing a nail bed laceration under the hematoma but, even if present, splinting the wound by its own nail plate should help heal the underlying laceration.

When there are associated lacerations, open hemorrhage, broken nails, or disruption of the nail plate borders, perform a digital block and remove the nail to inspect the nail bed and repair any lacerations as necessary (see Chapter 146).

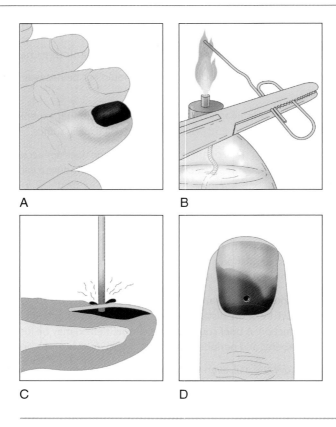

Figure 156-3 Trephination with a red-hot paper clip. **A,** Subungual hematoma. **B,** Heating metal. **C,** Nail trephination. **D,** Result.

Suggested Readings

Batrick N, Hashemi K, Freij R: Treatment of uncomplicated subungual haematoma, *Emerg Med J* 20:65, 2003.

Bonisteel PS: Practice tips. Trephining subungual hematomas, *Can Fam Physician* 54:693, 2008.

Kastle RK, Bothner J: *Subungual hematomas.* [*UpToDate* website]. Available at http://www.uptodate.com. Accessed August 2011.

Seaberg DC, Angelos WJ, Paris PM: Treatment of subungual hematomas with nail trephination: a prospective study, *Am J Emerg Med* 9:209–210, 1991.

Skinner PB: Jr: Management of traumatic subungual hematoma, *Am Fam Physician* 71:856, 2005.

Wang QC, Johnson BA: Fingertip injuries, *Am Fam Physician* 63:1961–1966, 2001.

Torn/Split Earlobe

Presentation

A patient comes to the emergency department or clinic with an earlobe torn by a sudden pull on an earring. Contributing factors might include previous lengthening of the earlobe hole because of long-term use of relatively heavy or dangling ear jewelry, or the original earring hole may have been placed in an excessively low position.

What To Do:

✓ Discuss the options: attempting to salvage the original piercing track (which may tend to elongate more easily) or removing the track entirely and providing for a new piercing at a later time. Inform the patient of the possibility of future inclusion cyst formation (caused by any hidden remnants of the old epithelial track) as well as the potential for postoperative scar contracture with resultant notching or scalloping of the lobe.

✓ **If cosmetic appearance is of great concern, it may be advisable to consult with a plastic surgeon before attempting the primary repair.**

✓ Always perform a thorough evaluation based on the patient's presentation. If there has been direct trauma to the ear, make sure to perform a thorough evaluation for signs of other clinically significant injuries, including intracranial, facial, and cervical.

✓ **Before repair, provide anesthesia,** either by infiltrating the lobe with 1% lidocaine (Xylocaine) until the lobe becomes firmer and pale or by performing a block of the greater auricular nerve. The use of anesthetic formulations that contain epinephrine in the ear is somewhat controversial because of the potential for excessive vasoconstriction, although these formulations are advocated by some authors. **Once the area is anesthetized, use a No. 11 or No. 15 blade to excise and undermine the wound edges as well as to make any required incisions for a Z-plasty repair.**

✓ Tears in the upper two thirds of the lobe may be excised and reapproximated. Tears in the lower third of the lobe should be converted to a full-thickness tear for easier management and better cosmetic results.

✓ **For repairs that attempt to salvage the original piercing track, excise the wound edges below the old track, including the lower segment of any elongated partial cleft** (Figure 157-1, *A* and *B*). **To encourage wound edge eversion, undermine the anterior and posterior skin edges to 1 mm** (Figure 157-2).

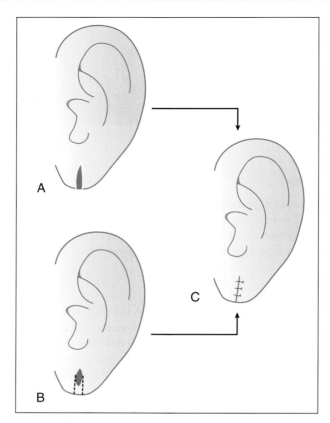

Figure 157-1 A, Incomplete excision of skin lining a full cleft. **B,** Excision of skin at the inferior lobe margin to convert a partial cleft to a full cleft. Apex epithelium is preserved. **C,** Straight-line closure of both cleft conditions, with preservation of the original hole. (Adapted from Watson D: Torn earlobe repair. *Otolaryngol Clin North Am* 35:187-205, vii-viii, 2002.)

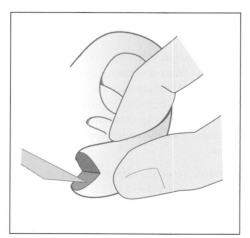

Figure 157-2 One-millimeter undermining of skin edges. (Adapted from Watson D: Torn earlobe repair. *Otolaryngol Clin North Am* 35:187-205, vii-viii, 2002.)

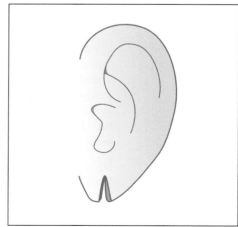

Figure 157-3 Inverted V-shaped excision of cleft. (Adapted from Watson D: Torn earlobe repair. *Otolaryngol Clin North Am* 35:187-205, vii-viii, 2002.)

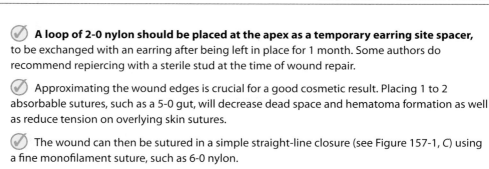

✅ **A loop of 2-0 nylon should be placed at the apex as a temporary earring site spacer,** to be exchanged with an earring after being left in place for 1 month. Some authors do recommend repiercing with a sterile stud at the time of wound repair.

✅ Approximating the wound edges is crucial for a good cosmetic result. Placing 1 to 2 absorbable sutures, such as a 5-0 gut, will decrease dead space and hematoma formation as well as reduce tension on overlying skin sutures.

✅ The wound can then be sutured in a simple straight-line closure (see Figure 157-1, *C*) using a fine monofilament suture, such as 6-0 nylon.

✅ **Place a single suture at the most inferior portion of the lobe before placing the other sutures.** This will ensure precise approximation and facilitate the remainder of the repair.

✅ **For repairs that remove the old track, excise the wound edges using an inverted V-shaped excision** (Figure 157-3), removing all remnants of any cleft. Undermine the skin edges as previously (see Figure 157-2), and make a similar straight-line closure (Figure 157-4).

✅ **To reduce the risk for scar contracture with earlobe deformity, the straight-line closure can be replaced by a simple Z-plasty** (Figure 157-5), closing the skin with the same fine (6-0) monofilament suture material.

✅ **Aftercare should include** daily showering and/or gentle wound cleansing with soap and water followed by application of bacitracin ointment or petroleum jelly is recommended.

✅ Sutures should be removed in approximately 5 days. Consider using tissue adhesive (Dermabond) after the sutures are removed to reduce tension on the healing wound.

✅ **Patients should be instructed that repiercing, if desired, should not be done through the scar but should be placed adjacent to the repair site. This will create a stronger piercing that is less prone to cleft formation. Preferably, replacement of the earring site should be delayed by 3 months.**

✅ Provide tetanus prophylaxis if needed (see Appendix H).

What Not To Do:

❌ Do not close an earlobe tear when remnants of the old earring track are known to be inside. This old epithelial track will eventually form an inclusion cyst, which will often require excision later.

❌ Do not use ointment containing neomycin. The neomycin provides no advantage and can often produce severe contact dermatitis.

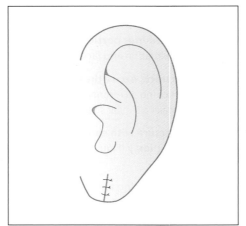

Figure 157-4 Straight-line closure. (Adapted from Watson D: Torn earlobe repair. *Otolaryngol Clin North Am* 35:187-205, vii-viii, 2002.)

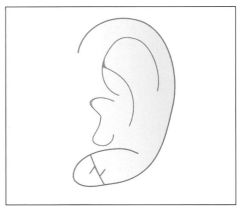

A

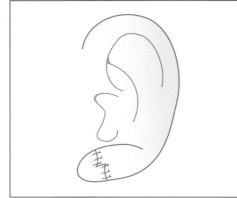

B

Figure 157-5 Straight-line closure with inferior rim modification by Casson. **A,** Incisions for a Z-plasty on inferior margin. **B,** Z-plasty flap transposition and closure. (Adapted from Watson D: Torn earlobe repair. *Otolaryngol Clin North Am* 35:187-205, vii-viii, 2002.)

Discussion

Piercing the earlobes is a practice that has persisted since ancient times and is common throughout the world today. Current cultural and fashion trends have encouraged an increase in earlobe piercing for men and multiple ear piercings for women, which has led to a greater incidence of piercing complications, including torn earlobes.

Torn earlobes also are referred to as split or cleft earlobes in the literature. A variety of techniques

have been described to repair torn earlobes. Some of these methods incorporate reconstruction of the original earring hole during earlobe repair, but many authors still recommend repiercing the earlobe at a later time.

Repiercing can be done safely by a physician or other qualified healthcare professional. The new piercing site should be placed in a nonscarred area of the lobe, preferably in a central location.

Discussion continued

Patients who have had multiple infections at the piercing site should not have the earlobe repierced.

Cleanse the earlobe with isopropyl alcohol or povidone-iodine (Betadine). Let the earlobe dry, and mark the desired piercing site approved by the patient.

Less than 0.5 mL of 1% lidocaine (Xylocaine) with epinephrine can be injected into the site using a 30-gauge needle. Then, take an 18-gauge sterile needle and insert it through the full thickness of the earlobe from the posterior surface through to the anterior surface. The needle tip must exit the anterior surface at the previously marked position.

The earring is slipped into the barrel of the 18-gauge needle. (Fitting the post into the lumen of the needle should be tested beforehand.) As the needle is backed out of the lobule, the earring post is guided into position through both the anterior and posterior punctures. Preferably, the post should be surgical grade or stainless steel and nickel free.

The backing piece should not squeeze the earlobe when it is slid into position on the post.

Patients should be instructed to gently cleanse the site with mild soap and water once or twice daily, followed by careful drying.

Patients should be instructed not to twist and turn the earring post, because this can increase the risk for irritation or infection.

The earring posts that are inserted initially should not be exchanged for at least 6 weeks to allow enough time for epithelialization in the new hole.

Avoidance of heavy and pendulous earrings is prudent.

Suggested Readings

Niamtu J: Eleven pearls for cosmetic earlobe repair, *Derm Surg* 28:180–185, 2002.

Ramakrishnan K: Surgical repair of the torn ear lobe, *Internet J Fam Pract* 2(2), 2003. Available at http://www.ispub.com/journal/the-internet-journal-of-family-practice/volume-2-number-2/surgical-repair-of-the-torn-ear-lobe.html.

Salam G, Amin J: The basic Z-plasty, *Am Fam Physician* 67:2329–2332, 2003.

Taher M, Metelitsa A, Salopek TG: Surgical pearl: earlobe repair assisted by guidewire punch technique: a useful method to remove unwanted epithelial tracks caused by body piercing, *J Am Acad Dermatol* 51:93–94, 2004.

Watson D: Torn earlobe repair, *Otolaryngol Clin North Am* 35:187–205, 2002. vii-viii.

Traumatic Tattoos and Abrasions

Presentation

The patient has fallen onto a coarse surface, such as a blacktop or macadam road. Most frequently, the skin of the face, forehead, chin, hands, and knees is abraded. When pigmented foreign particles are impregnated within the dermis, tattooing will occur. An explosive form of tattooing can also be seen with the use of firecrackers, firearms, and homemade bombs.

What To Do:

✓ Cleanse the wound with tap water, normal saline, or other products (e.g., poloxamer 188 or Shur Clens,) that are not destructive to epidermal and dermal skin cells.

✓ Provide tetanus prophylaxis (see Appendix H).

✓ **With explosive tattooing, particles are generally deeply embedded and will require plastic surgery consultation.** Any particles embedded in the dermis may become permanent tattoos. Abrasions that are large (more than several square centimeters), deep into the dermis, or into the subcutaneous tissues may also require consultation and/or skin grafts.

✓ **With superficial abrasions and abrasive tattooing, the area can usually be adequately anesthetized by applying 2% viscous lidocaine, 4% lidocaine solution, or gauze soaked with LET (lidocaine 4%, epinephrine 1:2000, tetracaine 0.5%) directly onto the wound for approximately 5 minutes.**

✓ If this is not successful, locally infiltrate with buffered 1% or 2% lidocaine using a 25- to 27-gauge, 1½- to 3-inch spinal needle for large areas. **Before infiltrating painful local anesthetics over large areas, consider parenteral opioid analgesia, or even procedural sedation.**

✓ For wounds containing tar or grease, application of bacitracin ointment before cleaning will help dissolve and loosen these contaminants.

 ✓ **The wound should then be cleaned with a gauze sponge with saline or 1% povidone-iodine (Betadine solution). For heavily contaminated wounds, use a surgical scrub brush, even one impregnated with chlorhexidine (as long as the chlorhexidine is rinsed thoroughly from the injured areas, because, over time, it is associated with mild tissue toxicity in wounds). If there is concern for tissue toxicity with povidone-iodine or chlorhexidine, consider using a poloxamer 188–impregnated sponge. When entrapped material remains, use a sterile stiff toothbrush to clean the wound or use the side of a No. 10 or 15 scalpel blade to scrape away any debris** (Figure 158-1). While working, continuously cleanse the wound surface with gauze soaked in normal saline to reveal any additional foreign particles. Large granules may be removed with the tip of the scalpel blade.

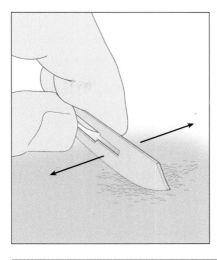

Figure 158-1 Dermabrasion with a No. 10 scalpel blade.

✓ **Small wounds should be left open and bacitracin ointment or petroleum jelly applied. The patient should be instructed to gently wash (not scrub) the area two or three times per day and continue applying the ointment until the wound becomes dry and comfortable under a new coat of epithelium, which may require a few weeks.** Use of ointments over excessively long periods can lead to maceration of tissue, rather than normal healing.

✓ **When a larger wound has been adequately cleansed, one alternative is to use a closed dressing with Adaptic (oil emulsion) gauze, ointment, and a scheduled dressing change within 2 to 3 days.**

What Not To Do:

✗ Do not ignore embedded particles. If they cannot be completely removed, inform the patient about the probability of permanent tattooing and arrange a plastic surgery consultation.

Discussion

The technique of tattooing involves painting pigment on the skin and then injecting it through the epidermis into the dermis with a needle. As the epidermis heals, the pigment particles are ingested by macrophages and permanently bound into the dermis. The best approach in managing patients with traumatic tattoos is the immediate removal of particles during the initial care. Immediate care is important because once the particles are embedded and healing is complete, it becomes much more difficult to remove them. It is advisable for a patient to protect a dermabraded area from sunlight for approximately 1 year to minimize excessive melanin pigmentation of the site.

Traditionally, destructive methods of delayed tattoo removal, including surgical excision, dermabrasion,

cryosurgery, and chemical peels, have all produced disappointing cosmetic results, with unacceptably high rates of scarring. With the development of Q-switched laser technology, however, tattoo removal has become much safer and more reliable, and the tattoos typically clear within a few laser treatments. The wavelengths emitted by these lasers are absorbed by pigmented particles, breaking them into smaller pieces that are less visible. The smaller particles are then taken up by inflammatory cells and eliminated by the lymphatic system or transepidermally. Tattoo removal with Q-switched lasers is moderately painful; a local anesthetic may be necessary. Transient or permanent hypopigmentation can occur, especially in dark-skinned patients.

Suggested Readings

El Sayed F: Treatment of fireworks tattoos with the Q-switched ruby laser, *Dermatol Surg* 31:706–708, 2005.

Graudenz K: Diffused traumatic dirt and decorative tattooing. Removal by Q-switched lasers, *Hautarzt* 54:756–759, 2003.

Tanzi EL, Lupton JR, Alster TS: Lasers in dermatology: four decades of progress, *J Am Acad Dermatol* 49:1–31, 2003.

Zipper Entrapment

(Penis or Chin)

Presentation

Usually a child has dressed too quickly and, possibly not wearing underpants, has accidentally pulled penile skin into his zipper. The skin becomes entrapped and crushed between the teeth and the actuator (slide) of the zipper, thereby painfully attaching the article of clothing to the body part involved (most often, the penis, or less often, the area beneath the chin) (Figure 159-1). There is generally little or no bleeding.

What To Do:

✓ **First, lubricate the entrapped skin and zipper with mineral oil.** In a significant percentage of cases, the entrapped skin may be released with lubrication and gentle lateral traction. This obviates the need for painful local anesthesia, systemic analgesia, and more complicated interventions.

✓ **If this is unsuccessful, consider systemic analgesics before local infiltration, which will be distressing and painful, especially in children.** Intranasal fentanyl may be a good option. In some cases, procedural sedation may be necessary.

✓ **Paint the area with a small amount of povidone-iodine (Betadine), and infiltrate the skin with 1% buffered lidocaine (without epinephrine).** As an alternative, perform a dorsal penile block. This will allow comfortable manipulation of the zipper and the article of clothing

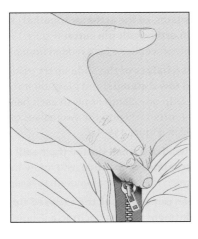

Figure 159-1 Penis caught in zipper.

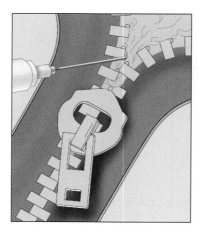
Figure 159-2 Injection of lidocaine.

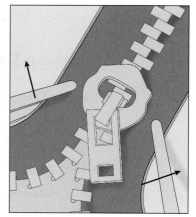
Figure 159-3 Opening zipper from rear.

(Figure 159-2). A more time-consuming alternative that sometimes may be more acceptable to the patient is to use a eutectic mixture of lidocaine and prilocaine (EMLA) to provide dermal anesthesia through the intact skin. This may take 45 to 60 minutes to become effective and therefore should be applied as soon as the patient arrives.

✅ **Cut the zipper away from the article of clothing.** This will improve access/visualization and will reduce the pain associated with the weight of the clothing on the entrapped skin.

✅ **The method of removal selected will depend on where in the zipper the skin is entrapped.**

○ **Between the teeth of the zipper:** this technique may work without elaborate pain control strategies. Simply cut across the zipper above and below the area of entrapment. **It may even be possible just to cut the closed zipper teeth below the actuator, permitting the unzipping of the zipper from the rear.** Pull the teeth gently apart to release the skin (Figure 159-3).

○ **Within the slide (actuator): cut the median bar (which holds the anterior and posterior halves, or faceplates, of the actuator together) with a pair of metal snips, a bone cutter, or an orthopedic pin cutter** (Figure 159-4, *A*). The patient is less likely to be frightened if this procedure is kept hidden from his view.

○ **If unable to break the two halves of the slide apart using a metal cutter, take two heavy-duty surgical towel clamps,** and place their tongs into the side grooves at both ends of the slide. Grip one clamp firmly in each hand, and twist your wrists in opposite directions. This often will pop the two halves of the actuator apart, releasing the entrapped skin (Figure 159-4, *B*).

○ **Alternatively, insert the head of a small slotted (flathead) screwdriver between the anterior and posterior faceplates of the slide,** and rotate the head 90 degrees. This may increase the gap between the faceplates enough to facilitate release of the skin.

✅ **After the zipper slide has been removed, pull the exposed zipper teeth apart, cleanse the crushed skin, and apply an ointment such as bacitracin** (Figure 159-5).

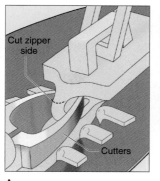
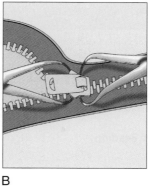

A　　　　　　　　B

Figure 159-4 Cut zipper actuator bar with a metal snip bone cutter or an orthopedic pin cutter (**A**), or use two heavy-duty surgical towel clamps to break the actuator apart (**B**).

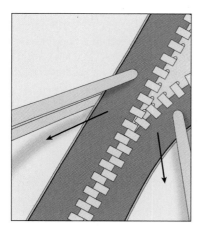

Figure 159-5 Pull exposed zipper teeth apart.

(✓) Tetanus prophylaxis should be administered as needed (see Appendix H).

(✓) **In the rare case when none of the described maneuvers is effective, consult a urologist.** The urologist may elect to perform an elliptic incision, or emergency circumcision in the operating room.

What Not To Do:

(✗) Do not cut clothing if mineral oil releases the zipper.

(✗) Do not fail to provide appropriate pain control.

(✗) Do not destroy the entire article of clothing by cutting into it. Only the zipper needs to be cut away, allowing repair of the clothing.

(✗) Do not excise an area of skin or perform a circumcision; it only creates unnecessary morbidity for the patient.

Discussion

Penile injuries (trauma) are relatively uncommon, but when they occur, zipper entrapment is involved in 3% to 14% of the cases. This injury usually occurs in a child who is between 3 and 6 years of age, and many of the victims are not wearing underpants.

Newer plastic zippers have made this problem less common than in the past, but it still occurs, and it is a very grateful patient who is released from this entrapment.

Suggested Readings

Bothner J: *Management of zipper injuries*. [*UpToDate* website]. Available at http://www.uptodate.com. Accessed October 2011.

Burns E: *Penile Zipper entrapment! In Life in the fast lane blog*. November 2010, Available at http://www. Lifeinthefastlane.com. Accessed December 2010.

Dubin J, Davis JE: Penile emergencies, *Emerg Med Clin North Am* 29:485–499, 2011.

Inoue N, Crook SC, Yamamoto LG: Comparing 2 methods of emergent zipper release, *Am J Emerg Med* 23:480–482, 2005.

Kanegaye JT, Schonfeld N: Penile zipper entrapment: a simple and less threatening approach using mineral oil, *Pediatr Emerg Care* 9:90–91, 1993.

Nolan JF, Stillwell TJ, Sands JP: Acute management of the zipper-entrapped penis, *J Emerg Med* 8:305–307, 1990.

Raveenthiran V: Releasing of zipper-entrapped foreskin: a novel nonsurgical technique, *Pediatr Emerg Care* 23:463–464, 2007.

Stone DB, Levine MR: Foreign body removal. In Roberts JR, Hedges JR, editors: *Roberts and Hedges clinical procedures in emergency medicine*, ed 5, Philadelphia, 2010, WB Saunders, pp 651–653.

Strait RT: A novel method for removal of penile zipper entrapment, *Pediatr Emerg Care* 15:412–413, 1999.

PART 11

Dermatologic Emergencies

■ Philip Buttaravoli ■ Page Hudson

CHAPTER 160

Allergic Contact Dermatitis

Presentation

The patient complains of a very pruritic, eczematous-like rash at sites of skin exposure to allergens. Lesions may consist of small papules, vesicles, or bullae that can be confluent at times. Inflammation may exist, with erythema, edema, oozing, or crusting. This dermatitis may remain localized at contact sites or, in severe cases, can spread to involve distant body areas. Sites with thin skin (e.g., eyelids [Figure 160-1], lateral neck, dorsum of hands, genitals) show greater susceptibility, whereas areas with a thick stratum corneum (palms and soles) have more resistance. Because this is a delayed hypersensitivity reaction, the pruritus and rash may not become evident for 24 to 48 hours or longer after exposure to the allergenic substance. Although a substance new to the patient in the past few weeks is more likely to be the precipitating agent, patients have been known to react to personal products that they have been using for years.

The one uniformly present feature of allergic contact dermatitis (ACD) is pruritus, without which the diagnosis of ACD is virtually excluded.

What To Do:

⊘ **Attempt to determine the offending agent.** Skin lesion distribution often provides a clue to the offending allergen. Question patients about potential exposure to topical medications (such as neomycin and benzocaine) or other potential allergens (such as sunscreens, moisturizing

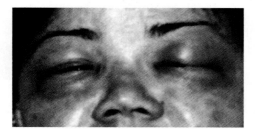

Figure 160-1 Marked eyelid swelling may mimic the angioedema of anaphylaxis, but with ACD there is only localized pruritus and no associated systemic signs or symptoms. This case was caused by contact with the allergen in hair dye. (Adapted from Mark BJ, Slavin RG: Allergic contact dermatitis. *Med Clin North Am* 90:169-185, 2006.)

639

lotions, perfumes and other fragrances, nail polish, artificial nails, cosmetics, soaps, shampoos, hair dyes, household cleaners, laundry products, paints, rubbers, latex, adhesives, footwear, clothing, and plants such as poison ivy [*Rhus toxicodendron*]) (see Chapter 182). Metals in jewelry (e.g., nickel, chromium, cobalt) (Figure 160-2) and chemicals in clothing and footwear (e.g., resins, crease resistant finishes, leather dyes, rubber accelerators) (Figure 160-3, *A* and *B*) can be sources of cutaneous allergens. Vulvitis and balanitis may occur in patients who have an allergy to latex in condoms or ingredients in douches, contraceptive jellies, feminine hygiene products, or toilet paper.

⊘ **Also evaluate for possible occupational exposure.** Industries in which workers are at the highest risk for occupational skin diseases include food production, construction, printing, metal plating, machine tool operation, engine service, leatherwork, healthcare, cosmetology, and forestry. Specific chemical agents encountered on the job may reveal the underlying cause.

⊘ **On physical examination, the appearance of the lesion in ACD often corresponds to the stage at which the patient presents.** During the acute stage, there is marked erythema, edema, and vesicle formation. Edema predominates in areas of loose connective tissue, such as the eyelids or genitalia. Vesicles are usually multiple, may coalesce, and eventually will rupture during the subacute stage, leading to oozing and eroded skin with a characteristic eczematous appearance. Vesicles may be replaced by papules, crusting and scaling become more prominent than the erythema and edema, and, over time, lichenification and further scaling predominate during the chronic stage. These stages often overlap, and there is no sharp delineation between them.

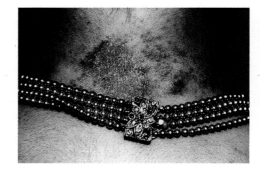

Figure 160-2 The classic erythematous papulovesicular eruption of ACD on the back of this patient's neck is caused by contact from nickel-plated jewelry. (Adapted from Mark BJ, Slavin RG: Allergic contact dermatitis. *Med Clin North Am* 90:169-185, 2006.)

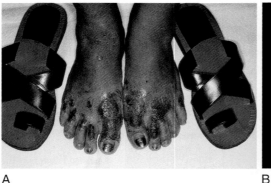
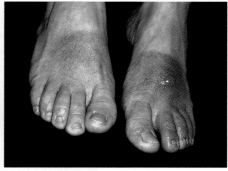

A   B

Figure 160-3 A and **B,** Allergic contact dermatitis to leather shoes. Note the correspondence to sites of exposure. (Adapted from Bolognia J, Jorizzo J, Rapini R: *Dermatology*. St Louis, 2003, Mosby.)

✅ Have the patient remove the offending allergen from the environment to avoid reexposure, and thoroughly wash the skin with a hypoallergenic soap such as Neutrogena.

✅ **For acute reactions with considerable edema and erythema—especially those with inflamed, oozing, or crusted lesions—frequent cool or cold compresses soaked with a 1:20 aluminum acetate (Burow) solution (Domeboro powder packets, two per pint of water) have cooling, soothing, and antiseptic effects.** Cool baths can also help (Aveeno Colloidal Oatmeal, 1 cup, or 1 cup each of cornstarch and baking soda in half a bathtub of water).

✅ **For severe reactions,** if there are no contraindications or relative contraindications (tuberculosis, peptic ulcer, diabetes, herpes, or severe hypertension), **prescribe systemic corticosteroids, such as triamcinolone (Kenalog-40), 40 mg IM, or oral prednisone, 60 mg (or 1 mg/kg) for approximately 5 days, and then taper slowly over at least 2 weeks.**

✅ Systemic oral antihistamine therapy, such as hydroxyzine (Atarax, Vistaril), 25 to 50 mg q6h prn, helps control pruritus. The benefits may be nominal in the delayed-type reactions of ACD, but any reduction in pruritus, along with its soporific effects, will be appreciated by the patient.

✅ **For mild and localized reactions, corticosteroid ointments or gels, such as desoximetasone (Topicort) 0.25% ointment, 0.05% gel, or fluocinonide (Lidex) 0.05% cream, gel, or ointment, applied twice per day, have anti-inflammatory and antipruritic effects. They are usually effective within a few days and should be continued for 2 weeks. More severe local reactions can be treated with the very potent topical ointment or gel clobetasol (Temovate, Clobex), 0.05% bid. Topical steroids may be potentiated with occlusive dressings.** Avoid long-term use (longer than 10 to 14 days) of these fluorinated corticosteroids on the face and genitalia, where they can cause atrophy. In general, higher potency steroids should be reserved for the extremities and torso.

✅ Steroid creams may have greater cosmetic appeal than steroid ointments, but creams typically contain more potentially allergenic preservatives and fragrances. Ointments, on the other hand, penetrate more deeply into the skin, increasing their potency.

✅ **Impetigo resulting from superimposed bacterial infection** (see Chapter 172) **should be treated with systemic antibiotics,** such as dicloxacillin (Dynapen), amoxicillin/clavulanate (Augmentin), 875 mg bid, cephalexin (Keflex), 500 mg qid, or erythromycin (Eryc), 250 mg qid × 10 days, or azithromycin (Zithromax), 500 mg, then 250 mg qd × 4 days. Consider antibiotics effective against community-acquired methicillin-resistant *Staphylococcus aureus* (CA-MRSA) when these organisms are prevalent in your area. **Avoid topical medications, because these are frequent allergic sensitizers.**

✅ When a precipitating agent cannot be determined, the patient should be referred for epicutaneous patch testing, which is considered the gold standard for diagnosing ACD. If patch testing fails to incriminate a likely allergen, and the diagnosis of ACD is still strongly considered, a detailed diary of the patient's daily activities may help discover patterns of allergen exposure.

✅ When the allergen cannot be avoided, wearing protective barriers is the next best preventive option. Gloves may be the most effective means of allergen protection. The ideal gloves are vinyl. They are waterproof and can be worn atop cotton gloves for greater comfort.

✓ The contacted objects sometimes can be modified to become less allergenic themselves, such as nickel-plated fasteners and jewelry that is painted with a clear polyurethane varnish.

What Not To Do:

✗ Do not allow patients to apply fluorinated corticosteroids for more than 10 to 14 days to the face or genital area, where they can produce premature aging of the skin with thinning and striae.

✗ Do not prescribe a prepackaged steroid dose pack that is tapered over 6 days. It is usually inadequate for treatment of ACD and frequently results in rebound dermatitis.

✗ Do not prescribe systemic steroids for secondary infections, such as cellulitis or erysipelas. Also, do not start steroids if there is a history of tuberculosis, diabetes, herpes, or severe hypertension, unless absolutely necessary and preferably in consultation with an appropriate specialist.

✗ Do not recommend desensitization protocols (allergy shots). They have no role in treating delayed-type hypersensitivities to contact allergens.

Discussion

Allergic contact dermatitis is a delayed cutaneous hypersensitivity or cell-mediated immune reaction to small-molecular-weight chemicals, which act as haptens. To date, more than 3000 chemicals have been described to cause allergic dermatitis in human beings. Approximately 50 chemicals cause 80% of the reactions seen in clinical practice. ACD begins with a sensitization phase, in which these small molecules pass through the stratum corneum and are processed by Langerhans cells in the epidermis. Antigen-coupled Langerhans cells then leave the epidermis and migrate to the regional lymph nodes via the afferent lymphatics and present this antigen to naïve CD4+ T cells. These T cells proliferate into memory and effector T cells, which are capable of inducing ACD after repeat exposure to the allergen. This elicitation phase has a latency period that corresponds to the travel time for Langerhans cells to present the allergen to T cells plus the time for these T cells to proliferate, secrete cytokines, and home with other inflammatory cells to the site of contact. A contact allergic reaction normally appears 12 to 72 hours after exposure in a previously sensitized individual.

In addition to the history and appearance of the rash, its anatomic distribution may help distinguish ACD from other types of dermatitis. Because the more exposed areas of skin are more open to allergen encounter, the hands and face are the most common body parts presenting with ACD.

Head and Neck

The skin of the scalp tends to be thicker and have greater resistance to ACD than the face, ears, and neck. Hair dyes and shampoos often spare the scalp but involve the thin skin of the eyelids, ears, cheeks, and neck. Facial cosmetics may cause similar symptoms, and products applied to the hands, particularly nail polish, may be inadvertently transmitted to the face. Metals from jewelry piercings anywhere on the face and ears and topical antibiotics for the eyes and ears are common triggers of ACD.

Extremities

More than half of all cases of contact dermatitis involve the hands. The list of household and occupational materials that are frequently handled is extensive but should include supposed innocuous items, such as foods, moisturizers, musical instruments, and protective gloves. ACD frequently occurs on the dorsal side of the hands, where the skin is thinner and the density of Langerhans cells is greater than on the palmar side. Bracelets, watches, and rings may lead to ACD from metal exposure or

Discussion continued

exotic wood. Metals from keys and coins, and even the striking surfaces of matchboxes in pants pockets, may be the culprits in ACD of the upper legs.

Torso and Groin

Fragrances from deodorants may cause ACD involving the entire axillary vault, whereas formaldehyde, detergents, and dyes from clothes may preferentially involve the torso and axillary folds, with sparing of the vault. Rubber chemicals in the elastic of undergarments may affect the bra line and waistline. ACD of the periumbilical region is often caused by the metallic fasteners of belts and pants. Medicines, douches, and spermicides may cause contact dermatitis in the genital area, principally the vulva and adjacent thighs rather than the vaginal mucosa.

Knowledge of the common contact allergens will also be helpful in identifying a source of an ACD rash.

Poison Ivy

See Chapter 182.

Metals

Nickel is the most common metal allergen in the United States. Other frequent causes of metal allergy include chromium, cobalt, gold (gold sodium thiosulfate), and organic forms of mercury.

Medications

Topical antibiotics, such as neomycin and, to a much lesser extent, bacitracin, induce more ACD than any other class of medicines. Mupirocin may be a safe alternative. Topical anesthetics of the ester class (benzocaine and tetracaine) are frequently implicated in ACD. The amide class of anesthetics (lidocaine, dibucaine, and mepivacaine) is a rare sensitizer. Surprisingly, topical corticosteroids may be altered to induce allergenicity through both metabolism in the skin and degradative reactions within the pharmaceutical preparation. A preservative with the highest prevalence of positive skin patch tests is thimerosal, found principally in vaccines and numerous topical medicines for the eyes, ears, and nose.

Formaldehyde and Fragrances

Formaldehyde and formaldehyde releasers, such as quaternium-15, are the most common preservatives

responsible for ACD other than thimerosal. These two preservatives are found in numerous cosmetics, moisturizers, and fabrics. Fragrances are widely used in cosmetics, fabrics, and topical medicines; in flavorings of foods, drinks, spices, and oral hygiene products; and in perfumes and colognes. Balsam of Peru is the fragrance most often implicated in ACD. In addition to the previously mentioned products, balsam of Peru is also found in sunscreens and shampoos.

Latex and Rubber Chemicals

Chemical accelerators and antioxidants are added to natural rubber latex during its vulcanization process. These chemicals are the primary sensitizers of ACD in rubber products. Of all the rubber products manufactured, latex gloves are the leading cause of ACD reactions.

Until patch testing can identify the specific offending agent, the patient should be instructed about avoidance of the most likely source of allergen that is inferred by the history and the distribution of the rash. A patient with facial dermatitis should be advised to avoid all cosmetics, hair products, facial creams, and lotions until the exact allergen has been identified.

Contact with blister fluid does not spread the allergen, but transfer of allergen remaining under the fingernails or reexposure to allergen persisting on fomites, such as clothing, can continue to spread the dermatitis.

Because corticosteroids halt lymphocyte proliferation and decrease cytokine production, they have become the mainstay of ACD therapy.

Local corticosteroid therapy is not necessary when systemic therapy is used. **When using a topical steroid on the face,** however, a less potent agent, such as hydrocortisone ointment 2.5% or desonide (Tridesilon) ointment 0.05%, is recommended.

It has been reported that 80% of cases of occupational contact dermatitis are attributable to irritant contact dermatitis (ICD) and 20% to allergic contact dermatitis (ACD). ICD results from skin-barrier disruption and subsequent release of inflammatory mediators without the requirement of previous sensitization. Mild irritants, such as water, soaps and detergents, typically cause chronic subclinical irritation, which is cumulative and

(continued)

Discussion continued

eventually leads to clinically perceptible dermatitis. Work that requires frequent immersion in water causes maceration, and with frequent wetting and drying, proteins leach from the stratum corneum, which, in turn, causes breaks with chapping, scaling, and fissuring. Wetting and drying alone is a common cause of ICD, and soaps and detergents accentuate these reactions. Other industrial materials that may cause ICD include petroleum distillates, alkalis, acids, organic solvents, alcohols, chlorinated hydrocarbons, and glycols.

It is often impossible to use appearance to differentiate between allergic and irritant contact reactions. Acute ICD may present within minutes to hours after exposure, with sharply delineated areas of erythema, vesicles, and/or bullae. Chronic cumulative ICD presents with more scaling, fissuring, and lichenification (thickening of the epidermis with marked accentuation of the skin creases).

The mainstay of treating ICD is frequent moisturization and avoidance of irritants. The best agents for this purpose include plain petrolatum (Vaseline), Neutrogena Norwegian Formula Hand Cream, and Cetaphil Cream by Neutrogena. Data regarding the efficacy of topical steroids on ICD has been mixed in the past, but the results of a recent study support the traditional use of topical steroids to treat the inflammation associated with ICD.

Photocontact dermatitis is caused by the interaction between an exogenous chemical in the skin and the ultraviolet (UV) component of sunlight. The photosensitive agent may be a recently ingested drug, such as a sulfonamide, fluoroquinolone, tetracycline, oral contraceptive, or nonsteroidal anti-inflammatory drug, or may be a topically applied substance, such as cold tar extract. Clinically, only sun-exposed areas, such as the face, arms, and upper chest, are affected, whereas the skin under the chin, behind the ears, and on the upper eyelids is noticeably spared. A **phototoxic reaction** manifests as macular and tender erythema, which can resemble severe sunburn. With a **photoallergic reaction,** a delayed hypersensitivity reaction is induced by UV light, which chemically alters the sensitizing allergen in the skin. This reaction may produce a pruritic, papulovesicular, eczematous dermatitis similar to ACD.

Two types of contact urticaria have recently been recognized as subsets of contact dermatitis. In its nonallergic form, the urticaria remains localized to the site of contact and may be caused by direct mast-cell mediator release from fragrances, food preservatives, insect stings, caterpillar hairs, or topical medicines. Allergic contact urticaria requires previous exposure to sensitizing allergens, such as foods, metals, animal saliva, latex, industrial products, or topical medicines. Both forms of contact urticaria resemble noncontact urticaria, and their classic wheal and flare response usually appears within 30 minutes of exposure and may be relieved or reduced by simple washing. Although allergic contact urticaria may become generalized and even progress to angioedema or anaphylaxis, most cases of generalized urticaria, angioedema, and anaphylaxis result from ingested or internal causes rather than from contact or physical triggers (see Chapter 183).

Suggested Readings

Antezana M, Parker F: Occupational contact dermatitis, *Immunol Allerg Clin North Am* 23:269–290, vii, 2003.

Belsito DV: Occupational contact dermatitis: etiology, prevalence, and resultant impairment/disability, *J Am Acad Dermatol* 53:303–313, 2005.

Cohen DE: Contact dermatitis: a quarter century perspective, *J Am Acad Dermatol* 51:S60–S63, 2004.

Gober MD, Decapite TJ, Gasppari AA: Contact dermatitis. In Adkinson NF, editor: *Middleton's allergy: principles and practice*, ed 7, Philadelphia, 2009, Mosby Elsevier, pp 1105–1116.

Leung DYM, Diaz LA, DeLeo V, et al: Allergic and immunologic skin disorders, *JAMA* 278:1914–1923, 1997.

Mark BJ, Slavin RG: Allergic contact dermatitis, *Med Clin North Am* 90:169–185, 2006.

Williams SR, Clark RF, Dunford JV: Contact dermatitis associated with capsaicin: Hunan hand syndrome, *Ann Emerg Med* 25:713–715, 1995.

Arachnid Envenomation

(Spider Bite)

Presentation

Occasionally patients will come in with a dead or captured spider after having rolled over it in bed or finding it in their clothing while dressing. They may have felt a minor pinprick sensation or no discomfort at all. Early, there may be mild erythema at the suspected bite site. Burning pain, pruritus, and swelling may develop within a few hours of the bite.

More commonly, patients come in with a raised erythematous painful lesion with central vesiculation, possibly hemorrhagic, or a darkened or bluish area of early skin necrosis. The patient or a friend or relative suspects that this might be a "spider bite," even though a biting spider was never observed.

True brown recluse spider bites vary from mild local reactions to severe ulcerative necrosis with eschar formation (necrotic arachnidism) (Figure 161-1, *A* and *B*). The bite often appears as a central blister with mottling and a blanched halo, with surrounding erythema that sometimes makes it look "red, white, and blue." Bites usually are found under clothing and on the thigh,

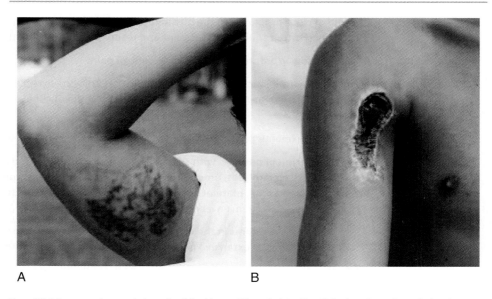

A   B

Figure 161-1 Appearance of presumptive loxoscelism. **A,** Local damage 48 hours after being bitten. **B,** Another patient seeking medical care for necrotic scab 26 days after a suspected spider bite. (Adapted from Hogan CJ, Barbaro KC, Winkel K: Loxoscelism: old obstacles, new directions. *Ann Emerg Med* 44:608-624, 2004.)

lateral torso, or upper arm. They are uncommon on the neck and are rare on the hands, feet, or face. Transient and mild constitutional signs and symptoms, such as myalgias, malaise, fever, chills, nausea, vomiting, generalized rashes, and headaches, may accompany these bites. A small subset of patients can have a more severe systemic response.

Lesions from other arthropod species and a variety of medical conditions may mimic bites of the brown recluse spider.

What To Do:

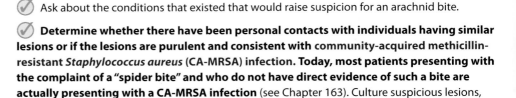 Ask about the conditions that existed that would raise suspicion for an arachnid bite.

Determine whether there have been personal contacts with individuals having similar lesions or if the lesions are purulent and consistent with community-acquired methicillin-resistant *Staphylococcus aureus* (CA-MRSA) infection. Today, most patients presenting with the complaint of a "spider bite" and who do not have direct evidence of such a bite are actually presenting with a CA-MRSA infection (see Chapter 163). Culture suspicious lesions, and provide appropriate antibiotic coverage.

Consider other possible diagnoses (especially outside areas endemic to the brown recluse spider), such as burns, cutaneous anthrax, erythema nodosum, focal vasculitis, foreign body, hemorrhagic gonococcal lesion, herpes simplex, Lyme disease (erythema migrans), malignancy, and necrotizing fasciitis.

Cleanse the bite site, and thoroughly irrigate any open wound.

When there is suspicion that a spider bite has actually occurred, provide and recommend cold compresses, immobilization, and elevation.

Confirmed bites are defined as bites associated with a captured or recovered spider found in close proximity to the bite and correctly identified by a qualified person. Most confirmed bites require no treatment and resolve without incident.

Provide appropriate analgesics to control pain.

Provide antibiotics for any secondary infection. True brown recluse spider bites only infrequently become infected; therefore prophylactic antibiotics have not been found to be useful.

Provide tetanus prophylaxis if indicated.

Evaluation of patients with systemic symptoms should include a complete blood count, electrolytes, blood urea nitrogen, creatinine, prothrombin time, partial thromboplastin time, platelet count, and urinalysis. There is no cost- or time-effective diagnostic test to confirm envenomation.

Systemic symptoms in the very young and very old most often require admission, and severe symptoms or extensive necrosis in any patient requires admission.

Patients with mild to moderate local findings can be managed as outpatients with close follow-up in 24 to 48 hours.

Warn patients of the potential for skin necrosis, with resultant scars requiring possible surgery. The absence of a lesion 2 to 3 days after the bite usually indicates that

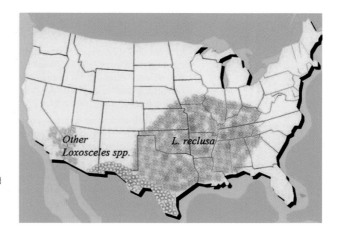

Figure 161-2 Reported distribution of *Loxosceles* species in the United States. (Adapted from Furbee RB, Kao LW, Ibrahim D: Brown recluse spider envenomation. *Clin Lab Med* 26:211-226, 2006.)

necrosis will not develop. **Necrotic wounds can take weeks to heal, the average time being 15 days (range, 0 to 78 days). Appropriate referral to a general or plastic surgeon should be considered.**

What Not To Do:

Ⓧ Do not apply heat or recommend hot compresses to suspected spider bites. Application of heat to these wounds results in more severe damage.

Ⓧ Do not inject the wound with antihistamines, corticosteroids, and/or vasodilators. This has not been shown to be of any benefit.

Ⓧ Do not perform early skin excision or débridement. Any débridement and/or skin grafting should be delayed until the wound has stabilized (6 to 8 weeks).

Discussion

Throughout the United States, dermonecrotic wounds of uncertain cause are often attributed to the brown recluse spider, *Loxosceles reclusa*. Many such diagnoses occur in parts of the country where the spider is not native and its populations are not known. The brown recluse has a fairly limited range (see map, Figure 161-2). Even inside endemic areas, these bites are very uncommon. Unfortunately, this spider has gotten a lot of press and has thereby inspired a lot of fear in the general population.

Necrotic wounds can be caused by many different factors. Today, patients frequently present with CA-MRSA skin infections that they have self-diagnosed

as a spider bite. Misdiagnosing a necrotic wound as a brown recluse spider bite can lead to delays in appropriate care, with adverse outcomes. In general, spider bites have been overdiagnosed as the cause of necrotic lesions. In addition to CA-MRSA, other important misdiagnosed conditions include neoplasms, Lyme disease (see Chapter 180), cutaneous anthrax, gonococcemia, and perhaps the worst case scenario—necrotizing fasciitis.

Corroborative evidence should be sought before attributing the cause to a spider or other arthropod bite. Although general wound care may be sufficient

(continued)

Discussion continued

for most similar wounds, it will be ineffective for conditions such as CA-MRSA, neoplasms, Lyme disease, cutaneous anthrax, gonococcemia, and necrotizing fasciitis, in which case a delay in treatment can have grave consequences.

Although all spiders are harmful to their prey, few are dangerous to human beings, and even fewer are capable of causing significant morbidity or mortality.

The brown recluse is a nonaggressive spider and will seek out shelter in undisturbed places, such as attics, closets, and storage areas for bedding and clothing. Humans may be bitten after donning clothing that has recently been taken out of storage.

Loxosceles spiders are the only globally distributed arachnid species capable of causing necrotizing skin lesions. Rarely, a more severe systemic reaction can occur, causing hemolysis, with subsequent renal failure and significant morbidity. There is no definitive treatment. Diagnosis remains difficult at best, with no specific test available to ensure that a lesion is attributable to the bite of a brown recluse.

***Loxosceles reclusa* has several distinguishing characteristics** that may not be visible without magnification. The dark-colored violin-shaped markings on the dorsal aspect of the cephalothorax (hence the name "fiddleback") (Figure 161-3) may not always be visible because of the variable color of the spider. A helpful identifying feature is the presence of six eyes arranged in three pairs (dyads) as opposed to the more common eight eyes found in most spiders.

The current mainstay of therapy is supportive care. Even in the rare case of a confirmed bite, treatment should be expectant. Despite multiple trials, early surgical excision, electric shock, steroids, hyperbaric oxygen therapy, colchicine, antihistamines, vasodilator drugs, anticoagulants, prophylactic antibiotics, and dapsone remain unproven therapies for brown recluse envenomation. All have variable degrees of risk. Antivenin and specific Fab fragments have been shown to be of some benefit but are not available commercially. Furthermore, given the inaccuracy of brown recluse bite diagnosis, much better documentation of the cause than is usually available would be required before assuming the risk of administration of these agents.

In areas of high *Loxosceles* density, the public should be educated about avoidance of bites (inspecting clothing and bed linen) and should be reminded to bring the suspected organism for identification, even if crushed. Should a person find a spider on himself or herself, it should be brushed off, not crushed.

Like the brown recluse, the maligned black widow spider (most commonly *Latrodectus mactans*) is a shy creature that bites only when provoked. Most of the 26 species of widow spiders are jet black and often can be identified from their characteristic red "hourglass" marking on the undersides of their abdomens. Because webs can be found around outdoor toilet seats, bites may occur on or near the genitalia. These bites may be painful but are usually associated with only mild dermatologic manifestations. Black widow venom causes depletion of acetylcholine at motor nerve endings and release of catecholamine at adrenergic nerve endings. Consequently, black widow bites may produce agonizing abdominal pain and muscle spasm, which may mimic acute abdomen. Other signs and symptoms include headache, paresthesias, nausea, vomiting, hypertension, and sometimes paralysis; fortunately, death is not common. Black widow bites may be misdiagnosed as drug withdrawal, appendicitis, meningitis, or tetanus, to name a few conditions. Treatment is supportive, with intravenous opioids for the pain and a muscle relaxant for the spasms. Wound care is usually minimal. At one time, calcium gluconate was recommended, but it has now been shown to be ineffective.

Equine-derived black widow antivenin is the only nonsnake antivenin approved in the United States. It is highly effective, even when given late. However, it has also been reported to cause hypersensitivity reactions. In one case series of 163 bite patients, 1 of the 58 treated patients died of bronchospasm. Therefore some experts will never use antivenin, whereas others may give it only for severe cases, when the patient is very old or very young.

With the increasing trend toward having exotic pets, a practitioner may find a patient presenting with a **tarantula** bite. While dramatic in size and appearance, these patient spiders are not likely to bite, and their envenomation is generally no worse than that of a hymenoptera sting. Several species do have irritant hairs on their abdomen, which they may fling outward, causing cutaneous or ophthalmic irritation.

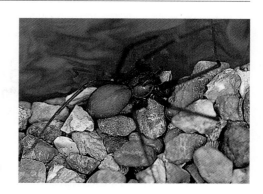

Figure 161-3 *L. reclusa* displays classic violin markings on the cephalothorax. (Adapted from Furbee RB, Kao LW, Ibrahim D: Brown recluse spider envenomation. *Clin Lab Med* 26:211-226, 2006.)

Suggested Readings

Boyer LV, Binford GJ, McNally JT: Spider bites. In Aurbach PS, editor: *Wilderness medicine: management of wilderness and environmental emergencies*, ed 5, St Louis, 2007, Mosby-Year Book, pp 1008–1033.

Furbee RB, Kao LW, Ibrahim D: Brown recluse spider envenomation, *Clin Lab Med* 26:211–226, 2006.

Hogan CJ, Barbaro KC, Winkel K: Loxoscelism: old obstacles, new directions, *Ann Emerg Med* 44:608–624, 2004.

Osterhoudt KC, Zaoutis T, Zorc JJ: Lyme disease masquerading as brown recluse spider bite, *Ann Emerg Med* 39:558–561, 2002.

Steen CJ, Carbonaro PA, Schwartz RA: Arthropods in dermatology, *J Am Acad Dermatol* 50:819–842, 2004.

Swanson DL, Vetter RS: Bites of brown recluse spiders and suspected necrotic arachnidism, *N Engl J Med* 352:700–707, 2005.

Vetter RS, Bush SP: The diagnosis of brown recluse spider bite is overused for dermonecrotic wounds of uncertain etiology, *Ann Emerg Med* 39:544–546, 2002.

Vetter RS, Isbister GK: Do hobo spider bites cause dermonecrotic injuries? *Ann Emerg Med* 44:605–607, 2004.

Arthropod Bites

(Bug Bites, Insect Bites)

Presentation

Patients with bug or insect bites seek medical help, because they are miserable with itching or secondary infection, or they are fearful of being infected with tiny creatures or exposed to a serious illness.

Skin lesions generally consist of single or multiple pruritic wheals or papules, which may include excoriations from scratching (Figure 162-1).

Mosquito bites most often occur on skin-exposed areas on warm summer nights in mosquito-infested environments (Figure 162-2). Other biting flies include midges, horse flies, deer flies, and black flies.

In tropical and subtropical regions of developing countries, as well as in hovels, homes, and high-class hotels throughout North America and Europe, bedbugs (true bugs) come out of hiding when their victim has retired to bed. The bites are painless, and unlike lice, the bedbug does not remain on the body after feeding. Bites are usually multiple and may be arranged in an irregular linear fashion. The wheals and papules that are formed have a small hemorrhagic punctum at the center. Blood that oozes from the wounds may be seen as flecks on the bed sheets. Bullous reactions are not uncommon (Figures 162-3 and 162-4). There is an apparent recrudescence of bedbugs in the United States recently. They are hard to avoid, because they may survive months, even in apparently hygienic circumstances. Avoiding residences with frequent turnover (shelters, hostels, etc.) may be prudent but perhaps impossible. Permethrin-sprayed bedclothes or sheets may be effective in prevention.

Kissing bugs (also true bugs) are found in the southwest United States, especially from Texas to California. These large (3 cm in diameter) winged insects are brown to black, with small stripes of red or orange in some species. The bites of these nocturnal insects occur almost exclusively in rural areas. The painless bite occurs only while the host is sleeping, because the blood meal takes 10 or more minutes to complete. Bites have been associated with papular, urticarial, and bullous reactions; hemorrhagic wounds that resemble bites of the brown recluse spider have also been reported.

Fleas are small (3 mm long), wingless bloodsuckers capable of jumping to a height of 7 inches. Flea saliva is highly antigenic and is capable of producing a pruritic papular rash. Cat and dog fleas also readily bite people, and therefore, pets infested with fleas are generally the source of the human rash (Figure 162-5).

Chigger bites are caused by the harvest mite or red bug, which commonly is found in grasslands of the southeastern United States. The larval form of the mite attaches to the patient's skin

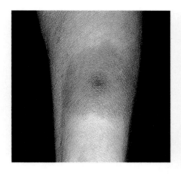

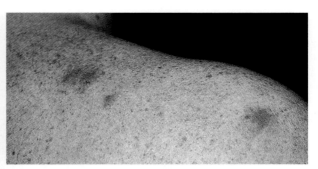

Figure 162-1 General arthropod bite. (From White G, Cox N: *Diseases of the skin,* ed 2. St Louis, 2006, Mosby.)

Figure 162-2 Mosquito bite. (From White G, Cox N: *Diseases of the skin,* ed 2. St Louis, 2006, Mosby.)

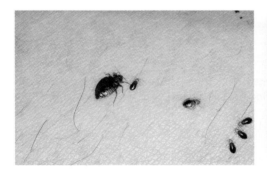

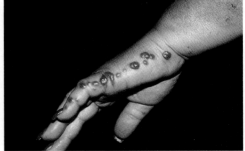

Figure 162-3 Bedbugs. (From Bolognia J, Jorizzo J, Rapini R: *Dermatology.* St Louis, 2003, Mosby.)

Figure 162-4 Bedbug bite. (From White G, Cox N: *Diseases of the skin,* ed 2. St Louis, 2006, Mosby.)

(usually during summer and fall) and sucks up lymph and tissue dissolved by the mite's proteolytic saliva. Frequently, the only signs of exposure are intensely pruritic, 1- to 2-mm papules on the ankles, legs, or belt line, because the bright red mites typically fall off after feeding. The erythematous papules may persist for up to 3 weeks.

A common hypersensitivity response to arthropod bites (most often caused by fleas or bedbugs) is papular urticaria. The condition consists of small, 3- to 10-mm pruritic urticarial papules that are present on exposed areas and affect predominantly children between the ages of 2 and 7 years. The papules form in clusters and are characteristically distributed on the extensor surfaces of the arms and legs. The lesions generally persist for 2 to 10 days and may result in temporary hyperpigmentation once they resolve.

Caterpillars have hairs (setae) with irritant and allergenic properties that can cause stinging pruritic erythematous papules, often arranged in linear streaks. Symptoms last a few days to 2 weeks. Whereas pruritus is characteristic of caterpillar dermatitis, the hallmark of the sting of the asp or puss caterpillar is intense pain out of proportion to the size of the lesion produced. A characteristic train-track pattern of purpura often appears at the site of the sting (Figure 162-6).

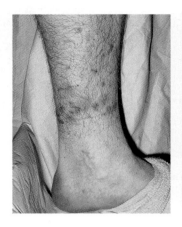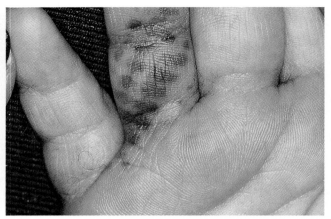

Figure 162-5 Flea bite. (From White G, Cox N: *Diseases of the skin,* ed 2. St Louis, 2006, Mosby.)

Figure 162-6 Caterpillar bite. (From Bolognia J, Jorizzo J, Rapini R: *Dermatology.* St Louis, 2003, Mosby.)

The range of the puss caterpillar is from Maryland down the eastern seaboard to Florida and across the states bordering the Gulf of Mexico.

What To Do:

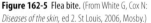 Take a careful history that includes any underlying medical conditions or medications that might produce a papular rash. Also perform a physical examination that provides a detailed description of the rash and its distribution. Attempt to uncover specific circumstances of biting arthropods, from the patient's history as described previously.

✓ **Pruritic lesions can be treated with local application of mild to moderate topical steroids (hydrocortisone cream 1% to 2.5%).**

✓ **An antipruritic, such as hydroxyzine (Atarax, Vistaril), 25 to 50 mg qid, may be comforting.**

✓ Treat any infectious complications with appropriate topical or systemic therapy (see Chapters 163, 166, and 172).

✓ **Mosquito bites and other fly bites can be prevented outdoors by covering exposed skin with clothing and by the use of insect repellents on skin and clothing.** Clothing is most protective if it has a tight weave and is loose and baggy. Diethyltoluamide (DEET) remains a highly effective repellent. The American Academy of Pediatrics recommends concentrations of 30% or less in products intended for use in children. DEET (Ultrathon) 25% (in aerosol) or 33% (in cream) is a polymer formulation that provides complete protection against mosquitoes for 6 to 12 hours. DEET can be sprayed on clothing, but permethrin, in a formula that can be sprayed on clothing (Duranon, Permanone), remains effective for several weeks through at least 5 or 6 launderings and can be used in combination with DEET for increased protection. **A 20% solution of Picaridin has recently become available in the United States. It is tolerated better than DEET and will probably replace DEET in the future (see Discussion, this chapter).**

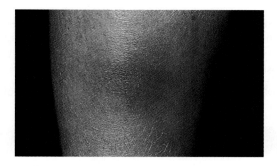

Figure 162-7 Erythema nodosum. (From White G, Cox N: *Diseases of the skin*, ed 2. St Louis, 2006, Mosby.)

✓ Using permethrin-impregnated mosquito nets while sleeping can be helpful when rooms are not screened or air-conditioned. **"No-see-ums" and sand flies are biting flies that are small enough to pass through the mesh of standard window screens and mosquito nets, but they may be blocked with fine-mesh screens or with ones that have been treated with permethrin.**

✓ **Eradication of bedbugs often requires protracted and costly treatments for the infested premises.**

✓ **Fleas must be eradicated from the environment to effectively end the problem of flea bites.** Eliminating cat and dog fleas depends on treating the animal hosts and premises, not the transient human host.

✓ **To prevent chigger bites, your patient should avoid sitting or lying in grass or weeds in the warm months of the year. Using DEET or spraying clothes with permethrin will also help.**

✓ **Caterpillar dermatitis may require moderate- to high-potency topical steroids to help alleviate itching in some cases.** Systemic steroids should be reserved for severe reactions. **Caterpillar hairs (setae) can be removed from the skin by "stripping" with adhesive tape, or, at home, have the patient apply nontoxic household glue (such as Elmer's Glue, not Krazy Glue) with a cotton swab and top it with a single layer of gauze. Instruct him to let the glue dry, then remove the gauze and glue. The setae will usually come out with the glue and gauze. Alternatively, the patient can use blackhead-removal strips (e.g., Bioré), following the same directions they would use to remove blackheads.**

✓ Intractable pain caused by the sting of the puss caterpillar may require oral or parenteral narcotic analgesics.

What Not To Do:

✗ Do not mistake the multiple painful nodules of erythema nodosum for bug bites (Figure 162-7). These erythematous nodules are not pruritic and usually develop over the anterior legs, occasionally over the torso, and infrequently over the extensor surfaces of the arms. This condition requires a special medical investigation.

✗ Do not recommend antihistamine creams. They are probably of no value and can irritate the skin.

(X) Do not recommend non-DEET insect repellents (excluding Picaridin). They provide little if any protection. An exception is the current availability of permethrin sprays as mentioned above. They may be viewed as complementary to DEET applications, but are likely more helpful at protecting against ticks or bugs that may stay hidden in clothing.

(X) Do not apply DEET near eyes or mouth, on broken skin, or under clothing.

Discussion

In general, the diagnosis of arthropod bites is dependent on maintenance of a high index of suspicion and familiarity with the arthropod fauna, not only in one's region of practice but also in the travel regions of one's patients. Taking a thorough history and determining the distribution of the rash will aid in the diagnosis.

Mosquitoes are responsible for the recent outbreaks of West Nile virus in the United States. **West Nile fever** develops in approximately 20% of infected humans and is accompanied by a flulike illness. A rash occurs in 20% of patients. Fortunately, severe neurologic manifestations of West Nile fever, including meningitis and encephalitis, are rare. Patients should be so informed and reassured.

Bedbugs are spread chiefly through the clothing and baggage of travelers and visitors, secondhand beds, and laundry.

DEET **has been found to be safe and effective, but some patients dislike its odor and find it irritating or uncomfortably oily or sticky on the skin. DEET can damage clothes made from synthetic fibers, such as spandex or rayon, and can also damage leather and plastics on eyeglass frames and watch crystals. Sawyer Premium Insect Repellent 20% Picaridin (3-oz spray) is now available on the internet in the United States. It is recommended as an alternative to DEET. Unlike DEET, it is odorless, does not feel greasy or sticky, is less likely to irritate the skin, and does not damage plastics or fabrics. Picaridin should now replace DEET because of its superior tolerability.**

Suggested Readings

Advice for travelers, *Med Lett Drugs Ther* 44:33–38, 2002.

Elston DM: Prevention of arthropod-related disease, *J Am Acad Dermatol* 51:947–954, 2004.

Goddard J, deShazo R: Bed bugs (*Cimex lectularius*) and clinical consequences of their bites, *JAMA* 301:1368–1366, 2009.

Pollack RJ, Marcus LC: A travel medicine guide to arthropods of medical importance, *Infect Dis Clin North Am* 19:169–183, 2005.

Porter A, Lang P, Huff R: Persistent pruritic papules, *Am Fam Physician* 69:2640–2642, 2004.

Steen CJ, Carbonaro PA, Schwartz RA: Arthropods in dermatology, *J Am Acad Dermatol* 50:819–842, 2004.

Cutaneous Abscess or Pustule

Presentation

A patient with an abscess may or may not have a history of minor trauma (such as an embedded foreign body or a small skin puncture) but has localized pain, swelling, and redness of the skin. The area is tender, warm, firm, and usually fluctuant to palpation. Sometimes there is surrounding cellulitis or lymphangitis and, in the more serious case, fever. There may be a spot where the abscess is close to the skin surface ("pointing"), where the skin is thinned, and pus may eventually break through to drain spontaneously. With the advent of community-acquired methicillin resistant *Staphylococcus aureus* (CA-MRSA), there may be a central or underlying darkened necrotic area, with the patient falsely assuming that he has a "spider bite." These abscesses generally are extremely tender and inflamed.

A pustule will appear only as a cloudy tender vesicle surrounded by some redness and induration, and occasionally, it will be the source of ascending lymphangitis.

What To Do:

✅ A history and physical examination should include inquiries about immunocompromise, artificial joints or heart valves, valvular heart disease, previous occurrence of similar abscesses, and close contact with people having similar lesions, as well as evidence of systemic symptoms, such as fever and tachycardia.

✅ **A pustule should not require any anesthesia for drainage. Very small pustules can be opened or unroofed using an 18-gauge needle.** For larger pustules, simply snip open the cutaneous roof with fine scissors or an inverted No. 11 scalpel blade, grasp an edge with pickups, and excise the entire overlying surface (Figure 163-1). Cleanse the open surface with normal saline and cover it with ointment and a dressing. The patient should be instructed to use warm compresses or soapy soaks at home.

✅ **When a simple abscess is suspected but the location of the abscess cavity is uncertain, the clinician can attempt to locate it using ultrasonography or by trying to aspirate pus from the cavity with a No. 18-gauge needle after preparing the area with povidone-iodine.** When using ultrasonography, if practical, placing the suspected abscess site in a water bath (you can use a bedpan filled with water) will eliminate the need for ultrasound gel or contact between the ultrasound transducer and the patient's skin, thus eliminating discomfort. **If an abscess cavity cannot be located, release the patient on antibiotics and intermittent warm, moist compresses. Have him seen in 24 hours to again check for abscess cavity formation.**

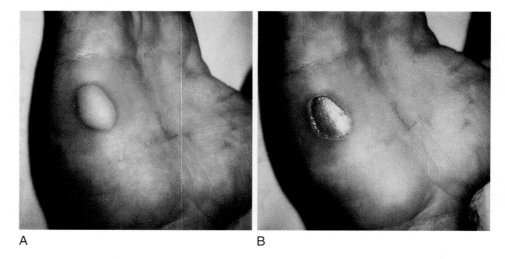

A   **B**

Figure 163-1 A, Large pustule before débridement. Local anesthesia is not required. **B,** Pustule after débridement and cleansing.

Figure 163-2 Anesthetizing the incision site of a small abscess. The anesthetic is injected in the subcutaneous plane under the area of the planned incision. (Adapted from Singer AJ, Hollander JE: *Lacerations and acute wounds.* Philadelphia, 2003, FA Davis.)

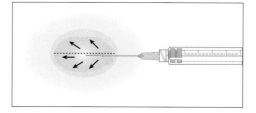

✅ In patients who are immunocompromised, have valvular heart disease, or have artificial heart valves or joints, administer empirical antibiotic prophylaxis before performing an incision and drainage (I&D). (See upcoming text for antibiotic choices.)

✅ **When the abscess is small with a thin roof or is beginning to point, prepare the overlying skin for incision and drainage with povidone-iodine solution. Inject lidocaine superficially into the roof of the abscess along the line of the projected incision** (Figure 163-2).

✅ **Incise with a No. 11 or 15 scalpel blade at the most dependent and thin-roofed area of fluctuance.** The incision should be large but directed along the relaxed skin-tension lines to reduce future scarring.

✅ **In larger, more complex abscesses, provide systemic analgesia or procedural sedation** (see Appendix E). **In addition to infiltration across the dome of the abscess, perform a field block by injecting a ring of subcutaneous 1% lidocaine around the abscess, approximately 1 cm peripheral to the erythematous border. As previously, an incision is made across the entire length of the fluctuant area.** A hemostat may then be inserted into the cavity to break up any loculated collections of pus. The cavity may be gently irrigated with normal saline and, when deep or expansive, loosely packed with iodoform or plain gauze (Figure 163-3). Leave a small wick of this gauze protruding through the incision to allow continued drainage and easy removal after 48 hours. Some authors have suggested that packing a wound is superfluous, but

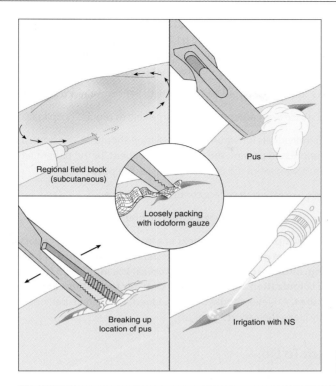

Regional field block
(subcutaneous)

Pus

Loosely packing
with iodoform gauze

Breaking up
location of pus

Irrigation with NS

Figure 163-3 Abscess drainage procedure. *NS,*
Normal saline.

this should be decided on a case-by-case basis. **The practitioner should at least be aware that
the purpose of packing is to keep a wound open and that a small amount of gauze suffices.
Overpacking an abscess is both painful and counterproductive;** it fails to allow the wound to
drain. In addition, iodoform gauze may cause the patient excessive pain.

✓ **To prevent recurrence, patients who have infected epidermoid (or sebaceous) cysts
containing foul-smelling cheesy material should be referred for complete excision of the
cyst after the infection and inflammation have resolved.**

✓ **Instruct the patient to use intermittent warm water soaks or compresses for a few
days when there is no packing used or after the packing is removed. This will encourage
further drainage when needed.**

✓ **With the new prevalence of CA-MRSA, it is now appropriate to obtain aerobic cultures
and sensitivities on most pus-containing lesions.**

✓ **Antimicrobials that cover CA-MRSA should now be prescribed for all wounds that require
antibiotic coverage (i.e., when extensive cellulitis is present).** Most abscesses in immune-
competent individuals, if not associated with lymphangitis or extensive cellulitis, probably do
not need antibiotics at all: incision and drainage is curative. This is as true of MRSA infections
as it is of non-MRSA lesions.

✓ **Empirical treatment currently includes 10 days of trimethoprim-sulfamethoxazole
(Bactrim DS), 1 to 2 tablets q12h, alone or in combination with rifampin, 300 mg q12h;**

doxycycline (Vibramycin), 100 mg q12h; clindamycin (Cleocin), 300 to 600 mg q6-8h; or minocycline (Minocin), 100 mg q12h. Linezolid (Zyvox), 600 mg q12h, is also recommended, but it is prohibitively expensive in most cases ($1000 to $1500 for 10 days). Resistance to these drugs may develop in the future.

✓ Severe infections should be treated with vancomycin, 1 g q12h, or 10 mg/kg q6h IV.

✓ Large abscesses (larger than 5 cm) are likely to require hospitalization and surgical drainage.

✓ Other individuals for whom hospitalization should be considered include the immunosuppressed patient, the toxic febrile patient, or the patient who has a large area of cellulitis, involvement of the central face, or severe pain.

✓ Provide a dressing to collect continued drainage.

✓ Have outpatients reexamined within 48 hours.

✓ **When multiple family members are involved or the abscesses are recurrent, stress the importance of good personal hygiene, recommend use of hexachlorophene soap for bathing, and prescribe 6 weeks of topical 2% mupirocin (Bactroban) for the nares to eradicate colonization and the carrier state for the patient and any contacts with positive nasal cultures.** Athletes should be encouraged not to share personal equipment or towels and to regularly clean their sports gear.

What Not To Do:

✗ Do not incise an abscess that is pulsatile or lies in close proximity to a major vessel, such as in the axilla, groin, or antecubital space, without first confirming its location and nature by needle aspiration or, preferably, ultrasonography.

✗ Do not treat deep infections of the hands as simple cutaneous abscesses. When significant pain and swelling exist or there is pain on range of motion of a finger, seek surgical consultation.

✗ Do not fully "pack" an abscess cavity with ribbon gauze. This may actually trap pus within the cavity, inhibit drainage, and enlarge the eventual scar. The goal is to insert the gauze across all the surfaces of the cavity and provide some degree of débridement when the gauze is removed.

✗ Do not use rifampin alone because of the rapid selection of resistant organisms.

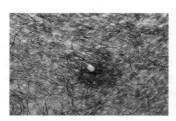

Figure 163-4 Folliculitis. (From White G, Cox N: *Diseases of the skin,* ed 2. St Louis, 2006, Mosby.)

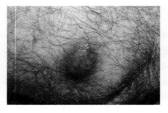

Figure 163-5 Furuncle. (From White G, Cox N: *Diseases of the skin,* ed 2. St Louis, 2006, Mosby.)

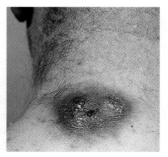

Figure 163-6 Carbuncle. (From White G, Cox N: *Diseases of the skin,* ed 2. St Louis, 2006, Mosby.)

Discussion

Either trauma or obstruction of glands in the skin can lead to cutaneous abscesses. In the past, incision and drainage were considered the definitive therapy for most of these lesions, and therefore routine cultures and antibiotics were generally not indicated. In the past few years, however, there has been an increasing incidence worldwide of CA-MRSA skin infections, and now the rules have changed.

Strains of CA-MRSA usually carry a gene encoding the Panton-Valentine leukocidin toxin, which causes necrosis. These strains of *S. aureus* are able to colonize the skin or nares and can produce spontaneous lesions.

There have been **community outbreaks of CA-MRSA** among prisoners and athletic teams. Direct transmission of the skin infection may occur through poor hygiene practices, close living quarters, and shared contaminated objects, such as athletic equipment, towels, and benches. Other risk factors include skin trauma from turf burns and shaving.

Currently, there are few research data to provide a scientifically proven regimen for managing these infections. I&D is still a basic tenet for managing an abscess. However, most experts suggest that cultures should always be obtained and CA-MRSA–specific antimicrobials be prescribed if antibiotics are needed. Early follow-up is also recommended. Over time, most of these recommendations most certainly will change.

Folliculitis is a superficial infection of the hair follicle that results in mild pain or itching with a small red papule or pustule surrounding a hair shaft (Figure 163-4). Common sites for folliculitis usually include areas where short, coarse hair predominates, such as the beard, upper back, chest, buttocks, and forearms. Minor uncomplicated cases can be treated with warm compresses, gentle cleansing with antibacterial soap, and, if this alone is ineffective, 2% mupirocin ointment. **Refractory folliculitis** will require CA-MRSA–specific antimicrobials. Advising the patient to avoiding shaving these areas may be warranted.

Hot tub folliculitis is caused by *Pseudomonas aeruginosa.* A patient usually presents within 72 hours after being in a hot tub with itchy red papules that will be most prominent on parts of the body covered by a bathing suit. Local treatment will usually suffice, but for severe cases, 7 to 10 days of ciprofloxacin (Cipro), 500 mg q12h, will usually clear up this rash.

A furuncle or boil is an extension of a folliculitis infection into the subcutaneous tissue. This forms a deep red, painful nodule that surrounds the hair shaft (Figure 163-5). Furunculosis is the most frequently reported presentation of CA-MRSA infections. The syndrome is characterized by the spontaneous development of primary necrotic lesions of the skin and soft tissues. These are the lesions that are often mistaken for spider bites by the patient. Crusted lesions and plaques progress to abscesses or cellulitis but may also present as impetigo, nodules, or pustules. Abscesses may become fluctuant and may drain spontaneously or require I&D and warm compresses. CA-MRSA–specific antimicrobials are now generally initiated.

A carbuncle results when individual furuncles coalesce, resulting in a large painful nodule with deep interconnected sinus tracts and multiseptate abscesses that often are draining pus from a cluster of pores (Figure 163-6). These are usually found on the back of the neck and generally require I&D with blunt dissection using a hemostat to break up the interconnected loculations of pus. Warm compresses and antibiotics are required as noted.

Hidradenitis suppurativa is a chronic inflammatory condition of the apocrine glands in the axilla and groin. Treatment for early lesions includes intralesional steroid injections, oral antibiotics, and isotretinoin (Accutane). Secondary infection typically results in abscess formation and fistulization requiring I&D and antibiotics. Local care with cleansers and compresses of Burow solution (Domeboro) is recommended, and patients should be encouraged to stop the use of antiperspirants. Recurrent I&Ds cause significant scarring, and extensive surgical procedures are eventually indicated.

A pilonidal cyst abscess is a relatively common finding in the sacrococcygeal region. Drainage should include a search for and removal of hair and follicular tissue at the base of the abscess cavity. Because *Escherichia coli* is a frequent infecting organism, these lesions may require broad-spectrum antibiotic coverage. To prevent recurrence after the initial infection has cleared, excision of the entire cyst cavity with marsupialization will eventually be required. Surgical referral is therefore necessary.

True brown recluse spider bites are actually very rare (see Chapter 161).

Suggested Readings

Barrett TW, Moran CJ: Methicillin-resistant *Staphylococcus aureus* infections among competitive sports participants—Colorado, Indiana, Pennsylvania, and Los Angeles County, 2000-2003, *Ann Emerg Med* 43:43–45, 2004.

Bhumbra NA, McCullough SG: Skin and subcutaneous infections, *Prim Care* 30:1–24, 2003.

Blaivas M, Lyon M, Brannam L, et al: Water bath evaluation technique for emergency ultrasound of painful superficial structures, *Am J Emerg Med* 22:589–593, 2004.

Frazee BW, Lynn J, Charlebols ED, et al: High prevalence of methicillin-resistant *Staphylococcus aureus* in emergency department skin and soft tissue infections, *Ann Emerg Med* 45:311–320, 2005.

Iyer S, Jones DH: Community-acquired methicillin-resistant *Staphylococcus aureus* skin infection, *J Am Acad Dermatol* 50:854–858, 2004.

Llera JL, Levy RC: Treatment of cutaneous abscess: a double-blind clinical study, *Ann Emerg Med* 14:15–19, 1985.

Naimi TS, LeDeell KH, Como-Sabetti K, et al: Comparison of community- and health care–associated methicillin-resistant *Staphylococcus aureus* infection, *JAMA* 290:2976–2984, 2003.

Palavecino E: Community-acquired methicillin-resistant *Staphylococcus aureus* infections, *Clin Lab Med* 24:403–418, 2004.

Treatment of community-associated MRSA infections, *Med Lett Drugs Ther* 48:13–14, 2006.

Zetola N, Francis JS, Nuermberger EL, Bishai WR: Community-acquired methicillin-resistant *Staphylococcus aureus*: an emerging threat, *Lancet Infect Dis* 5:275–286, 2005.

Cutaneous Larva Migrans 164

(Creeping Eruption)

Presentation

The patient has an intensely pruritic, thin, erythematous, serpiginous, raised eruption on the sole of the foot, hand, or buttock (Figure 164-1). The patient may remember recently walking barefoot or sitting in the sand or soil in an area frequented by dogs or cats. Most commonly, this is seen in travelers returning from tropical or subtropical locations in the Caribbean, Central America, and South America, as well as in the southeastern United States.

This is a dog or cat hookworm infection. Beaches and sandboxes provide excellent reservoirs for these parasites. Humans become a dead-end host for the microorganisms by walking through contaminated areas with bare feet or with open footwear, or by sitting in the tainted sand or soil.

What To Do:

✅ **Prescribe ivermectin (Stromectol), 200 µg/kg, one single dose (supplied as 3-mg tablet). Alternatively, prescribe albendazole (Albenza), 200 mg PO bid, or 400 mg qd (supplied as 200-mg tablet or in a 200 mg/mL suspension) × 3 days, or topical thiabendazole lotion, tid × 7 to 10 days (pharmacist formulated—these dosages are the same for both adults and pediatric patients).**

✅ Although it is only mildly effective, it may still be helpful to prescribe hydroxyzine (Atarax, Vistaril), 25 to 50 mg qid, or diphenhydramine (Benadryl), 25 to 50 mg qid prn to reduce itching.

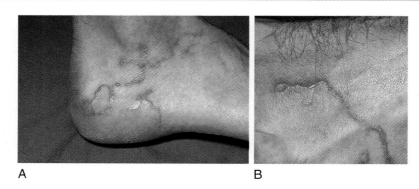

A   B

Figure 164-1 A and **B,** Cutaneous larva migrans. (From White G, Cox N: *Diseases of the skin,* ed 2. St Louis, 2006, Mosby.)

What Not To Do:

(X) Do not refer patients for cryotherapy. This was a historic treatment but has been shown to be ineffective and sometimes locally harmful.

Discussion

This disease is now usually referred to as creeping eruption, cutaneous larva migrans, or both. To be more precise, it has been proposed that the term "hookworm-related cutaneous larva migrans" be used to describe the cutaneous migration of larvae of animal hookworms in humans.

These lesions result from infestation by the skin-penetrating filiform larvae of hookworms (*Ancylostoma braziliense, Ancylostoma caninum, Uncinaria stenocephala*, and others) that hatch from eggs that are passed in dog and cat feces. If a human accidentally comes into contact with soil or sand contaminated by these animal droppings, these larvae may then penetrate through the skin. The incidence of this rash is greatest in warm, moist, sandy areas, such as tropical beaches.

Migration of the larvae at several millimeters per day results in the characteristic meandering, snakelike burrows in the epidermis. During larval migration, a local inflammatory response is provoked, which causes moderate to intense pruritus. Man is not the normal host for these parasites, and therefore,

the microorganisms lack the necessary collagenase to disrupt the basement membrane beneath the epithelial cells. Therefore the larvae usually die within 2 to 8 weeks, even without treatment, but may persist for up to 1 year. Lesions are mostly localized on the feet, but they also appear on the buttocks and thighs, trunk, and knees. The diagnosis of this parasitosis is essentially clinical and relies entirely on history and physical findings.

The use of topical compounds (e.g., 10% thiabendazole) is all too frequently accompanied by irritation, recurrence, and poor patient compliance. Ivermectin and albendazole, on the other hand, are effective and fast: 24 to 48 hours are enough to stop the larvae from migrating, with consequent regression of pruritus. The skin heals in 2 to 3 weeks, and adverse reactions are rare. Therefore, although hookworm-related cutaneous larva migrans is self-limited, medical treatment shortens the duration and may prevent complications such as impetigo that results from scratching.

Suggested Readings

Albanese G, Venturi C: Albendazole: a new drug for human parasitoses, *Dermatol Clin* 21:283–290, 2003.

Chen TM, Paniker P: An unpleasant memento, *Am J Med* 118:604–605, 2005.

Caumes E, Danis M: From creeping eruption to hookworm-related cutaneous larva migrans, *Lancet* 4:659–660, 2004.

del Mar Sáez-De-Ocariz M, McKinster CD, Orozco-Covarrubias L, et al: Treatment of 18 children with scabies or cutaneous larva migrans using ivermectin, *Clin Exp Derm* 27:264–267, 2002.

Healy CP, Thomas DE: Leg rash, *Am Fam Physician* 69:2429–2431, 2004.

Moon TD, Oberhelman RA: Antiparasitic therapy in children, *Pediatr Clin North Am* 52:917–948, 2005.

Diaper Dermatitis

(Diaper Rash)

Presentation

Irritant Diaper Dermatitis

An infant, most commonly between 8 and 10 months of age, may be left too long between diaper changes or, during a diarrheal illness, develops irritation and erythema that is most evident on the prominent parts of the buttocks, medial thigh, and vulva or scrotum. Margins are not always evident. There may be papules or small superficial erosions, and skin folds are spared or involved last (Figure 165-1).

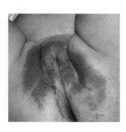

Figure 165-1 Irritant diaper dermatitis. (Adapted from White G, Cox N: *Diseases of the skin*, ed 2. St Louis, 2006, Mosby.)

Candidal Diaper Dermatitis

Following a course of antibiotics, a mild diaper rash may suddenly worsen, with clusters of erythematous papules and pustules coalescing into a beefy red confluent painful rash with sharp borders that are surrounded by small satellite lesions. The skin folds are commonly involved (Figure 165-2).

What To Do:

✓ **For a mild irritant rash, recommend frequent diaper changes (the most important intervention) and have the parents avoid excessive rubbing, especially with baby wipes that contain alcohol or fragrance, which may actually add to the irritation.** Have the parents rinse the baby's bottom with clear water at each diaper change. They can use a sink, tub, or water bottle for this purpose. Gentle cleansing with soft moist washcloths and cotton balls also can be helpful. Have them pat the baby dry rather than rubbing her down with a towel.

✓ **Tell the parents to loosen their baby's diapers** or use oversized diapers to allow airflow and prevent chafing at the waist and thighs.

✓ **They may also apply a barrier over-the-counter (OTC) agent such as petroleum jelly (Vaseline), A and D Ointment, Triple Paste, Diaperene, Desitin, or Balmex.** Zinc oxide is the active ingredient in many diaper rash creams. These products are usually applied in a thin layer to the irritated region several times throughout the day.

✓ **For a more severe or persistent rash, also instruct the parents to allow the child to go "bare" and wear no diapers as much as possible, but especially at nap time, until the rash has healed.** To avoid messy accidents, the parents may try laying the baby on a large towel and engaging her in some playtime while going bare-bottomed. This may increase the laundry load, but it allows the skin to dry, avoids physical trauma, and restores natural defenses.

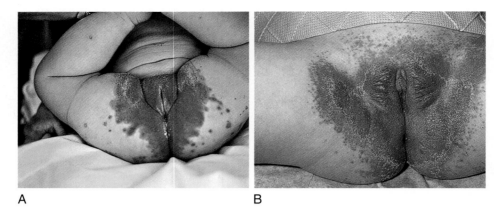

A   B

Figure 165-2 Two examples of *Candida* diaper rash. (Adapted from White G, Cox N: *Diseases of the skin,* ed 2. St Louis, 2006, Mosby.)

✓ **These more severe cases will also benefit from the application of an OTC 1% hydrocortisone cream or ointment bid.**

✓ **For a mild candidal infection, or for a diaper rash lasting more than 3 days, have the parents apply a topical antifungal cream or ointment, such as 2% miconazole (Micatin), 1% clotrimazole (Lotrimin), 2% ketoconazole (Nizoral), or 1% naftifine after each diaper change.**

✓ **With increased inflammation, a combination antifungal-steroid agent, such as triamcinolone/nystatin (Mycolog II), can be applied bid.**

✓ **For a severe *Candida* diaper rash, or if there is oral thrush, perianal candidiasis, or repeated bouts of candidal infection, prescribe oral treatment with nystatin to clear the gastrointestinal tract. Use nystatin oral suspension (60-mL bottle, 100,000 units/mL), 4 to 6 mL PO qid, 2 mL qid for infants.**

✓ **Recommend the same local measures as noted previously for irritant diaper rash.**

✓ **For secondary bacterial infection (e.g., crusting, vesicles, bullae), prescribe mupirocin (Bactroban) 2% ointment tid for 10 days.** For severe infections, a broad-spectrum systemic antibiotic, such as amoxicillin/clavulanate (Augmentin), will be required.

✓ **Encourage parents to practice hand washing after changing diapers to prevent the spread of bacteria or yeast to other parts of their baby or to other children.**

✓ Make sure that the family has a pediatrician or family practitioner for further follow-up.

What Not To Do:

✗ Do not recommend talcum powder or "talcum-free" powders for use when diapers are changed. They add little in terms of medication or absorbency and are occasionally aspirated by infants as their diapers are being changed.

✗ Do not recommend using cornstarch to protect the baby's skin. Cornstarch helps promote the growth of yeast and bacteria.

Discussion

Irritant contact diaper dermatitis is a very common disorder during infancy and predisposes the baby to developing a secondary infection with *Candida* organisms. Excessive moisture accompanied by chafing, elevated ammonia and pH levels within the diaper, and proteolytic enzymes present in the stool all irritate and damage the baby's skin. **Superinfection with *Candida* organisms is probably common enough to treat presumptively in every case of a diaper rash present for longer than 72 hours and severe enough to bring the baby for medical treatment.**

Patients with atopic dermatitis are more susceptible to *Staphylococcus aureus* infection. A culture may help guide therapy in complicated cases. Cases not responding to the usual treatments warrant investigation for psoriasis, nutritional deficiencies, and allergic or irritant contact dermatitis.

Suggested Reading

Stephan MR, Kirby MB, Blackwell KM: Common newborn dermatologic conditions, *Clin Fam Pract* 5:535–555, 2003.

Erysipelas, Cellulitis, Lymphangitis

Presentation

Erysipelas is a superficial cutaneous infection that commonly is found on the legs or face and generally does not have an inciting wound or skin lesion. It appears as a painful, bright fiery-red induration with raised, sharply demarcated borders, at times giving the skin a pitted appearance like an orange peel (peau d'orange) (Figure 166-1). *Cellulitis*, on the other hand, is deeper, involves the subcutaneous connective tissue, and has an indistinct advancing border. This deeper infection is characterized by pain and tenderness and by warmth and edema, which give the skin a light red or pink appearance (Figure 166-2). Cellulitis can occur on any part of the body but is most commonly found on the legs, face, feet, and hands. *Lymphangitis* has minimal induration and an unmistakable erythematous linear pattern ascending along lymphatic channels (Figure 166-3).

These relatively superficial skin infections (Figure 166-4) are often preceded by minor trauma, such as an abrasion or the presence of a foreign body, and are most common in patients who have predisposing factors, such as diabetes, drug addiction, alcoholism, immunosuppression, arterial or venous insufficiency, and lymphatic drainage obstruction. They may be associated with an abscess or other dermatologic abnormality, such as tinea pedis, impetigo, or folliculitis. Often they have no clear-cut origin. With any of these skin infections, the patient may have tender lymphadenopathy proximal to the site of infection and may or may not have signs of systemic toxicity (fever, chills, rigors, and listlessness).

What To Do:

✅ Perform a careful history and physical examination to determine if there are any underlying factors that would predispose the patient to such an infection. History of a previous injury, suspicion of a retained foreign body, or knowledge of previous infections may help clarify a possible cause. Underlying illness, such as diabetes, renal failure, chronic dependent edema, immunosuppression, or postoperative lymphedema, will give clues to an underlying predisposition to developing these infections and the need for hospitalization.

✅ **Look for a possible source of infection and remove it. Débride and cleanse any wound, remove any foreign body, and drain any abscess.**

✅ When the patient is very sick with high fever or severe pain, or the area of skin involvement is greater than 50% of limb or torso or greater than 10% of total body surface, obtain medical consultation, if needed, and prepare the patient for hospitalization and IV antibiotics. Other indications for hospitalization include a rapidly advancing edge of cellulitis that exceeds 5 cm

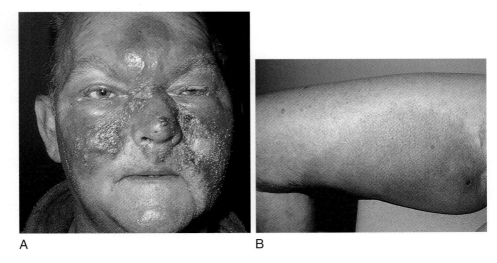

Figure 166-1 Erysipelas on the face (**A**); erysipelas of the leg (**B**). (Adapted from White G, Cox N: *Diseases of the skin*, ed 2. St Louis, 2006, Mosby.)

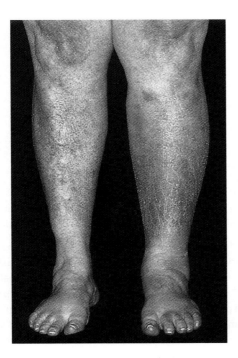

Figure 166-2 Cellulitis with tender erythema, swelling, and warmth of the patient's left leg. (Adapted from Knoop K: *Atlas of emergency medicine*, ed 2. New York, 2002, McGraw-Hill.)

per hour or coexisting morbidity, as noted. Obtain a complete blood count (CBC) and blood cultures, and consider obtaining radiographs to look for gas-forming organisms. Air in the soft tissues may represent necrotizing fasciitis, and rapid surgical débridement is indicated. Obtain cultures from any associated wounds. If there is no wound to culture in these complicated cases, it is reasonable to attempt a needle aspiration of fluid from the leading edge of the involved area. These fluid cultures, however, are often unsuccessful in establishing a bacteriologic diagnosis.

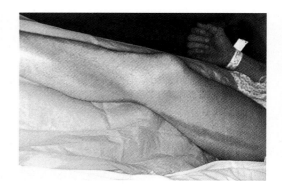

Figure 166-3 Lymphangitis. (From Knoop K: *Atlas of emergency medicine,* ed 2. New York, 2002, McGraw-Hill.)

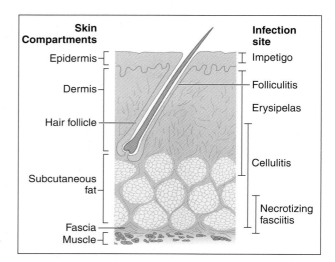

Figure 166-4 Cutaneous anatomy and sites of infection. (Adapted from Gorbach SL: *Infectious diseases,* ed 3. Philadelphia, 2003, Lippincott Williams & Wilkins.)

Hospitalization should also be strongly considered for central facial erysipelas or cellulitis, a deep infection of the hand, or failure to respond after 72 hours of oral antibiotic therapy.

✓ **If there is little or no fever and the patient is nontoxic and has no significant comorbidity, it is appropriate to treat the patient on an outpatient basis. For other than mild infections, it may be most effective to give an initial IV dose of nafcillin (Unipen), 1 to 2 g, or cefazolin (Ancef), 1 to 2 g; or, if the patient is highly allergic to penicillin, vancomycin (Vancocin), 1 to 2 g. Then prescribe dicloxacillin (Dynapen), 500 mg qid × 10 to 14 days; cephalexin (Keflex), 500 mg tid × 10 to 14 days; cefadroxil (Duricef), 1 g qd × 10 to 14 days; or, in penicillin-allergic individuals, azithromycin (Zithromax), 500 mg, then 250 mg qd × 4 days.**

✓ **Community-acquired methicillin-resistant *Staphylococcus aureus* (CA-MRSA) has become a common source of infection. Although it more typically forms abscesses, cellulitis is also common. Obtaining cultures is even more important, and opening any pocket of purulence is essential to successful treatment. Antibiotic coverage should consist of vancomycin, 1 to 2 g IV, or clindamycin (Cleocin), 900 mg IV. In the most**

worrisome infections, order linezolid (Zyvox), 600 mg IV (highly expensive), followed by a prescription for clindamycin (Cleocin), 300 mg q6h × 10 to 14 days, or trimethoprim-sulfamethoxazole (Bactrim DS), 160 TMP q12h × 10 to 14 days (alone or in combination with rifampin, 300 mg q12h), or linezolid, 600 mg q12h × 10 to 14 days (highly expensive). Oral antibiotics alone may be used in less worrisome infections.

✓ Provide tetanus prophylaxis as indicated, and prescribe analgesics for pain as needed.

✓ **Always outline the leading edges of the infection with a pen or marker so that the patient and follow-up clinician can monitor the effectiveness of the treatment.**

✓ Instruct the patient to keep the infected part at rest and elevated and to use intermittent warm (some experts recommend cool) moist compresses.

✓ Follow up within 24 to 48 hours to ensure that the therapy has been adequate. Infections still worsening after 24 to 48 hours of outpatient treatment will either need a change in antibiotic therapy or require hospital admission for better immobilization, elevation, and IV antibiotics.

What Not To Do:

✗ Do not obtain blood cultures or try to aspirate the border of a lesion for bacterial culture in uncomplicated cases. The yield is very low, and it produces unnecessary pain and expense.

✗ Do not overlook a case of necrotizing fasciitis, myonecrosis, or pyomyositis. These patients generally have comorbid conditions, systemic toxicity, and, in the case of pyomyositis, a prolonged course (see Discussion).

Discussion

Erysipelas (known in the Middle Ages as St. Anthony's Fire) is a rapidly progressing, erythematous, indurated, painful, and sharply demarcated area of superficial skin infection that is usually caused by *Streptococcus pyogenes*. Other causes include *Staphylococcus aureus* (including MRSA) and *Streptococcus pneumoniae*. The initial site of entry is often trivial or not apparent. Systemic symptoms, such as chills and fever, are common. Predisposing factors include venous stasis, diabetes mellitus, alcoholism, and chronic lymphatic obstruction. Erysipelas may progress to cellulitis.

Cellulitis is a deeper skin infection extending through the subcutaneous tissue. It appears as a painful, tender, erythematous, warm area that spreads along indistinct borders. Fever, chills, rigors, and sweats are frequent. There is often an extension via the lymphatic system, producing lymphangitis (once referred to as blood poisoning). Causative organisms include group A beta-hemolytic streptococci, *S. aureus* (including MRSA), and *Streptococcus pyogenes*.

Predisposing factors are similar to erysipelas, but also look for tinea pedis with fissures, which can serve as a common portal of entry.

All of these infections are typically diagnosed by clinical presentation and treated empirically. **The recent increase in CA-MRSA infections must influence the clinician to maintain a cautious skepticism regarding the use of a traditional antibiotic regimen for treatment of erysipelas, cellulitis, and lymphangitis. Penicillinase-resistant penicillins and cephalosporins would not be expected to be effective against these microorganisms. Clindamycin and trimethoprim-sulfamethoxazole are more effective choices currently, but these choices will certainly change in the future.**

Alternative conditions exist that can mimic uncomplicated cutaneous infections and may not be apparent until follow-up. These may include abscess, herpes zoster, septic bursitis, gout, and septic arthritis.

(continued)

Discussion continued

Three conditions that should never be confused with uncomplicated cellulitis are necrotizing fasciitis, myonecrosis, and pyomyositis.

Necrotizing fasciitis is a deep-seated polymicrobial infection that results in the progressive destruction of fascia and fat. It most commonly is found in patients with impaired circulation, immune compromise, or in intravenous drug users. When this infection is caused by group A streptococci, it is often referred to as **"flesh-eating bacteria"** by the press. These patients rapidly become very ill with signs and symptoms of systemic toxicity. The affected area (most often the extremities, particularly the legs) is initially erythematous, swollen, hot, shiny, exquisitely tender, and painful. Skin changes progress from red-purple to patches of blue-gray, then to bullae (with clear fluid) associated with marked swelling and edema. These patients develop anesthesia over the affected area, the result of destruction of superficial nerves caused by thrombosis of small blood vessels. It is essential to distinguish necrotizing fasciitis from the less dangerous cellulitis or erysipelas. Urgent surgical débridement and antibiotic therapy are required if the patient is to survive. The presence of marked systemic toxicity, severe pain, numb skin surface, color changes (red to blue-gray), tendon or nerve impairment, crepitation, and bullae formation point to necrotizing fasciitis.

Myonecrosis or gas gangrene is a pure *Clostridium perfringens* infection characterized by gas in a gangrenous muscle group. (*Escherichia coli* and *Klebsiella* spp. can also produce gas under anaerobic conditions.) Currently, this is an unusual infection but remains devastating and also requires rapid surgical intervention, IV antibiotics, and hyperbaric oxygen, if available. Pain is the earliest and most common symptom and is accompanied by fever and tachycardia. The patient appears pale, sweaty, and sick. Edema and tenderness may be the only local symptoms. The wound discharge, if present, typically is serosanguineous and dirty and has a foul odor.

Pyomyositis is often referred to as "tropical pyomyositis," because it is endemic in the tropics. These patients will also often have a predisposing condition or comorbidity, such as diabetes mellitus, alcoholic liver disease, concurrent corticosteroid therapy, or immunosuppression. This is an infection of skeletal muscle, usually caused by *S. aureus*. One or more muscles may be affected, most frequently the thigh and buttocks. The muscles initially feel achy or crampy, and examination reveals a woody, deep induration of the muscle belly. This is usually a slowly progressive disease; if untreated, within 2 weeks fluctuation, erythema, and then boggy swelling will develop. Tenderness is minimal initially, but fever and marked muscle tenderness develop as the infection progresses. MRI shows enlargement of the involved muscles along with any fluid collection. Surgical drainage is essential for treatment, along with empirical antibiotic therapy.

Suggested Readings

Bisno AL, Stevens DL: Streptococcal infections of skin and soft tissues, *N Engl J Med* 334:240–245, 1996.

El-Daher N, Magnussen CR: Skin and soft tissue infections: superficial lesions versus deadly disease, *J Crit Illness* 20:18–23, 2005.

Mills AM, Chen EH: Are blood cultures necessary in adults with cellulitis? *Ann Emerg Med* 45:548–549, 2005.

Moran GJ, Krishnadasan A, et al: Methicillin-resistant *S. aureus* infections among patients in the emergency department, *N Eng J Med* 355:666–674, 2006.

Perl B, Gottehrer NP, Raveh D, et al: Cost-effectiveness of blood cultures for adult patients with cellulitis, *Clin Infect Dis* 29:1483–1488, 1999.

Powers RD: Soft tissue infections in the emergency department: the case for the use of "simple" antibiotics, *South Med J* 84:1313–1315, 1991.

Stulberg DL, Penrod MA, Blatny RA: Common bacterial skin infections, *Am Fam Physician* 66:119–124, 2002.

Fire Ant Stings

Presentation

Usually the patient has experienced multiple burning stings (the "fire" in fire ant) and is seeking help because of local swelling, itching, and/or pain. Twenty-four hours after the initial wheal and flare at the sting site, there is formation of a small (2 mm), sterile, round pustule on an erythematous base, which is virtually pathognomonic for a fire ant sting (Figure 167-1). These lesions often occur in clusters. Sometimes there are large local reactions, and it is not unusual for an entire extremity to be affected. Systemic reactions in previously sensitized individuals are analogous to those caused by hymenopteran stings (see Chapter 171).

The appearance of the sting site changes over time. Within 1 week, the pustule often ruptures, forming a small crust or superficial ulcer, which then may become secondarily infected. After 1 month, small visible scars will be persistent (Figure 167-2).

What To Do:

✓ Examine the patient for any signs of an immediate systemic allergic reaction (anaphylaxis), such as decreased blood pressure, generalized urticaria or erythema, or wheezing. Treat with 0.3 to 0.5 mL of intramuscular epinephrine 1:1000 (may repeat every 10 to 15 minutes, as needed, to reverse the symptoms) along with boluses of IV normal saline (see Chapter 171).

✓ Reassure patients who present for treatment after 12 to 24 hours that anaphylaxis is no longer a cause for concern.

✓ **Relieve itching and burning with cold compresses.**

✓ **Treat minor reactions with topical steroids, such as triamcinolone (Aristocort A), 0.1% or 0.5% cream, or desoximetasone (Topicort) emollient cream, 0.25% or gel 0.05%. Dispense 15 g to apply tid or qid.**

✓ For pruritus, prescribe an antihistamine, such as hydroxyzine (Atarax, Vistaril), 25 to 50 mg PO qid.

✓ **When swelling is severe or there are other signs and symptoms of an allergic component to the stings, and there are no signs of infection or other contraindications to systemic corticosteroids, prescribe a brief course of prednisone, 40 to 60 mg qd for 4 to 5 days, or give one dose of triamcinolone (Aristocort Forte, Kenalog-40), 40 mg IM.**

✓ Have the patient return or seek follow-up immediately at any sign of infection.

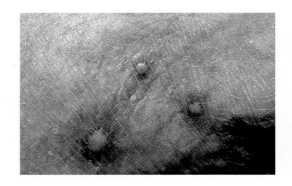

Figure 167-1 Fire ant sting. (Adapted from White G, Cox N: *Diseases of the skin,* ed 2. St Louis, 2006, Mosby.)

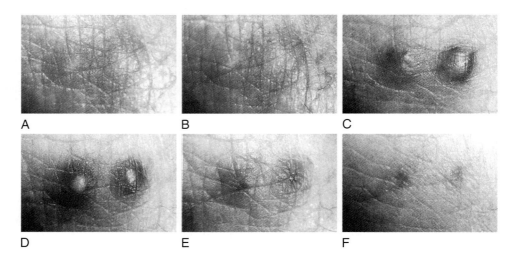

Figure 167-2 A, Thirty minutes poststing. **B,** One hour poststing. **C,** Twenty-four hours poststing. **D,** Seventy-two hours poststing. **E,** One week poststing. **F,** One month poststing. (Adapted from Goddard J, Jarratt J, de Castro FR: Evolution of the fire ant lesion. *JAMA* 284:2162-2163, 2000.)

✅ If there are signs of infection with surrounding swelling, tenderness, heat, and erythema, treat aggressively with cephalexin (Keflex), 500 mg qid, cefadroxil (Duricef), 500 mg bid × 10 days, or azithromycin (Zithromax), 500 mg, then 250 mg qd × 4 days. Always consider the possibility of community-acquired methicillin-resistant *Staphylococcus aureus* (CA-MRSA) infection (see Chapter 166).

✅ **Advise all these patients about avoiding future fire ant stings by wearing shoes (not sandals) when walking outside and to add socks, long pants, and work gloves when working outside. If there are infestations of fire ants around homes or businesses, have professional exterminators help with their removal.**

What Not To Do:

❌ Do not open pustules. They are initially sterile, and opening them only increases the chance that they will become infected.

Do not send a patient out less than 1 hour after the initial sting. Observe for possible anaphylaxis.

Do not apply heat, even if an infection is suspected. The swelling and discomfort will worsen.

Discussion

The term "imported fire ant" refers to several members of the genus *Solenopsis* (order Hymenoptera), which includes *Solenopsis invicta,* the most widespread of the species. They were first introduced to Mobile, Alabama, from Brazil in the late 1930s. They rapidly migrated and now occupy approximately 310 million acres in at least 12 states. Their current territory covers much of the South Atlantic seaboard from North Carolina to Florida, extends throughout the southern United States and across Texas, and stretches into portions of New Mexico, Arizona, and California. Compared with most native ants, imported fire ants are aggressive and will actively sting intruders.

When their anthill is disturbed, they will swarm and sting any passerby with the venomous apparatus at the tail end of their abdomens. They can inflict several painful burning stings within seconds, and each ant can inflict multiple stings. They use their mandibles to grasp the skin, then sting and pivot around their mandibles, inflicting stings that eventually produce the distinctive circular pustules. Unlike stings from bees and wasps, fire ant venom contains hemolytic factors that induce the release of vasoactive amines from mast cells and thereby create these sterile lesions. In heavily infested areas, approximately 30% of the population is stung by fire ants each year, with consequences ranging from local reactions to rare life-threatening anaphylaxis. Secondary infection, which can be severe, especially in diabetics and other infection-prone individuals, is an additional threat, even when the immediate reaction is relatively minor.

Increasingly, fire ants have been implicated in indoor attacks on persons in extended care facilities, where patients typically have sustained hundreds or thousands of stings. Immobility is also a risk factor for infants and persons who are inebriated and who fall asleep on or near an ant mound. Patients who are not allergic have sustained thousands of stings without complication.

Studies have shown, on the basis of allergic-specific IgE, that imported fire ants may be the arthropod posing the greatest risk for anaphylaxis to adults who live in endemic areas. Systemic reactions typically occur in patients previously sensitized to fire ant stings, but because their venom contains allergenic proteins that are antigenically similar to other hymenopteran venom, initial sensitization may occur with a bee or wasp sting. Densensitization may be helpful to protect patients who have experienced generalized allergic reactions. Conventional and rush immunotherapy performed with imported fire ant whole-body extract has proved effective and safe for the treatment of this form of hypersensitivity.

The fire ant gets its name from the fierce burning discomfort caused by its sting, not from its color, which ranges from dark red to brown or black. Most stings occur during the late spring and early summer, when the ants are most active and their venom is most potent.

Suggested Readings

Caplan EL, Ford JL, Young PF, et al: Fire ants represent an important risk for anaphylaxis among residents of an endemic region, *J Allerg Clin Immunol* 111:1274–1277, 2003.

Goddard J, Jarratt J, de Castro FR: Evolution of the fire ant lesion, *JAMA* 284:2162–2163, 2000.

Moffitt JE, Golden DB, Reisman RE, et al: Stinging insect hypersensitivity: a practice parameter update, *J Allerg Clin Immunol* 114:869–886, 2004.

Nugent JS, More DR, Hagan LL, et al: Cross-reactivity between allergens in the venom of the common striped scorpion and the imported fire ant, *J Allerg Clin Immunol* 114:383–386, 2004.

Steen CJ, Carbonaro PA, Schwartz RA: Arthropods in dermatology, *J Am Acad Dermatol* 50:819–842, 2004.

Friction Blister

Presentation

After wearing a pair of new or ill-fitting shoes or having gone on an unusually long hike or run, the patient complains of an uncomfortable open or intact blister on the posterior heel or ball of the foot. Occasionally, these blisters will be hemorrhagic. Secondary infection may be the cause of the visit, after painful pustules, cellulitis, or lymphangitis develops.

What To Do:

✅ **For torn or open blisters or blisters that have become infected, remove the overlying cornified epithelium with fine scissors and forceps. Clean the area thoroughly with a nontoxic skin cleanser (e.g., 1% povidone-iodine solution). Cover the wound with antibiotic ointment that does not contain neomycin and with a simple strip bandage. Have the patient wash the area and repeat the dressings until complete healing has taken place.** It usually takes about 5 days for a new stratum corneum to form.

✅ When cellulitis or lymphangitis is present, provide appropriate antibiotics (see Chapter 166).

✅ **For small (less than 1 cm) untorn or closed blisters that are not infected, the skin may be left intact and covered with a protective dressing.**

✅ **To provide comfort for lesions larger than 1 cm, the blister can be decompressed. Cleanse the area with povidone-iodine; then, using a 25-gauge needle, aspirate the blister fluid until the blister has completely collapsed. To prevent contamination and infection, either provide continuous antibacterial ointment (bacitracin) and strip bandage protection, or cover the punctured blister with a polyurethane film (such as OpSite) or a hydrogel dressing (such as Spenco 2nd Skin or Vigilon), or seal the needle puncture with cyanoacrylate (Dermabond).** Other acceptable protective coverings include the hydrocolloid, Duoderm; the occlusive dressing, moleskin; or the over-the-counter (OTC) liquid bandage, New-Skin. Additional padding may also be protective and comforting.

✅ **Instruct the patient about friction blister prevention.** A properly fitting shoe is essential, and even comfortable shoes need to be broken in gradually. Walking and running activities should be slowly increased day by day. Good socks with moisture wicking and padded insoles can also help prevent friction blisters. Wearing two pairs of socks that are made of different materials may reduce skin friction and prevent blisters. United States Military Academy cadets who applied an antiperspirant solution containing 20% aluminum chloride to their feet for at least 3 consecutive days reduced their risk for developing foot blisters during a 21-km hike by approximately half. The use of such antiperspirants unfortunately causes a high incidence of skin irritation.

What Not To Do:

⊗ Do not use neomycin-containing ointments because of the potential for allergic reactions.

⊗ Do not unroof sterile blisters. This will lead to unnecessary discomfort from the denuded area as well as increase the risk for infection.

Discussion

Blisters result from frictional forces—compounded by perspiration—that mechanically separate epidermal cells at the level of the stratum spinosum. This usually occurs when there is inadequate time to develop the protective epidermal hyperplasia that normally occurs with gradual increases in friction stress. Hydrostatic pressure causes the resultant separation to fill with a fluid that is similar in composition to plasma but has a lower protein level.

Active people often develop friction blisters on their feet. Although such blisters rarely cause significant medical problems, they can be quite painful and hinder athletic performance. Treatment goals include maintaining comfort, promoting healing, and preventing infection.

Suggested Readings

Freiman A, Barankin B, Elpern DJ: Sports dermatology part 1: common dermatoses, *Can Med Assoc J* 171:851–853, 2004.

Heymann WR: Dermatologic problems of the endurance athlete, *J Am Acad Dermatol* 52:345–346, 2005.

Pratte MK, Mustafa MA, Stulberg D: Common skin conditions in athletes, *Clin Fam Pract* 5:653–666, 2003.

Frostnip, Frostbite, and Mild Hypothermia

Presentation

Frostnip occurs when skin surfaces, such as the tip of the nose and ears, are exposed to an environment cold enough to freeze the epidermis. These prominent, exposed surfaces become blanched and develop paresthesias and numbness but remain pliable. As they are rewarmed, they become hyperemic and are usually very painful.

Superficial frostbite can be either a partial- or a full-thickness freezing of the dermis. The frozen surfaces appear white or mottled, feel doughy or hard, and are insensitive. With rewarming, these areas become erythematous and edematous, with severe pain (Figure 169-1). Blistering occurs within 24 to 48 hours with deeper partial-thickness frostbite.

Patients who have core body temperatures between 32° C and 35° C are considered to suffer from **mild hypothermia** and may demonstrate tachypnea, tachycardia, dysarthria, and shivering.

What To Do:

Obtain an accurate history of the severity and length of exposure as well as a history of any underlying preexisting medical disorders. Examine the sensitivity of any affected parts of the body. The ability to sense light touch and noxious stimuli helps determine the prognosis. **Favorable prognostic indicators suggesting superficial injury are normal**

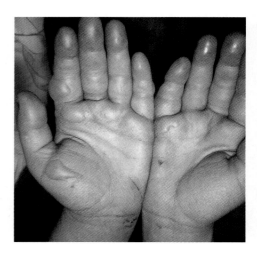

Figure 169-1 Early frostbite. (Adapted from Marx JA, Hockberger RS, Walls RM: *Rosen's emergency medicine,* ed 6. Philadelphia, 2006, Mosby.)

skin color, development of clear fluid in blisters, and the ability of the skin to deform under pressure. Dark color, hemorrhagic blisters, cyanosis, and hard nondeforming skin suggest deep injury.

✓ **Prior to rewarming, give ibuprofen (Motrin), 400 mg PO, or aspirin, 325 mg PO. This may improve tissue salvage.**

✓ **When there is no longer any danger of reexposure and refreezing, rapidly warm the affected part with heated blankets (or someone else's warm skin in the case of frostnip) or, preferably, in a warm whirlpool bath (at 40° C to 42° C [104° F to 108° F]) for 15 to 30 minutes or until capillary refill returns and the tissue is supple.**

✓ A strong parenteral analgesic, such as morphine or hydromorphone (Dilaudid), may be required to control pain.

✓ **Mild hypothermia can be treated with passive external rewarming, which consists of placing the patient in a warm dry environment after removal of wet clothing. The patient is then covered with blankets.** This alone can be expected to raise the core temperature approximately 0.5° C to 2° C per hour. Adding heating blankets or a forced heated air system (active external rewarming) will increase the rate of recovery.

✓ **When blistering occurs, bullae should not be ruptured, although this is somewhat controversial. If the blisters are open, however, they should be débrided and gently cleansed with 1% povidone-iodine and normal saline. Silvadene cream may be applied, followed by a sterile absorbent dressing.** Although topical aloe vera is now often recommended, it has not been proven to improve tissue viability. Injured tissue should be handled gently, and dressings must be loose, noncompressive, and nonadherent.

✓ More extensive involvement (often anything more than first-degree injury) requires hospitalization. Hands and feet should be splinted and elevated to reduce edema, and the digits must be separated by nonadherent gauze.

✓ Intravenous hydration with crystalloid will theoretically reduce blood viscosity and capillary sludging.

✓ Tetanus prophylaxis should be instituted when indicated (see Appendix H).

✓ Outpatients should be provided with follow-up care and warned that healing of the deeper injuries may be slow and produce skin that remains sensitive for weeks. Late sequelae of superficial frostbite include cold hypersensitivity (53%), numbness (40%), decreased sensation (33%), and impaired ability to work (13%).

What Not To Do:

✗ Do not warm the injured skin surface while in the field, if there is a chance that refreezing will occur. Reexposing even mildly frostbitten tissue to the cold without complete rewarming can result in additional damage.

✗ Do not rub the injured skin surface in an attempt to warm it by friction. This can also create further tissue destruction.

⊗ Do not allow the patient to smoke. Smoking causes vasoconstriction and may further decrease blood flow to the frostbitten extremity.

⊗ Do not confuse frostnip and superficial frostbite with deep frostbite. Severe frostbite, when the deep tissue or extremity is frozen with a woody feeling and lifeless appearance, requires inpatient management and could be associated with life-threatening hypothermia.

Discussion

Current scientific knowledge suggests that localized cold injury represents a continuous spectrum ranging from minimal to severe tissue destruction and loss. Frostbite has been categorized into four degrees of severity. First-degree frostbite is characterized by an anesthetic central white plaque with peripheral erythema. Second-degree injury reveals blisters filled with clear or milky fluid surrounded by erythema and edema, which appear in the first 24 hours. Third-degree injury is associated with hemorrhagic blisters that result in a hard black eschar, seen over the course of 2 weeks. Fourth-degree injury produces complete necrosis and tissue loss.

In general, treatment for the four categories of frostbite is the same until demarcation occurs within 3 to 4 weeks after injury.

Hypothermia is classified as being either mild (as previously described) or moderate—with temperatures between 28° C and 32° C, loss of shivering, and diminished level of consciousness—or severe, with core temperatures below 28° C and loss of reflexes, coma, and, eventually, ventricular fibrillation and death. Moderate to severe hypothermia is a medical emergency necessitating maintenance of airway, breathing, and circulation.

Most victims of hypothermia and localized cold injuries are in one of three categories: the urban poor, wilderness enthusiasts, and winter sports participants.

Frostbite is more common in persons exposed to cold at high altitudes. The areas of the body most likely to suffer are those farthest from the trunk or large muscles: ear lobes, nose, cheeks, fingers, hands, toes, and feet. Touching cold metal with bare hands can cause immediate frostbite, as can the spilling of gasoline or other volatile liquids on the skin when the temperature is very low. Factors contributing to hypothermia as well as localized cold injuries include alcohol intoxication, homelessness, and major psychiatric disorders. For those who participate in winter outdoor recreational and sports activities, direct exposure of skin and wearing constricting clothing, such as tight-fitting footwear, will predispose them to frostbite.

Frostnip is a superficial freezing of the skin, a precursor to frostbite, and produces reversible skin changes, including blanching and numbness that resolve with warming. It is important to treat frostnip early to avoid progression to frostbite. With gentle rewarming, the frostnip-affected area becomes hyperemic, and the sensation of pain returns rapidly.

Frostbite occurs when tissue freezes and crystals form in the extracellular space between cells. This occurs at ambient temperatures below 32° F (0° C). With dehydration, vasoconstriction, and low epidermal temperature, circulation is limited as blood viscosity increases, and water, hydrostatically pulled out of cells, begins to freeze. Close to 60% of frostbite injuries involve the lower extremities, in particular the great toe and feet. Predisposing diseases can include Raynaud disease, peripheral vascular disease, and diabetes mellitus. Tobacco smoking is another factor that can increase the likelihood of developing frostbite.

Planning for the threat of hypothermia can prevent cold injury. Individuals in cold and isolated areas should never be alone, or they should carry communication devices, such as cell phones or walkie-talkies. They should limit heat loss by insulating and dressing appropriately. Many layers are better than one thick layer. Waterproofed outer clothing is essential. Clothing materials should be wool, wool blends, or polypropylene. Cotton is not recommended. All extremities and the head should be covered. The face should be covered, especially with high wind chill. The feet should be protected with two layers of socks. The first layer should be made of polypropylene and the second layer made of wool.

Suggested Readings

Biem J, Koehncke N, Dosman J: Out of the cold: management of hypothermia and frostbite, *Can Med Assoc J* 168:305–311, 2003.

Petrone P, Kuncir E, Asensio JA: Surgical management and strategies in the treatment of hypothermia and cold injury, *Emerg Med Clin North Am* 21:1165–1178, 2003.

Seto GK, Way D, O'Connor N: Environmental illness in athletes, *Clin Sports Med* 24:695–718, 2005.

Ulrich AS, Rathlev NK: Hypothermia and localized cold injuries, *Emerg Med Clin North Am* 22:281–298, 2004.

Herpes Zoster

(Shingles)

Presentation

There may be prodromal symptoms that include malaise, nausea and vomiting, headache, and photophobia. Less commonly, there may be fever. During this prodromal stage, which can last several days, there may be accompanying preherpetic neuralgia.

Patients complain of symptoms that range from an itch or tingling to severe lancinating pain, tenderness, dysesthesias, paresthesia, or hypersensitivity that covers a specific dermatome. This discomfort may be precipitated by minor skin stimulation from the patient's clothes and is characteristic of this type of neurologic pain. After 1 to 5 days, the patient may develop a characteristic unilateral rash. The discomfort may be difficult for the patient to describe, often alternating between an itch, a burning, and even a deep aching pain. Prior to the onset of the rash, zoster can be confused with pleuritic or cardiac pain, cholecystitis, or ureteral colic. The pain may precede the eruption by as much as a few weeks, and occasionally, pain alone is the only manifestation (zoster sine herpete). Although almost exclusively a unilateral disease, in one study, approximately 1% of patients had bilateral involvement.

The early rash consists of an eruption of erythematous macules and papules that usually appear posteriorly first and then spread anteriorly along the course of an involved nerve segment. In most instances, clusters of clear vesicles on an erythematous base will appear within the next 24 hours (Figures 170-1 to 170-3). These continue to form for 3 to 5 days and then evolve through states of pustulation, ulceration, and crusting.

The skin eruption usually is limited to a single dermatome; the most commonly involved dermatomes are the thoracolumbar region and the face. Lesions may involve more than one dermatome and occasionally may cross the midline. With seventh cranial nerve involvement (causing weakness of all facial muscles on one side), the rash will be found in the ipsilateral external ear (called zoster oticus), or vesicles may be seen on the hard palate.

What To Do:

✅ **If it has been 3 days or less since the onset of the rash, prescribe valacyclovir (Valtrex), 1000 mg tid × 7 days; famciclovir (Famvir), 500 mg tid × 7 days; or the much less expensive but more inconvenient acyclovir (Zovirax), 800 mg five times per day × 7 days. If a patient presents later than 72 hours after onset, antivirals may still be considered if new lesions are being formed.**

✅ **Prescribe analgesics appropriate for the level of pain the patient is experiencing.**
NSAIDs may help, but narcotics are often required (e.g., oxycodone [Oxycontin, Roxicodone]

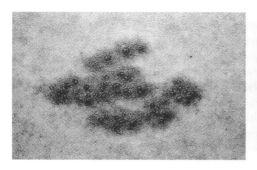

Figure 170-1 Herpes zoster. Classic appearance of grouped vesicles. (From White G, Cox N: Diseases of the skin, ed 2. St Louis, 2006, Mosby.)

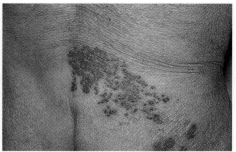

Figure 170-2 The vesicles of herpes zoster may at times be hemorrhagic. (From White G, Cox N: Diseases of the skin, ed 2. St Louis, 2006, Mosby.)

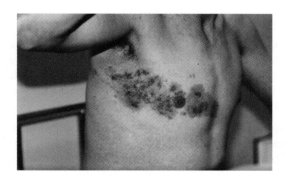

Figure 170-3 Herpes zoster infection, typically involving a single unilateral dermatome. (From White G, Cox N: Diseases of the skin, ed 2. St Louis, 2006, Mosby.)

q6-12h or Percocet q4h). When prescribing narcotics for the elderly, remember to warn them that they are likely to suffer constipation as a side effect (see Chapter 67). Other side effects of opioids include nausea, decreased appetite, and sedation. If the pain is severe, consider referring the patient for an epidural nerve block, which has been successful in relieving the acute pain and may decrease the incidence of postherpetic neuralgia.

✓ **There is evidence that treating older patients (60 years of age and older) with amitriptyline (Elavil), 25 mg qd × 90 days, will reduce the risk for postherpetic neuralgia. (There was a 50% decrease in pain prevalence at 6 months compared with placebo.) Coordinate such treatment with a follow-up physician.**

✓ **Cool compresses** with Burow solution will be comforting (e.g., Domeboro powder, 2 packets in 1 pint of water).

✓ Dressing the lesions with gauze and splinting them with an elastic wrap may also help bring relief. Superficial infection may be prevented by the use of a topical antibiotic ointment, such as mupirocin (Bactroban) 2% ointment (1 tube, 22 g), applied bid.

✓ Secondary infection should be treated with systemic antibiotics, such as cephalexin, 500 mg qid × 7 to 10 days, or azithromycin, 500 mg, then 250 mg qd × 4 days. Always keep in mind the possibility of an infection with community-acquired methicillin-resistant *Staphylococcus aureus* (CA-MRSA) (see Chapter 172).

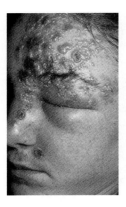

Figure 170-4 Ophthalmologic zoster vesicles and crusting of the top and side of the nose in herpes zoster implies involvement of the nasociliary branch of the trigeminal nerve and eye involvement. (From White G, Cox N: Diseases of the skin, ed 2. St Louis, 2006, Mosby.)

✅ Ocular lesions should be evaluated by an ophthalmologist and treated with topical ophthalmic corticosteroids. Although topical steroids are contraindicated in herpes simplex keratitis, because they allow deeper corneal injury, this does not appear to be a problem with herpes zoster ophthalmicus (Figure 170-4). If the rash extends to the tip of the nose (the Hutchinson sign), the eye will probably be involved, because it is served by the same nasociliary branch of the trigeminal nerve. Look for punctate keratopathy on slit-lamp examination with fluorescein staining, although patients may have only pain, lacrimation, conjunctivitis, or scleritis. Herpes zoster ophthalmicus can result in corneal scarring, uveitis, glaucoma, corneal perforation, or blindness. Patients with AIDS are at risk for developing acute retinal necrosis.

✅ Until all lesions are crusted, instruct patients to stay away from immunocompromised individuals and pregnant women who have not had chickenpox. Explain that they can transmit varicella (chickenpox) to a susceptible individual.

What Not To Do:

❌ Do not prescribe systemic steroids to prevent postherpetic neuralgia, especially for patients who are at high risk (i.e., with latent tuberculosis, immunocompromise, peptic ulcer, diabetes mellitus, hypertension, or congestive heart failure). Although they are sometimes recommended to reduce acute symptoms, oral corticosteroids given during the acute phase of the illness have not been shown to reduce the incidence or severity of postherpetic neuralgia.

❌ Do not initiate a comprehensive diagnostic workup to look for an occult malignancy simply on the basis of zoster. The incidence of cancer among patients with zoster is no greater than that of the general population. Patients with cancers, particularly lymphomas, are, however, at increased risk for zoster. Usually the cancer diagnosis is already known when zoster occurs.

❌ Do not use topical antiviral agents. They are not effective and are not recommended.

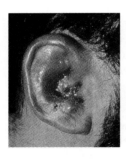

Figure 170-5 Ramsay Hunt syndrome. (From White G, Cox N: Diseases of the skin, ed 2. St Louis, 2006, Mosby.)

Discussion

Herpes zoster can usually be readily diagnosed from its clinical appearance of typical lesions in a dermatomal distribution. One well-known diagnostic caveat is that the pain and rash do not cross the midline; however, it is not impossible for the disease to be bilateral and involve more than one dermatome, and multidermatomal zoster may be the presenting finding for human immunodeficiency virus (HIV).

Bell's palsy (see Chapter 5) following zoster dermatitis of the external ear canal is well known and can be part of the Ramsay Hunt syndrome (Figure 170-5). The virus invades the facial nerve, especially the geniculate ganglion, and occasionally the auditory nerve, and can produce the peripheral seventh-nerve palsy, along with hearing loss, vertigo, and taste dysfunction.

Antiviral therapy has been shown to shorten the duration of viral shedding, halt the formation of new lesions more quickly, accelerate the rate of healing, and reduce the severity of acute pain. Herpes zoster ophthalmicus is a particularly important variant, and these patients should definitely receive antiviral therapy early with the goal of preventing ocular complications.

Antiviral treatment is generally recommended for all patients of any age with severely symptomatic herpes zoster and for patients older than age 50 years with zoster of any severity. Most authors on the subject do not advocate the use of antiviral therapy for immunocompetent patients who are younger than 50 years of age and who have mild acute symptoms.

Discussion continued

When the diagnosis is in doubt, the Tzanck test can help. Select an intact early vesicular lesion, unroof it, and, using the belly of a No. 15 scalpel blade, scrape the floor of the vesicle to obtain as much exudate as possible. Gently transfer this material to a clean glass slide and allow it to air dry. A Wright or Giemsa stain will reveal multinucleated giant cells.

If available, polymerase chain reaction (PCR) techniques are the most sensitive and specific diagnostic tests for detecting the varicella DNA in fluid taken from the vesicles. The direct immunofluorescence antigen-staining test provides an alternative diagnostic modality when PCR is not available, but it carries a lower sensitivity (77% to 82% vs. 94% to 95% with PCR) and a lower specificity (70% to 76% vs. 100% with PCR).

Herpes zoster affects 10% to 20% of the U.S. population. It results from reactivation of latent herpes varicella-zoster (chickenpox) virus residing in dorsal root or cranial nerve ganglion cells. The virus migrates peripherally along axons into the skin. Two thirds of the patients are older than 40 years of age. Herpes zoster is contagious to those who have not had varicella or have not received the varicella vaccine. Although shingles is not as contagious as chickenpox, it can be transmitted by contact with secretions from the vesicles. A patient with zoster can give chickenpox to a susceptible individual. A patient with chickenpox cannot give any other patient herpes zoster.

In addition to increasing age, other risk factors for reactivation of varicella zoster virus include conditions in which there is altered cell-mediated immunity, including diabetes, cancer, administration of immunosuppressive drugs (including corticosteroids), HIV, and organ transplantation. In immunocompetent patients, zoster is usually a self-limiting localized disease and heals within 3 to 4 weeks. Most patients can be reassured that their disease will abate without permanent problems. The incidence in immunocompromised patients is up to 10 times higher than in immunocompetent hosts, and usually their treatment must be more aggressive.

In these immunocompromised patients, herpes zoster can become disseminated, with lesions appearing outside the primary dermatomes and with visceral involvement. These patients generally require hospital admission for IV antiviral therapy.

The most common complication of herpes zoster is postherpetic neuralgia (i.e., pain along cutaneous nerves, persisting more than 30 days after the lesions have healed). This is more likely to occur in older patients (60 years of age or older), those in whom the degree of skin surface involved is larger, and those with severe pain at time of presentation. Both the incidence and the duration of postherpetic neuralgia are directly correlated with the patient's age; nearly half of patients 60 years of age or older will develop enduring neuropathic pain. Pain can persist for months and in some patients for many years and can be the source of debilitating neuropathic pain, with considerable physical and psychosocial morbidity.

The tricyclic antidepressant amitriptyline (Elavil) can be used to treat such pain. It can be started at 12.5 to 25 mg daily and increased by 12.5 to 25 mg every 3 to 5 days, to a maximum of 250 mg daily. The most common side effects are dry mouth, constipation, and sedation, which are generally not a major problem at the relatively low doses needed for effect (average dosage being 70 mg daily).

At present, the most promising analgesic approaches for reducing the risk for postherpetic neuralgia, beyond that achieved by antiviral agents, is treatment with an opioid analgesic or with one of the anticonvulsant drugs, such as gabapentin (Neurontin) and pregabalin (Lyrica). These are drugs that already have demonstrated efficacy in treating postherpetic neuralgia (PHN).

PHN can be treated with oxycodone (Oxycontin), titrating the dosage from 10 mg bid to effect or a maximum of 60 mg bid or until the patient experiences intolerable side effects. Common side effects include constipation, sedation, and nausea.

The anticonvulsant gabapentin is an alternative choice for treating PHN. The dosage can be started at 300 mg daily divided tid and titrated over 2 weeks to a maximum of 1800 mg daily divided tid (although dosages up to 3600 mg have been used). Side effects include sedation and dizziness. Pregabalin can also be used, initially starting with 75 mg bid and increasing within 1 week to 100 to 150 mg bid. Always take into consideration that dosage is to be adjusted to a patient's medical history and tolerance.

(continued)

Discussion continued

Topical treatment of PHN includes the relatively inexpensive capsaicin cream (Zostrix) 0.075%, which needs to be applied four times per day and can cause burning and stinging that usually subsides after the first week. An alternative is the more expensive 5% lidocaine patch (Lidoderm), which is applied to intact skin covering the most painful area. These topical treatments may be used to complement systemic analgesia.

Intrathecal methylprednisolone is an option for PHN patients with persistent pain.

It is interesting that most immunosuppressed individuals who develop zoster, even those with disseminated disease, do not develop PHN.

The new live attenuated varicella-zoster vaccine (Zostavax), which is a more powerful version of the vaccine currently given to children for chickenpox, is approved for adults age 60 years and older. It is expected to reduce the incidence of herpes zoster by about 50% and greatly reduce the severity and duration of the disease in those cases that do occur after vaccination. Its efficacy overall in preventing postherpetic neuralgia was 67%. The duration of protection and the need for booster vaccination remain to be determined.

Suggested Readings

Alper BS, Lewis PR: Does treatment of acute herpes zoster prevent or shorten postherpetic neuralgia? *J Fam Pract* 49:255–264, 2000.

Berry JD, Peterson KL: A single dose of gabapentin reduces acute pain and allodynia in patients with herpes zoster, *Neurology* 65:444–447, 2005.

Dworkin RH, Johnson RW, Breuer J, et al: Recommendations for the management of herpes zoster, *Clin Infect Dis* 44(Suppl 1):S1–S26, 2007.

Gabapentin (Neurontin) for chronic pain, *Med Lett Drugs Ther* 46:29–31, 2004.

Goh CL, Khoo L: A retrospective study on the clinical outcome of herpes zoster in patients with acyclovir or valaciclovir vs. patients not treated with antiviral, *Internat J Derm* 37:544–546, 1998.

Grant DM, Mauskopf JA, Bell L, et al: Comparison of valacyclovir and acyclovir for the treatment of herpes zoster in immunocompetent patients over 50 years of age, *Pharmacotherapy* 17:333–341, 1997.

Herpes zoster vaccine (Zostavax), *Med Lett Drugs Ther* 48:73–74, 2006.

Holten KB: Treatment of herpes zoster, *Am Fam Physician* 73:882–884, 2006.

Leung AKC, Rafaat M: Vesicular rash on the flank and buttock, *Am Fam Physician* 67:1045–1046, 2003.

Mounsey AL, Matthew LG, Slawson DC: Herpes zoster and postherpetic neuralgia: prevention and management, *Am Fam Physician* 72:1075–1080, 2005.

Pascuzzi RM: Peripheral neuropathies in clinical practice, *Med Clin North Am* 87:697–724, 2003.

Rowbotham M, Harden N, Stacey B, et al: Gabapentin for the treatment of postherpetic neuralgia: a randomized controlled trial, *JAMA* 280:1837–1842, 1998.

Shafran SD, Tyring SK, Ashton R, et al: Once, twice, or three times daily famiciclovir compared with acyclovir for the oral treatment of herpes zoster in immunocompetent adults, *J Clin Virol* 29:248–253, 2004.

Smith KJ, Roberts MS: Antiviral therapies for herpes zoster infections, *Pharmacoeconomics* 18:95–104, 2000.

Tenser RB, Dworkin RH: Herpes zoster and the prevention of postherpetic neuralgia: beyond antiviral therapy, *Neurology* 65:340–350, 2005.

Thomas SL, Hall AJ: What does epidemiology tell us about risk factors for herpes zoster? *Lancet Infect Dis* 4:26–33, 2004.

Tyring S, Barbarash RA, Nahlik JE, et al: Famciclovir for the treatment of acute herpes zoster: effects on acute disease and postherpetic neuralgia, *Ann Intern Med* 123:89–96, 1995.

Whitley RJ, Weiss H, Gnann JW, et al: Acyclovir with and without prednisone for the treatment of herpes zoster, *Ann Intern Med* 125:376–383, 1996.

Wood MJ, Johnson RW, McKendrick MW, et al: A randomized trial of acyclovir for 7 days or 21 days with and without prednisolone for treatment of acute herpes zoster, *N Engl J Med* 330:896–900, 1994.

Hymenoptera (Bee, Wasp, Hornet) Envenomation

(Bee Sting)

Presentation

Sometimes a patient comes to a hospital emergency department (ED) or urgent care center immediately after a painful sting, because he is alarmed at the intensity of the pain or worried about developing a serious life-threatening reaction. Sometimes he seeks help the next day because of swelling, redness, and itching. Parents may not be aware that their child was stung by a bee and may be concerned only about the local swelling.

The usual local reaction to a hymenopteran sting is immediate burning and pain, followed by an intense local erythematous wheal, which usually subsides within several hours. Often there is a central punctate discoloration at the site of the sting, or, uncommonly, a stinger may be protruding (only honeybees leave a stinger). A more extensive delayed hypersensitivity reaction can occur, producing varying degrees of edema and induration, which can be quite dramatic when present on the face and may involve all of an arm or leg (Figure 171-1). These local hypersensitivity reactions can last as long as 7 days. Tenderness and, occasionally, ascending lymphangitis can occur.

Symptoms of a severe anaphylactic reaction may include generalized urticaria, angioedema, generalized pruritus, shortness of breath, chest constriction, wheezing, stomach pain, dizziness, nausea, hoarseness, thickened speech, inspiratory stridor, weakness, confusion, and feelings of impending doom or even loss of consciousness. Milder forms of acute anaphylaxis subside within 20 minutes in most cases.

What To Do:

✅ **If an imbedded honeybee stinger is present at the time the patient is stung, it is most important to remove the stinger quickly,** even if it is grasped and pulled off, rather than delaying to find a hard edge to scrape it off with. The entire honeybee venom load is injected in less than 20 seconds. Because of regulation valves on the sting apparatus, the venom does not flow freely when the sting bulb is compressed.

✅ **Examine the patient for any signs of an immediate systemic allergic reaction (anaphylaxis),** such as decreased blood pressure, generalized urticaria or erythema, wheezing, tongue swelling, pharyngeal edema, or laryngeal spasm. Treat any of these findings aggressively with epinephrine, 1:1000 (0.01 mL/kg, maximum 0.5 mL IM [with severe reactions, every 10 to 20 minutes]; airway support; supplemental O_2; IV fluids (20 mL/kg normal saline bolus infused rapidly); corticosteroids (e.g., methylprednisolone [Solu-Medrol], 0.2 mg/kg or 125 mg IV); antihistamines (e.g., diphenhydramine [Benadryl], 1 to 2 mg/kg, or 25 to 50 mg/dose IV); an H_2

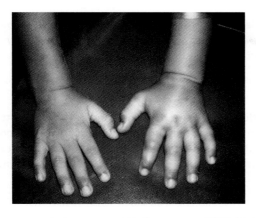

Figure 171-1 Edema due to local reaction to bee sting.

blocker (e.g., ranitidine [Zantac], 0.7 mg/kg or 50 mg IV); and glucagon in patients with beta-blockade (0.05 mg/kg, maximum 1 mg IV every 5 to 10 minutes). Glucagon's catecholamine-like action occurs by directly increasing cellular cyclic adenosine monophosphate (cAMP). **Epinephrine is the keystone of management. It halts the further release of mediators and reverses many of the effects of released mediators.**

Patients with milder generalized reactions that rapidly clear after treatment with epinephrine, steroids, antihistamines, and H_2 blockers may be observed for 3 to 6 hours and released if their symptoms have completely cleared. Patients with more serious reactions or with recurrent signs and symptoms of anaphylaxis should be admitted to the hospital for continued treatment and further observation.

On discharge from acute care after an anaphylactic reaction, prescribe a sting kit to carry at all times (e.g., an epinephrine autoinjector [EpiPen, 0.3 mg; Epi Pen Jr., 0.15 mg]) and refer the patient to an allergist for possible desensitization. Also provide a short course of steroids in addition to antihistamines and an H_2 receptor antagonist (see Chapter 183). Inform patients that if stung in the future, subsequent reactions are more likely to be less severe, but if generalized symptoms occur, they should use their epinephrine and report to a medical care facility.

Apply a cold pack to an acute sting to give pain relief and reduce swelling. Try ibuprofen or acetaminophen for analgesia.

For a minor sting, give an oral antihistamine, such as diphenhydramine, 25 to 50 mg, or hydroxyzine (Atarax, Vistaril), 25 to 50 mg, to reduce subsequent itching.

Prescribe additional antihistamine qid for further itching. A minor reaction will also benefit from a topical steroid cream, such as hydrocortisone, 1% to 2.5%, or triamcinolone (Kenalog, Aristocort), 0.1% to 0.5%.

For a severe local reaction with no contraindications, you may prescribe a systemic corticosteroid, such as prednisone, 50 mg qd for 3 to 4 days. This is a common practice and a reasonable treatment, although steroids have no proven benefit. Be aware of common side affects from steroids: insomnia, agitation, some immune suppression, and a slightly higher incidence of tendon rupture.

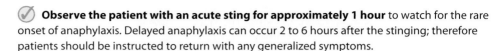

✅ **Observe the patient with an acute sting for approximately 1 hour** to watch for the rare onset of anaphylaxis. Delayed anaphylaxis can occur 2 to 6 hours after the stinging; therefore patients should be instructed to return with any generalized symptoms.

✅ Reassure the patient who has come in after 12 to 24 hours that anaphylaxis is no longer a potential problem.

✅ **Large local reactions often have the appearance of cellulitis with swelling, erythema, and, on occasion, warmth and ascending lymphangitis. These reactions most often represent chemical cellulitis and are pruritic and nontender. Reactions such as these do not require antibiotics but only elevation and soothing, cooling compresses in addition to the antihistamine.**

✅ When there is tenderness and pain, and therefore true bacterial cellulitis is a possibility (although uncommon), it is reasonable to treat the patient with an appropriate antibiotic, such as cefadroxil (Duricef), 1 g qd; cephalexin (Keflex), 500 mg tid; dicloxacillin (Dynapen), 500 mg qid for 5 to 10 days; or azithromycin (Zithromax), 500 mg, then 250 mg qd for 4 days.

✅ Provide tetanus prophylaxis (see Appendix H) as for a clean minor wound.

✅ **In all situations, if an extremity is involved, have the patient keep it elevated and instruct him that the swelling may worsen if the hand or foot is held in a dependent position. Warn patients who have been recently stung that swelling and redness may increase over the next 24 to 48 hours** and may involve a large area and continue for several days. Preparing them for this potentially alarming development may prevent unnecessary worry and an unneeded revisit. Reassure them that even the worst swelling will resolve with time and elevation.

✅ **Promptly remove any rings** (see Chapter 152) **in cases of hand or arm stings.**

✅ To help prevent future stings, instruct patients to wear shoes and avoid wearing brightly colored clothing and using fragrances when outside, and to avoid recreational activities when yellow jackets or hornets are nearby. Hives and nests around a home should be exterminated, and good sanitation should be practiced, because garbage and outdoor food, especially canned drinks, attract yellow jackets. Unfortunately, insect repellents have little or no effect.

What Not To Do:

❌ Do not send the patient with an acute sting home less than 1 hour after the sting.

❌ Do not apply heat, even if an infection is suspected—the swelling and discomfort will worsen.

❌ Do not prescribe the Epi-Pen or another anaphylaxis treatment for patients who have only had a localized reaction.

Discussion

Only stinging insects of the Hymenoptera order cause anaphylaxis with any frequency. A sting is an injection of venom by the female of each species through a modified ovipositor. Honeybees and bumblebees are relatively nonaggressive and generally sting only when caught underfoot. The barbs along the shaft of the honeybee stinger cause it to remain embedded at the sting site. Africanized honeybees have expanded northward and by 2002 were present in most of Texas and Arizona and southern areas of Nevada, California, and New Mexico. Referred to as "killer bees," they do not have increased venom potency or allergenicity but rather a tendency to attack en masse. Fortunately, even massive stinging incidents of 50 to 100 stings are not usually fatal. Most deleterious effects are estimated to occur in the range of 500 to 1200 stings. Older victims are more susceptible to the toxic effects of the venom.

The family Vespidae includes the yellow jackets, hornets, and wasps, which make papier-mâché–like nests of wood fiber. Yellow jackets, which cause most of the allergic sting reactions in the United States, usually nest in the ground or in decaying logs. Hornets build teardrop-shaped nests that hang in trees or bushes. Both yellow jackets and hornets are extremely aggressive, especially in the late summer when crowded conditions develop in the nests. Not quite as aggressive as the other vespids, the thin-bodied paper wasps build nests in the eaves of buildings.

Hymenopteran venoms contain a number of interesting constituents. Most of the venoms contain histamine, dopamine, acetylcholine, and kinins, which cause the characteristics of burning and pain. The allergens in the venoms are mostly proteins with enzyme activity.

Systemic allergic reactions (anaphylaxis) may be mild with only cutaneous symptoms (pruritus, urticaria, and angioedema of the eyes, lips, hands) or severe with potentially life-threatening symptoms of laryngeal edema, bronchospasm, and hypotension. Systemic allergic reactions are, in general, less severe in children than adults, although children are more likely to develop isolated cutaneous reactions.

Large local reactions are usually late-phase IgE-mediated allergic reactions with severe swelling developing over 24 to 48 hours and resolving in 2 to 7 days.

Bee stings by themselves are very painful and frightening. There are many misconceptions about the danger of bee stings, and many patients with previous localized reactions have been instructed unnecessarily to report to an emergency department or clinic immediately after being stung. Patients who have suffered only localized hypersensitivity reactions in the past are not at a significantly greater risk than the general public for developing anaphylaxis, which is defined as an immediate generalized reaction. Other than some relief of pain and itching for the acute sting, there is little more than reassurance to offer these patients.

Anaphylactic reactions generally occur within a few minutes to 1 hour after the sting. Most victims have no history of bee sting allergy.

Patients with a history of systemic sting reactions have been found on average to have a 50% risk for experiencing another systemic reaction to a challenge sting. Some patients who do not react to a first sting challenge react to a subsequent sting. Systemic reactions usually do not become progressively more severe with each sting. Often, the stinging insect allergy is self-limited. The risk for reaction declines from more than 50% initially to 35% 3 to 5 years after the sting reaction, and to approximately 25% 10 years or more after the sting reaction. In some instances, unfortunately, the risk for anaphylaxis persists for decades, even with no intervening stings.

Patients with a history of systemic reactions should carry a kit containing injectable epinephrine and chewable antihistamines to be used at the first sign of a generalized reaction. Venom-specific immunotherapy for hymenopteran allergy can markedly reduce the risk for repeat systemic reaction approximately 30% to 60%. Patients who have had extensive local reactions, but not general ones, tend to react the same way to subsequent stings despite venom immunotherapy.

Although at times it may seem most prudent to treat ascending lymphangitis with an antibiotic, it should be realized that after a bee sting, the resultant local cellulitis and lymphangitis are usually chemically mediated inflammatory reactions and are not affected by antibiotic therapy.

Suggested Readings

Anchor J, Settipane RA: Appropriate use of epinephrine in anaphylaxis, *Am J Emerg Med* 22:488–490, 2004.

Chiu AM, Kelly KJ: Anaphylaxis: drug allergy, insect stings, and latex, *Immunol Allerg Clin North Am* 25:389–405, 2005.

Golden DBK: Stinging insect allergy, *Am Fam Physician* 67:2541–2546, 2003.

Graft DF: Insect sting allergy, *Med Clin North Am* 90:211–232, 2006.

Jerrard DA: Emergency department management of insect stings, *Am J Emerg Med* 14:429–433, 1996.

Simons FE: Anaphylaxis: Recent advances in assessment and treatment, *J Allergy Clin Immunol* 124:625–635, 2009.

Visscher PK, Vetter RS, Camazine S: Removing bee stings, *Lancet* 348:301–302, 1996.

Impetigo

Presentation

Parents will usually bring their children (most commonly aged 2 to 5 years) to be checked, because they are developing unsightly skin lesions. The lesions are usually painless but may be pruritic and are found most often on the face (Figure 172-1) or other exposed areas. Parents may be worried that their young child has "infant-tigo" (the common lay misnomer). Nonbullous lesions consist of irregular or somewhat circular red oozing erosions (sores), often covered with a yellow-brown honey-like crust (Figure 172-2). These may be surrounded by smaller erythematous macular or vesiculopustular areas. Bullous lesions (Figure 172-3) present as large thin-walled bullae, which quickly rupture and are replaced by a thin shiny varnish-like coating over the denuded area on an erythematous base. More than one area may be involved, and a mix of bullous and nonbullous findings can exist.

What To Do:

✅ **For a few lesions involving a relatively small area, prescribe mupirocin 2% (Bactroban) cream or ointment to be applied to the rash tid for 10 days.** Have parents soften and cleanse crusts with warm soapy compresses before applying the antibiotic cream or ointment. There is little scientific evidence regarding the value of any disinfecting measures, such as the use of povidone-iodine and chlorhexidine. A newer antibiotic, retapamulin (Altabax) (ointment 1% [available in 5-, 10-, and 15-g tubes], apply bid × 5 days), was approved by the Food and Drug Administration (FDA) in 2007 and although expensive, appears to be effective even against MRSA strains.

✅ **For large areas of involvement or resistant cases, add an oral antibiotic with activity against *Staphylococcus aureus* and group A beta-hemolytic streptococcal infections:** azithromycin (Zithromax), 500 mg, then 250 mg qd (10 mg/kg, then 5 mg/kg/day) × 4 days, or cephalexin (Keflex), 250 to 500 mg tid to qid (25 to 50 mg/kg/day). Alternatives include amoxicillin/clavulanate (Augmentin), 250 to 500 mg/125 mg q8h (25 to 45 mg/kg/day divided q12h) × 10 days, or dicloxacillin, 250 to 500 mg qid (12.5 to 25 mg/kg/day divided q6h) × 10 days. In communities where community-acquired methicillin-resistant *Staphylococcus aureus* (CA-MRSA) is prevalent, prescribe trimethoprim/sulfamethoxazole (Bactrim, Septra), 160 mg TMP bid (8 to 10 mg/kg/day divided q12h) × 10 days, or clindamycin (Cleocin), 150 to 300 mg qid (10 to 30 mg/kg/day divided q8h) × 10 days. Alternative options should be based on local susceptibility results.

✅ **Consider obtaining cultures if CA-MRSA is prevalent in your area.**

✅ To prevent the spread of this infection, have the patient and his family wash their hands frequently, change towels and bed linens every day, and keep infected schoolchildren home

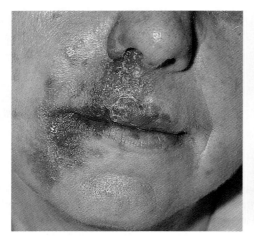

Figure 172-1 Impetigo of the face. (From White G, Cox N: *Diseases of the skin*, ed 2. St Louis, 2006, Mosby.)

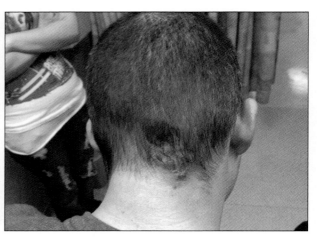

Figure 172-2 Kerion with surrounding impetigo.

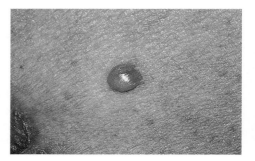

Figure 172-3 Bullous impetigo. (From White G, Cox N: *Diseases of the skin*, ed 2. St Louis, 2006, Mosby.)

until the acute phase has cleared. Nasal carriage of *S. aureus* has been implicated as a source of recurrent disease and can be reduced by the topical application of mupirocin within the nares twice daily for 5 days (nasal ointment 2% [1-g single-use tubes]); apply ½ tube in each nostril bid.

What Not To Do:

Ⓧ Do not use bacitracin, neomycin, or similar antibacterial ointments on these lesions. They are less effective than mupirocin and may cause unnecessary contact dermatitis.

Discussion

Impetigo is a common superficial skin infection that is mostly seen during the summer in temperate climates and throughout the year in warm, humid tropical regions worldwide.

Nonbullous impetigo was previously thought to be a group A streptococcal process, and bullous impetigo was primarily thought to be caused by *S. aureus*. Studies now indicate that both forms of impetigo are primarily caused by *S. aureus*, with *Streptococcus* usually being involved in the nonbullous form. If the infection is a toxin-producing phage group II type 71 *Staphylococcus* (the same toxin seen in scalded skin syndrome), large bullae will form as the toxin produces intradermal cleavage. Otherwise, smaller bullae develop, and the honey-crusted lesions predominate.

Impetigo is thought to be self-limiting, but studies on its natural history do not exist.

It is thought that antibiotic treatment does not alter the subsequent low incidence of **secondary glomerulonephritis,** especially in children aged 2 to 6 years. Presenting signs and symptoms of glomerulonephritis include edema and hypertension; about one third of patients have smoky or tea-colored urine.

Impetigo is very contagious among infants and young children and may be associated with poor hygiene, a break in the skin, or predisposing skin eruptions, such as herpes simplex, angular cheilitis, insect bites, scabies, and atopic and contact dermatitis. When lesions occur singly, they may be mistaken for herpes simplex. *S. aureus* can directly invade the skin and cause a de novo infection.

Suggested Readings

Bass JW, Chan DS, Creamer KM, et al: Comparison of oral cephalexin, topical mupirocin, and topical bacitracin for treatment of impetigo, *Ped Infect Dis J* 16:708–710, 1997.

Bhumbra NA, McCullough SG: Skin and subcutaneous infections, *Prim Care* 30:1–24, 2003.

Iyer S, Jones DH: Community-acquired methicillin-resistant *Staphylococcus aureus* skin infection, *J Am Acad Dermatol* 50:854–858, 2004.

Kosowka-Schick K, Clark C, Credito K, et al: Single- and multistep resistance selection on the activity of retapamulin compared to other agents against *Staphylococcus aureus* and *Streptococcous pyogenes*, *Antimicrob Agents Chemother* 50:765–769, 2006.

Kraus SJ, Eron LJ, Bottenfield GW, et al: Mupirocin cream is as effective as oral cephalexin in the treatment of secondarily infected wounds, *J Fam Pract* 47:429–433, 1998.

McVicar J: Oral or topical antibiotics for impetigo, *J Accid Emerg Med* 16:364, 1999.

Sanfilippo AM, Barrio V, Kulp-Shorten C: Common pediatric and adolescent skin conditions, *J Pediatr Adolesc Gynecol* 16:269–283, 2003.

Stulberg DL: Common bacterial skin infections, *Am Fam Physician* 66:119–124, 2002.

Taylor JS: Interventions for impetigo, *Am Fam Physician* 7:1680–1681, 2004.

Partial-Thickness (Second-Degree) Burns and Tar Burns

Presentation

Partial-thickness burns can occur in a variety of ways. Spilled or splattered hot water and grease are among the most common causes, along with hot objects, explosive fumes, and burning (volatile) liquids. The patient will complain of excruciating pain, and the burn will appear erythematous with vesicle formation. Some of these vesicles or bullae may have ruptured before the patient's arrival, whereas others may not develop for 24 hours. Tar burns are special in that the tar adheres aggressively to the burned skin and therefore makes the burns look very unsightly.

What To Do:

✓ **To stop the pain, immediately cover the burned area with sterile towels that have first been soaked in iced normal saline, or just use cold tap water.** Continue irrigating the burn with the iced or cold solution for the next 20 to 30 minutes or until the patient can remain comfortable without the cold compresses.

✓ Determine the mechanism of injury and the extent and severity of the burn. The patient's palm represents approximately 1% of his total body surface and can be used to estimate the total area of the body surface burned. Examine the patient for any associated injuries. Transfer to a burn center and/or initiate generous fluid resuscitation if there are third-degree (full-thickness) burns over 5% of the total body surface, second-degree (partial-thickness) burns (alone or in combination with the third-degree burns) of over 10% to 15% of the total body surface (5% to 10% in children under 10 years of age), or extensive burns involving the face, hands, feet, joints, or genitalia. Special consideration should be given to the elderly or patients with significant comorbidity.

✓ **Consider and report any burn injuries suggestive of child abuse.** A supposed mechanism of injury that does not fit the injury or is not consistent with the child's level of development warrants investigation. Specific injuries that usually should be reported as suspected abuse include burns to the face, dorsum of the feet, and genitalia; cigarette burns; imprint burns, such as those from a hot iron or grill; stocking burns with a sharp line of demarcation from immersion in hot water; or glove burns to the hand as well as any circumferential burns or symmetric extremity burns.

✓ Provide the patient with any necessary tetanus prophylaxis (see Appendix H).

✓ **Administer potent pain medication (e.g., hydromorphone [Dilaudid], morphine, fentanyl [Sublimaze]) as required.**

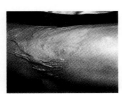

Figure 173-1 Open second-degree burn bullae may be left in place as a physiologic burn dressing.

✓ When the pain has subsided, gently cleanse the burn, with intact vesicles, with povidone-iodine scrub and rinse this off with normal saline. If bullae or vesicles are open, gently cleanse with plain normal saline.

✓ The providers participating in débridement and wound dressing should wear sterile gowns, gloves and masks, generally following "universal precautions" for wound care. This protects the wounds from potential infection and protects the providers as well.

✓ **If the bullae or vesicles are not perforated, they should be left intact. With small burns, patients can be sent home to continue cold compresses for comfort.** Otherwise, these vesicles should be protected from future rupture and contamination with a bulky sterile dressing.

✓ **Open bullae or vesicles that are fresh and uncontaminated can be easily pulled back into their original position to cover the burn surface** (Figure 173-1) **and then may be left in place as a physiologic burn dressing.** This should be covered with nonadherent oil emulsion gauze, such as Adaptic, and then protected with a bulky sterile dressing (e.g., fluffed 4 × 4 gauze pads wrapped with Kerlex). This will hold the thin layer of epithelium in place and absorb any leaking plasma while protecting the burn from contamination and providing comfort.

✓ **Bullae or vesicles that are open and contaminated, old, or whose walls are so friable and damaged that they cannot be used as a biologic burn dressing should be completely débrided. Then the burn surface should be flushed with saline.** Using fine scissors and forceps, strip away any of this loose epithelium from the burn.

✓ **For small clean burns that have been débrided, covering them with a transparent film of polyurethane with an adhesive coating (OpSite, Bioclusive, Tegaderm) provides a moist environment that enhances reepithelization and is comfortable.** There needs to be intact skin surrounding the area being dressed so that the dressing will adhere. Exudate collects under these film dressings and frequently leaks out. An outer absorbent dressing with dressing changes is required when this occurs. The synthetic film is left in place.

✓ **For larger débrided areas, a simple dressing with oil emulsion gauze (Adaptic) covered with sterile fluffed gauze is an effective acceptable burn dressing. A new soft silicone dressing (Mepitel, Mölnlycke Healthcare, Norcross, Ga.) can also be applied directly to the burn, with an overlying sterile dressing that will provide adequate padding to exclude voids beneath this polyamide net. Mepitel may be left in place for up to 7 to 10 days, but the outer absorbent layer should be changed more frequently as required. One study showed that burn wounds covered with Mepitel healed significantly faster with less eschar formation and less pain than with the standard control dressings.**

✓ **Although unnecessary for most superficial partial-thickness burns in outpatients, silver sulfadiazine (Silvadene) cream is most commonly used to cover these open burn wounds.** When this cream is used, it is only necessary to provide an absorbent protective gauze dressing over the burn area (without Adaptic); alternatively, the area can be left open and gently washed twice daily, followed by reapplication of the cream.

✓ **For greater patient convenience, an alternative is to use a silver-impregnated dressing (Acticoat), which is occlusive, promotes a moist healing environment, and eliminates the need for frequent dressing changes.** The Acticoat dressing is placed on the wound and is kept moist by applying sterile water, which activates the release of the silver ions into the wound. An outer layer of gauze bandage, such as Kerlix or Kling, can be used to protect the wound and keep the Acticoat in place. The Acticoat dressing does not have to be changed more frequently than every 3 days.

✓ **Biobrane collagen Silastic is an alternative synthetic dressing that is designed to be placed tightly against the wound with a compressive gauze dressing wrapped over it.** Within 2 days, as long as the wound is clean and has no seroma formation, the collagen side of the dressing adheres to the surface of the burn and effectively seals it. The dressing acts as a skin substitute and allows the underlying skin to heal and reepithelialize more comfortably. Biobrane may be left in place for 1 month.

✓ Dressings in general are used to absorb secretions, protect the burn from bacterial contamination, and prevent the wound from rubbing against clothing or other objects. When simple sterile dressings are used with Adaptic gauze or Mepitel, the frequency of dressing changes will vary depending on the amount of secretions. When Silvadene cream is used, washing and reapplication require that the dressing be changed once daily. The first dressing change should be done at a return visit to provide teaching instructions and additional dressing material. If available, continued burn management can be provided at a local burn clinic.

✓ **Facial and neck burns** cannot be easily dressed and generally require only the soothing topical application of bacitracin ointment. These burns will do well without any topical agents and require only gentle washing with a mild soap twice a day.

✓ **Tar burns** do not require removal of solidified residual tar. The tar is not toxic to the skin and often forms a sterile wound dressing. By covering the burn and tar with bacitracin ointment and performing daily washing and repeated dressing changes with more ointment, the tar will gradually dissolve away. Neomycin sulfate/polymyxin cream (Neosporin) has been recommended as a preferred tar emulsifier, but it carries the potential of causing allergic contact dermatitis. When tar burns on the face are unsightly, the hardened tar can usually be mechanically débrided or cleaned off with repeated applications of creams or ointments. Petrolatum jelly (Vaseline) and mineral oil can also be used to slowly wipe away the tar. The facial burns are then treated like any other facial burn.

✓ **Radiator and brief flash burns** (when patients attempt to light a gas stove) of the face are not associated with inhalation injuries (even with singed facial hair) and are also treated in the standard manner.

✓ Patients should be instructed to keep extremity and facial burns elevated to reduce swelling.

✓ **Prescribe adequate narcotic analgesics to provide adequate pain relief over the next 24 hours.**

✓ Patients can be reassured that superficial partial-thickness burns will generally heal in 7 to 21 days with full function, and, unless there are complications (such as infection), patients do not have to worry about scarring. Most superficial burns heal within 2 weeks, and long-term follow-up is unnecessary.

What Not To Do:

❌ Do not use large ice-containing packs or compresses that might increase tissue damage. Iced compresses should also be avoided on large burns (greater than 15% of total body surface), because they may lead to problems with hypothermia. When pain cannot be controlled with compresses, use strong parenteral analgesics, such as morphine sulfate.

❌ Do not provide prophylactic systemic antibiotics. They have not been shown to reduce the incidence of wound infection and are generally not indicated.

❌ Do not use neomycin-containing creams or ointments. They have the potential to cause a very unpleasant allergic contact dermatitis.

❌ Do not confuse partial-thickness burns with full-thickness burns. With full-thickness burns, there is no sensory function or skin appendages, such as hair follicles, remaining. They do not form vesicles and may have evidence of thrombosed vessels. If areas of full-thickness burn are present or suspected, seek surgical consultation, because these areas will later require skin grafting.

❌ Do not discharge patients with suspected respiratory burns or extensive burns of the hands, feet, or genitalia. These patients require special inpatient observation and management.

❌ Do not use caustic solvents in an attempt to remove tar from burns. It is unnecessary and painful and will cause further tissue destruction.

❌ Do not use synthetic dressings on old or contaminated burns, which have a high risk for infection.

Discussion

First-degree or superficial burns involve only the epidermis. These burns are usually painful and erythematous and do not blister. The pain usually resolves in 1 to 2 days and generally does not require anything more than cool compresses. These burns usually occur with brief contact with hot liquids.

Second-degree or partial-thickness burns involve the epidermis and portions of the dermis. Damaged dermal vessels leak serum into the stratum spinosum layer of the epidermis, forming the identifiable blisters or bullae. These burns are particularly painful. They heal spontaneously by reepithelization within 10 days to 2 weeks, providing that no infection occurs.

Third-degree or full-thickness burns involve all layers of the epidermis and dermis. These burns take on a "waxy white" appearance, and, with prolonged heat exposure, the skin takes on a yellow-brown "leathery" appearance. These burns are painless because of the damaged nerve endings, but the penumbra of partial-thickness burns may still cause the patient to have significant pain.

Simple partial-thickness burns will do well with nothing more than cleansing, débridement, and a sterile dressing. All other therapy, therefore, should be directed at making the patient more comfortable. Silvadene cream is not always necessary, but it is soothing and may reduce the risk for infection. Bacitracin ointment may also be used on small burns. **When it is possible to leave vesicles intact, the patient will have a shorter period of disability and will require fewer dressing changes and follow-up visits. Studies suggest that leaving the burn blisters intact results in more rapid reepithelization than when the blisters are débrided.** If the wound must be débrided, the closed-dressing technique may be more convenient and less of a mess than the open technique of washings and cream applications.

Some physicians believe that it is important to remove all traces of tar from a burn. Removal can be accomplished relatively easily by using a petroleum-based antibiotic ointment such as bacitracin, which

(continued)

Discussion continued

will dissolve the tar. This can be mixed with an equal amount of Unibase (ingredients: water, cetyl alcohol, stearyl alcohol, white petrolatum, glycerin, sodium citrate, sodium laurel sulfate, propylparaben). Others have found the citrus-and–petroleum distillate industrial cleanser Medi-Sol (Orange-Sol, Chandler, Ariz.) effective, as well as nontoxic and nonirritating.

Other effective solvents include polysorbate and Tween 80.

It is interesting to note that raw honey has been used as a successful burn dressing for centuries. One study demonstrated that honey was actually better than Silvadene for superficial burns.

Suggested Readings

American Burn Association: Guidelines for service standards and severity classicfications in the treatment of burn injury, *Am Coll Surg Bull* 69:24, 1984.

Gotschall CS, Morrison MI, Eichelberger MR: Prospective, randomized study of the efficacy of Mepitel on children with partial-thickness scalds, *J Burn Care Rehabil* 19:279–283, 1998.

Levy DB, Barone JA, York JM, et al: Unibase and triple antibiotic ointment for hardened tar removal, *Ann Emerg Med* 15:765–766, 1986.

Lionelli GT, Lawrence WT: Wound dressings, *Surg Clin North Am* 83:617–638, 2003.

Stratta RJ, Saffle JR, Kravitz M, et al: Management of tar and asphalt injuries, *Am J Surg* 146:766–769, 1983.

Subrahmanyam M: A prospective randomized clinical and histological study of superficial burn wound healing with honey and silver sulfadiazine, *Burns* 24:157–161, 1998.

Pediculosis

(Lice, Crabs)

Presentation

Patients arrive with emotions ranging from annoyance to sheer disgust at the discovery of an infestation with lice or crabs and request acute medical care. There may be extreme pruritus, and the patient may bring in a sample of the creature to show you. Head lice generally affect children, primarily girls, aged 3 to 12 years. The adult forms of head lice can be very difficult to find, but their oval, light gray eggs (nits) can be readily found firmly attached to the hairs above the ears and toward the occiput. Secondary impetigo and furunculosis can occur.

The adult forms of pubic lice (*Phthirus* organisms or crab lice) are more easily found, but their light yellow-gray color still makes them difficult to see. Small black dots present in infested areas represent either ingested blood in adult lice or their excreta. Maculae ceruleae (bluish-brown macules), which represent intradermal hemorrhage at sites where lice have fed, can sometimes be found. Pubic lice are not limited to the pubic region and may be found on other short hairs of the body, such as body hair, eyebrows, and eyelashes (pediculosis ciliaris).

Identification of lice, larvae, or viable nits with a magnifying glass makes the diagnosis (Figure 174-1).

What To Do:

✓ **For head lice, instruct the patient and other close contacts regarding the use of nonprescription louse treatments. The most effective is 1% permethrin (Nix), which should be applied undiluted to clean, towel-dried hair until the affected area is entirely wet.** After 10 minutes, shampoo and rinse with warm water. It is not necessary to remove nits. To kill newly hatched nymphs, a second treatment should be given 7 to 10 days later.

✓ Itching or mild burning of the scalp caused by inflammation of the skin in response to topical therapeutic agents can persist for many days after lice are killed, and the condition is not a reason for re-treatment. Topical corticosteroids and oral antihistamines may be beneficial for relieving these signs and symptoms.

✓ **For severe or resistant infestations, combining 1% permethrin treatment with oral trimethoprim/sulfamethoxazole (TMP/SMX), 5 mg/kg bid for 10 days, will have a higher cure rate than permethrin alone at 4 weeks (93% vs. 72%).** TMP/SMX is not toxic to the louse; instead, it acts by killing essential bacterial flora in the insect's gastrointestinal tract.

✓ A second over-the-counter (OTC) choice is a preparation combining piperonyl butoxide and pyrethrin extracts (RID), which is applied in the same fashion. This product does not kill all of the unhatched eggs and has no residual activity, is less effective, and is more allergenic than permethrin.

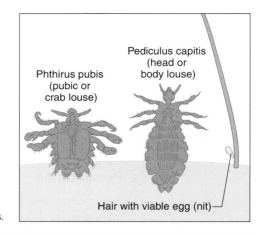

Figure 174-1 Pediculosis.

✅ **As lice have become resistant to OTC treatments, some clinicians have had to escalate to prescription strength 5% permethrin cream (Elimite) applied to clean, dry hair and left on overnight (8 to 14 hours) under a shower cap.** Resistance still occurs even at these higher concentrations of permethrin.

✅ **Benzyl alcohol lotion 5% (Ulesfia [Sciele Pharma, Atlanta, Ga.]) is a prescription medicine** that was approved by the U.S. Food and Drug Administration (FDA) in April 2009 for treatment of head lice in children older than 6 months. The product is not neurotoxic and kills head lice by asphyxiation. Patients receive two 10-minute treatments 1 week apart, but consideration should be given to re-treating in 9 days or using three treatment cycles (days 0, 7, and 13 to 15).

✅ **Resistant infestations with treatment failures are most commonly treated with the prescription formula of malathion (Ovide) 0.5% lotion.** Apply it to dry hair and then shampoo. It may be reapplied 7 to 9 days later if necessary. Although a lengthy application time is specified on the product's label (8 to 12 hours), a recent study found that malathion 0.5% was 98% effective with just one or two 20-minute applications. Because of potential flammability, patients should be instructed to avoid using a hair dryer or curling iron during treatment with malathion. **Malathion can only be used in people who are 24 months of age or older, when resistance to permethrin or pyrethrins is documented, or when treatment with these products fails despite their correct use.**

✅ **Removal of all topical pediculicides should be accomplished by rinsing the hair over a sink** rather than in the shower or bath. This limits skin exposure. Using warm, rather than hot water, will minimize absorption attributable to vasodilation.

✅ **For head lice that are resistant to all other treatments, give a single oral dose of ivermectin (Stromectol), 200 to 400 µg/kg PO once, repeated once after 7 to 10 days.** Most recently, a single oral dose of 400 µg/kg repeated in 7 days has been shown to be more effective than 0.5% malathion lotion. Ivermectin should not be used for children who weigh less than 15 kg.

✅ **Instruct families** to disinfect sheets and clothing by machine washing in hot water, machine drying on the hot cycle for 20 minutes, ironing, dry cleaning, or just storing in plastic bags for 2 weeks. Combs and brushes should be soaked in 2% Lysol or heated in water to about 65° C for 10 minutes.

✅ **Nit removal is recommended for aesthetic reasons and can help identify if there is a later recurrence.** Removal of the eggs is not necessary to prevent spreading the infestation. Application of a 1:1 solution of white vinegar and water may help to loosen nits before removal with a fine-toothed comb.

✅ **Pubic lice are most commonly sexually transmitted, and sexual contacts must also be treated. In addition, this finding should prompt an evaluation for other sexually transmitted diseases. Treatment is the same as that for pediculosis capitis, with the exception that pediculosis of the eyelashes should be treated with an occlusive ophthalmic ointment** applied to the eyelid margins for 10 days.

✅ **Patients often want to use "natural," less toxic products or techniques** for their children or themselves. Some occlusive products, such as petroleum jelly (Vaseline), mayonnaise, and olive oil, have been used in place of traditional pediculicides, but their effectiveness has not been established in controlled trials. **One OTC product, HairClean 1-2-3, consisting of anise oil, ylang ylang oil, coconut oil, and isopropyl alcohol, was more effective than 1% permethrin in an uncontrolled study.**

✅ **A "nonneurotoxic" suffocation-based pediculicide ("Nuvo lotion," which is actually Cetaphil Gentle Skin Cleanser) produced a high cure rate in children with head lice in one small nonblinded study.**

✅ One author is an enthusiastic advocate of the LiceGuard Robi Comb, a fine-toothed metal comb that is connected to a single AA battery. When used on dry hair for 5 to 10 minutes daily for 2 weeks, it is said to eliminate head lice by essentially electrocuting them.

✅ **When cosmetically acceptable, head shaving is effective.**

✅ **When one is facing a persistent case of lice,** several explanations must be considered, including misdiagnosis, noncompliance with treatment protocol, reinfestation, lack of adequate ovicidal properties of the treatment product, and resistance to the pediculicide. All household members should be checked for lice, but only those with live lice or eggs within 1 cm of the scalp should be treated.

What Not To Do:

❌ Do not mistake a hair cast for a nit (which is firmly attached to a hair shaft). Hair casts are freely movable along the hair shaft.

❌ Do not apply pediculicides to wet hair. Water dilutes the product and protects lice as they reflexively close their respiratory spiracles when exposed to water.

❌ Do not recommend comprehensive cleaning of the whole house. Adult lice cannot survive for more than 1 day if they cannot find a meal of blood.

❌ Do not have the family use commercial sprays (R&C Spray or Li-Ban Spray) to control lice on inanimate objects. Their use is no more effective than vacuuming.

❌ Do not prescribe lindane (Kwell) shampoo. It is an organochloride compound that is absorbed and can be toxic to the central nervous system and cause anemia. In view of reports of lindane resistance and the availability of products with more favorable safety profiles, it is no longer recommended.

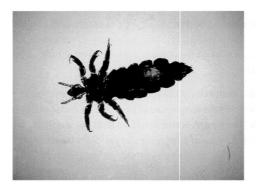

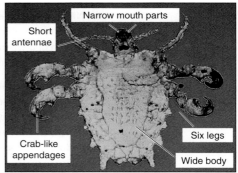

Figure 174-2 Identifying characteristics of a head louse. (Adapted from Ko CJ, Elston DM: Pediculosis, *J Am Acad Dermatol* 50:1-12, 2004.)

Figure 174-3 Identifying characteristics of crab louse. (Adapted from Ko CJ, Elston DM: Pediculosis, *J Am Acad Dermatol* 50:1-12, 2004.)

(X) Do not use flammable or toxic substances, such as gasoline or kerosene.

(X) Do not use products intended for animal use.

Discussion

Blood-sucking lice have long been successful obligate parasites of humans. The three major lice that infest humans are *Pediculus humanus capitis* (head louse) (Figure 174-2), *Pthirus pubis* (crab louse) (Figure 174-3), and *Pediculus humanus humanus* (body louse). Patients with louse infestation present with pruritus, excoriations, and lymphadenopathy. A hypersensitivity rash, or pediculid, may mimic a viral exanthem.

Head lice infestation crosses all economic and social boundaries. The head louse is the size of a sesame seed, 1 to 2 mm in length. After attaching to the patient, the louse inserts its mouth parts and injects saliva with vasodilatory properties. An inflammatory reaction to injected louse saliva has been suggested as the most likely cause of bite reactions. Transmission in most cases occurs by direct contact with the head of another infested individual. Head lice move by grasping hairs, generally remaining close to the scalp. Head lice can crawl rapidly, traveling up to 23 cm/min. Lice egg cases are referred to as nits. They are firmly cemented to human hair and are thus difficult to remove (Figure 174-4). Except in very humid climates, lice lay nits (ova within a chitinous case) within 1 to 2 mm of the scalp. Young lice hatch within 1 week and pass through three nymphal stages, maturing to adults over a period of 1 week. Lice must generally eat every 4 to 6 hours. In most climates, they survive only several hours off the scalp, although they may live for up to 4 days in favorable conditions. In the United States, blacks have a lower incidence of infestation, possibly because lice are better adapted to grasp the more cylindrical hairs of whites or Asians.

The diagnosis of head lice is definitive when crawling lice are seen in the scalp hair or are combed from the scalp. Because head lice avoid light and can crawl quickly, the use of louse combs increases the chances of finding live lice. Nits alone are not diagnostic of active infestation, but if the nits are within 1 cm (¼ inch) of the scalp, active infestation is likely. Hair casts may closely resemble nits stuck to hair shafts. A parent, teacher, or school nurse generally notices them and mistakes them for nits. In contrast to nits, hair casts are freely movable along the hair shaft. Among presumed "lice" and "nits" submitted by physicians, nurses, teachers, and parents to a laboratory for identification, many were found to be artifacts such as dandruff, hairspray droplets, scabs, dirt, or other insects (e.g., aphids blown by the wind and caught in the hair).

The female louse lives about 3 to 4 weeks and lays approximately 10 eggs a day. The eggs are incubated

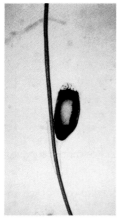

Figure 174-4 Lice nit firmly cemented to human hair. (Adapted from Ko CJ, Elston DM: Pediculosis, *J Am Acad Dermatol* 50:1-12, 2004.)

Discussion continued

by body heat and hatch in 7 to 10 days. If newly hatched eggs that survived the initial therapy are not re-treated, the cycle may repeat itself every 3 weeks.

Although there is no proven transmission from fomites, such as brushes, hats, combs, linens, and stuffed animals, head lice and ova have been found on such items; therefore it is probably expedient to eradicate these lice by vacuuming, washing, dry cleaning, or isolating items in sealed plastic bags for 2 weeks. These insects do not hop, jump, or fly.

No healthy child should be excluded from or allowed to miss school time because of head lice. "No nit" policies for return to school should be discouraged.

Pubic lice are distinct in appearance from head and body lice; they have short crablike bodies. They are challenging to eradicate, because they often inhabit several hair areas on an individual patient (Figure 174-5). A major concern in treating crab lice is the lack of appreciation for their tendency to reside in rectal hairs. **If one treats patients with *P. pubis* with topical preparations, one must instruct patients to liberally treat the groin and rectal regions; otherwise, treatment failures will occur. Some dermatologists prefer to treat pubic lice using ivermectin as their first-line therapy.** Besides sexual transmission, pubic lice may also be acquired by sharing a bed with an infested person. Children with pubic lice have usually been infected through contact with an adult. Always demand investigation for possible child abuse.

Fortunately, head and pubic lice do not transmit systemic disease.

In the United States, the body louse has become less common in the general population. **Body lice** infestation in all developed countries is generally seen among the homeless in urban areas. It also is common among refugees and those who live in crowded conditions or cannot launder their clothing. Worldwide, body lice are important vectors for louse-borne relapsing fever, trench fever, and epidemic typhus, especially among refugees. The body louse and nits are generally found in the clothing seams of a parasitized individual, but the louse grabs onto body hairs to feed. Clothing may be stained with serum, blood, or louse feces. Body lice are eradicated by means of proper hygiene and laundering of clothing. A pediculicide may be helpful to treat any lice adherent to body hairs.

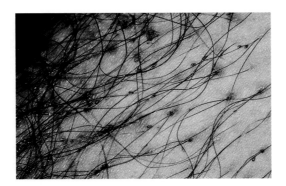

Figure 174-5 Crab louse nits at the base of lower abdominal hairs. (Adapted from Ko CJ, Elston DM: Pediculosis, *J Am Acad Dermatol* 50:1-12, 2004.)

Suggested Readings

Frankowski BL, Bocchini JA Jr: Council on School Health and Committee on Infectious Diseases: head lice, *Pediatrics* 126:392–403, 2010.

Burkhart CG, Burkhart CN: Asphyxiation of lice with topical agents, not a reality ... yet, *J Am Acad Dermatol* 54:721–722, 2006.

Burkhart CG, Burkhart CN: Oral ivermectin for *Phthirus pubis*, *J Am Acad Dermatol* 51:1037, 2004.

Drugs for head lice: *Med Lett Drugs Ther* 39:6–7, 1997.

Fischer TF: Lindane toxicity in a 24-year-old woman, *Ann Emerg Med* 24:972–974, 1994.

Flinders DC, De Schweinitz P: Pediculosis and scabies, *Am Fam Physician* 69:341–348, 2004.

Huynh TH, Norman RA: Scabies and pediculosis, *Dermatol Clin* 22:7–11, 2004.

Jones KN, English JC 3rd: Review of common therapeutic options in the United States for the treatment of pediculosis capitis, *Clin Infect Dis* 36:1355–1361, 2003.

Ko CJ, Elston DM: *Pediculosis. J Am Acad Dermatol* 50:1–12, 2004.

Meinking TL, Clineschmidt CM, Chen C, et al: An observer-blinded study of 1% permethrin crème rinse with and without adjunctive combing in patients with head lice, *J Pediatr* 141:665–670, 2002.

Meinking TL, Taplin D, Kalter DC, et al: Comparative efficacy of treatments for pediculosis capitis infestations, *Arch Dermatol* 122:267–271, 1986.

Pearlman DL: A simple treatment for head lice: dry-on, suffocation-based pediculocide, *Pediatrics* 114:e275–e279, 2004.

Resnick KS: A non-chemical therapeutic modality for head lice, *J Am Acad Dermatol* 52:374, 2005.

Ressel GW: AAP releases clinical report on head lice, *Am Fam Physician* 67:1391–1392, 2003.

Steen CJ, Carbonaro PA, Schwartz RA: Arthropods in dermatology, *J Am Acad Dermatol* 50:819–842, 2004.

Pityriasis Rosea

Presentation

Patients with this rash often seek acute medical help because of the worrisome sudden spread of a rash that began with one local skin lesion. This "herald patch" may develop anywhere on the body, but it is typically on the trunk and appears as an ovoid, 2 to 6 cm in diameter, mildly erythematous and slightly raised scaling plaque with a collarette of scale at the margin (Figure 175-1). There is no change for a period of several days to a few weeks; then the generalized rash appears, composed of crops of small (0.5 to 2 cm), pale, salmon-colored, oval, raised macules or plaques with a coarse surface surrounded by the same rim of fine scales as the herald patch (Figure 175-2). The distribution is usually truncal (face, hands, and feet being spared), with the long axis of the oval lesions running in the planes of cleavage of the skin (Langer lines, which are parallel to the ribs), giving it a typical "Christmas tree" appearance and making the diagnosis (Figure 175-3).

The condition may be asymptomatic or accompanied by varying degrees of pruritus (25% of patients have mild to severe itching). No systemic symptoms typically are present during the rash phase of pityriasis rosea (PR). The lesions will gradually extend in size and may become confluent with one another. The rash persists for 6 to 8 weeks and then completely disappears. Transient worsening of the rash or a second wave of lesions is not uncommon until eventual spontaneous resolution of the eruption. Recurrence of the condition later in life is rare.

Pityriasis rosea can have a distinctly different appearance on patients with brown skin or dark skin. The herald patch, as well as the diffuse rash that follows, may have a gray, dark brown, or even black appearance. There may be either hypopigmented or hyperpigmented areas visible after the lesions resolve.

What To Do:

✅ **After performing a careful history and physical examination, reassure patients about the benign self-limited nature of this disease. Be sympathetic, and let them know that it is understandable how frightening it can seem. Inform them that the rash will last for 6 to 8 weeks. In addition, inform them about the need to contact their physician if the rash or pruritus lasts more than 3 months.**

✅ **Encourage sun exposure, because it hastens resolution of individual lesions.**

✅ **Acyclovir may be effective in the treatment of pityriasis rosea, especially in patients treated within the first week of onset of the generalized rash. Prescribe acyclovir (Zovirax), 800 mg given five times daily for 7 days.** This dosage hastened the clearance of lesions in one placebo-controlled study. A single patient has been reported, however, who developed PR

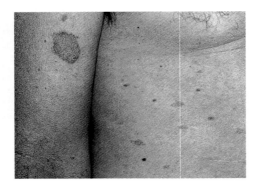

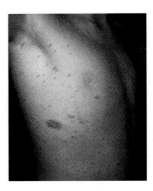

Figure 175-1 Herald patch on the arm with a collarette of scale at the margin. (From White G, Cox N: *Diseases of the skin,* ed 2. St Louis, 2006, Mosby.)

Figure 175-2 Pityriasis rosea with herald patch and subtle smaller spots on trunk.

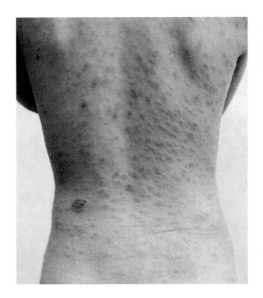

Figure 175-3 Typical "Christmas tree" pattern of pityriasis rosea. (From Leung AKS, Wong BE, Chan PYH: Pediatrics review. *Resident Staff Physician* 43:109, 1997.)

while taking low doses of acyclovir. Early high doses of acyclovir should probably be prescribed in pregnancy to prevent miscarriage or premature births, especially when PR develops during the first weeks of gestation, when the lesions have an unusual extension and long duration, and when constitutional symptoms are present. At the moment, however, no treatment can be recommended on the basis of evidence-based medicine.

If the diagnosis is uncertain, especially if the palms and soles are affected and the patient is sexually active, draw blood for serologic testing for syphilis (e.g., rapid plasma reagin [RPR], Venereal Disease Research Laboratory [VDRL]). Secondary syphilis can mimic pityriasis rosea. Make a note to track down the results of the test.

Microscopy with potassium hydroxide (KOH) preparation may be helpful to distinguish a herald patch from a tinea infection.

✓ **Provide relief from pruritus by prescribing hydroxyzine (Atarax), 25 to 50 mg q6h, or an emollient, such as Lubriderm.** Tepid cornstarch baths (1 cup in ½ tub of water) may also be comforting.

What Not To Do:

✗ Do not have a biopsy performed when findings are typical for pityriasis rosea. A biopsy is not indicated.

✗ Do not routinely use topical or systemic steroids. These are effective only in the most severe inflammatory varieties of this syndrome. Topical steroids may cause the eruption to generalize to erythroderma.

✗ Do not send off a serologic test for syphilis without ensuring that the results will be seen and acted on.

Discussion

Pityriasis rosea (PR) is a common, acute exanthem of uncertain cause. PR most commonly affects adolescents, with a concentration of cases in the 10- to 35-year-old age range, peaking in persons 20 to 29 years of age. PR occurs in pregnancy more frequently than in the general population (18% vs. 6%). The diagnosis of PR can usually be made based on the appearance of the lesions and the history. It has been described in the medical literature for more than 200 years but was given its current name by Camille Gilbert in 1860. Viral and bacterial causes have been sought, but convincing answers have not yet been found. PR shares many features with the viral exanthemas of childhood, and cases tend to cluster in the fall and winter.

Recently, an increasing number of studies have focused on human herpes virus 6 (HHV-6) and, primarily, on HHV-7 as causative agents. The skin lesions would not be a result of a direct infection of skin cells but, rather, would occur as a reactive response to the systemic HHV-6 and HHV-7 replication, alone or through the interaction with other viruses. The higher proportion of pregnant women with PR is probably related to the altered maternal immunity, the innate proinflammatory immune responses being tightly regulated to prevent immunologic rejection of the fetal allograft. In fact, HHV-6 reactivation seems common during pregnancy, and this fact may be one of the causes of spontaneous abortions.

Results of a controlled trial (neither randomized nor double-blind) with oral acyclovir suggest that early treatment with this antiviral is justified, because it apparently reduces the duration and severity of symptoms.

Up to 69% of patients with PR have a **prodromal illness** before the herald patch appears. Malaise, nausea, loss of appetite, headache, difficulty in concentration, irritability, gastrointestinal and upper respiratory symptoms (up to 69%), joint pain, swelling of lymph nodes, sore throat, and mild fever are often, although inconsistently, reported.

The **herald patch** often is misdiagnosed as eczema. PR is difficult to identify until the appearance of the characteristic smaller secondary lesions. When these secondary lesions are not on the patient's back, where they form the typical "Christmas tree" pattern, the lesions follow the cleavage lines in the following patterns: transversely across the lower abdomen and back, circumferentially around the shoulders, and in a V-shaped pattern on the upper chest.

The "herald patch" may not be seen in 20% to 30% of cases, and there are many variations from the classic presentation described. Atypical cases make up 20% of the total and occur more commonly in children. Lesions can exhibit urticarial, vesicular, pustular, or purpuric characteristics. Infrequently, oral lesions will accompany the skin rash and resolve along with it: These include punctate hemorrhages, erosions, ulcerations, erythematous macules, annular lesions, and plaques.

(continued)

Discussion continued

There are no noninvasive tests that confirm the diagnosis of PR. **Other diagnostic considerations** besides syphilis include tinea corporis, seborrheic dermatitis, guttate psoriasis, and tinea versicolor.

Numerous drugs have been implicated in a severe prolonged exanthem that resembles PR. Some of the medications that have been associated with a PR-type rash include bismuth, bacillus Calmette-

Guérin (BCG) vaccine, captopril, clonidine, diphtheria toxoid, gold, isotretinoin, ketotifen, metronidazole, and omeprazole.

Persistence of a rash beyond 3 months should prompt a clinician to reconsider the original diagnosis, to consider biopsy to confirm the diagnosis, and to check for the use of medications that may cause a rash similar to that of PR.

Suggested Readings

Brangman SA: Appearance of pityriasis rosea in patients with dark skin (letter), *Am Fam Physician* 70:821, 2004.

Drago F, Vecchio F, Rebora A: Use of high-dose acyclovir in pityriasis rosea, *J Am Acad Dermatol* 54:82–85, 2006.

Drago F, Broccolo F, Alfredo Rebora A: Pityriasis rosea: an update with a critical appraisal of its possible herpesviral etiology, *J Am Acad Dermatol* 61:303–318, 2009.

Habif T: *Clinical dermatology*, ed 3, St Louis, 1996, Mosby-Year Book.

Handbook of adolescent medicine: dermatology, *Adolesc Med* 14:183–524, 2003.

Jones D: The young adult: common inflammatory skin disorders, *Clin Fam Pract* 5:627–652, 2003.

Stulberg DL, Wolfrey J: Pityriasis rosea, *Am Fam Physician* 69:87–91, 2004.

Wolfrey JD, Billica WH, Gulbranson SH, et al: Pediatric exanthems, *Clin Fam Pract* 5:557–588, 2003.

Pyogenic Granuloma or Lobular Capillary Hemangioma

(Proud Flesh)

Presentation

Often there is a history of a laceration or minor trauma to the skin or mucous membrane several days to a few weeks before presentation, but in most cases there is no apparent cause. The head, neck, and extremities are most commonly involved, especially the lips, oral mucosa, and fingers. An unsightly lesion forms, beginning as an extremely friable red or yellow papule or polyp, which now bleeds with every slight trauma. Objective findings usually include a crusted, sometimes purulent-appearing collection of erythematous, well-demarcated, red granulation tissue arising from a moist, sometimes hemorrhagic, skin ulceration, often with a collarette of scale at the base. There are usually no signs of a deep tissue infection (Figure 176-1).

What To Do:

✓ Cleanse the area with an agent such as hydrogen peroxide or povidone-iodine solution.

✓ **For small lesions (≤0.75 cm), cauterize the granulation tissue with a silver nitrate stick until it is completely discolored.** Excess granulation tissue may first be shaved away using a No. 15 scalpel blade. The base of the lesion can be injected with 1% lidocaine with epinephrine to minimize the resulting hemorrhage. Thermal cautery may also be used, but local anesthesia will probably be required because of the potential inadvertent contact with intact dermis.

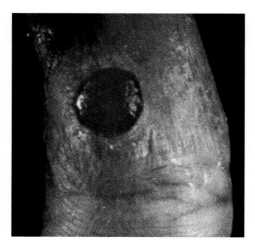

Figure 176-1 Pyogenic granuloma.

✅ **Dress the wound after applying an antibacterial ointment, and have the patient gently wash and repeat ointment and dressings two to three times per day until healed.**

✅ **For pedunculated lesions, an atraumatic, simple, fast, and cost-effective alternative that does not require anesthesia is to ligate the base of the granuloma using a soft, absorbable, surgical suture material.** This maneuver can be facilitated by lifting the pyogenic granuloma with forceps. The tissue is ligated with knots that are as tight as possible. The suture material is then snipped short. This can be covered by a simple wound dressing, and the tumor can be expected to become necrotic and fall off in several days. Inform patients or parents that although uncommon, bleeding could occur, and simple continuous compression for several minutes will control any minor hemorrhage. If the ligature does not reach far enough down to include the nurturing vessel, part of the granuloma may persist. This smaller lesion can then be easily treated with silver nitrate or thermal cautery.

✅ Patients with large lesions can be referred for treatment with a pulsed-dye laser.

✅ Warn the patient about the potential signs of developing infection and the need to return for treatment.

✅ Patients and parents should also be alerted to the possibility of recurrence after removal.

✅ Dermatology referral is recommended if the lesion recurs or multiple satellite lesions occur after excision.

What Not To Do:

❌ Do not cauterize or ligate any lesion that by history and appearance might be neoplastic in nature. Only treat clinically obvious cases. Pyogenic granuloma is occasionally confused with amelanotic melanoma, basal cell carcinoma, and squamous cell carcinoma. Periungual malignant melanoma can mimic pyogenic granuloma. Suspicious lesions should be referred for complete excision and pathologic examination.

❌ Do not cauterize a recurrent, large, or extensive lesion. These should also be considered for complete excision.

Discussion

Pyogenic granulomas, also known as lobular hemangiomas, are common vascular tumors of the skin and mucous membranes usually seen in children and young adults. They are usually smaller than 1 cm but can be up to 2 cm. Their cause is unknown, but pyogenic granuloma is a misnomer, because it is probably not infectious (pyogenic) in origin. It has been argued to be inflammatory and hyperplastic rather than a true neoplasm. Rapid growth is in response to an unknown stimulus that triggers endothelial proliferation and angiogenesis. They can be solitary or multiple and can arise within preexisting lesions, such as spider angioma and port wine stain.

Although a minority of pyogenic granulomas involute spontaneously within 6 months, most patients seek treatment because of bleeding. Pyogenic granulomas recur if any abnormal tissue remains.

Gingival lesions are common in **pregnant women,** in whom these lesions are called epulis gravidarum. Spontaneous resolution occurs after delivery.

It is not uncommon for secondary cellulitis to develop after the pyogenic granuloma is cauterized. It is therefore reasonable to place a patient on a short course (3 to 4 days) of a high-dose antibiotic (dicloxacillin or cephalexin, 500 mg qid, or cefadroxil, 500 mg bid) when the wound is located on a distal extremity.

Scabies

(Human Itch Mite)

Presentation

Patients may rush to the emergency department or call for medical help shortly after having gone to bed, unable to sleep because of intense itching. (Severe pruritus, which is the hallmark of this disease, is intensified at night for no known reason.) These patients have skin lesions that include mite burrows, which appear as short (about 2 to 3 mm in length), elevated, gray, threadlike, serpiginous tracks. A small papule or vesicle may appear at the end of the burrow or may occur independently (Figure 177-1). These papules and burrows are chiefly found in the interdigital web spaces (Figure 177-2), as well as on the volar aspects of the wrists, axillae, olecranon area, nipples, waistline, genitalia, and gluteal cleft (Figure 177-3). Nipple pruritus in females is a useful historical clue. Pruritic erythematous papules on the glans penis are characteristics of scabies infestation in males (Figure 177-4). The head and neck are usually spared, but scabies lesions can occur anywhere on the body (Figure 177-5), including the face and scalp. Infants and young children may also have palm and sole involvement with vesicular and pustular lesions. Secondary bacterial infection is often present. Scabies in the elderly may be difficult to diagnose because the cutaneous lesions are often very subtle.

What To Do:

✓ **Attempt to confirm the diagnosis of scabies by placing mineral oil over five or six nonexcoriated suspicious papules or burrows, and scrape or shave them with a No. 15 scalpel blade onto a microscope slide. Examine under low magnification for the mite, its oval eggs, or fecal concretions (scybala). Any one of these findings clinches the diagnosis** (Figure 177-6).

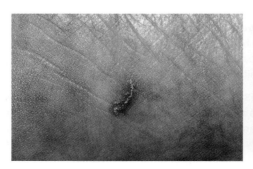

Figure 177-1 Scabies burrow on the side of the foot. (From White G, Cox N: *Diseases of the skin,* ed 2. St Louis, 2006, Mosby.)

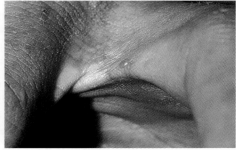

Figure 177-2 Lesions are commonly found in the interdigital web spaces and the sides of the fingers. (From White G, Cox N: *Diseases of the skin,* ed 2. St Louis, 2006, Mosby.)

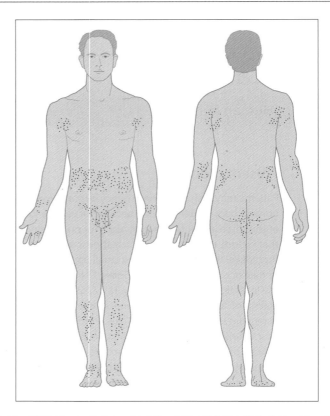

Figure 177-3 Characteristics of distribution of scabies lesions. (Adapted from Goldstein BG, Goldstein AO: *Practical dermatology,* ed 2. St Louis, 1997, Mosby.)

Burrows can be made more visible by first liberally covering the area with liquid ink and then removing excess ink with an alcohol swab, leaving the burrows stained. If the clinical picture alone is convincing, especially if there is someone else at home (a source) who is itching, treatment should be instituted without the help of microscopic examination, or even in the face of negative scrapings.

✅ **Prescribe prescription-strength permethrin (Elimite) 5% insecticidal cream, 60 g, for the patient to massage from his head to the soles of his feet at bedtime, and have him leave it on for 8 to 14 hours before washing it off the next morning.** Mites tend to persist in subungual areas. The patient should trim fingernails, scrub beneath them, and then apply the scabicide under the nails. Patients should apply a second treatment 1 week later.

✅ **Oral ivermectin (Stromectol), 0.2 mg/kg as a single oral dose repeated within an interval of 2 weeks, is as effective as a single application of 5% topical permethrin cream.** It should be taken on an empty stomach with water. A total of two or more doses at least 7 days apart may be necessary to eliminate a scabies infestation. Ivermectin is currently available in the form of a 3-mg tablet. The safety of ivermectin in children weighing less than 15 kg and in pregnant women has not been established. (Although permethrin is still perhaps the treatment of choice for scabies, this may not be so in future practice. The high cost and extensive surface area of application that is necessary lead to poor compliance, especially in elderly patients.

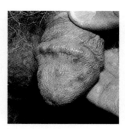

Figure 177-4 Scabies of the penis causes intense itching and red papules on the glans, which is nearly diagnostic of the disease. (From White G, Cox N: *Diseases of the skin*, ed 2. St Louis, 2006, Mosby.)

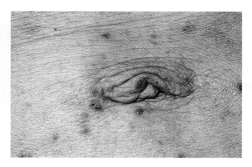

Figure 177-5 Lesions about the umbilicus. (From White G, Cox N: *Diseases of the skin*, ed 2. St Louis, 2006, Mosby.)

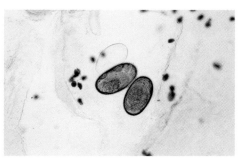

Figure 177-6 Microscopic examination of burrow scrapings showing two oval eggs and multiple brown feces (scybala). (From White G, Cox N: *Diseases of the skin*, ed 2. St Louis, 2006, Mosby.)

Because of this, ivermectin may soon be considered the drug of choice. Currently, it is still not approved by the U.S. Food and Drug Administration [FDA] for treating scabies.)

Crotamiton lotion 10% (60, 480 mL) and crotamiton cream 10% (60 g) (Eurax; Crotan) are approved by the FDA for the treatment of scabies in adults; they are considered safe when used as directed. Massage cream/lotion into entire body from chin down, repeat 24 hours later and then bathe 48 hours later. Crotamiton is not FDA-approved for use in children. Frequent treatment failure has been reported with crotamiton.

Sulfur is the oldest known treatment of scabies, and it is the drug of choice for infants younger than 2 months of age and for pregnant or lactating women. It is available as 5% and 10% precipitated sulfur in petrolatum. The cream is applied nightly for three consecutive nights and washed off 24 hours later. The major drawback to sulfur treatment is the unpleasant odor; also, the treatment will often stain clothes.

Secondary infection from scratching, such as impetiginized excoriations, can be treated with mupirocin (Bactroban) cream 2%. Folliculitis, abscess formation, lymphangitis, and cellulitis should be treated with appropriate drainage and antibiotics (see Chapters 163, 166, and 172).

Tell the patient that the **itching will not go away immediately** and that this does not mean that the treatment was ineffective. Dead mites and eggs continue to cause an immune response but will eventually be eliminated during normal cutaneous turnover.

An antipruritic agent, such as hydroxyzine (Atarax, Vistaril), 25 to 50 mg q6h, can be prescribed for comfort. Adding a short course of oral prednisone may be most effective when pruritus is severe.

Clothing, bedding, and towels should be washed with hot water or dry cleaned or placed through the heat cycle of a dryer to prevent reinfection. An alternative method is to place all bedding and clothing that might be infested in sealed plastic bags for at least 72 hours. Thorough cleaning of the patient's room is recommended.

Family members, frequent household guests, and close physical and sexual contacts should also be treated simultaneously, whether or not symptoms are present.

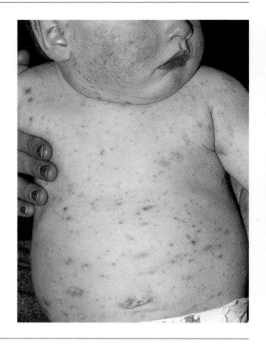

Figure 177-7 Scabies in an infant involving the face. (From White G, Cox N: *Diseases of the skin*, ed 2. St Louis, 2006, Mosby.)

 Reexamine patients 1 to 2 weeks after initiating therapy to ensure that there is no recurrence.

What Not To Do:

Do not use lindane (Kwell) on infants, young children, or pregnant women or in widespread "Norwegian" scabies, because enough of this pesticide may be absorbed percutaneously to produce seizures or central nervous system (CNS) toxicity. For this reason, lindane is generally no longer recommended for any patient with scabies.

Discussion

Scabies should be suspected in any patient with pruritus.

Scabies has been a scourge among humans for thousands of years. The condition is caused by the mite *Sarcoptes scabiei,* var. *hominis.* The adult is barely visible to the naked eye. The organism is an obligate parasite, requiring an appropriate host for survival. The mites subsist on a diet of dissolved human tissue but do not feed on blood. An adult female mite has a tortoise shape and is only about 0.3 to 0.4 mm in size. The male mite is about half the female size. Although mites cannot fly or jump, they can crawl as fast as 2.5 cm/min on warm skin. After mating on the surface of the skin, the gravid female mite dissolves the stratum corneum with proteolytic secretions and then burrows headfirst into the skin. Eggs are laid at a rate of 2 to 3 per day. Both male and female mites have a lifespan of about 1 month. Young mites develop quickly, leaving the burrows to enter hair follicles and skinfolds in which to hide and feed. They mature within 10 to 14 days, after which mating takes place, beginning a new cycle. Mites can live only up to 3 days off a host's body environment.

A delayed hypersensitivity reaction to the mites, their eggs, saliva, and scybala (packets of feces) occurs within approximately 2 to 6 weeks of infestations. This

Discussion continued

inflammatory reaction is responsible for the intense pruritus (the hallmark of this disease). Although scabietic lesions are uncommon above the neck in children and adults, infants may have involvement of the face (Figure 177-7). Scabies in an infant usually means that a close adult contact is the source of the infection.

A distinctive highly contagious form of scabies, known as "Norwegian scabies" or "crusted or keratotic scabies," has a predilection for individuals who are immunocompromised, elderly, debilitated, or mentally impaired. The patient becomes infected with thousands to millions of mites, in contrast to the usual case of scabies, where the average infected adult human has 10 to 15 live adult female mites on his or her body at any given time. Skin manifestations of keratotic scabies are much more severe, but the latter is usually not very pruritic.

Scabies is transmitted principally through close personal contact but may be transmitted through clothing, linens, or towels.

Less than 25% of cases show the characteristic 2- to 3-mm serpiginous tracks. Another method of detecting scabies, other than skin scrapings, is video dermatoscopy. This is noninvasive in vivo visualization of the skin at magnifications of up to 600× to detect signs of infestation (mites, eggs, and feces).

Families may acquire **canine scabies** when a puppy is brought into the home. The distribution of lesions on humans infected with dog scabies is distinctively different from that of the human variety. A child who hugs an infested family pet will make greatest contact with his trunk and arms, and most eruptions are thereby seen in this distribution. Canine scabies manifests itself within 24 to 96 hours. It is generally self-limiting in humans, because the mites cannot complete their life cycle and therefore do not survive for more than a few days on a foreign host. For those patients who are unwilling to wait for this form of scabies to resolve on its own, 5% permethrin applied topically is the treatment of choice. The assistance of a veterinarian is recommended for treating the pet.

Suggested Readings

Centers for Disease Control and Prevention: *Parasites—Scabies.* Available at http://cdc.gov/parasites/scabies/health_professionals/meds.html. Accessed March 13, 2012.

Huynh TH, Norman RA: Scabies and pediculosis, *Dermatol Clin* 22:7–11, 2004.

Madan V, Jaskiran K, Gupta U, et al: Oral ivermectin in scabies patients: a comparison with 1% topical lindane lotion, *J Dermatol* 28:481–484, 2001.

Steen CJ, Carbonaro PA, Schwarz RA: Arthropods in dermatology, *J Am Acad Dermatol* 50:819–842, 2004.

Sea Bather's Eruption

(Sea Lice)

Presentation

Patients seek help because of an intense pruritic or painful eruption of red raised welts, sometimes like mosquito bites. They are at times confluent, appearing in areas that had been covered by swimwear (Figure 178-1). This will occur within a few hours after bathing in the Caribbean or off the coasts of Mexico, Florida, or Long Island during periods when "sea lice" are active. Exposed areas of skin are spared. Symptoms may have started as a tingling sensation while in the water, with itching and burning becoming more pronounced if a freshwater shower was taken while still wearing the same suit. Symptoms usually resolve spontaneously in a few days; however, some individuals (especially children) experience a more severe delayed hypersensitivity reaction occurring approximately 10 days after exposure. This rash extends to exposed areas of the body not previously affected, and victims may also experience severe itching, fatigue, fever, chills, nausea, and headache. Outbreaks occur between March and August, with a peak incidence in May.

What To Do:

✓ **At the onset of symptoms, the patient should remove the bathing suit before showering and, if possible, decontaminate the affected areas using vinegar for 30 minutes.**

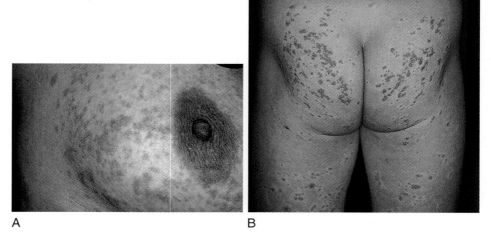

A   B

Figures 178-1 A and **B,** Sea bather's eruption with multiple edematous pink papules found in areas previously covered by a bathing suit. (A, From White G, Cox N: *Diseases of the skin.* St Louis, 2006, Mosby; **B,** from Bolognia J, Jorizzo J, Rapini R: *Dermatology.* St Louis, 2003, Mosby.)

Inform the patient about the nature of this rash and that it will usually last for 3 to 5 days.

Prescribe a topical steroid in combination with a topical anesthetic to be applied tid to qid. Pramosone cream or lotion 1% and 2.5% is supplied in 1- and 2-ounce tubes and in bottles of 2, 4, and 8 fluid ounces.

Prescribe an oral antihistamine, such as hydroxyzine (Atarax, Vistaril), 25 to 50 mg qid, to help with itching.

If systemic symptoms are present or if the rash is extensive and severe, prescribe 4 to 5 days of a systemic steroid, such as prednisone, 60 to 80 mg qd (1 mg/kg).

Instruct the patient to wash swimwear in detergent and fresh water and to dry it before wearing it again, because nematocysts may remain in the bathing suit after drying. Without washing and drying, any unreleased nematodes can be triggered and discharged, producing lesions without additional exposure to ocean water.

Instruct the patient about future prevention, either by avoiding ocean bathing during known outbreaks or by immediately removing swimwear after sea bathing, cleansing the skin with vinegar (to prevent the triggering of nematocysts) and then showering. Showering with fresh water while still wearing swimwear may cause a discharge of nematocysts and worsening of symptoms.

Safe Sea Sunblock Jellyfish Sting Protective Lotion, sold by Seavenger (Walnut, Calif.) and available on Amazon.com, reportedly prevents stings from sea lice, stinging corals, and jellyfish. A 4-ounce bottle gives roughly four adult full-body applications, each giving approximately 1 hour of protection. One small randomized, controlled study demonstrated a relative risk reduction of 82% (95% confidence interval: 21% to 96%; $P = .02$). No sea bather's eruption or side effects occurred.

What Not To Do:

Do not prescribe systemic steroids for patients in whom there are strong contraindications. This is a self-limiting condition.

Discussion

Sea bather's eruption typically occurs 4 to 24 hours after exposure, although some persons may develop a "prickling" sensation or urticarial lesions while still in the water. The larval forms of certain sea anemones and thimble jellyfish, *Linuche unguiculata*, are implicated as the cause. Water flows through bathing suits and traps the larvae, which discharge nematocysts when they contact skin. Lesions also occur on uncovered skin surfaces subjected to friction, such as axillae and inner thighs. Surfers develop lesions on the chest and abdomen that were in contact with surfboards. Sea lice do not infest humans.

Cercarial dermatitis, or "swimmer's itch," is a different condition that occurs sporadically in fresh water as well as ocean water. It occurs in exposed skin rather than under bathing suits and is thought to be caused by an avian schistosome, *Microbilharzia variglandis*. An over-the-counter topical steroid is generally all that is required to treat this problem.

Suggested Readings

Boulware DR: A randomized, controlled field trial for the prevention of jellyfish stings with a topical sting inhibitor, *J Travel Med* 13:166–171, 2006.

Singletary EM, Rochman AS, Bodmer JC, Holstege CP: Envenomations, *Med Clin North Am* 89:1195–1224, 2005.

Tomchik RS, Russell MT, Szmant AM, et al: Clinical perspectives on sea bather's eruption, also known as "sea lice", *JAMA* 269:1669–1672, 1993.

Sunburn

Presentation

Patients generally seek help only if their sunburn is severe. There will be a history of extended exposure to sunlight or to an artificial source of ultraviolet radiation, such as a sunlamp. Patients at highest risk typically have fair skin, blue eyes, and red or blond hair. The burns will be accompanied by intense pain, and the patient will not be able to tolerate anything touching the skin. Most exposure is limited to sun-exposed areas of the body (Figure 179-1, *A* and *B*). There may be systemic complaints of "sun poisoning" that include nausea, vomiting, chills, and fever. The affected areas are erythematous and are accompanied by mild edema. Erythema develops after 2 to 6 hours and peaks at 12 to 24 hours. The more severe the burn, the earlier it will appear and the more likely that it will progress to edema and blistering. Signs and symptoms usually resolve over 4 to 7 days, often with skin scaling and peeling (Figure 179-2).

What To Do:

✓ Inquire whether the patient is using a photosensitizing drug (e.g., tetracyclines, thiazides, sulfonamides, phenothiazines, sulfonylurea hypoglycemic agents, griseofulvin, and vitamin B$_6$); if so, have her discontinue its use and avoid the sun for at least 3 weeks.

✓ **Have the patient apply cool compresses of skim milk and water or Burow solution (Domeboro Powder Packets, two packets in 1 pint of water) as often as desired to relieve pain. This is the most comforting therapy.** Cool baths or showers will also help.

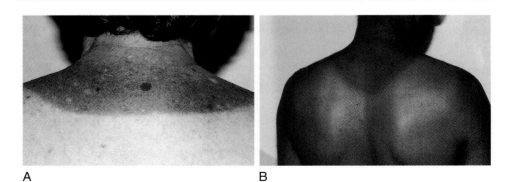

A   B

Figure 179-1 A and **B,** Sunburn on the upper back. Note the sharp cut-off at the line of clothing (**A**) and the relative sparing further up the neck because of shielding by the hair. (From White G, Cox N: *Diseases of the skin,* ed 2. St Louis, 2006, Mosby.)

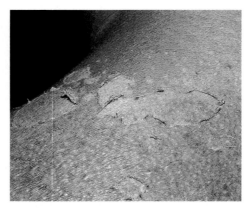

Figure 179-2 Sunburn typically causes peeling as it resolves, even if frank blistering has not been an early feature. (From White G, Cox N: *Diseases of the skin,* ed 2. St Louis, 2006, Mosby.)

✓ **If there is no contraindication, nonsteroidal anti-inflammatory drugs (NSAIDs), such as ibuprofen (Motrin), 400 mg q6h, or naproxen (Naprosyn), 500 mg bid, will help reduce pain and inflammation. When pain is severe, prescribe narcotics, such as hydrocodone or oxycodone.**

✓ **Suggest an emollient, such as Lubriderm or cold cream for topical treatment.** The patient may also be helped by a topical steroid spray, such as dexamethasone (Decaspray), although some investigators have not found topical steroids to be of any significant value. Most recommend not using them unless there is coexistent contact dermatitis. Products with *Aloe vera* are increasingly popular.

✓ **With a more severe burn or when a photosensitizing drug is involved, especially with the systemic symptoms of "sun poisoning," prescribe a short course of systemic steroids (50 to 100 mg of prednisone [1 mg/kg] qd × 3 days)** to reduce inflammation, swelling, pain, and itching. Add a mild sedative and antipruritic, such as hydroxyzine (Vistaril), 50 mg qid.

✓ **Instruct the patient to avoid the sun for a minimum of 3 weeks.**

What Not To Do:

✗ Do not allow the patient to use over-the-counter (OTC) sunburn medications that contain local anesthetics (benzocaine, dibucaine, or lidocaine). They are usually ineffective or provide only very transient relief. In addition, there is the potential hazard of sensitizing the patient to these ingredients.

✗ Do not trouble the patient with unnecessary burn dressings. These wounds have a very low probability of becoming infected, and most cases resolve spontaneously with no significant sequelae. Treatment should be directed at making the patient as comfortable as possible.

✗ Do not overlook toxic shock syndrome in the hypotensive patient with fever, diarrhea, vomiting, altered mental status, or abnormal liver functions. The generalized rash looks like sunburn.

ⓧ Do not forget that sunburns may trigger recurrence of herpes simplex, lupus, porphyria, and other cutaneous disorders. (Easy sunburning during infancy may indicate a serious underlying disease, such as porphyria or xeroderma pigmentosum.)

Discussion

Sunburn is an acute cutaneous inflammatory reaction that follows excessive exposure of the skin to ultraviolet radiation (UVR).

UVR from the sun that reaches the earth is divided into UVB (290 to 320 nm) and UVA (320 to 400 nm). The ratio of UVA to UVB is 20:1. UVR is strongest between 10 AM and 4 PM. The acute response of human skin to UVB irradiation includes erythema, edema, and pigment darkening, followed by delayed tanning, thickening of the epidermis and dermis, and synthesis of vitamin D; chronic UVB effects are photoaging, immunosuppression, and photocarcinogenesis. UVB-induced erythema occurs approximately 4 hours after exposure, peaks around 8 to 24 hours, and fades over a day or so; in fair-skinned and older individuals, UVB erythema may be persistent, sometimes lasting for weeks. To produce the same erythemal response, approximately 1000 times more UVA dose is needed compared with UVB. UVA is more efficient in inducing tanning, whereas UVB is more efficient in inducing erythema and sunburn.

Once the signs and symptoms of sunburn are present, no treatment, including systemic corticosteroids, has unequivocally been shown to be effective. Prevention is the most effective therapy for sunburn.

Seeking shade and minimizing sun exposure during peak UVR times (10 AM to 4 PM) is recommended. This should be combined with the use of appropriate clothing, a wide-brimmed hat, sunglasses, and broad-spectrum sunscreen to achieve the optimal protection.

Clothing is an excellent photoprotectant. UV protectiveness of fabrics is expressed as "UV protection factor" (UPF), which is analogous to the SPF of sunscreens. Adequate UV protection is provided by a UPF greater than 30. Denim provides a UPF of 1700. Typical summer cotton T-shirts provide a UPF of 5 to 9; when wet, the UPF decreases to only 3 to 4. The introduction of UV-cutting agent (UVCA) compounds, which increase the absorption of UV radiation by the fabrics to which they are applied, has increased the ability of cotton and cotton blend fabrics to

protect against the most harmful wavelengths of UV radiation.

SPF-15 sunscreen can filter out 94% of UVB radiation, and SPF-30 sunscreen provides greater than 97% protection. It is known that, in actual use, most people apply less than the amount used in testing (2 mg/cm^2). The overall median application thickness in general is only 0.5 mg/cm^2. **Most sunscreen activity failure is caused by inadequate application and by less-than-adequate frequency of reapplication.** As a rule of thumb, sunscreens provide only 33% of the protection value stated on a label, because of this lack of proper compliance. Sunscreen on the skin may shed easily with rubbing, sweating, or water immersion. It has been recommended that sunscreen be applied 20 minutes before sun exposure and be reapplied every 2 to 3 hours or after swimming or sweating. Sensitivity to the sun increases on the second day of exposure; therefore a higher SPF sunscreen is important for individuals who are expected to have multiday sun exposure. **In general, use of a sunscreen with an SPF of 30 is sufficient. Approximately 1 ounce is enough for each application for an average-sized adult in an average-sized swimsuit.**

Sunscreen use alone, no matter how substantive or durable the product, should not be trusted to prevent all of the possible harmful effects of sun exposure. For example, most sunscreens offer less protection against UVA, which may be more important in causing melanoma than UVB. Multiple studies demonstrate a major impact of UVA in skin photodamage and emphasize the need for a broad protection covering the entire solar UV spectrum. When they are trusted, it is important to read and follow the label directions on these sunscreen products.

The U.S. Food and Drug Administration (FDA) has recently approved a sunscreen containing ecamsule (Mexoryl), which is more protective against the deeper penetrating UVA than any other sunscreen ingredient. Mexoryl SX has been demonstrated to play a central beneficial role in broad-spectrum sunscreen formulations. Its

(continued)

Discussion continued

efficacy has been brought out in numerous clinical trials.

Several preparations combine avobenzone, which blocks UVA, with UVB blocking agents. They are sold by numerous companies, and patients should be directed to check labels to ensure the presence of a UVA blocking component. Mexoryl SX was developed for use in combination with avobenzone and octocrylene for broad-spectrum protection. In this formulation, octocrylene acts to stabilize avobenzone. **Available in Europe and Canada since 1993, Mexoryl SX is the first new photostable short-UVA filter in a sunscreen formula to be approved by the U.S. FDA and is now available in the United States in the new sunscreen product Anthelios SX.** Anthelios SX is an SPF15 lightweight moisturizing cream that is intended for daily use. The product protects against both UVB and UVA. Fragrance-free and allergy tested, it is suitable for sensitive skin and is oil-free and noncomedogenic.

Photosensitivity reactions occur often with drug ingestion in combination with exposure to the sun. The reaction occurs in sun-exposed areas, primarily of the face, arms, and chest. It resembles sunburn and is usually not pruritic (Figures 179-3 and 179-4). Reactions are divided into phototoxic and photoallergic. Phototoxic reactions are more common and are not truly allergic, because previous exposure is not necessary. The severity of the reaction is drug- and UVA-dose dependent and usually occurs within hours. Photoallergic reactions represent delayed-type hypersensitivity and require previous exposure to a drug plus UVA exposure. This reaction is typically pruritic and eczematous and occurs within 1 to 2 days of exposure.

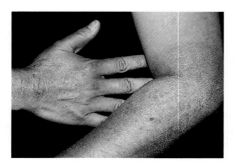

Figure 179-3 Photodermatitis showing a typical distribution pattern. There is a cut-off from short sleeves, and relative sparing of the ulnar side of the hand and distal fingers. (From White G, Cox N: *Diseases of the skin*, ed 2. St Louis, 2006, Mosby.)

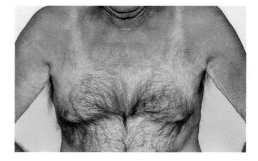

Figure 179-4 Photosensitivity resulting from a thiazide diuretic, showing sparing under clothing. (From White G, Cox N: *Diseases of the skin*, ed 2. St Louis, 2006, Mosby.)

Suggested Readings

Agin PP: Water resistance and extended wear sunscreens, *Dermatol Clin* 24:75–79, 2006.

Duteil L, Queille-Roussel C, Lorenz B, et al: A randomized controlled study of the safety and efficacy of topical corticosteroid treatments of sunburn in healthy volunteers, *Clin Exp Dermatol* 27:314–318, 2002.

Eide MJ, Weinstock MA: Public health challenges in sun protection, *Dermatol Clin* 24:119–124, 2006.

Faurschou A: Topical corticosteroids in the treatment of acute sunburn: a randomized, double-blind clinical trial, *Arch Dermatol* 144:620–624, 2008.

Fourtanier A, Moyal D, Seité S: Sunscreens containing the broad-spectrum UVA absorber, Mexoryl SX, prevent the cutaneous detrimental effects of UV exposure: a review of clinical study results, *Photodermatol Photoimmunol Photomed* 24:164–174, 2008.

Hatch KL, Osterwalder U: Garments as solar ultraviolet radiation screening materials, *Dermatol Clin* 24:85–100, 2006.

Kullavanijaya P, Lim HW: Photoprotection, *J Am Acad Dermatol* 52:937–958, 2005.

Lim HW, Rigel DS: UVA: Grasping a better understanding of this formidable opponent, *Skin Aging* 15:62–67, 2007.

Prevention and treatment of sunburn, *Med Lett Drugs Ther* 46:45–46, 2004.

Saffle JR: What's new in general surgery: burns and metabolism, *J Am Coll Surg* 196:267–289, 2003.

Sunscreens: An update, *Med Lett Drugs Ther* 50:70–72, 2008.

Wolfrey JD, Billica WH, Gulbranson SH, et al: Pediatric exanthems, *Clin Fam Pract* 5:557–588, 2003.

Tick Bite, Tick Removal

Presentation

The patient arrives with a tick attached to the skin (Figure 180-1), often the scalp. He is often frightened or disgusted and concerned about developing Lyme disease, Rocky Mountain spotted fever (RMSF), or "tick fever." Alternatively, the patient may only have a history of having removed a tick within the past week or so and now has developed a spreading erythematous rash at the previous site of attachment (Figure 180-2, A to C). By this time, systemic signs and symptoms consisting of myalgia, arthralgia, fever, headache, and fatigue may be present.

What To Do:

✓ When there is no tick present, obtaining a history of tick exposure in the recreational, occupational, and travel history can be essential for diagnosis.

✓ Carefully examine the patient for an individual tick or multiple ticks. Ticks can attach themselves to any part of the body, but certain species appear to prefer particular locations. Dog ticks may favor the head and neck, while the Lone Star tick may favor the lower extremities, buttocks, and groin. Although tick bites can be painful, the ticks are often not detected when they crawl, attach, feed, or depart from human skin.

✓ **When an embedded tick is present, apply protective gloves if available, and promptly remove the tick. Grasp the tick as close to the skin as possible with a pair of narrow-tipped forceps and slowly but firmly pull straight up until the tick mouth parts separate from the skin** (Figure 180-3). Be careful not to squeeze the tick's body or twist the tick's head. Alternatively, the tick's jaws may be pried away from the skin using a 20-gauge needle tip as a wedge.

✓ **Although not proven, it has been suggested that by injecting and infiltrating lidocaine with epinephrine beneath the attached tick, removal by traction is made easier.** Also, covering the tick with 2% viscous lidocaine has led to spontaneous detachment within 5 minutes in a very small series.

✓ **After removal of the tick, disinfect the attachment site and wash your hands with soap and water. Save the tick in a container of alcohol for future identification, or flush it down the toilet after it has been properly identified.**

✓ If the mouth parts appear to remain embedded, anesthetize the area with an infiltration of 1% Xylocaine, and use the tip of a No. 15 scalpel blade to scrape (dermabrade) these fragments away.

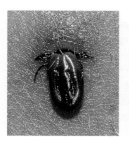

Figure 180-1 Embedded tick *Ixodes pacificus* (western blacklegged tick). (From White G, Cox N: *Diseases of the skin*, ed 2. St Louis, 2006, Mosby.)

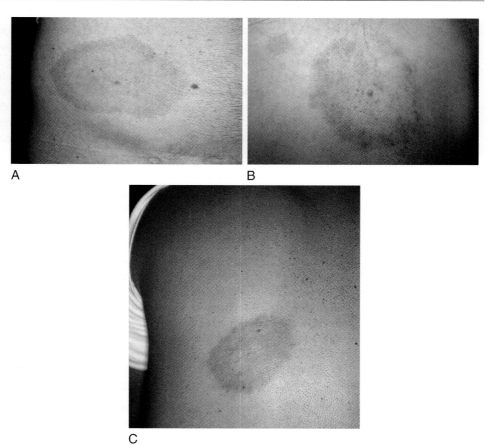

A

B

C

Figure 180-2 A to C, Erythema migrans. The causative organism is *Borrelia burgdorferi.* (From White G, Cox N: *Diseases of the skin*, ed 2. St Louis, 2006, Mosby.)

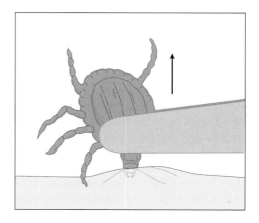

Figure 180-3 Remove tick with narrow-tipped forceps.

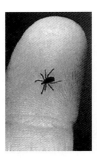

Figure 180-4 Life-sized deer tick. (From Gorman C: Deer tick turns deadly. *Time,* July 24, 1995, p 56.)

✅ **If it is an *Ixodes scapularis* or deer tick** (Figure 180-4) **(or *Ixodes pacificus,*** see Figure 180-1**), but it has been attached for less than 72 hours and was not engorged, there is minimal risk for disease transmission. There is no need for prophylaxis.** The patient or family can be reassured, but instruct them to record the patient's temperature daily for the next 4 weeks and to notify a physician or return at the first sign of a fever. In addition, over the same time period, instruct the family to watch for a pink patch at the site, which could be the beginning of erythema migrans. Also, if any rash, fever, cranial or peripheral neuropathies, or systemic symptoms, such as headache, myalgia, malaise, sweats, chills, or joint pains ("flu symptoms") occur, have them return to evaluate for possible tick-borne illness, and initiate treatment as noted later.

✅ **If an *Ixodes* tick has been attached for less than 72 hours, but the tick appears to be engorged with blood, treat prophylactically for Lyme disease with doxycycline, 200 mg PO in 1 dose. Patients who are very anxious and cannot be reassured may also be given a single preventative dose.**

✅ **If this was an *Ixodes* tick that was attached for more than 72 hours, the patient presents with a focal rash at the site where the tick had been attached, or there are signs and symptoms as noted earlier, prescribe antibiotics to prevent or treat early Lyme disease (see later, this chapter). In a patient with typical erythema migrans, in an endemic area, laboratory confirmation is not required. Doxycycline, 100 mg bid × 2 to 3 weeks, is the agent of choice.** For pregnant or nursing women and children younger than 8 years of age, amoxicillin, 500 mg tid or 25 to 50 mg/kg/day in divided doses for 2 to 3 weeks, can be used. Cefuroxime (Ceftin), 500 mg bid for adults and 250 mg bid for children for 2 to 3 weeks, is an alternative for patients who are allergic to doxycycline and amoxicillin.

✅ **If a wood tick (in the western United States) or a dog tick (in the eastern United States) has been removed** (Figure 180-5)**, reassure the patient and family that the likelihood of developing Rocky Mountain spotted fever (RMSF) is very small (1%), and that if it should occur, prompt treatment will be quite effective on development of fever and/or headache.** It is not recommended to give prophylactic antibiotics in an attempt to prevent RMSF. If transmission of infection has occurred, within 1 to 2 weeks after the tick bite, acute onset of fever, chills, severe headache, and myalgias will develop. **Patients should seek immediate care at the onset of their symptoms.** In most patients, fever and severe headache precede the characteristic rash that generally appears on the fourth day, starting on the wrists, ankles, and forearms as blanching red macules that progress to form papules centrally to the arms, thigh, trunk, and face. **Therapy should be started when the disease is suspected and should never be delayed for confirmatory tests.** Tetracyclines and chloramphenicol are the only drugs proven to be effective for the treatment of RMSF. Because of its effectiveness, broad margin of safety, and convenient dosing schedule, doxycycline is currently considered the drug of choice for nearly all patients, including young children. The current recommended regimens of treatment with doxycycline are 100 mg per dose given twice daily for adults, and 2.2 mg/kg body weight per dose given twice daily for children weighing less than 45 kg. These recommended doses may be given orally or intravenously, and treatment should be maintained for 5 to 7 days. Doxycycline therapy should be continued until the patient is afebrile for at least 2 or 3 days. Intravenous therapy is often indicated for hospital inpatients, particularly for those with vomiting, unstable vital signs, and neurologic symptoms. Chloramphenicol remains the

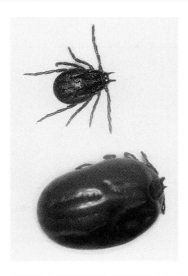

Figure 180-5 Dog ticks showing normal morphology *(upper photo)* and after being fully engorged with blood *(lower photo).* (From Bolognia J, Jorizzo J, Rapini R: *Dermatology.* St Louis, 2003, Mosby.)

recommended therapy for RMSF in pregnant women, despite the risk of grey baby syndrome. The indicated dose of chloramphenicol is 50 to75 mg/kg/day, divided into four doses, given for 7 days, or until 2 days after the fever has subsided. In life-threatening situations, the use of tetracyclines might be warranted during pregnancy.

Provide information about prevention of tick exposure. Measures to help prevent tick exposure include avoiding tick-infested areas (especially during the summer months); avoiding the grassy, overgrown areas favored by ticks; staying to the center of a trail while hiking; and avoiding sitting on logs or leaning against trees. Other measures include wearing long pants and tucking pant legs into socks, using tick repellents containing diethyltoluamide (DEET) for exposed skin and permethrin (Duranon) for clothing, and using bed nets sprayed with permethrin when sleeping on the ground or camping. Wearing light-colored clothing and checking the skin carefully at the end of the day for ticks (especially the head, scalp, and genital area—"tick checks") will help in spotting a tick before it bites. Special graspers for removing ticks are available and can be handy in the field (e.g., Tick Nipper).

What Not To Do:

Do not use heat, occlusion, or caustics to remove a tick. Many techniques have been promoted, but they are generally ineffective and may increase the chance of infection or may potentially do harm.

Do not contaminate fingers with potentially infected tick products.

Do not mutilate the skin by attempting to remove the tick's "head." Usually what is left behind is cementum secreted by the tick, which is easily scraped off. Retained mouth parts (Figure 180-6) can produce local inflammation or minor bacterial infection, but they do not transmit Lyme disease.

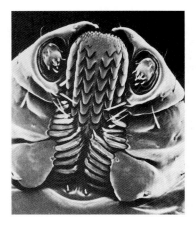

Figure 180-6 Tick mouth parts.

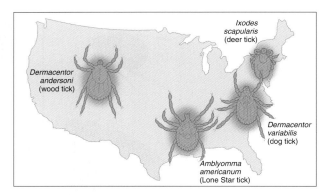

Figure 180-7 Ticks by region.

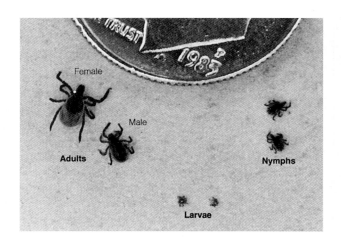

Figure 180-8 Three phases in the life cycle of *Ixodes scapularis,* or deer tick. (From Marzouk JB: Tick-borne diseases: where to expect and how to detect such bite-caused syndromes. *Consultant* 25:21-44, 1985.)

(X) Do not prescribe prophylactic antibiotics for RMSF.

(X) Do not prescribe prophylactic antibiotics for Lyme disease if its prevalence is very low in your geographic area (Figure 180-7).

(X) Do not initiate serologic testing in the asymptomatic patient with suspected Lyme disease or early in the course of the disease. It is costly, inaccurate, and unnecessary. Serologic testing may be more useful in later stages of the disease, when sensitivity and specificity of the test is improved.

Discussion

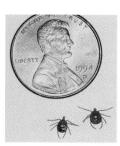

Figure 180-9 Lone star ticks. (From Bolognia J, Jorizzo J, Rapini R: *Dermatology.* St Louis, 2003, Mosby.)

Ixodes scapularis (previously *I. dammini*) (Figure 180-8), the tiny deer tick of the eastern United States, and *I. pacificus* of the western United States (Pacific coast states) can carry babesiosis, human granulocytic ehrlichiosis, and Lyme disease. **Most patients presenting in the summer with a viral syndrome have just that; however, there are other important considerations. Tick-borne diseases may present in this fashion. The clinician must maintain a high index of suspicion in the appropriate epidemiologic setting. Treatment with doxycycline or tetracycline is indicated for RMSF, Lyme disease, ehrlichiosis, and relapsing fever. In patients with clinical findings suggestive of tick-borne disease, empirical treatment should not be delayed. The same tick may harbor different infectious pathogens and may transmit several with one bite.**

Ticks are divided into three families, only two of which are capable of causing infection: soft ticks (Argasidae) and hard ticks (Ixodidae), the latter being responsible for most tick-related diseases. In the United States, the most common Ixodidae genera to transmit disease to humans include *Amblyomma, Ixodes,* and *Dermacentor.* Among the most common in the United States are *I. scapularis* (deer tick, formerly known as *I. dammini*), *I. pacificus, Amblyomma americanum* (Lone Star tick) (Figure 180-9), *Dermacentor andersoni* (American wood tick), and *D. variabilis* (American dog tick).

Tick-borne diseases in the United States include Lyme disease, RMSF, ehrlichiosis, tularemia, babesiosis, Colorado tick fever, and relapsing fever.

Lyme disease is the most common vector-borne disease in the United States. It has been reported in 49 of the 50 United States, but most cases occur in the Northeast to Midwest and North Central regions of the United States. Nine states account for more than 90% of the nationally reported cases, with Connecticut leading the group. The other states (in decreasing order) are Rhode Island, New York, Pennsylvania, Delaware, New Jersey, Maryland, Massachusetts, and Wisconsin. The etiologic agent is the slow-growing, motile spirochete *Borrelia burgdorferi,* which is transmitted by ticks. Deer tick nymphs appear to be the most important vector for transmission of Lyme disease. This nymph stage is when they are tiny and likely to be missed. A minimum of 36 to 48 hours of attachment of the tick is required for transmission. Most cases occur between May and August, which corresponds with increased outdoor human activity and nymphal

activity. The risk for developing Lyme disease after a tick bite is low, even in endemic areas. It should also be noted that less than half of affected patients recall receiving a tick bite because of the small size of the tick.

The incubation period is typically 1 week, but the rash might develop as late as 16 weeks after the tick bite. The rash develops centrifugally as an erythematous, annular, round to oval, well-demarcated plaque (erythema migrans) and has a median diameter of 15 cm. Typically oval or round in shape, this is variable, with a morphology that usually consists of a flat erythema. The phenomenon of central clearing, previously emphasized, actually occurs in a minority of cases. The color may be uniform or centrally darker, and there may be induration or vesiculation.

Within days to a few weeks after the infection, hematogenous and lymphatic dissemination of the spirochete to distant sites commonly occurs. Other annular plaques develop in up to half of patients. The most common neurologic feature is unilateral or bilateral facial paralysis (unilateral paralysis mimicking Bell's Palsy (see Chapter 5). Late-stage disease can occur months to years after the initial infection.

The diagnosis of Lyme disease is usually based on the history of a tick bite in an endemic area, with characteristic clinical findings. Serology using enzyme-linked immunosorbent assay (ELISA) is the most common laboratory test to screen for antibodies; however, the test is not standardized, and false negatives, especially with active or recent infections (or, more commonly, false positives), are common. When a positive or equivocal test is obtained using ELISA, a Western blot (immunoblot) test should be performed on the same serum sample. If the immunoblot is negative, the ELISA is likely a false positive; if the immunoblot is positive, a diagnosis of Lyme disease can be confirmed in a patient with clinical evidence of Lyme disease.

One bout of Lyme disease will not confer immunity to future infections.

RMSF, the most common acute rickettsial infection in the United States, is caused by *Rickettsia rickettsii*. In the United States, the disease is most commonly seen in the Southeast, West, and South Central states. The infection typically occurs in spring and summer,

(continued)

Discussion continued

and the exposure is usually in rural or suburban areas. Primary offenders in the western United States are the wood tick *(D. andersoni),* and, in the eastern United States, the dog tick *(D. variabilis).* The diagnosis of RMSF is based largely on clinical presentation in a patient with history of tick exposure. **Various serology tests are available to confirm the diagnosis. When administered early in the disease, tetracycline and chloramphenicol (orally and intravenously) are extremely effective.** The use of tetracyclines in the treatment of tick-borne rickettsial diseases in children was controversial in the past because of the risk of permanent tooth discoloration. Today, there is a consensus that doxycycline is the drug of choice for treating presumptive or confirmed RMSF in children of any age. A prospective study reported that children treated with doxycycline for RMSF did not show substantial discoloration of permanent teeth compared with those who had never received the drug.

Ehrlichieae are a group of small, gram-negative, obligate intracellular pleomorphic bacteria that are closely related to rickettsiae. In the United States, human monocytic ehrlichiosis (HME) has been seen mainly in the Mid-Atlantic, South Central, and Southeast states as well as in California. *A. americanum* (Lone Star tick) is the primary vector. Most cases occur during summer and autumn, and more than 80% of patients have a history of tick exposure. The clinical manifestations of HME are similar to those of RMSF, with a lesser likelihood of rash. In general, the treatment of choice for ehrlichiosis is a tetracycline. Human granulocytic ehrlichiosis (HGE) has been reported in the Northeast, the upper Midwest, and regions of northern California. Ticks of the *I. persulcatus* complex serve as the principal vector. Other principal vectors are *I. scapularis* (northeastern America) and *I. pacificus* (western United States). The clinical presentation for HGE is indistinguishable from HME, and the treatment is similar.

Tularemia is caused by *Francisella tularensis,* a short, gram-negative, nonmotile coccobacillus. In the United States, the disease is most commonly seen in southern and western states. Inoculation of organisms into the skin most frequently occurs from bites of deer flies or ticks and from direct contact with infected animals, primarily wild rabbits, especially after skinning their hides. The tick in the Southeast and South Central United States is *A. americanum* (Lone Star tick), and in the West, it is

D. andersoni (wood tick); the most widely distributed is *D. variabilis* (dog tick). Tularemia is characterized by acute onset of fever, headache, chills, myalgias, fatigue, and leukocytosis. The typical incubation period is 3 to 5 days. The most common clinical presentation is the ulceroglandular type, which begins at the site of the tick bite, usually on the lower extremities or perineum, as a papule or nodule that rapidly ulcerates. A lymphatic spread occurs with painful regional lymphadenopathy, usually inguinal or femoral, which might progress to ulceration. Streptomycin given intramuscularly is the treatment of choice.

Babesiosis is a malaria-like disease caused by an intracellular parasite that invades red blood cells. The major endemic areas in the United States are Massachusetts (Martha's Vineyard, Nantucket), New York (eastern and southern Long Island), Connecticut, and other offshore islands of the Northeast. The causative agent is *Babesia microti,* which is transmitted by the larvae of *I. scapularis* (deer tick). The illness usually occurs in older patients or in asplenic or immunocompromised patients. The incubation period after a tick bite is about 1 week. The classic clinical presentation is high fever, drenching sweats, myalgias, and hemolytic anemia. Blood smear may be confusing: The tetrad of merozoites of babesiosis can be confused with the ring forms of *Plasmodium falciparum*–induced malaria. A 7- to 10-day concomitant course of quinine and intravenous clindamycin is used most commonly to treat the infection.

Colorado tick fever is caused by an RNA orbivirus transmitted by the *D. andersoni* wood tick. It is predominantly found in the Rocky Mountain region. Influenza-like symptoms usually begin within 1 week after inoculation. The disease usually lasts 7 to 10 days. Treatment is supportive, but at the onset of symptoms, most patients will be treated empirically with tetracycline, doxycycline, or chloramphenicol to cover other tick-borne diseases.

Tick-borne relapsing fever is caused by the spirochete within the genus *Borrelia.* It is transmitted by species of the soft tick genus, *Ornithodoros.* The tick species capable of transmitting the disease in the United States tends to exist in remote undisturbed settings in most regions. After an incubation period of 1 week, the disease is characterized by acute onset of high fever with chills, headache, myalgias, tachycardia, arthralgias, and malaise. If untreated, the primary episode

Discussion continued

lasts 3 to 6 days; rapid defervescence followed by drenching sweats marks resolution of disease. If left untreated, a second shorter course and as many as three to five relapses per year can occur. Tick-borne relapsing fever warrants treatment with either tetracycline or erythromycin for 5 to 10 days.

Tick paralysis rarely occurs in humans; when it does, it usually affects children. Most cases in the United States occur in the Northwest in the spring or summer months, and the ticks usually attach to the scalp or neck. In the United States, most cases are attributed to wood ticks, dog ticks, Lone Star ticks, and deer ticks. Paralysis usually occurs 4 to 7 days after attachment of the tick and is caused by the production of a neurotoxin secreted in the saliva of the tick. An acute ascending lower motor neuron paralysis develops, beginning in the legs and sparing sensory function. Definitive therapy is simply to remove any ticks attached to the patient's body. However, symptoms can progress after tick removal. In general, improvement is much faster in cases in North America than in Australia. Normally, once the tick is removed in the former setting, symptoms begin to rapidly resolve within hours and are completely resolved 24 hours later. Patients who are minimally symptomatic can be observed

for several hours and discharged if no progression occurs. In Australian cases, where symptoms can dramatically progress after the tick is removed, patients should be observed for a longer period, until the clinical course is clearly steadily and unequivocally improving.

Fever and a rash following a tick bite can signify a true medical emergency. Recent findings show that Rocky Mountain spotted fever continues to be the most lethal tick-borne illness in the United States and is emerging as an important disease in South America. Other important emerging diseases include human anaplasmosis, southern tick-associated rash illness, human monocytic ehrlichiosis, and a variety of rickettsial fevers, including those caused by *Rickettsia parkeri* and *Rickettsia amblyommii*.

In summary, most tick-borne illnesses respond readily to doxycycline therapy. In the case of Rocky Mountain spotted fever, therapy should be started when the disease is suspected and should never be delayed for confirmatory tests. Accurate identification of tick vectors can help establish a diagnosis and can help guide preventive measures.

Suggested Readings

Aberer E: What should one do in case of a tick bite? *Curr Probl Dermatol* 37:155–166, 2009.

Bolognia EA, Reed KD, Mitchell PD, et al: Tickborne infections as a cause of nonspecific febrile illness in Wisconsin, *Clin Infect Dis* 32:1434–1439, 2001.

Bratton RL, Corey GR: Tick-borne disease, *Am Fam Physician* 71:2323–2330, 2005.

Brown L, Hansen SL, Langone JJ, et al: Lyme disease test kits: potential for misdiagnosis, *FDA Med Bull* 3, (Summer), 1999.

Clark RP, DO, Hu LT: Prevention of Lyme disease and other tick-borne infections, *Infect Dis Clin North Am* 22:381–396, vii, 2008.

Dantas-Torres F: Rocky Mountain spotted fever, *Lancet Infect Dis* 7:724–732, 2007.

Dedeoglu F, Sundel RP: Emergency department management of Lyme disease, *Clin Pediatr Emerg Med* 5:54–62, 2004.

Edlow JA: Lyme disease and tick-borne illnesses, *Ann Emerg Med* 33:680–693, 1999.

Elston DM: Tick bites and skin rashes, *Curr Opin Infect Dis* 23:132–138, 2010.

Edlow JA, McGillicuddy DC: Tick paralysis, *Infect Dis Clin North Am* 22:397–413, vi, 2008.

Karras DJ: Letter to the editor: tick removal, *Ann Emerg Med* 32:4, 1998.

Kirkland KB, Wilkinson WE, Sexton DJ: Therapeutic delay and mortality in cases of Rocky Mountain spotted fever, *Clin Infect Dis* 20:1118–1121, 1995.

Magid D, Schwartz B, Craft J, Schwartz JS: Prevention of Lyme disease after tick bites, *N Engl J Med* 327:534–541, 1992. (Letters, *N Engl J Med* 328:1418-1420, 1993.)

McGinley-Smith DE, Tsao SS: Dermatoses from ticks, *J Am Acad Dermatol* 49:363–392, 2003.

Nadelman RB, Nawakowski J, Fish D, et al: Prophylaxis with single-dose doxycycline for the prevention of lyme disease after an *Ixodes scapularis* tick bite, *J Med* 345:79–84, 2001.

Nadelman RB, Nowakowski J, Forseter G, et al: The clinical spectrum of early Lyme borreliosis in patients with culture-confirmed erythema migrans, *Am J Med* 100:502–508, 1996.

Needham GR: Evaluation of five popular methods for tick removal, *Pediatrics* 75:997–1002, 1985.

Singh-Behl D, La Rosa SP, Tomecki KJ: Tick-borne infections, *Dermatol Clin* 21:237–244, 2003.

Smith RP, Schoen RT, Rahn DW: Clinical characteristics and treatment outcome of early Lyme disease in patients with microbiologically confirmed erythema migrans, *Ann Intern Med* 136:421–428, 2002.

Treatment of Lyme disease, *Med Lett Drugs Ther* 47:41–43, 2005.

Volovitz B, Shkap R, Amir J, et al: Absence of tooth staining with doxycycline treatment in young children, *Clin Pediatr* 2007;121–126, 2007.

Wormser GP, Ramanathan R, Nowakowski J, et al: Duration of antibiotic therapy for early Lyme disease, *Ann Intern Med* 138:697–704, 2003.

Tinea Pedis, Tinea Cruris, Tinea Corporis

(Athlete's Foot, Jock Itch, Ringworm)

Presentation

Patients usually seek medical care for "athlete's foot," "jock itch," or "ringworm" when pruritus is severe or when secondary infection causes pain and swelling. Worrisome spreading of the rash, along with an unsightly and annoying appearance, will also motivate these patients to seek medical treatment.

Tinea pedis: There are three general clinical presentations: interdigital, moccasin, and vesicobullous. Interdigital disease is most common. Often there is fissuring, scaling, and maceration of the interdigitial or subdigital areas, particularly the fourth-to-fifth toe web space (Figure 181-1, *A* and *B*). Moccasin-type tinea is characterized by fine silvery scales, with underlying pink to red skin that most commonly affects areas of the soles, heels, and sides of the feet (moccasin distribution) (Figure 181-1, *C*). Vesicobullous tinea pedis is the least common form. There may be acute and highly inflammatory vesicular or bullous lesions that are pruritic and commonly found at the instep of the foot; however, inflammation may spread over the entire sole (Figure 181-1, *D*).

Tinea cruris: This is a dermatophyte infection of the inguinal folds, inner thighs, perineum, and buttocks that usually spares the scrotum and penis (unlike *Candida intertrigo*). There is an erythematous scaling eruption that is often annular in appearance (Figure 181-2). Pruritus is a common symptom, and pain may be present if the involved area is moist and macerated or secondarily infected. More commonly seen in men, tinea cruris often occurs in patients with tinea pedis and onychomycosis (dermatophyte infection of the toenails) and is thought to spread to the groin from contaminated underpants.

Tinea corporis: This dermatophyte infection of the glabrous (hairless) skin elsewhere on the body typically presents as an erythematous, scaling, annular eruption with central clearing on the extremities or trunk (Figure 181-3). The classic ringworm pattern is a flat scaly area with a raised border that advances circumferentially. Vesicles or pustules may form as the lesion becomes inflamed.

What To Do:

✓ When microscopic examination of skin scrapings in potassium hydroxide (KOH) is readily available, definite identification of the lesion can be made by looking for the presence of hyphae or spores. Using a No. 10 scalpel blade, scrape flakes or scales from the active leading edge of the lesion (or from the web space) onto a glass slide. Sweep the particles toward the center of the slide and add a drop of 10% to 20% KOH and a cover slip. Warm with a flame, and then view

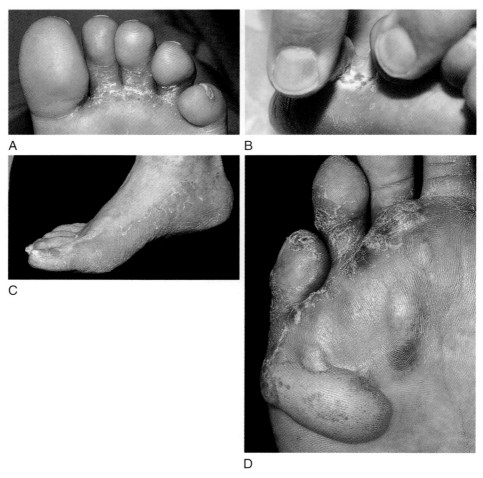

Figure 181-1 A, Interdigital tinea pedis. **B,** White macerated web between fourth and fifth toes. **C,** Moccasin distribution of tinea pedis. **D,** Bullous tinea. (From White G, Cox N: *Diseases of the skin,* ed 2. St Louis, 2006, Mosby.)

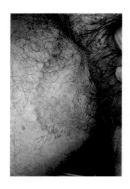

Figure 181-2 Tinea cruris. (From Bolognia J, Jorizzo J, Rapini R: *Dermatology.* St Louis, 2003, Mosby.)

under low (100×) magnification with the microscope light condenser lowered. Branching fungal filaments (hyphae and myceliae) identify superficial dermatophytes (Figure 181-4). Budding cells and pseudohyphae ("spaghetti and meatballs") suggest yeast, particularly *Candida* organisms. Fungal cultures are rarely necessary for acute uncomplicated lesions. Treatment can be started presumptively when microscopic examination is not easily accomplished, but always consider the "herald patch" of pityriasis rosea (see Chapter 175), nummular dermatitis, secondary and tertiary syphilis, lichen planus, seborrheic dermatitis, psoriasis, impetigo (see Chapter 172), and neurodermatitis in the differential diagnosis.

✅ **Terbinafine (Lamisil AT cream or spray), clotrimazole (Lotrimin or Lotrimin Ultra 1% cream, solution, or lotion), and miconazole (Micatin) 2% cream, spray, lotion, or powder, as well as butenafine (Mentax) 1% cream applied qd to bid are available over the counter and can be applied bid. Naftifine (Naftin 1% cream applied qd or 1% gel applied qd to bid) requires a prescription.** If applied to the rash, they will cause involution of most superficial

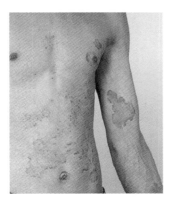

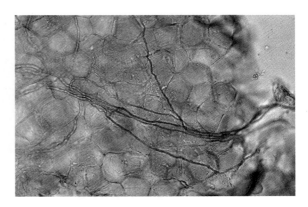

Figure 181-3 Tinea corporis. (From White G, Cox N: *Diseases of the skin,* ed 2. St Louis, 2006, Mosby.)

Figure 181-4 Potassium hydrochloride (KOH) preparation of a dermatophyte demonstrating branching hyphae. (From Bolognia J, Jorizzo J, Rapini R: *Dermatology.* St Louis, 2003, Mosby.)

lesions within 1 to 2 weeks but may need to be continued for up to 4 weeks. They should be continued for 7 to 14 days beyond symptom resolution to prevent relapse. Advise the patient to apply the topical medication 2 cm past the border of the skin lesion.

✓ Sertaconazole nitrate (Ertaczo) cream 2% [30, 60 g] is a newer imidazole agent that possesses both fungicidal and fungistatic properties to eradicate existing infections. In addition to antifungal properties, it exhibits anti-inflammatory and antipruritic effects. Apply bid (not approved for children younger than 12 years of age).

✓ Rarely, more severe or extensive lesions can be treated with oral antifungals. Terbinafine (Lamisil), 250 mg qd × 2 weeks; ketoconazole (Nizoral), 200 mg qd × 4 weeks; or fluconazole (Diflucan), 150 mg weekly for 2 to 4 weeks, can be used. (See the *Physicians' Desk Reference [PDR]* for adverse side effects and interactions.)

✓ **With signs of secondary infection, begin treatment first with wet compresses of Burow solution (2 packets of Domeboro powder in 1 pint water) for a half hour every 3 to 4 hours. Use mupirocin (Bactroban) 2% cream for superficial bacterial infections (impetigo).** With signs of deep infection (cellulitis, lymphangitis), begin systemic antibiotics with streptococcal coverage, such as cefadroxil (Duricef), 500 mg bid × 7 to 10 days; cephalexin (Keflex) or dicloxacillin (Dynapen), 250 to 500 mg qid × 7 to 10 days; or azithromycin (Zithromax), 500 mg, then 250 mg qd × 4 days. **Always consider coverage for community-acquired methicillin-resistant *Staphylococcus aureus* (CA-MRSA) if it is prevalent in your area** (see Chapter 166).

✓ **With inflammation and weeping lesions, a topical antifungal and steroid cream combination, such as Lotrisone in addition to the wet compresses, will be most effective.** Warn patients that this medication has a potent steroid that can lead to skin atrophy or striae if used for an extended period, especially in the groin. **An alternative is to use the recommended antifungals and add a low-dose over-the-counter (OTC) corticosteroid (e.g., 2.5% hydrocortisone cream [Cortaid]) for the first few days.**

✓ For tinea pedis, instruct patients to wear nonocclusive footwear, such as sandals, that allow the foot to "breathe." Have them put on socks before underwear to avoid spreading the fungus from feet to groin. **A gel formulation of naftifine may be helpful for moist web spaces.**

735

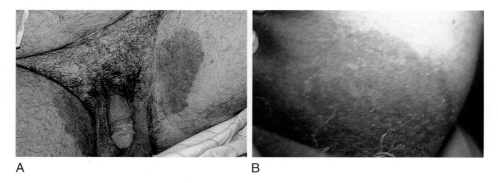

Figure 181-5 A and **B,** Erythrasma appears as red-brown patches of the groin or axilla that fluoresce coral-pink under Wood light examination. (From White G, Cox N: *Diseases of the skin,* ed 2. St Louis, 2006, Mosby.)

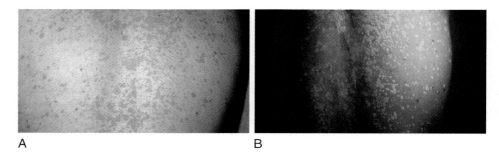

Figure 181-6 A, Tinea versicolor on the upper back of a young adult. **B,** Wood light examination of the same patient. (From White G, Cox N: *Diseases of the skin,* ed 2. St Louis, 2006, Mosby.)

✓ For tinea cruris, suggest loose undergarments made of absorbent materials, such as cotton rather than synthetics. Skin should be dried well with a towel or hair dryer. Absorbent powders and drying agents, such as Zeasorb-AF and Drysol, can be applied lightly.

✓ To prevent reinfection when onychomycosis is present, nail infections should be treated (see later, this chapter).

What Not To Do:

✗ Do not attempt to treat fungal infections of the scalp (tinea capitis) with local therapy. A boggy swelling (tinea kerion) or patchy hair loss with inflammation and scaling requires systemic antifungals, such as griseofulvin.

✗ Do not use Nystatin, a drug familiar for its usefulness against *Candida* infections. Tinea infections are not killed by this drug.

✗ Do not treat with corticosteroids alone. They will reduce signs and symptoms (tinea incognito) but allow increased fungal growth.

Discussion

Tinea infections are caused by superficial fungi known as dermatophytes, which are true saprophytes that take all their nutrients from dead keratin in the stratum corneum of the skin and the keratinized tissue of hair and nails. They cannot invade live epidermis. Some of these infections cause circular lesions that result from the inflammatory reaction, forcing the dermatophytes outward to an inflammation-free area. As long as the infection persists, so does the outward migration.

Tinea pedis or athlete's foot is the most common fungal infection. It is seen most in those who wear occlusive footwear because shoes promote warmth and sweating, which encourage fungal growth. Tinea must be differentiated from allergic and irritant contact dermatitis (see Chapter 160). **In several studies, application of the allylamine terbinafine bid resulted in a higher cure rate than twice-daily application of the imidazole clotrimazole, and at a quicker rate (1 week vs. 4 weeks).**

All superficial dermatophytes of the skin, except those involving the scalp, beard, face, hands, feet, groin, and nails, are known as **tinea corporis,** or ringworm of the body. Contact with pets is often the source of the infection. Systemic diseases (e.g., diabetes, leukemia, acquired immunodeficiency disease [AIDS]) predisposes patients to tinea corporis.

Candidiasis and erythrasma may resemble tinea cruris, but candidal lesions are usually more moist, red, and tender (see Chapter 165). Pustules may be seen within the indistinct border, and satellite lesions may be scattered over adjacent skin. Candidiasis also may involve the scrotum or penis, which are usually spared by tinea. ***Candida* organisms may be treated topically with naftifine (Naftin), ciclopirox (Loprox), or clotrimazole (Lotrimin, Mycelex).**

Erythrasma is a skin infection caused by *Corynebacterium minutissimum,* a gram-positive bacterium. The rash characteristically consists of asymptomatic, reddish-brown, superficial dull patches with well-defined margins and no central clearing. The peripheral edge is not usually any more raised than the center (Figure 181-5, *A*). When illuminated with an ultraviolet Wood lamp, the infected skin glows with coral-pink fluorescence (Figure 181-5, *B*). **Erythrasma is treated with oral erythromycin, 250 mg qid × 14 days.**

Tinea versicolor is a misnomer, because it is not caused by a dermatophyte fungus but by lipophilic yeast. Pityriasis versicolor is the more correct name. It is asymptomatic, and its presentation to an acute care facility usually is incidental to some other problem. There is, however, no reason to ignore this chronic superficial skin infection, which causes cosmetically unpleasant irregular patches of varying pigmentation that tend to be lighter than the surrounding skin in the summer and darker than the surrounding skin in the winter. Wood light examination sometimes reveals a white or yellow fluorescence (Figure 181-6).

Differential diagnosis includes tinea corporis, pityriasis alba, pityriasis rosea, vitiligo, leprosy, and secondary syphilis.

Prescribe a 2.5% selenium sulfide lotion (Selsun) to be applied as lather, leave on 10 to 15 minutes, then wash off daily for 10 to 14 days and then qhs monthly, or use three to five times weekly for 2 to 4 weeks (which also should be followed with monthly re-treatments). Alternatively, use terbinafine 1% solution (spray) twice daily for 1 week or ketoconazole (Nizoral) cream 2% daily for 2 weeks, or ketoconazole or fluconazole (Diflucan) as a single 300-mg oral dose to be repeated in 4 weeks. Also, itraconazole can be taken 200 mg qd × 3 to 7 days. (See the *PDR* for adverse side effects and interactions.) Superficial scaling should resolve in a few days, and the pigmentary changes will slowly clear over a period of several months. Tinea versicolor has a recurrence rate of 80% after 2 years; patients are therefore likely to need periodic re-treatment or preventive maintenance.

Tinea capitis is mainly a disease of infants, children, and young adolescents, usually involving black or Hispanic preschoolers. Tinea capitis presents in numerous ways: The primary lesions may be scales, papules, pustules, plaques, or nodules on the scalp. Inflammation and secondary infection lead to secondary processes, such as alopecia, erythema, exudate, and edema (Figure 181-7). A kerion forms as a result of increased cell-mediated immune response, demonstrated by an inflamed, exudative, nodular, boggy swelling with associated hair loss and cervical lymphadenopathy (Figure 181-8). Tinea capitis can be diagnosed on KOH examination of extracted hair. Culture must involve the extracted hair, not simply scales.

(continued)

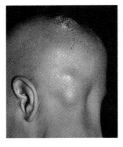

Figure 181-8 Kerion with swollen regional lymph nodes. (From White G, Cox N: *Diseases of the skin*, ed 2. St Louis, 2006, Mosby.)

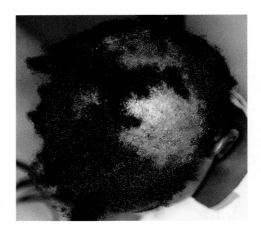

Figure 181-7 Tinea capitis. (From Bolognia J, Jorizzo J, Rapini R: *Dermatology*. St Louis, 2003, Mosby.)

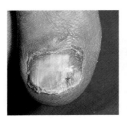

Figure 181-9 Tinea unguium or subungual onychomycosis. (From White G, Cox N: *Diseases of the skin*, ed 2. St Louis, 2006, Mosby.)

Discussion continued

Oral antifungals are the mainstay of treatment for tinea capitis. Griseofulvin is the only drug approved by the United States Food and Drug Administration for use in children, although other medications have been used. Terbinafine (Lamisil) is now considered the primary drug of choice for the treatment of tinea capitis. Prescribe 250 mg qd × 4 to 8 weeks. Prescribe 6 to 12 mg/kg/day qd × 4 to 8 weeks for children. Griseofulvin is given as 20 to 25 mg/kg/day qd × 8 weeks (or 2 weeks beyond cure), or liquid microsized griseofulvin (Grifulvin V), 15 to 25 mg/kg every day for 8 weeks. Ketoconazole shampoo and cream can be used to reduce fungal shedding. To prevent spread to other family members, contaminated combs and brushes should be cleaned, and family members can use selenium sulfide lotion or shampoo for 5 to 10 minutes (then rinse) three times per week.

Onychomycosis (also known as tinea unguium) is an infection of the nail plate or nail bed that interferes with normal nail function (Figure 181-9). Patients with this infection often have concomitant fungal infections at other sites. Because onychomycosis requires expensive prolonged therapy (6 weeks for fingernail infections and 12 weeks for toenail infections), the diagnosis should be confirmed before treatment is initiated. This can be achieved by clipping off the distal edge of the affected nail, placing it in formalin along with attached subungual debris, and sending it for periodic acid–Schiff staining with histologic examination in a hospital or reference laboratory.

Terbinafine, at a dosage of 250 mg per day for 12 weeks, has a better mycologic cure rate than "pulse" therapy, in which 500 mg of terbinafine is given once daily for 7 days of each of 2 months (fingernails) or 4 months (toenails). It should be noted, though, that follow-up must be arranged with a patient's primary doctor or dermatologist. Long-term dosage with this drug has caused some significant liver disease. Terbinafine is considered the drug of choice for dermatophyte onychomycosis, with greater mycologic cure rates, less serious and fewer drug interactions, and a lower cost than continuous itraconazole therapy. Adjunct débridement may improve the clinical and complete cure rates compared with terbinafine alone.

Newer oral antifungal agents have greatly improved the management of dermatomycoses, but not without consequence. Some are very expensive, have side effects and organ toxicity that may or may not be tolerable, and have significant adverse drug interactions. Laboratory monitoring is recommended during treatment with all oral antifungal medications. Liver function tests for itraconazole should be done at baseline, at 1 month, and if any signs or symptoms of liver dysfunction present. Terbinafine use warrants liver function tests at baseline, at 6 weeks, if signs or symptoms present, and then 4 weeks later. In general, one should monitor patients more closely if taking medications that impair renal or hepatic function.

Suggested Readings

Fleece D, Gaughan JP, Aronoff SC: Griseofulvin versus terbinafine in the treatment of tinea capitis, *Pediatrics* 114:1312–1315, 2004.

Gupta AK, Chaudhry M, Elewski B: Tinea corporis, tinea cruris, tinea nigra, and piedra, *Dermatol Clin* 21:395–400, 2003.

Gupta AK, Chow M, Daniel CR, et al: Treatments of tinea pedis, *Dermatol Clin* 21:431–462, 2003.

Gupta AK, Cooper EA, Lynde CW: The efficacy and safety of terbinafine in children, *Dermatol Clin* 21:511–520, 2003.

Gupta AK, Cooper EA, Montero-Gei F: The use of fluconazole to treat superficial fungal infections in children, *Dermatol Clin* 21:537–542, 2003.

Hainer BL: Dermatophyte infections, *Am Fam Physician* 67:101–108, 2003.

Janniger CK, Schwartz RA, Szepietowski JC, et al: Intertrigo and common secondary skin infections, *Am Fam Physician* 72:833–838, 2005.

Loo DS: Onychomycosis in the elderly drug treatment options, *Drugs Aging* 24:293–302, 2007.

Martin ES, Elewski BE: Cutaneous fungal infections in the elderly, *Clin Geriatr Med* 18:59–75, 2002.

Nandedkar-Thomas MA, Scher RK: An update on disorders of the nails, *J Am Acad Dermatol* 52:877–887, 2005.

Patel GA, Wiederkerh M, Schwartz RA: Tinea cruris in children, *Cutis* 84:133–137, 2009.

Ribotsky BM: Sertaconazole nitrate cream 2% for the treatment of tinea pedis, *Cutis* 83:274–277, 2009.

Sanfilippo AM, Barrio V, Kulp-Shorten C, et al: Common pediatric and adolescent skin conditions, *J Pediatr Adolesc Gynecol* 16:269–283, 2003.

Vander Straten MR, Hossain MA: Ghannoum MA: Cutaneous infections, *Infect Dis Clin North Am* 17:101–108, 2003.

Warshaw EM, Fett DD, Bloomfield HE, et al: Pulse versus continuous terbinafine for onychomycosis, *J Am Acad Dermatol* 53:578–584, 2005.

Toxicodendron (Rhus) Allergic Contact Dermatitis

(Poison Ivy, Oak, or Sumac)

Presentation

The patient is troubled with an intensely pruritic rash that often consists of raised lesions that develop into vesicles and are usually formed in a streaked or linear pattern. Eventually, there is a weeping, honey-colored crust, confluence of vesicles, and, sometimes, large bullae (Figure 182-1, *A* and *B*). If involvement is severe, there may be marked edema, particularly on the face, periorbital areas (Figure 182-2), and genital areas. The thick protective stratum corneum of the palms and the soles generally protects these areas. Inflammation usually peaks in 5 days, evolving into a subacute phase in which the swelling and blistering subside, replaced by drier crust and scaling. Redness and itching persist. Secondary bacterial infection can develop, often caused by the patient's scratching.

The patient is often not aware of having been in contact with poison ivy, oak, or sumac but may recall working in a field or garden from several hours to 4 days before the onset of symptoms. In general, the shorter the reaction time, the greater is the degree of the individual's sensitivity, which decreases with age. Most cases of *Toxicodendron* dermatitis begin to dissipate after 10 to 14 days.

What To Do:

✓ **If it is available, have the patient cleanse all affected areas with Zanfel Poison Ivy Wash (www.zanfel.com), an over-the-counter (OTC) product that can actively bind the allergen, reduce its load in the skin, and provide some relief from the itching.**

✓ **To reduce pruritus, have the patient apply cool or cold compresses of aluminum subacetate (Burow solution; Domeboro Powder Packets [2 packets in**

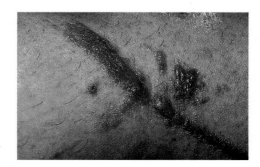

Figure 182-1 Classic *Toxicodendron* allergic contact dermatitis demonstrating linear streaking of vesicles and bullae. (From White G, Cox N: *Diseases of the skin*, ed 2. St Louis, 2006, Mosby.)

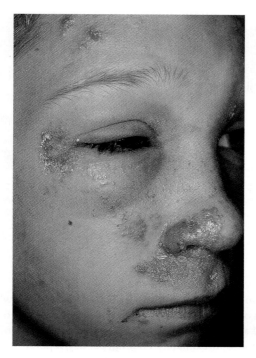

Figure 182-2 In addition to crusted and weeping plaques, there is periorbital edema in this case of acute allergic dermatitis to poison ivy. (From Bolognia J, Jorizzo J, Rapini R: *Dermatology.* St Louis, 2003, Mosby.)

1 pint of refrigerated water]) for approximately 20 minutes every 3 to 4 hours (more often if needed for comfort). Anything that cools the skin, including ice, will reduce itching.

✓ **Small areas on the trunk or extremities can be treated with potent topical steroids, such as fluocinonide (Lidex) or desoximetasone (Topicort) 0.05% cream or gel, two to three times per day,** after using cool compresses. Topical steroids can be enhanced at night with an occlusive plastic (Saran) wrap dressing. A severe local reaction can be treated with clobetasol (Temovate) 0.05% cream bid, a very powerful topical steroid. These severe reactions may require 2 days of application before itching subsides significantly. These agents must be continued for 2 weeks or the dermatitis will reappear.

✓ Diphenhydramine (OTC, Benadryl) or hydroxyzine (Atarax, Vistaril), 25 to 50 mg PO q6h, may help mild itching between application of compresses but will probably provide nothing more than a soporific effect. There is no evidence to support the efficacy of nonsedating antihistamines.

✓ **Tepid tub baths with Aveeno colloidal oatmeal (one cup in half-full bathtub) or cornstarch and baking soda (1 cup of each in half-full bathtub) will provide soothing relief for more extensive lesions.** To prevent ground oatmeal from caking in pipes, place it in a tied sock before dropping it into the bathtub.

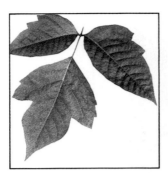

Figure 182-3 Poison ivy. (From Cruz PD: *Toxicodendron* dermatitis. Paper presented by Extension Services in Pharmacy, School of Pharmacy, University of Wisconsin–Madison, April 2003.)

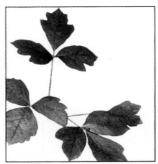

Figure 182-4 Poison oak. (From Cruz PD: *Toxicodendron* dermatitis. Paper presented by Extension Services in Pharmacy, School of Pharmacy, University of Wisconsin–Madison, April 2003.)

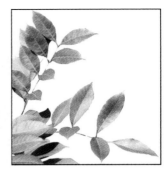

Figure 182-5 Poison sumac. (From Cruz PD: *Toxicodendron* dermatitis. Paper presented by Extension Services in Pharmacy, School of Pharmacy, University of Wisconsin–Madison, April 2003.)

✅ **When there is involvement of the face, eyes, hands, or genitalia; when there are severe generalized reactions or a history of severe reactions; or when the patient's livelihood is threatened, early and aggressive treatment with systemic corticosteroids should be initiated. Prednisone (60 to 80 mg [approximately 1 mg/kg] per day, tapered over 2 to 3 weeks) will be necessary to prevent a late flare-up or rebound reaction. One 40-mg dose of triamcinolone acetonide (Kenalog) intramuscularly will be equally effective.** For pediatric patients, use prednisolone syrup, 15 mg/5 mL (Prelone), 1 mg/kg/day, tapered over 2 to 3 weeks.

✅ **Inform patients about** preventing future exposures **by using IvyBlock, an OTC lotion containing bentoquatam 5%, which binds with plant allergens, preventing them from penetrating the skin. This is of no use for patients who already have a rash.**

✅ **Avoidance of the offending agent is the key to prevention.** Instruct patients regarding how to recognize poison ivy and its close relatives (Figures 182-3 to 182-5). Also have them cover up in the future with long pants, a long-sleeved shirt, vinyl gloves, and boots. They should wash with water (and soap if available) immediately after suspecting contact with a *Toxicodendron*. After 10 minutes, only 50% can be removed; after 15 minutes, only 25%; after 30 minutes, only 10%; and after 60 minutes, none of the urushiol can be removed using soap and water. **After 60 minutes, Zanfel may be the only cleansing agent that can effectively bind and remove *Toxicodendron* sap from the skin.**

✅ Treat secondary infections with antibiotics, such as dicloxacillin, 500 mg qid; cephalexin, 500 mg tid for 10 days; or azithromycin, 500 mg, then 250 mg qd 4 days, or, when appropriate, provide coverage for community-acquired methicillin-resistant *Staphylococcus aureus* (CA-MRSA) (see Chapters 166 and 172).

✅ Although hyperpigmentation can occur in dark-skinned individuals and may last a few weeks after resolution of the dermatitis, patients can usually be reassured that even severe lesions will not leave any visible skin markings when healing is complete. Scarring occurs only if scratching leads to damage beneath the epidermis.

What Not To Do:

(X) Do not have the patient use heavy-duty skin cleansers, alcohol, or other strong solvents to remove any remaining antigen. This would be ineffective and may do harm. Strong soap and scrubbing merely irritate the skin and are not more effective than mild soap and gentle washing.

(X) Do not try to substitute prepackaged steroid regimens (Medrol Dosepak, Aristopak). The course is not long enough and may lead to a flare-up.

(X) Do not allow patients to apply fluorinated corticosteroids, such as Lidex or Valisone, for more than 3 weeks to the face or intertriginous areas, where they can produce thinning of skin and telangiectasias. A 10- to 14-day course should not be a problem. Any significant involvement of the face should be treated with systemic corticosteroids.

(X) Do not institute systemic steroids in the presence of severe secondary infections, such as cellulitis or erysipelas. Also, do not start steroids if there is a history of tuberculosis, peptic ulcer, diabetes, herpes, or severe hypertension without careful monitoring and/or specialty consultation.

(X) Do not recommend OTC topical steroid preparations. They are not potent enough to be effective.

(X) Do not prescribe topical steroids if systemic steroids are being given. They should no longer be necessary.

(X) Do not recommend the use of topical antihistamines (which do not reduce itching) or topical benzocaine because of the added risk for the development of a second allergic contact dermatitis. Topical antibiotics with neomycin should be avoided for the same reason.

Discussion

Poison ivy is the most ubiquitous of the four species of the *Toxicodendron* genus of the Anacardiaceae plant family, which also includes poison sumac and two species of poison oak. In the United States, these four species of plants are responsible for more cases of allergic contact dermatitis than all other contact allergens combined. The strongly sensitizing allergen of *Toxicodendron* plants is urushiol, a catechol derivative found in the plants' sap. It is also found in the Japanese lacquer tree, mango rinds, cashew shell oil, and the seed coat of the ginkgo tree. When exposed to oxygen, urushiol easily oxidizes and, after polymerizing, becomes a shiny black lacquer. Urushiol is found not only in the leaves but also in vines (aerial roots), stems, and root systems.

In an area where *Toxicodendron* grows, *Toxicodendron* dermatitis should be suspected in anyone with severe acute allergic contact dermatitis. In the summer, any contact dermatitis of unknown cause should be considered *Toxicodendron* dermatitis until proven otherwise.

This is an allergic contact dermatitis that is T cell–mediated and develops in genetically susceptible individuals following skin contact with urushiol. This allergen induces sensitization in more than 70% of the population, may be carried by pets, and is frequently transferred from hands to other areas of the body that may, unfortunately, include the

(continued)

Discussion continued

genital area. Broad areas of redness and dermatitis are generally the result of rubbing. There is always pruritus, which most often is intense. **If there is no itching, it is almost certainly not** *Toxicodendron* **dermatitis.**

The gradual appearance of the eruption over a period of several days is a reflection of the amount of antigen deposited on the skin and the reactivity of the site, not an indication of any further spread of the allergen. The vesicle fluid is a transudate, does not contain antigen, and will not spread the eruption to elsewhere on the body or to other people. The rash only seems to spread because different areas of the body have different thicknesses of stratum corneum, leading to different rates of absorption of antigen and, therefore, different rates of eruption. The allergic skin reaction usually runs a course of about 2 weeks, sometimes longer, and is not shortened by any of the previously mentioned treatments (except possibly in the case of Zanfel). The aim of therapy is to reduce the severity of symptoms. It is not currently clear whether we are able to shorten the course of this reaction. Those skin areas with the greatest degree of initial reaction tend to be affected the longest. In a dry environment, the allergen can remain under fingernails for several days and on clothes for longer than 1 week.

Urushiol is degraded by soap and water. Once urushiol touches the skin, however, it begins to penetrate in minutes. It is completely bound to the skin within 8 hours and is probably no longer affected by normal soap and water after 1 to 6 hours. Zanfel Poison Ivy Wash is an OTC soap mixture of ethoxylate and sodium lauryl sarcosinate surfactants that is claimed, by its manufacturer, to render urushiol totally inactive by complementing the polarity of the urushiol to form a micelle. This is said to allow the urushiol to be rinsed away with water at any point during the dermatitis cycle. During the first 3 days, multiple washings may be necessary. Clinical trials to support the manufacturer's claims are in progress. A 1-ounce tube costs approximately $40.00 and is supposed to be enough for 15 applications to an area the size of an adult forearm. The manufacturer also claims that often Zanfel will eliminate the itching of *Toxicodendron* dermatitis with no further treatment. Zanfel is specific for urushiol; it does not work on other causes of allergic contact dermatitis.

Washing skin immediately after exposure can abort the rash. Washing clothes in a standard washing machine will inactivate the antigen remaining on the patient's clothing, as long as they have no black lacquer deposits causing visible staining. Shoes, tools, and sports equipment may require separate cleansing and can be the source of late spread. They should at least be rinsed with copious amounts of water. Pets suspected of harboring urushiol should be bathed.

Poison ivy dermatitis can sometimes be confused with **phytophotodermatitis,** which is a nonallergic skin reaction to psoralens, which react with ultraviolet (UV) light to cause blister formation and burning pain in the skin rather than pruritus. The most common causes are lime juice, weeds, or plants of the Apiaceae family (parsley, celery, parsnip) and other members of the Rutaceae family (includes citrus fruits). Redness, swelling, blisters, and bizarre configurations appear 24 hours after contact with the psoralens and ultraviolet light from the sun or a tanning booth. Within 1 to 2 weeks, patients will develop dark streaks wherever the initial rash occurred. This color will last for months to years, and the involved skin will often remain very sensitive to UV light.

Suggested Readings

Cruz PD: *Toxicodendron dermatitis. Paper presented by Extension Services in Pharmacy,* School of Pharmacy, April 2003, University of Wisconsin–Madison.

Davila A, Laurora M, Fulton J, et al: A new topical agent, Zanfel, ameliorates urushiol-induced *Toxicodendron* allergic contact dermatitis, *Ann Emerg Med* 42:98, 2003.

Froberg B, Ibrahim D, Furbee RB: *Emerg Med Clin North Am* 25:375–433, 2007.

Mark BJ, Slavin RG: Allergic contact dermatitis, *Med Clin North Am* 90:1–5, 2006.

Saary J, Qureshi R, Palda V, et al: A systematic review of contact dermatitis treatment and prevention, *J Am Acad Dermatol* 53:845–855, 2005.

Stankewicz H, Cancel G, Eberhardt M, Melanson S: Effective topical treatment and post exposure prophylaxis of poison ivy: objective confirmation (abstract), *Ann Emerg Med* 50(Suppl):S26–S27, 2007.

Urticaria, Acute

(Hives)

Presentation

The patient is generally very uncomfortable with intense itching. There may be a history of similar episodes and perhaps a known precipitating agent (bee or fire ant sting, food, or drug). More often, the patient will only have a rash. Sometimes this is accompanied by nonpitting edematous swelling of the lips, face, hands, and/or genitalia (angioedema). In the more severe cases, patients may have associated abdominal pain and vomiting (especially if an offending allergen was ingested), wheezing, laryngeal edema, and/or frank cardiovascular collapse (anaphylaxis).

Lesions may occur anywhere on the body. The urticarial rash consists of sharply defined, slightly raised wheals surrounded by erythema and tends to be circular or appear as incomplete rings (Figures 183-1 to 183-3). Each eruption is transient, lasting no more than 8 to 12 hours, but may be replaced by new lesions in different locations. It is not unusual to see these characteristic wheals appear or disappear from areas on the patient's body, even during a brief encounter. The edematous central area can be pale in comparison with the erythematous surrounding area. These eruptions may occur immediately after exposure to an allergen, or they may be delayed for several days. Allergic reactions to foods or medications are self-limited, typically 1 to 3 days, but will recur with repetitive exposures to cross-reactive substances. Urticaria can sometimes last for 1 to 3 weeks with some drug reactions.

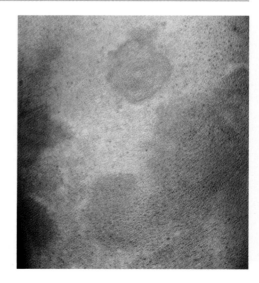

Figure 183-1 Hives. The most characteristic presentation is uniformly red edematous plaques surrounded by a faint white halo. (From Habif T: *Clinical dermatology,* ed 4. St Louis, 2004, Mosby.)

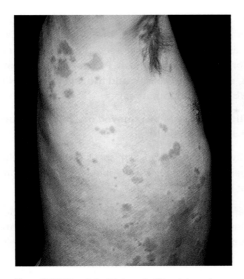

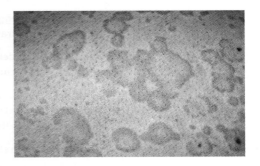

Figure 183-3 Superficial hives vary in color. (From Habif T: *Clinical dermatology*, ed 4. St Louis, 2004, Mosby.)

Figure 183-2 Hives. Urticarial plaques in different stages of formation. (From Habif T: *Clinical dermatology*, ed 4. St Louis, 2004, Mosby.)

Contact urticaria (in which contact of the skin with an allergen, such as latex, causes hives at the site of contact) may be complicated by angioedema and even severe anaphylaxis (see Chapter 160).

What To Do:

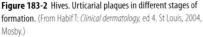 If the respiratory tract is involved, the first priority must be to secure the airway, which occasionally may require intubation. Administer oxygen and establish an intravenous line. For these and other severe systemic reactions, administer intramuscular adrenaline to reduce the edema. A dose of 0.3 to 0.5 mg of epinephrine (0.3-0.5 mL of a 1:1000 dilution) should be given IM every 10 to 15 minutes until symptoms subside, and normal saline should be given intravenously in generous boluses to correct hypotension. Diphenhydramine (Benadryl), 50 mg, should be given IV (or IM if there is no venous access). Solu-Medrol, 40 mg, given intravenously will not provide immediate relief but may reduce the possibility of relapse. Patients with severe angioedema should be admitted for at least 24 hours of observation and further treatment as required. Glucagon may have a role in refractory anaphylaxis when the patient is taking a beta-blocker. The recommended dose is 1 to 5 mg IV over 5 minutes. H_2 blockers, such as Pepcid or Zantac may be useful in some patients (responders are unpredictable), and IV epinephrine can be given on very rare (vascular collapse) situations.

In all cases, **attempt to elicit a hidden precipitating cause, including stings, drugs, or foods.** Obtain the patient's medical history, focusing on a history of allergy, asthma, or any other preexisting, atopic conditions (i.e., allergic rhinitis and atopic dermatitis). **Question patients about their use of all drugs, especially penicillin and sulfa drugs and their derivatives, aspirin (which they may not think of as a drug or which may be hidden in Alka-Seltzer or**

other over-the-counter [OTC] remedies), oral contraceptives, herbal and vitamin supplements, and foods or drugs containing tartrazine (FD&C yellow dye #5), nitrates, nitrites, sulfites, monosodium glutamate, and aspartame (NutraSweet), among others. **Inquire about the foods eaten 6 to 12 hours before developing the rash. Pay particular attention to tree nuts, peanuts, shellfish, eggs, soy, dairy products, and fish, as well as fresh fruits (e.g., kiwi fruit, banana, avocado, strawberries, and tomatoes).**

✓ **If the cause is identified, it should be removed or avoided. In food or drug hypersensitivity, future avoidance is critical.**

✓ Perform a general physical examination, with special attention to the skin, to determine the location of lesions and their morphology. Urticaria should present as nontender erythematous cutaneous elevations that blanch with pressure.

✓ **For immediate relief of severe pruritus, especially if accompanied by systemic symptoms, such as wheezing or hoarseness (although not life threatening as noted previously), give 0.3 mL of epinephrine (1:1000) intramuscularly;** this may need to be repeated. If the lesions do not clear with epinephrine, the patient most likely does not have urticaria. Because of the potential for unpleasant side effects, **epinephrine use can be omitted for most urticarial reactions that are less intense.**

✓ **For relief of rash and itching, administer H_1 blockers—diphenhydramine (Benadryl), 25 to 50 mg IV, or hydroxyzine (Vistaril, Atarax), 50 mg PO or IM stat—followed by a prescription for 25 to 50 mg PO qid, or cyproheptadine hydrochloride (Periactin), 4 mg tid (all of which can be sedating). Alternatively, give nonsedating cetirizine (Zyrtec), 10 mg qd to bid or fexofenadine (Allegra), 60 to 180 mg qd for the next 48 to 72 hours.** Patients might prefer nonsedating antihistamines during the day and sedating antihistamines at night to help with sleep.

✓ **Adding H_2 blockers to H_1 antagonists results in improved clearing of urticaria. Therefore combine one of the antihistamines mentioned with cimetidine (Tagamet), 300 mg IV/IM/PO, ranitidine (Zantac), 50 mg IV or 150 mg PO, or famotidine (Pepcid), 20 mg bid. Follow this with a prescription for cimetidine, 400 mg bid, or ranitidine, 150 mg bid, for the next 48 to 72 hours.**

✓ **To help reduce the likelihood of recurrence, give prednisone, 60 mg PO stat, and prescribe 20 to 50 mg qd for 4 days. When possible, avoid systemic corticosteroids in patients with diabetes, active peptic ulcers, or other steroid risks.**

✓ In chronic resistant cases, the tricyclic antidepressant doxepin (Sinequan) can be used in doses of 10 to 50 mg qhs. This drug has activity against both H_1 and H_2 histamine receptors and is 700 times more potent than diphenhydramine. Sedation is common. Leukotriene modifiers, such as montelukast (Singulair), 10 mg qd, and zafirlukast (Accolate), 20 mg bid, in combination with antihistamines may also provide additional benefit in chronic cases.

✓ **Inform the patient that the cause of hives cannot be determined in most cases.** Let him know that the condition is usually of minor consequence but can at times become chronic and, under unusual circumstances, is associated with other illnesses. Therefore, with recurrent symptoms, the patient should be provided with elective follow-up care, preferably by an allergist.

✓ **Patients with suspected food allergies can be referred to the Food Allergy and Anaphylaxis Network at (800) 929-4040 (www.foodallergy.org).**

✅ Patients who experience a more severe reaction should be given a prescription for injectable epinephrine (EpiPen or EpiPen Jr., Ana-Kit), which should be available to them at all times, and they should be advised to wear a MedicAlert bracelet inscribed with this information.

✅ When angioedema of the lips, tongue, pharynx, and larynx is the predominant finding and pruritic urticaria is absent, consider angiotensin-converting enzyme (ACE) inhibitors (e.g., Capoten, Vasotec, Lotensin, Prinivil, Zestril) as the precipitating cause. For a patient who is not taking ACE inhibitors, consider hereditary angioedema (see Chapter 60).

✅ If the urticarial lesions are tender and accompanied by fever or arthralgias, consider an underlying infection or illness (e.g., collagen vascular disease with vasculitis, viral infections of children and adolescents, anicteric hepatitis, cytomegalovirus, or infectious mononucleosis).

What Not To Do:

❌ Do not perform a comprehensive medical and laboratory investigation in simple straightforward cases of acute urticaria. These studies are expensive and unnecessary. Even with chronic idiopathic urticaria, the evaluation should generally be limited to a complete blood count (CBC), erythrocyte sedimentation rate (ESR), thyroid testing, and liver function tests.

❌ Do not let the patient take aspirin or consume excessive alcohol. Some patients experience precipitation or worsening of their symptoms with the use of aspirin, other nonsteroidal anti-inflammatory drugs (NSAIDs), or alcohol. Morphine and codeine as well as certain food additives, such as azo food dyes, tartrazine dye, and benzoates, are often allergens or potentiate allergic reactions and should probably also be avoided.

❌ Do not recommend or prescribe topical steroids, topical antihistamines, or topical anesthetic creams or sprays. They are ineffective and have no role in the management of urticaria.

❌ Do not overlook the possibility of an urticarial vasculitis when the presenting rash is more painful than itchy and there are systemic symptoms, such as purpura, arthralgias, fever, abdominal pain, and nephritis. Obtain an ESR, consider the diagnosis of systemic lupus erythematosus or Sjögren syndrome, and consult specialists appropriately.

❌ Do not restrict the use of iodinated contrast media for patients with a history of seafood allergy. There is no evidence that seafood allergy is a specific contraindication to use of ionic contrast. Most events occur randomly.

Discussion

Urticaria, also referred to as hives or wheals, is a common and distinctive skin reaction pattern that may occur at any age.

Urticaria present for less than 6 weeks is classified as acute, greater than 6 weeks is considered chronic. Simple urticaria affects approximately 20% of the population at some time. Most cases are acute. This local is the result, at least in part, to the release of histamines and other vasoactive peptides from mast cells following an IgE-mediated antigen-antibody reaction. This results in vasodilatation and

(continued)

Discussion continued

increased vascular permeability, with the leaking of protein and fluid into extravascular spaces. The heavier concentration of mast cells within the lips, face, and hands explains why these areas are more commonly affected. The edema of urticaria is found in the superficial dermis. The edema in angioedema is found in the deep dermis or subcutaneous/submucosal tissues. Angioedema is more common in children and young adults. Chronic urticaria is more common in middle-aged women. Acute urticaria is often allergic in origin; in the event that a particular cause can be identified, symptoms resolve rapidly after avoidance and do not recur without further exposure. **The ideal treatment for allergic urticaria is identification and elimination of its cause.** Because the cause is often obscure, however, only symptomatic treatment may be possible. The spontaneous resolution of symptoms obviates the need for an extensive evaluation.

It is well established that food allergies are common causes of acute urticaria. Although virtually any food can act as a food allergen, it is remarkable that most type I (IgE-mediated) food allergies are caused by a rather limited number of food categories. Specifically, milk (dairy), egg, wheat, legumes (including peanut, soybean, and pea), tree nuts, and seafood (fish, crustacean, and mollusk) account for more than 95% of all food allergies. It is also common for acute symptoms to have no obvious cause and spontaneously resolve over the course of a few weeks.

Chronic urticaria and angioedema, on the other hand, usually remain symptomatic for months to years, with periodic remissions and relapses. Although they look like an allergic reaction, they are rarely the result of an allergic process and instead are considered to be caused by an autoimmune or idiopathic mechanism. A significant proportion of chronic urticaria is triggered through particular physical stimuli. Most common among these is dermatographism, in which mast cell degranulation is caused by minor skin trauma (e.g., simple scratching). Cold-induced urticaria is another relatively common form of chronic physical urticaria.

Urticarial vasculitis should be considered if a single urticarial lesion (rather than being short-lived) lasts longer than 24 to 36 hours, if lesions are burning or painful, if they are more common in the lower extremities, or if they leave an area of hemosiderin pigment after they have resolved. Infection, drug sensitivity, serum sickness, chronic hepatitis, and systemic lupus erythematosus may cause urticarial vasculitis. These patients should be referred to a dermatologist for punch biopsy, further evaluation, and management.

The overall incidence of ACE inhibitor–induced angioedema is reported to be approximately 0.1% to 0.2% and is five times more common among black than among white patients. Although angioedema most typically occurs during the first week of therapy, some patients may have taken the ACE inhibitor without any problem for weeks or months before angioedema develops. Because of this, ACE inhibitors are often overlooked as a cause of angioedema, and this may lead to the unfortunate continuation of the edema-producing drug, along with more severe attacks. **A clue to the underlying cause is angioedema without urticaria.** Because of the risk for relapse and airway compromise and the slow response to standard therapy, some authors recommend that all of these patients should be admitted to a hospital for overnight observation. However, others believe that if patients experience significant improvement and are comfortable after treatment, it is reasonable to consider them for discharge. Symptoms tend to resolve within 24 to 48 hours of cessation of the ACE inhibitor, although the course may be more variable. **The use of fresh frozen plasma to replenish ACE stores has been used for the treatment of life-threatening angioedema, especially when it is resistant to other treatments.** Also, an airway specialist should be consulted as soon as possible before trouble develops. In general, angiotensin II receptor antagonists are tolerated by patients who have reacted to ACE inhibitors.

Suggested Readings

Alper BS: SOAP: solutions to often asked problems. Choice of antihistamines for urticaria, *Arch Fam Med* 9:748–751, 2000.

Alsrabi M, Shikh A: A comparison of international guidelines for the emergency medical management of anaphylaxis, *Allergy* 62:838–841, 2007.

Dibbern DA: Urticaria: selected highlights and recent advances, *Med Clin North Am* 90:187–209, 2006.

Dibbern DA Jr, Dreskin SC: Urticaria, *Immunol Allergy Clin North Am* 24:141–162, 2004.

Graft DF: Insect sting allergy, *Med Clin North Am* 90:211–232, 2006.

Horan RF, Schneider LC, Sheffer AL: Allergic skin disorders and mastocytosis, *JAMA* 268:2858–2868, 1992.

Kaplan AP, Greaves MW: Angioedema, *J Am Acad Dermatol* 53:373–388, 2005.

Kemp SF, Lockey RF, Wolf BL, et al: Anaphylaxis: a review of 266 cases, *Arch Intern Med* 155:1749–1754, 1995.

Lin RY, Curry A, Pesola GR, et al: Improved outcomes in patients with acute allergic syndromes who are treated with combined H1 and H2 antagonists, *Ann Emerg Med* 36:462–468, 2000.

Muller BA: Urticaria and angioedema: a practical approach, *Am Fam Physician* 69:1123–1128, 2004.

Pollack CV, Romano TJ: Outpatient management of acute urticaria: the role of prednisone, *Ann Emerg Med* 547–551, 1995.

Runge JW, Martinez JC, Caravati EM, et al: Histamine antagonists in the treatment of acute allergic reactions, *Ann Emerg Med* 21:237–242, 1992.

Rusli M: Cimetidine treatment of recalcitrant acute allergic urticaria, *Ann Emerg Med* 15:1363–1365, 1986.

Schlifke A, Geiderman JM: Medical mythology: seafood allergy is a specific and unique contraindication to the administration of ionic contrast media, *Can J Emerg Med* 5:166–168, 2003.

Thomas M: Glucagon infusion in refractory anaphylactic shock in patients on beta-blockers, *Emerg Med J* 22:272–273, 2005.

Warts

(Common Wart, Plantar Wart)

Presentation

Patients generally seek medical care when a wart has become painful, partially avulsed, or cosmetically unacceptable and annoying.

Common warts usually appear as one or more dome-shaped hyperkeratotic verrucous papules on the hands but may occur anywhere on the body. Plantar warts occur on the soles of the feet, interrupting the normal skin lines and frequently occurring at points of maximum pressure, such as over the heads of the metatarsal bones or on the heel. Plantar warts do not have a verrucous or cauliflower appearance but are surrounded by a thick painful callus that impairs walking. Both types of wart contain black dots within their substance, which represent thrombosed capillaries (Figures 184-1 and 184-2).

These lesions may appear at any age but commonly occur in children and young adults. Their course is highly variable; most resolve spontaneously in weeks or months, and others may last years or a lifetime.

What To Do:

✓ Confirm the diagnosis by obtaining a typical history, along with noting classic physical findings, which include the obscuring of normal skin lines. Shaving off the overlying hyperkeratotic surface with a No. 15 or No. 10 surgical blade may also reveal the typical black dots of thrombosed vessels, along with a uniform mosaic surface pattern. (The pattern can be seen with a hand lens.)

✓ **Inform patients that warts often require several treatments before a cure is realized and that, in general, the more rapid the wart removal technique, the more likely the process will cause pain.**

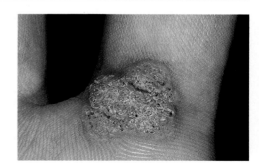

Figure 184-1 A common wart with black dots on the surface. (From Habif T: *Clinical dermatology,* ed 4. St Louis, 2004, Mosby.)

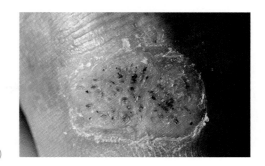

Figure 184-2 Thrombosed black vessels are trapped in the cylindrical projections. (From Habif T: *Clinical dermatology*, ed 4. St Louis, 2004, Mosby.)

✅ **If a slower, less painful treatment is selected, suggestive therapy generally works through the age of 10 years.** A banana peel, a potato eye, or a penny applied to the skin and covered with tape for a 1- to 2-week period has been effective in young children. Another technique is to draw the body part on a piece of paper and then draw a picture of the wart on the diagram. Finally, crumble the pictures and throw them away.

✅ **Other nonpainful techniques can be used on patients of any age. Duct tape occlusion therapy may be more effective than cryotherapy for common warts.** The patient completely covers the wart and the area around the wart with common duct tape. This is left on for 6 days; the wart is then soaked in warm water until its surface is softened; then the surface is scraped off using an emery board or pumice stone. After 12 hours, the patient puts on a new piece of tape for another 6 days and then repeats the process for 2 months or until the wart is gone. This technique is effective approximately 85% of the time. When the skin lines are reestablished, the warts are gone.

✅ **More traditional keratolytic therapy (40% salicylic acid plasters—Mediplast and others) can also be used on both common and plantar warts.** Shave excessive tissue from the surface of the wart using a No. 15 or No. 10 scalpel blade. Have the patient cut a piece of the salicylic acid plaster to a size and shape that will fit over the entire wart. (This is particularly useful for treating large plantar warts.) The sticky surface is applied to the wart and then secured with tape. The plaster is removed after 48 hours, and the white keratin is scraped off as described, using an emery board or a pumice stone. Another plaster is immediately applied, and the process is repeated every 2 days for many weeks or until the wart is completely gone.

✅ Salicylic acid liquid (DuoPlant gel, Occlusal-HP liquid and many others that are now available over the counter) is also effective but is more likely to cause inflammation and soreness.

✅ One single-blinded clinical trial performed on 60 patients with common hand warts compared cryotherapy with the application of an 80% phenol solution (which is a caustic agent). Thirty patients were treated with cryotherapy and 30 patients were treated with 80% phenol, on a once-weekly basis until complete clearance of the lesions or a maximum duration of 6 weeks occurred. Complete clearance of warts after 6 weeks was observed in 70% of patients who were treated with cryotherapy, and 82.6% of patients in the 80% phenol group; there was no statistically significant difference between the two methods ($P = .014$). This study showed that

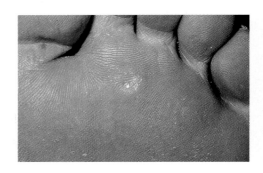

Figure 184-3 A pared corn shows a translucent core. (From White G, Cox N: *Diseases of the skin*, ed 2. St Louis, 2006, Mosby.)

80% phenol and cryotherapy were both effective and simple treatments for common warts of the hands, and patients do not experience any pain during the phenol treatment.

✓ For resistant lesions, the immunomodulating drug imiquimod 5% cream (Aldara) can be used in combination with a keratolytic agent. It is essential to débride the thick scale before applying imiquimod. The patient applies the cream daily before bedtime and covers the area with tape (for ≥12 hours). This may be used 3 days per week for 10 to 16 weeks. This treatment is quite expensive, costing from $200 to $250.

✓ The most rapid but most painful treatment for common warts is cryotherapy. The hyperkeratotic surface is reduced using a scalpel blade; then liquid nitrogen is applied to the wart using a cotton-tipped applicator until a 1- to 2-mm zone of frozen tissue is created and maintained around the lesion for about 5 seconds. The area is then allowed to thaw. A second or third freeze during the same treatment session may increase the cure rate. Severe pain may develop and last for minutes to hours; appropriate analgesia should be provided. Inform the patient that a small blister that is sometimes hemorrhagic will develop under the wart. If the wart does not completely resolve, freezing may be repeated in 2 to 4 weeks. One small randomized controlled trial provided evidence to support the use of cryotherapy over salicylic acid treatment for common warts only. For plantar warts, they found no clinically relevant difference between cryotherapy, salicylic acid treatment, or a wait-and-see approach after 13 weeks. It should also be noted that one study demonstrated that OTC refrigerants did not achieve results equivalent to liquid nitrogen when used for treating warts.

✓ Recalcitrant warts or periungual warts that may be difficult or painful to remove should be referred to a dermatologist. Carbon dioxide (CO_2) laser vaporization and pulsed-dye laser treatments may be used under certain circumstances, and they have a 51.1% to 90% success rate.

What Not To Do:

✗ Do not mistake corns (clavi) that form over the metatarsal heads for plantar warts. After paring warts with a No. 15 blade, they will reveal centrally located black vessels (dots) that will sometimes bleed with additional paring. Corns, on the other hand, have a hard, painful, well-demarcated translucent central core (Figure 184-3). Lateral pressure on a wart causes pain, but pinching a plantar corn is painless.

Discussion

Warts are common and usually benign. They are caused by human papillomaviruses. The virus infects keratinocytes, which proliferate to form a mass that remains confined to the epidermis. There are no "roots" that penetrate the dermis. Warts are transmitted simply by touch. Plantar warts may be acquired from moist surfaces in communal swimming areas.

Diagnosis is usually made by history and simple examination of these familiar-appearing growths.

Some warts respond quickly to routine therapy, whereas others are resistant. Subungual and periungual warts are more resistant to treatment than are warts located in other areas. There may be more to these warts than meets the eye, with a portion of the wart being hidden under the nail.

Because warts are confined to the epidermis, they can usually be removed with little, if any, scarring.

Suggested Readings

Banihashemi M: Efficacy of 80% phenol solution in comparison with cryotherapy in the treatment of common warts of hands, *Singapore Med J* 49:1035–1037, 2008.

Bruggink SC: Cryotherapy with liquid nitrogen versus topical salicylic acid application for cutaneous warts in primary care: randomized controlled trial, *Can Med Assoc J* 182:1624–1630, 2010.

Burkhart CG: An in vitro study comparing temperatures of over-the-counter wart preparations with liquid nitrogen, *J Amer Acad Dermatol* 57:1019–1020, 2007.

Park HS: Pulsed dye laser treatment for viral warts: a study of 120 patients, *J Dermatol* 35:491–498, 2008.

Sanfilippo AM, Barrio V, Kulp-Shorten C, et al: Common pediatric and adolescent skin conditions, *J Pediatr Adolesc Gynecol* 16:269–283, 2003.

Complete Eye Examination

What To Do:

✓ Record visual acuity, using a Snellen (wall) or Jaeger (hand-held) chart, first without and then with the patient's own corrective lenses. If glasses are not available, a pinhole will compensate for most refractory errors.

✓ Wearing gloves and using a bright light, inspect the lids, conjunctivae, sclera, cornea, iris, extraocular movements, and pupillary reflexes.

✓ Use a 10× magnification slit lamp to further examine the cornea and anterior chamber; look for any injection of ciliary vessels at the corneal limbus, which indicates iritis. When the slit lamp is stopped down to a pinhole, look for light reflected from protein exudate or suspended white cells in the normally clear aqueous humor of the anterior chamber (a late sign of iritis). Look for red cells (hyphema) or white cells (hypopyon) settling to the bottom of the anterior chamber after the patient has been sitting up for 15 minutes. The ophthalmoscope can be used to evaluate the optic nerve and retina.

✓ Demonstrate the integrity of the corneal epithelium with fluorescein dye, which is taken up by exposed stroma or nonviable epithelium and glows green in ultraviolet or cobalt blue light.

✓ Note the depth of the anterior chamber with tangential lighting.

Digital Block

It is necessary to provide complete anesthesia before treatment of most fingertip injuries. Many techniques for performing a digital nerve block have been described. The following technique is effective and rapid in onset. This type of digital block provides complete anesthesia distal to and including the distal interphalangeal joint, the site that most often demands a nerve block.

What To Do:

✓ Cleanse the finger and paint the area with povidone-iodine (Betadine) solution or equivalent antiseptic.

✓ Using a 27- to 30-gauge needle, slowly inject 1% lidocaine (Xylocaine) warmed to body temperature and buffered 10:1 with sodium bicarbonate (Neut) midway between the dorsal and palmar surfaces of the finger at the midpoint of the middle phalanx.

✓ Inject straight in along the side of the periosteum; then, pull back without removing the needle from the skin and fan the needle dorsally.

✓ Advance the needle dorsally and inject again. Pull the needle back a second time, and, without removing it from the skin, fan the needle in a palmar direction.

✓ Advance the needle and inject the lidocaine in the vicinity of the digital neurovascular bundle (Figure B-1).

✓ With each injection, instill enough lidocaine to produce visible soft tissue swelling.

✓ Repeat this procedure on the opposite side of the finger. This can be made less painful if, while injecting on the initial side of the finger, you inject across the dorsum of the digit to initiate anesthesia on the opposite side, thereby eliminating the sensation of the second needlestick.

✓ For anesthesia of the proximal finger as well, a similar block may be performed as far proximally as the middle of the metacarpal (a metacarpal block) with a dorsal approach. The connective tissue is looser there, and the needle need not be fanned into digital septa as described earlier. Be prepared to use larger amounts of lidocaine and to wait 3 to 10 minutes for adequate anesthesia.

✓ With fractures, burns, crush injuries, or other conditions in which the pain will be prolonged or when the procedure itself will be prolonged, substitute bupivacaine (Marcaine), 0.25% to 0.5%, for the lidocaine.

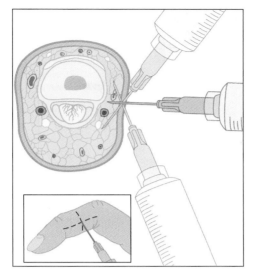

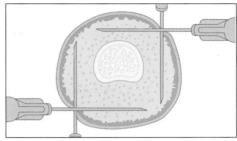

Figure B-2 Needle insertion for a modified ring block. (Courtesy Mary Albury-Noyes. From Gillette RD: Practical management of ingrown toenails. *Postgrad Med* 84:145-146, 1998.)

Figure B-1 Needle insertion points for a digital block.

What Not To Do:

Ⓧ Do not use lidocaine with epinephrine routinely. Although this combination has been shown to be safe, it causes more pain on injection, and it is usually unnecessary when there has been adequate infiltration with plain lidocaine. This mixture should not be used for injuries involving vascular compromise or in patients with peripheral arterial disease. The use of lidocaine with epinephrine can be better justified when performing a metacarpal block or when a tourniquet is required for a bloodless field but is unavailable. Use 1% to 2% lidocaine and 1:100,000 or 1:200,000 epinephrine.

Discussion

Digital nerve blocks are often described as being injected at the base of the proximal phalanx, but it is not necessary to block the whole digit when only the distal tip is injured. The first technique described here provides anesthesia faster than the traditional technique. Toes are difficult to separate, and it may be easier to perform a modified ring block at their base (Figure B-2). For injuries over the dorsum of the proximal phalanx and proximal interphalangeal joint, the connective tissue is loose enough for direct infiltration of anesthetic with minimal discomfort, and a digital block is not required.

Some studies have demonstrated adequate digital anesthesia by injecting 2 mL of buffered lidocaine directly into the flexor tendon sheath, using a 25- or 27-gauge needle at a 45-degree angle at the distal palmar crease of the hand.

Allergy to amide anesthetics such as lidocaine (Xylocaine) and bupivacaine (Marcaine) is rare, and when it does occur, it is usually caused by the preservative methylparaben. One way to circumvent a potential allergic reaction is to use preservative-free lidocaine, which is available in single-dose vials. History of an allergy to an ester anesthetic, such

(continued)

Discussion continued

as procaine (Novocain) or tetracaine (Pontocaine), is not a contraindication to the use of lidocaine or bupivacaine, because they are chemically different and cross-reaction is rare.

An alternative for avoiding any possibility of an allergic reaction is to use benzyl alcohol or benzyl alcohol with epinephrine as a substitute for both the amide and ester anesthetics.

Suggested Readings

Achar S, Kundu S: Principles of office anesthesia: part I. Infiltrative anesthesia, *Am Fam Physician* 66:91–94, 2002.

Chowdhry S, Seidenstricker L, Cooney DS, et al: Do not use epinephrine and digital blocks: myth or truth? Part II. A retrospective review of 1111 cases, *Plast Reconstr Surg* 126:2031–2034, 2010.

Denkler K: A comprehensive review of epinephrine in the finger: to do or not to do, *Plast Reconstr Surg* 108:114–124, 2001.

Wilhelmi BJ, Blackwell SJ, Miller JH, et al: Do not use epinephrine in digital blocks: myth or truth? *Plast Reconstr Surg* 107:393–397, 2001.

Fingertip Dressing, Simple

To provide a complete nonadherent compression dressing for an injured finger tip, first cut out an L-shaped segment from a strip of oil-emulsion (Adaptic) gauze. Cover the gauze with antibiotic ointment to provide occlusion and prevent adhesion to the wound surface, but making it possible for the gauze to stick to itself.

What To Do:

✓ Place the tip of the finger over the short leg of the gauze and then fold the gauze over the top of the finger (Figure C-1).

✓ Take the long leg of the gauze and wrap it around the tip of the finger.

✓ For absorption and compression, fluff a cotton gauze pad and apply it over the end of the finger.

✓ Cover with roller or tube gauze and secure with adhesive tape.

What Not To Do:

✗ Do not place tight circumferential wraps of tape around a finger, especially if swelling is expected. Such a wrap may act as a tourniquet and lead to vascular compromise. For the same reason, use caution applying tight layers of tube gauze—three or four layers will suffice.

Discussion

With small fingertip injuries or partially healed injuries, for convenience, the patient can apply his own simple homemade fingertip dressing. Have him use the two halves of an adhesive strip bandage cut lengthwise. One half is crossed over the finger tip, the adhesive portions of the cut strip being placed along the long axis of the finger. The second half of the cut strip is then placed at a right angle to the first, thereby covering the entire end of the finger. Finally, have him encircle the distal phalanx with a second uncut strip bandage to provide full fingertip coverage (Figure C-2).

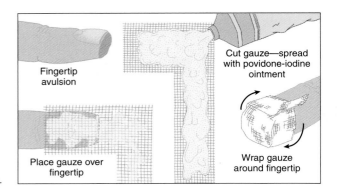

Figure C-1 Simple fingertip dressing.

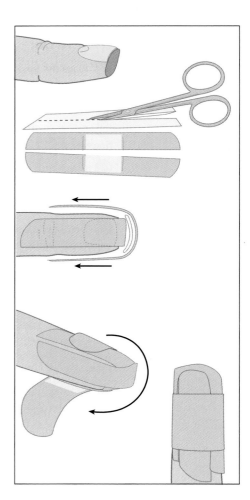

Figure C-2 Homemade fingertip dressing using two Band-Aids.

Oral Nerve Blocks

What To Do:

✓ **An inferior alveolar nerve block** provides anesthesia and rapid relief of pain in all teeth on one side of the mandible, the lower lip, and the chin via the mental nerve (Figure D-1).

✓ Stand on the side of the patient opposite the side you are injecting. Palpate the retromolar fossa with the index finger and identify the convexity of the mandibular ramus.

✓ Hold the syringe parallel to the occlusal surfaces of the teeth so that its barrel is in line between the first and second premolars on the opposite side of the mandible.

✓ With your nondominant hand, retract the cheek laterally and find the pterygomandibular triangle posterior to the molars. Leave your noninjecting thumb in the coronoid notch, on the anterior surface of the mandible.

✓ Puncture in this triangle 1 cm above the occlusive surface of the molars, ensuring that the needle passes through the ligaments and muscles of the medial mandibular surface (about 1 to 2 cm).

✓ Stop advancing the needle when it reaches the mandibular bone, withdraw it a few millimeters, aspirate to be sure the tip is not in a vein, and deposit 1 to 2 mL of local anesthetic (e.g., lidocaine 1% with epinephrine, bupivacaine 0.5%). Inject 3 to 5 mL if the needle is placed suboptimally.

✓ **A supraperiosteal block (apical block)** provides intraoral local anesthesia for pain arising from maxillary teeth. It is best suited for anesthesia of a single tooth or of a circumscribed portion of the maxilla.

✓ First, the mucosa of the upper lip is pulled downward and out. (The distraction technique of shaking the lip may decrease the pain of injection.) The mucobuccal fold is then punctured with a 27-gauge needle. Hold the bevel of the needle toward the bone and aspirate the area; then, if you are not in a vessel, inject 1.5 to 3 mL of anesthetic near the apex of the affected tooth. This technique usually produces full anesthesia in 5 to 10 minutes. For best results, inject as close as possible to the tooth-bearing maxillary bone (Figure D-2).

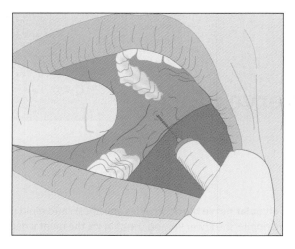

Figure D-1 Needle placement for an oral nerve block.

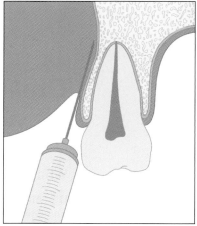

Figure D-2 Schematic illustration of supraperiosteal injection. (From *Manual of local anesthesia in dentistry*. New York, Cook-Waite Laboratories, Inc. Reprinted courtesy Eastman Kodak Company.)

Discussion

See Appendix B for a discussion of allergy to infiltrative analgesics.

For video examples of multiple mandibular nerve blocks, go to http://www.youtube.com/watch?v=eC K6K0YrjEQ&feature=related.

For video examples of multiple maxillary nerve blocks, go to http://www.youtube.com/watch?v=3h aklcbCWmw&NR=1.

Suggested Reading

Crystal CS, Blankenship RB: Local anesthetics and peripheral nerve blocks in the emergency department, *Emerg Med Clin North Am* 23:477–502, 2005.

Procedural Sedation and Analgesia

■ Alfred Sacchetti

The very nature of emergency medicine has led to emergency physicians (EPs) becoming experts in the control of pain for emergency department (ED) procedures. From children to seniors, EPs must be adept at minimizing pain, relieving anxiety, and providing cooperation for diagnostic studies. Effective procedural sedation and analgesia not only helps the patient but also makes it much easier for any qualified clinician to successfully complete a procedure.

No single procedural sedation and analgesia (PSA) policy is appropriate for every institution. It is well worthwhile for any department to design a specific policy that addresses its unique staffing, credentialing, monitoring and formulary characteristics. As a very general rule, every PSA case will require a minimum of two individuals, one to perform the procedure and one to monitor the patient.

Procedural sedation begins with a focused history and physical examination, with particular attention paid to the oral pharynx and respiratory tract. An American Society of Anesthesiologists (ASA) classification status should be assigned and documented for the patient. Most institutions now require a formal pause or "time out" before beginning any procedure. Regardless of how trivial you may believe this process to be, it has clearly been shown to reduce errors and complications for all procedures. In the ED setting, this is an excellent time to be certain all of the proper supplies are in place and functional. This should include all airway and suction equipment, supplies for the particular procedure, and monitoring equipment, including a pulse oximeter, cardiac monitor and blood pressure device.

There are many procedural sedations options, and no single agent is appropriate for every clinician or every patient. As such, anyone performing PSA should be familiar with multiple options for any procedure. All procedural sedation agents have unique pharmacologic characteristics, and the clinician using them should be familiar with them before their use. The following agents have all been used successfully in ED and ambulatory settings.

Medication	Dose	Maximum Unit Dose	Duration	Precautions
Fentanyl (Sublimaze)	Ped 1-3 yr, 2-3 µg/kg IV 3-12 yr, 1-2 µg/kg IV Adult 0.5-1 µg/kg IV given slowly over 1-2 min, titrate to effect	200 µg	0.5-1 hr	Rigid chest ,vomiting Decrease dose in infants
Methohexital (Brevital)	Adult 0.5-1 mg/kg IV Ped 18-25 mg/kg PR	100 mg	20-60 min	Respiratory depression Respiratory depression Avoid all barbiturates in children with porphyria
Midazolam (Versed)	0.05-0.2 mg/kg IV or 1 mg IV slowly q2 min up to 5 mg	5 mg	1-2 hr	Respiratory depression Agitation with low dose
Propofol* (Diprivan)	0.5-1 (mg/kg) slow IV bolus 1-3 mg/kg/hr; adult younger than 55 yr, give 40 mg IV q10 sec, titrate to effect, maintain with infusion 100-200 µg/kg/min	100 mg	6-10 min	Respiratory depression
Remifentanil (Ultiva)	0.15 µg/kg/min drip	0.2 µg/kg/min	5 min	Same as with fentanyl
Etomidate (Amidate)	0.1-0.3 mg/kg IV	300 mg	15-20 min	Myoclonic jerks
Ketamine* (Ketalar)	3-5 mg/kg IM 1-2 mg/kg IV		1-2 hr 0.5-1 hr	Airway secretions, avoid with URI
Naloxone (Narcan)	0.005-0.01 mg/kg (partial reversal), 0.1 mg/kg (total reversal); give 0.4-2 mg q2-3 min	10 mg	20 min	Opiate antagonist
Flumazenil (Romazicon)	0.01 mg/kg; give 0.2 mg IV over 15 sec, then 0.2 mg q1 min prn up to 1 mg total	1 mg	30 min	Local irritation can occur following vein extravasation

Ped, Pediatric; *URI*, upper respiratory infection.

*Propofol and ketamine may be combined in single syringe as ketofol, given IV with a dosage of ketamine 0.5 mg/kg and propofol 0.5 mg/kg, followed by propofol 0.5 mg/kg every 2 minutes, titrated to the desired depth of sedation. This combination produces slightly faster recoveries while also demonstrating less vomiting and higher satisfaction scores (with similar efficacy and airway complications) than either agent used alone. Another approach is to combine both drugs in the same syringe as a 1:1 mixture. The combination is then administered intravenously, beginning as 0.5 mg/kg of propofol and 0.5 mg/kg of ketamine and titrating up to a maximum dose of 1 mg/kg of each drug.

The advantage to giving ketamine separately as an IM injection is that, in children, it avoids any painful struggle in attempting to start an IV line before any analgesia and sedation has been provided.

Many procedural sedation cases require a combination of both a sedative and an analgesic. The most commonly used analgesic is fentanyl, which is generally combined with either midazolam or propofol. When using these combinations, the fentanyl is generally administered first, followed by the sedative.

Remifentanil is another new agent that is as potent as fentanyl but has a duration of action of only 5 minutes. It is administered as a continuous infusion of 0.15 μg/kg/min.

Reversal agents are available for both the narcotics (naloxone) and the benzodiazepines (flumazenil).

What Not To Do:

(X) Do not ignore proper monitoring. Almost all adverse events from procedural sedation are associated with inadequate monitoring. Proper monitoring begins before the procedure and ends only when the patient is awake and back to baseline, not simply when the procedure is complete.

Discussion

The most common and potentially most serious complications of PSA are adverse respiratory events, such as diminished pulse oximetry levels, hypoventilation, and apnea. Appropriate monitoring with pulse oximetry and a bedside observer, such as a nurse or technician, will identify these problems before any patient complications occur. The most current consensus recommends that capnometry should be used in all episodes of procedural sedation.

Most respiratory problems result from airway obstruction and can be resolved with simple maneuvers, such as head repositioning or jaw thrusts. More severe problems may require bag valve mask ventilations and or administration of a reversal agent.

Preoxygenation or use of oxygen during the procedure can avoid hypoxic episodes resulting from respiratory depression.

Adverse events from procedural sedation generally occur within minutes of administration of the medications; however, delayed problems have been documented.

With ketamine, provide a quiet area with dim lighting for recovery and advise the parents not to stimulate the patient prematurely.

Often, sedative medications alone will be adequate for performing brief, painful procedures. When significant pain relief is required, add an analgesic agent, such as morphine or fentanyl. Morphine is preferred rather than fentanyl when more prolonged pain relief is anticipated.

Intravenous isotonic saline solution can be administered to prevent or treat potential cardiovascular preload reduction and subsequent hypotension.

Suggested Readings

Agrawal D, Manzi SF, Gupta R, et al: Preprocedural fasting state and adverse events in children undergoing procedural sedation and analgesia in a pediatric emergency department, *Ann Emerg Med* 42:636–646, 2003.

Burton JH, Bock AJ, Strout TD, et al: Etomidate and midazolam for reduction of anterior shoulder dislocation, *Ann Emerg Med* 40:496–504, 2002.

EMSC Grant Panel: Clinical policy: evidence-based approach to pharmacologic agents used in pediatric agents used in pediatric sedation and analgesia in the emergency department, *Ann Emerg Med* 44:342–377, 2004.

Green SM: Fasting is a consideration—not a necessity—for emergency department procedural sedation and analgesia, *Ann Emerg Med* 42:647–650, 2003.

Green SM, Rothrock SG, Lynch EL, et al: Intramuscular ketamine for pediatric sedation in the emergency department: safety profile in 1022 cases, *Ann Emerg Med* 31:688–697, 1998.

Mace SE, Brown LA, Francis L, et al: Clinical policy: critical issues in the sedation of pediatric patients in the emergency department, *Ann Emerg Med* 51:378–399, 2008.

McGlone RG, Howes MC: The Lancaster experience of 2.0 to 2.5 mg/kg intramuscular ketamine for pediatric sedation, *Emerg Med J* 21:290–295, 2004.

Newman DH, Azer MM, Pitetti RD, Singh S: When is a patient safe for discharge after procedural sedation? *Ann Emerg Med* 42:627–635, 2003.

Roback MG, Bajaj L, Wathen JE, et al: Preprocedural fasting and adverse events in procedural sedation and analgesia in a pediatric emergency department: are they related? *Ann Emerg Med* 44:454–459, 2004.

Sacchetti A, Senula G, Strickland J, Dubin R: Procedural sedation in the community emergency department: initial results of the ProSCED registry, *Acad Emerg Med* 14:41–46, 2007.

Shah A, Mosdossy G, McLeod S, et al: A blinded, randomized controlled trial to evaluate ketamine/propofol versus ketamine alone for procedural sedation in children, *Ann Emerg Med* 57:425–433, 2011.

Treston G: Prolonged pre-procedure fasting time is unnecessary when using titrated intravenous ketamine for paediatric procedural sedation, *Emerg Med Australas* 16:145–150, 2004.

Rabies Prophylaxis

Presentation

A possibly contagious animal has bitten the patient, or the animal's saliva has contaminated an abrasion or mucous membrane. There may have only been a questionable exposure to a bat, but the nature of the contact (if there was any contact) is unknown.

What To Do:

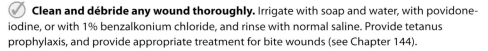 **Clean and débride any wound thoroughly.** Irrigate with soap and water, with povidone-iodine, or with 1% benzalkonium chloride, and rinse with normal saline. Provide tetanus prophylaxis, and provide appropriate treatment for bite wounds (see Chapter 144).

Know the local prevalence of rabies, or ask someone who knows (e.g., local health department).

If the offending animal was an apparently healthy dog or cat and is available for observation, arrange to have the animal confined for 10 days. During that period, an animal infected with rabies will show symptoms. If the animal has symptoms of rabies, it should be euthanized and examined using a fluorescent rabies antibody (FRA) technique. If the FRA test is positive for rabies, the patient must be treated with rabies immune globulin (RIG) and human diploid cell vaccine (HDCV) or another rabies vaccine.

If the animal is not available for observation, the decision whether to provide rabies prophylaxis depends on the local prevalence of rabies in domestic animals, rodents, and lagomorphs. It should be noted that international travelers to areas where canine rabies is still endemic have an increased risk for exposure to rabies.

An unprovoked attack is more likely than a provoked attack to indicate that the animal is rabid. Bites inflicted on a person attempting to feed or handle an apparently healthy animal should generally be regarded as provoked.

If the patient has been bitten by a wild animal (e.g., bat, coyote, fox, opossum, raccoon, skunk) capable of transmitting rabies, the animal should be caught, killed, and sent to the local public health department for brain examination with FRA. If the animal did not appear to be healthy or if the bite is on the patient's face, the patient should be started on RIG and HDCV in the meantime. Treatment should be stopped only if the FRA test is negative.

✓ **If the offending wild animal is not captured,** no matter how normal-appearing it was, assume that it was rabid and provide a full course of RIG and HDCV.

✓ **Postexposure prophylaxis should be considered when contact with a bat or a bite from a bat is possible but uncertain, such as when a bat is found near a sleeping person or a previously unattended child and the animal is unavailable for testing.** In the United States, bats have been the most common source of rabies among humans.

When Postexposure Prophylaxis Is Required

✓ Provide passive immunity with 20 IU/kg of RIG (Imogam Rabies-HT, BayRab). Infiltrate around the wound (if anatomically feasible) as much as possible and administer the remainder intramuscularly in the gluteus. Give two separate injections if the remaining volume is greater than 5 mL. This passive protection has a half-life of 21 days.

✓ **Begin immunization with rabies vaccine, HDCV (Imovax), or purified chick embryo cell vaccine (PCECV, RabAvert), 1 mL IM in the deltoid (or the anterolateral thigh in children), at a site distant from the immune globulin.** Both types of rabies vaccines are considered equally safe and efficacious.

✓ **Make arrangements for repeat doses of rabies vaccine at 3, 7 and 14 days postexposure, and obtain an antibody level after the series.**

What Not To Do:

✗ Do not treat patients who were only petting a rabid animal or only came into contact with blood, urine, or feces (e.g., guano) of a rabid animal. Because the rabies virus is inactivated by desiccation and ultraviolet irradiation, in general, if the material suspected of containing the virus is dry, the virus can be considered noninfectious.

✗ Do not treat the bites of rodents and lagomorphs (e.g., hamsters, rabbits, squirrels, rats) unless rabies is endemic in your area. To date, rodent and lagomorph bites have not caused human rabies in the United States.

✗ Do not defer prophylaxis because there has been a delay in seeking care for a documented or likely exposure unless clinical signs of rabies are present. Incubation periods of greater than 1 year have been reported.

✗ Do not omit RIG from treatment. Treatment failures have resulted from giving rabies vaccine alone.

✗ Do not withhold treatment because the exposed patient is pregnant. Although a theoretical risk exists for adverse effects from rabies immune globulin and killed rabies virus vaccines, several studies assessing the safety of this treatment have failed to identify these risks). Indeed, the consensus is that pregnancy is not a contraindication to rabies postexposure prophylaxis (PEP).

Discussion

Previously, the Advisory Committee on Immunization Practices (ACIP) recommended a five-dose rabies vaccination regimen with HDCV or PCECV. Their new recommendations reduce the number of vaccine doses to four. The reduction in doses recommended for PEP was based in part on evidence from rabies virus pathogenesis data, experimental animal work, clinical studies, and epidemiologic surveillance. These studies indicated that four vaccine doses in combination with RIG elicited adequate immune responses and that a fifth dose of vaccine did not contribute to more favorable outcomes.

The older (but still feared by some patients) duck embryo vaccine (DEV) for rabies required 21 injections and produced more side effects and less of an antibody response than the new HDCV. Sometimes, neurologic symptoms would arise from DEV treatment, raising the agonizing question of whether the symptoms represented early signs of rabies or side effects of the treatment and thus whether treatment should be continued or discontinued.

Currently, it is much easier to initiate immunization with HDCV or PCECV and provide follow-through, because side effects are minimal and antibody response is excellent. Approximately 25% of patients experience redness, tenderness, and itching around the injection site, and another 20% experience headache, myalgia, or nausea. The newer rabies vaccine that is prepared in purified chick embryo cell culture appears to be as effective as HDCV but does not cause the serum sickness–like hypersensitivity reactions, which include generalized urticaria, sometimes accompanied by arthralgia, arthritis, angioedema, and vomiting.

Patients with immunosuppressive illness or those taking immunosuppressive medications, corticosteroids, or antimalarials may have an inadequate response to vaccination. For such persons, PEP should continue to comprise a five-dose vaccination regimen (the fifth dose on day 28) with 1 dose of RIG.

Recommendations for preexposure prophylaxis remain unchanged, with three doses of vaccine administered on days 0, 7, and 21 or 28.

The incubation period of rabies varies from weeks to months, roughly in proportion to the length of the axons on which the virus must propagate to the brain, which is why prophylaxis is especially urgent in facial bites.

Suggested Readings

Abazeed M, Cinti S: Rabies prophylaxis for pregnant women, *Emerg Infect Dis* 13:1966–1967, 2007.

Human rabies prevention—United States: Recommendations of the Advisory Committee on Immunization Practices (ACIP), *MMWR* 48(RR-1):1–21, 1999.

Kauffman FH, Goldmann BJ: Rabies, *Am J Emerg Med* 4:525–531, 1986.

Noah DL, Drenzek CL, Smith JS, et al: Epidemiology of human rabies in the United States, 1980 to 1996, *Ann Intern Med* 128:922–930, 1998.

Rupprecht CE, Briggs D, Brown CM, et al: Use of a reduced (4-dose) vaccine schedule for postexposure prophylaxis to prevent human rabies, *MMWR Recomm Rep* 59(RR-2):1–9, 2010.

State and Regional Poison Control Centers

You can reach your local poison control center anywhere in the United States by calling 1-800-222-1222.

This page provides access to phone numbers and addresses for regional and state poison control centers. Please contact the following centers in case of emergency or for poison prevention information.

Alabama

Alabama Poison Center
2503 Phoenix Drive
Tuscaloosa, AL 35405
1-800-222-1222

Regional Poison Control Center–Children's
Hospital of Alabama
1600 7th Avenue South
Birmingham, AL 35233
1-800-222-1222

Alaska*

Oregon Poison Center
3181 S.W. Sam Jackson Park Road
Portland, OR 97239
1-800-222-1222

American Samoa*

Nebraska Regional Poison Center
8401 West Dodge Road, Suite 115
Omaha, NE 68114
1-800-222-1222

Arizona

Arizona Poison and Drug Information Center
445 N. 5th Street, Suite 120

Tucson, AZ 85004
1-800-222-1222

Banner Poison Control Center
1111 E. McDowell Road
Phoenix, AZ 85006
1-800-222-1222

Arkansas

Arkansas Poison and Drug Information Center
4301 West Markham, Slot 522-2
Little Rock, AR 72205
1-800-222-1222

California

California Poison Control System
School of Pharmacy–Department of Clinical Pharmacy
University of California, San Francisco
Box 1262
San Francisco, CA 94143
1-800-222-1222

California Poison Control System–Fresno/
Madera Division
Children's Hospital Central California
9300 Valley Children's Place
MB 15
Madera, CA 93638
1-800-222-1222

The information about U.S. poison control centers is also available at http://poisonhelp.hrsa.gov/poison-centers/text-only-resources/index.html.

California Poison Control System–Sacramento
Division
University of California Davis Medical
Center
2315 Stockton Boulevard
Sacramento, CA 95817
1-800-222-1222

California Poison Control System–San Diego
Division
University of California San Diego Medical
Center
200 West Arbor Drive
San Diego, CA 92103
1-800-222-1222

Colorado

Rocky Mountain Poison and Drug Center
777 Bannock Street, Mail Code 0180
Denver, CO 80204
1-800-222-1222

Connecticut

Connecticut Poison Control Center
263 Farmington Avenue
Farmington, CT 06030
1-800-222-1222

Delaware*

Poison Control Center at the Children's
Hospital of Philadelphia
34th and Civic Center Boulevard
Philadelphia, PA 19104
1-800-222-1222

District of Columbia

National Capital Poison Center
3201 New Mexico Avenue, NW,
Suite 310
Washington, DC 20016
1-800-222-1222

Federated States of Micronesia*

Nebraska Regional Poison Center
8401 West Dodge Road, Suite 115
Omaha, NE 68114
1-888-222-4516

Florida

Florida Poison Information
Center–Jacksonville
655 West Eighth Street, Box C-23
Jacksonville, FL 32209
1-800-222-1222

Florida Poison Information Center–Miami
University of Miami
Department of Pediatrics
P.O. Box 016960 (R-131)
Miami, FL 33101
1-800-222-1222

Florida Poison Information Center–Tampa
Tampa General Hospital
P.O. Box 1289
Tampa, FL 33601
1-800-222-1222

Georgia

Georgia Poison Center
80 Jesse Hill Jr. Drive, SE
Atlanta, GA 30303
1-800-222-1222

Guam*

Oregon Poison Center
3181 S.W. Sam Jackson Park Road
Portland, OR 97239
1-800-222-1222

Hawaii*

Rocky Mountain Poison and Drug Center
777 Bannock Street, Mail Code 0180
Denver, CO 80204
1-800-222-1222

Idaho*

Rocky Mountain Poison and Drug Center
777 Bannock Street, Mail Code 0180
Denver, CO 80204
1-800-222-1222

Illinois

Illinois Poison Center
222 South Riverside Plaza, Suite 1900
Chicago, IL 60606
1-800-222-1222

Indiana

Indiana Poison Center
Indiana University Health Methodist Hospital
I-65 at 21st Street
Indianapolis, IN 46206
1-800-222-1222

Iowa

Iowa Statewide Poison Control Center
401 Douglas Street, Suite 402
Sioux City, IA 51101
1-800-222-1222

Kansas

The University of Kansas Hospital Poison
Control Center
University of Kansas Medical Center
3901 Rainbow Boulevard, Room B-400
Kansas City, KS 66160
1-800-222-1222

Kentucky

Kentucky Regional Poison Center
Medical Towers South, Suite 847
234 East Gray Street
Louisville, KY 40202
1-800-222-1222

Louisiana

Louisiana Poison Center
LSUHSC–Shreveport
Department of Emergency Medicine
Section of Clinical Toxicology
1455 Wilkinson Street
Shreveport, LA 71130
1-800-222-1222

Maine

Northern New England Poison Center
22 Bramhall Street
Portland, ME 04102
1-800-222-1222

Maryland

Maryland Poison Center
220 Arch Street, Office Level 1
Baltimore, MD 21201
1-800-222-1222

National Capital Poison Center
3201 New Mexico Avenue, NW, Suite 310
Washington, DC 20016
1-800-222-1222

Massachusetts

Regional Center for Poison Control and
Prevention
Children's Hospital Boston
300 Longwood Avenue
IC Smith Building
Boston, MA 02115
1-800-222-1222

Michigan

VHS Children's Hospital of Michigan
3901 Beaubien Street
Detroit, MI 48201-2119

Minnesota

Hennepin Regional Poison Center
Hennepin County Medical Center
701 Park Avenue, Mail Code RL
Minneapolis, MN 55415
1-800-222-1222

Mississippi

Mississippi Poison Control Center
University of Mississippi Medical Center
2500 North State Street
Jackson, MS 39216
1-800-222-1222

Missouri

Missouri Poison Center at SSM Cardinal
Glennon Children's Medical Center
1465 S. Grand Boulevard
St. Louis, MO 63104
1-800-222-1222

Montana*

Rocky Mountain Poison and Drug Center
777 Bannock Street, Mail Code 0180
Denver, CO 80204
1-800-222-1222

Nebraska

Nebraska Regional Poison Center
8401 West Dodge Road, Suite 115
Omaha, NE 68114
1-800-222-1222

Nevada*

Rocky Mountain Poison and Drug Center
777 Bannock Street, Mail Code 0180
Denver, CO 80204
1-800-222-1222

New Hampshire*

Northern New England Poison Center
22 Bramhall Street
Portland, ME 04102
1-800-222-1222

New Jersey

New Jersey Poison Information and
Education System
University of Medicine and Dentistry of
New Jersey
140 Bergen Street, P.O. Box 1709
Newark, NJ 07107
1-800-222-1222

New Mexico

New Mexico Poison and Drug Information
Center
MSC09 5080
1 University of New Mexico
Albuquerque, NM 87131
1-800-222-1222

New York

New York City Poison Control Center
N.Y.C. Bureau of Public Health Labs
455 First Avenue
Room 123, Box 81
New York, NY 10016
1-800-222-1222

Upstate New York Poison Center
750 East Adams Street
Syracuse, NY 13210
1-800-222-1222

North Carolina

Carolinas Poison Center
Carolinas Medical Center
P.O. Box 32861
Charlotte, NC 28232
1-800-222-1222

North Dakota*

North Dakota Poison Center, Served by
Hennepin Regional Poison Center
North Dakota Department of Health
600 East Boulevard Avenue
Bismarck, ND 58505-0200
1-800-222-1222

Ohio

Central Ohio Poison Center
Nationwide Children's Hospital
700 Children's Drive
Columbus, OH 43205
1-800-222-1222

Cincinnati Drug and Poison Information
Center
Regional Poison Control System
3333 Burnet Avenue, MLC 9004
Cincinnati, OH 45229
1-800-222-1222

Northern Ohio Poison Control Center
University Hospitals Rainbow Babies and
Children's Hospital
11100 Euclid Avenue
Cleveland, OH 44106
1-800-222-1222

Oklahoma

Oklahoma Poison Control Center
940 NE 13th Street/Suite 3850/Nicholson
Tower
Oklahoma City, OK 73104-5008
1-800-222-1222

Oregon

Oregon Poison Center
3181 S.W. Sam Jackson Park Road
Portland, OR 97239
1-800-222-1222

Pennsylvania

Pittsburgh Poison Center
University of Pittsburgh Medical Center
200 Lothrop Street
Pittsburgh, PA 15213
1-800-222-1222

Poison Control Center at the Children's
Hospital of Philadelphia
34th and Civic Center Boulevard
Philadelphia, PA 19104
1-800-222-1112

Rhode Island*

Regional Center for Poison Control and
Prevention
Children's Hospital Boston
300 Longwood Avenue, IC Smith Building
Boston, MA 02115
1-800-222-1222

South Carolina

Palmetto Poison Center
South Carolina College of Pharmacy
University of South Carolina
Columbia, SC 29208
1-800-222-1222

South Dakota*

Sanford Poison Center, Served by Hennepin
Regional Poison Center
Sanford Health
1305 West 18th Street
Sioux Falls, SD 57117-5039
1-800-222-1222

Tennessee

Tennessee Poison Center
501 Oxford House
1161 21st Avenue South
Nashville, TN 37232
1-800-222-1222

Texas

Central Texas Poison Center
2401 South 31st Street
Temple, TX 76508
1-800-222-1222

North Texas Poison Center
5201 Harry Hines Boulevard
Dallas, TX 75235
1-800-222-1222

UT Health Science Center San Antonio Cancer
Therapy and Research Center
7979 Wurzbach Road
San Antonio, TX 78229
1-800-222-1222

Southeast Texas Poison Control
301 University Boulevard
3.112 Trauma Center
Galveston, TX 77555
1-800-222-1222

Texas Panhandle Poison Center
1501 South Coulter
Amarillo, TX 79106
1-800-222-1222

West Texas Regional Poison Center
Thomason Hospital
4815 Alameda Avenue
El Paso, TX 79905
1-800-222-1222

U.S. Virgin Islands*

Florida Poison Information
Center–Jacksonville
655 West Eighth Street, Box C-23
Jacksonville, FL 32209
1-800-222-1222

Utah

The Utah Poison Control Center
585 Komas Drive, Suite 200
Salt Lake City, UT 84108
1-800-222-1222

Vermont*

Northern New England Poison Center
22 Bramhall Street
Portland, ME 04102
1-800-222-1222

Virginia

Blue Ridge Poison Center
1222 Jefferson Park Avenue, P.O. Box 800774
Charlottesville, VA 22903
1-800-222-1222

National Capital Poison Center
3201 New Mexico Avenue, NW, Suite 310
Washington, DC 20016
1-800-222-1222

Virginia Poison Center
Virginia Commonwealth University Medical
Center
600 E. Broad Street, Suite 640
P.O. Box 980522
Richmond, VA 23298
1-800-222-1222

Washington

Washington Poison Center
155 NE 100th Street, Suite 100
Seattle, WA 98125
1-800-222-1222

West Virginia

West Virginia Poison Center
3110 MacCorkle Avenue, SE
Charleston, WV 25314
1-800- 222-1222

Wisconsin

Wisconsin Poison Center
P.O. Box 1997, Mail Station C660
Milwaukee, WI 53201
1-800-222-1222

Wyoming*

Nebraska Regional Poison Center
8401 West Dodge Road, Suite 115
Omaha, NE 68114
1-800-222-1222

*This state is served by an out-of-state Poison Center.

Tetanus Prophylaxis

Presentation

The patient may have stepped on a nail or sustained any sort of laceration, abrasion, or puncture wound when the question of tetanus prophylaxis arises.

What To Do:

✓ Always provide appropriate wound care with adequate cleansing, débridement, irrigation, and antibiotics when indicated.

✓ **Determine a patient's tetanus immunity status by asking if he has ever received a series of primary tetanus shots (or if he attended primary school in the United States or has been in the military), and if and when he received any booster shots since then.**

✓ If the patient's tetanus immunization is up to date, **no prophylaxis is required.**

✓ **If the patient has not had tetanus immunization in the past 5 years, give adult tetanus and diphtheria toxoid (Td), 0.5 mL IM.** For clean minor wounds, Td is not required unless it has been more than 10 years since the last booster. Give pediatric diphtheria and tetanus toxoid (DT), 0.5 mL, to children younger than 7 years of age if their history of previous immunization is unknown or includes less than three doses of DT; otherwise, no prophylaxis is necessary.

✓ **Individuals 19 years of age or older who never have received tetanus-diphtheria-pertussis vaccine (Tdap), now receive a *one-time* dose of Tdap, regardless of the interval since the most recent tetanus or diphtheria-containing vaccine. Then boost with Td every 10 years thereafter.**

✓ Administer a one-time dose of Tdap to adults aged less than 65 years who have not received Tdap previously or for whom vaccine status is unknown, to replace one of the 10-year Td boosters, and, as soon as feasible, to all (1) postpartum women, (2) close contacts of infants younger than age 12 months (e.g., grandparents and child-care providers), and (3) healthcare personnel with direct patient contact.

✓ Adults aged 65 years and older who have not previously received Tdap and who have close contact with an infant aged less than 12 months also should be vaccinated. Other adults aged 65 years and older may receive Tdap.

✓ **If there is any doubt whether the patient has had his original series of three tetanus immunizations, add tetanus immune globulin (Hyper-Tet), 250 mg IM, and make arrangements for him to complete the full series with additional immunizations**

at 4 to 8 weeks and 6 to 12 months. Administer the first two doses at least 4 weeks apart and the third dose 6 to 12 months after the second. If incompletely vaccinated (i.e., less than three doses), administer the remaining doses. Substitute a one-time dose of Tdap for one of the doses of Td, either in the primary series or for the routine booster, whichever comes first. (For children less than 7 years of age, give boosters 2 to 8 weeks after the first dose, 4 to 8 weeks after the second, and 6 to 12 months after the third). **Some experts advise using tetanus immune globulin (TIG) plus a tetanus toxoid booster for all patients older than age 65 years with a tetanus-prone wound, regardless of their "known" immunization status. TIG is also appropriate in individuals with immune deficiency.**

 If a woman is pregnant and received the most recent Td vaccination 10 or more years previously, administer Td during the second or third trimester. If the woman received the most recent Td vaccination less than 10 years previously, administer Tdap during the immediate postpartum period. At the clinician's discretion, Td may be deferred during pregnancy and Tdap substituted in the immediate postpartum period, or Tdap may be administered instead of Td to a pregnant woman after an informed discussion with the woman.

If there is a history of true hypersensitivity to tetanus toxoid, provide passive immunity with tetanus immune globulin, but instruct the patient that he or she does not have protection against future exposure. Tetanus immunoglobulin has had no reported adverse effect in pregnant patients but is classified as a category C drug in pregnancy. Consequently, it is recommended for pregnant women only if clearly indicated.

Provide the patient with written documentation of the immunizations given.

What Not To Do:

Do not assume adequate immunization. **The groups most at risk in the United States today are immigrants from outside of North America and Western Europe, patients older than 70 years, and particularly those of lower socioeconomic status without education beyond grade school. Persons with human immunodeficiency virus (HIV) infection, injecting-drug users, and those undergoing cancer therapy may also be at risk.** Many patients incorrectly assume that they were immunized during a surgical procedure. Although it occurs rarely, surviving tetanus does not confer immunity. Children attending school in the United States and active military personnel tend to be well protected against tetanus. Veterans usually have been immunized.

Do not give Tdap to a pregnant patient. Give Td and delay Tdap until the postpartum period.

Do not give tetanus immunizations indiscriminately. Besides being wasteful, too-frequent immunizations are more likely to cause reactions, probably of the antigen-antibody type. (Surprisingly, the routine of administering toxoid and immune globulin simultaneously in separate sites does not seem to cause mutual inactivation or serum sickness.) Most tetanus cases occur in individuals who are unvaccinated or whose history of vaccination is not known.

Do not believe every story of allergy to tetanus toxoid (which is actually quite rare). Is the patient actually describing a local reaction or a reaction to older, less pure preparations of toxoid? The only absolute contraindication is a history of immediate hypersensitivity (urticaria, bronchospasm, or shock or neurologic complications), polyneuropathy, Guillain-Barré syndrome, or encephalopathy. Tetanus toxoid is safe for use in pregnancy, but Tdap should be delayed until the postpartum period.

(X) Do not give pediatric tetanus and diphtheria toxoid (DT) to an adult. DT contains eight times as much diphtheria toxoid as Td and can cause adult patients to become very ill.

Discussion

The estimated worldwide incidence of tetanus is between 700,000 and 1 million cases annually. Tetanus is caused by the exotoxin of Clostridium tetani, a gram-positive, spore-forming anaerobic rod. Spores of C. tetani are ubiquitous in the soil and in the feces of animals. They are highly resistant to destruction and can survive on almost any surface for long periods of time. Once these spores enter a break in the skin, they germinate and begin to secrete the toxin tetanospasmin, a very potent neurotoxin. Spores become vegetative only in an anaerobic environment such as occurs in necrotic tissue and poorly vascularized areas. The incubation period for the disease averages 8 days, with a range of 24 hours to several months. A shorter incubation period corresponds to more severe disease.

Tetanospasmin irreversibly binds and blocks the release of inhibitory neurotransmitters, resulting in unrelenting muscle spasms, also known as tetany. Masseter muscle contractions cause trismus, also referred to as lockjaw, or the classic grinning expression, called risus sardonicus (the sardonic smile). Progression leads to diffuse muscle rigidity and autonomic dysfunction, resulting in death in up to 45% of cases.

There continue to be 50 to 100 cases of tetanus in the United States each year. From 1995 to 1997, puncture wounds were the major type of disease-producing injury, with 15% of all tetanus patients having stepped on a nail. Lacerations and abrasions comprised the great majority of the remaining cases. Other forms of inoculation include self-performed body piercing and tattooing, animal bites, insect bites, and splinters. About 18% of cases occurred in IV drug users, half of whom report a wound, such as an abscess at the injection site.

The Centers for Disease Control and Prevention (CDC) recommends that everyone older than 7 years of age should receive Td every 10 years, but somehow physicians and patients alike forget tetanus prophylaxis except after a wound. Because tetanus has followed negligible injuries, spontaneous infections, and chronic wounds, the concept of the "tetanus-prone wound" is not really helpful. The CDC recommends including a small dose of diphtheria toxoid (Td), but because this is more apt to cause local reactions, it is reasonable to revert back to plain tetanus toxoid in patients who have complained of such reactions. Adverse side effects of tetanus toxoid administration include local tenderness, erythema; swelling; and, at times, flulike illness; low-grade fever; Arthus-type sensitivity reaction; and, rarely, anaphylaxis. Other severe reactions may include Guillain-Barré syndrome and acute relapsing polyneuropathy.

Passive immunization using human TIG involves the administration of a bolus of antibody that becomes available immediately. Although the protection is temporary, it remains within the protective range throughout the time frame necessary to protect against tetanus related to a recent wound. TIG is generally associated with a lower incidence of adverse effects than tetanus toxoid. It is highly protective when given in a dose of 250 U IM, but if the wound is very high risk, including those that are more than 24 hours old and those that may have happened in areas with a very high level of bacterial contamination (such as barns or sewers), a higher dose of up to 500 U may be warranted.

For routine immunization, pediatric diphtheria-pertussis-tetanus vaccine is given at 2, 4, and 6 months, with a fourth dose at 12 to 18 months (6 months after the last dose), and a fifth dose at 4 to 6 years. Thereafter, tetanus toxoid with a reduced dose of diphtheria (Td) is given every 10 years, and boosters are given within 5 years for "tetanus-prone" wounds, which the CDC guidelines define as wounds contaminated with dirt, feces, or saliva; puncture wounds; tears; and wounds from bullets, crushing, burns, and frostbite.

Despite sustained high coverage for childhood pertussis vaccination, pertussis remains poorly controlled in the United States. A total of 16,858 pertussis cases and 12 infant deaths were reported in 2009. Although 2005 recommendations by the Advisory Committee on Immunization Practices (ACIP) called for vaccination with tetanus toxoid,

(continued)

Discussion continued

reduced diphtheria toxoid, and acellular pertussis (Tdap) for adolescents and adults to improve immunity against pertussis, Tdap coverage is 56% among adolescents and less than 6% among adults. In October 2010, ACIP recommended expanded use of Tdap.

ACIP recommends a single Tdap dose for persons aged 11 through 18 years who have completed the recommended childhood diphtheria and tetanus toxoids and pertussis/ diphtheria and tetanus toxoids and acellular pertussis (DTP/DTaP) vaccination series and also for adults aged 19 through 64 years. Two Tdap vaccines are available in the United States. Boostrix (GlaxoSmithKline Biologicals, Rixensart, Belgium) is licensed for use in persons aged 10 through 64 years, and Adacel (Sanofi Pasteur, Toronto, Canada) is licensed for use in persons aged 11 through 64 years. Both Tdap products are licensed for use at an interval of at least 5 years between the tetanus and diphtheria toxoids (Td) and Tdap dose. **On October 27, 2010, ACIP approved the following additional recommendations: (1) use of Tdap, regardless of interval since the last tetanus- or diphtheria-toxoid–containing vaccine, (2) use of Tdap in certain adults aged 65 years and older, and (3) use of Tdap in undervaccinated children aged 7 through 10 years.**

Suggested Readings

Alagappan K, Rennie W, Kwiatkowski T, et al: Antibody protection to diphtheria in geriatric patients: need for ED compliance with immunization guidelines, *Ann Emerg Med* 30:455–458, 1997.

Alagappan K, Rennie W, Kwiatkowski T, et al: Seroprevalence of tetanus antibodies among adults older than 65 years, *Ann Emerg Med* 28:18–21, 1996.

Alagappan K, Rennie W, Narang V, et al: Immunologic response to tetanus toxoid in geriatric patients, *Ann Emerg Med* 30:459–462, 1997.

Fernandes R, Valcour V, Flynn B, et al: Tetanus immunity in long-term care facilities, *J Am Geriatr Soc* 51:1116–1119, 2003.

Gergen PJ, McQuillan GM, Kiely M, et al: A population-based serologic survey of immunity to tetanus in the United States, *N Engl J Med* 332:761–766, 1995.

Giangrasso J, Smith RK: Misuse of tetanus immunoprophylaxis in wound care, *Ann Emerg Med* 14:573–579, 1985.

Halperin SA, Sweet L, Baxendale D, et al: How soon after a prior tetanus-diphtheria vaccination can one give adult formulation tetanus-diphtheria-acellular pertussis vaccine? *Pediatr Infect Dis J* 25:195–200, 2006.

Kruszon-Moran DM, McQuillan GM, Chu SY: Tetanus and diphtheria immunity among females in the United States: are recommendations being followed? *Am J Obstet Gynecol* 190:1070–1076, 2004.

Macko MB, Powell CE: Comparison of the morbidity of tetanus toxoid boosters with tetanus-diphtheria toxoid boosters, *Ann Emerg Med* 14:33–35, 1985.

Recommended adult immunization schedule, *MMWR* 60:1–4, 2011.

Talan DA, Abrahamian FM, Moran GJ, et al: Tetanus immunity and physician compliance with tetanus prophylaxis practices among emergency department patients presenting with wounds, *Ann Emerg Med* 43:305–314, 2004.

Updated recommendations for use of tetanus toxoid, reduced diphtheria toxoid and acellular pertussis (Tdap) vaccine from the Advisory Committee on Immunization Practices, *MMWR* 60:13–15, 2011.

Index

Note: Page numbers followed by *b* indicate boxed material. Page numbers followed by *f* indicate figures, and those followed by *t* indicate tables.